Skin Cancer: Recognition and Management

Skin Cancer: Recognition and Management

Edited by Elizabeth Burns

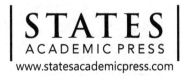

STATES
ACADEMIC PRESS
www.statesacademicpress.com

States Academic Press,
109 South 5th Street,
Brooklyn, NY 11249, USA

Visit us on the World Wide Web at:
www.statesacademicpress.com

ISBN: 978-1-63989-760-5

Cataloging-in-Publication Data

Skin cancer : recognition and management / edited by Elizabeth Burns.
p. cm.
Includes bibliographical references and index.
ISBN 978-1-63989-760-5
1. Skin--Cancer. 2. Skin--Cancer--Diagnosis. 3. Skin--Cancer--Treatment.
I. Burns, Elizabeth.
RC280.S5 D53 2023
616.994 77--dc23

Table of Contents

Preface

Skin cancer refers to the abnormal growth of skin cells. In most cases, skin cancer develops on skin exposed to the sun. However, skin cancer can also develop on skin that is not exposed to sunlight. It is the most common type of cancer. It is categorized into three types, namely, melanoma, squamous cell carcinoma, and basal cell carcinoma. Melanoma is a type of skin cancer that develops in the melanocyte cells. It has a high probability of invading surrounding tissues and can spread to other body parts. Major signs of skin cancer include skin lesions, ragged and uneven border of lesions, unusual color spots, size greater than 0.25 inches, etc. In certain cases, skin biopsy may be required to determine skin cancer. Its treatment depends on factors such as size and location of cancer, as well as its type and stage. Treatment options for skin cancer include cryosurgery, excisional surgery, Moh's surgery, curettage and electrodesiccation, chemotherapy, photodynamic therapy, radiation, biological therapy, and immunotherapy. This book unravels the recent studies on the recognition and management of skin cancer. It will serve as a reference to a broad spectrum of readers.

This book is a comprehensive compilation of works of different researchers from varied parts of the world. It includes valuable experiences of the researchers with the sole objective of providing the readers (learners) with a proper knowledge of the concerned field. This book will be beneficial in evoking inspiration and enhancing the knowledge of the interested readers.

In the end, I would like to extend my heartiest thanks to the authors who worked with great determination on their chapters. I also appreciate the publisher's support in the course of the book. I would also like to deeply acknowledge my family who stood by me as a source of inspiration during the project.

Editor

The Effectiveness of Different Treatment Modalities of Cutaneous Angiosarcoma: Results from Meta-Analysis and Observational Data from SEER Database

Siwei Bi[1], Shanshan Chen[2], Beiyi Wu[2], Ying Cen[1]* and Junjie Chen[1]*

[1] Department of Burn and Plastic Surgery, West China Hospital, Sichuan University, Chengdu, China, [2] West China School of Medicine, Sichuan University, Chengdu, China

*Correspondence:
Ying Cen
cenying0141@163.com
Junjie Chen
cjjemail@163.com

Introduction: Cutaneous angiosarcoma (cAS) is an aggressive vascular tumor that originates from vascular or lymphatic epithelial cells. To date, the cAS literature has been limited in a small number with single-center experiences or reports due to its rarity and the optimal treatment strategy is still in dispute. This study aimed to conduct a systematic review and compare the effect of available treatments retrieved from observational studies and Surveillance, Epidemiology, and End Results (SEER) program.

Methods: The authors performed a systematic review in the PubMed, Embase and MEDLINE database identifying the researches assessing the treatment for cAS patients. Clinical and treatment information of patients who had been diagnosed with a primary cAS were also obtained from the SEER program.

Results: Thirty-two studies were eligible but only 5 of which with 276 patients were included in meta-analysis since the unclear or unavailable information. The risk ratio of 5-year death for surgery, surgery with radiotherapy and surgery with chemotherapy were 0.84, 0.96, and 0.69. Meanwhile, in SEER database, there are 291 metastatic and 437 localized patients with cAS. The localized patients receiving surgery showed a significantly worse overall survival result when compared with the surgery combined with RT: hazard ratio: 1.6, 95% confidential interval: 1.05, 2.42, P = 0.03.

Conclusion: In conclusion, our study provided a detailed picture of the effectiveness of present treatments for localized and metastatic cAS patients. The CT could be inappropriate in localized patients. For metastatic patients, the surgery combined RT was recommended compared with surgery alone since its enhanced OS prognosis. Yet, more novel-designed clinical trials with specific targeted populations and rigorous conducting are needed for a solid conclusion on which would be a better treatment strategy.

Keywords: cutaneous angiosarcoma, SEER database, treatment modalities, meta-analysis, clinical efficacy, 5-year death rate, overall survival, cancer-specific survival

INTRODUCTION

Angiosarcomas are a group of vascular malignant tumors that are relatively rare and account for 1-2% of all soft tissue sarcomas (1). With an extremely poor prognosis, patients with angiosarcomas always ending within a year (2). They originate from vascular or lymphatic epithelial cells and can arise in various locations of the body (3, 4). About 60% of angiosarcomas present as cutaneous angiosarcomas (cAS) involving the head and neck predominantly. Others can exist in visceral organs, bones, and other soft tissues (4, 5). Multiple factors are proved to affect the survival rates of cAS, including age, tumor size, tumor site and so on (6).

The prognosis of cAS is relatively poor with a 5-year survival rate ranging from 26% to 51% (6, 7). There are many treatment options for cAS (8, 9), including surgery (10, 11), radiotherapy (RT) (12), chemotherapy (CT) (13), targeted therapy (14, 15) and more recently, immunotherapy (IT) (16). Mainstay therapy remains surgery with adjuvant RT (9). However, with the presence of new effective strategies, the treatment choice for cAS patients could be controversial. Besides, limited literature focused on the possible prognostic significance of treatments on different groups of patients such as metastatic or localized, which would be confusing in clinical practice.

Surveillance, Epidemiology, and End Results (SEER) Program of the National Cancer Institute (17) was initiated in 1973. SEER has now gained enough data that clinical and descriptive characteristics of uncommon tumors can be described at a population level. Based on the clinical characteristics, survival outcomes and corresponding therapy information retrieved from SEER program, we compared the therapeutic effect of different treatments of cAS patients. Moreover, we performed a systematic review and meta-analysis to summarize the previous observational studies evaluating the efficacy of different therapies in treating cAS, through which, independent results of the previous studies could be synthesized.

METHODS

Meta-Analysis: Data Sources and Search Strategy

The following English databases were searched systematically: PubMed, EMBASE and Medline Database with: (cutaneous angiosarcoma [Title/Abstract]) AND (treatment [Title/Abstract]). Only English articles published up to the searching date: 2020.5.17 were included. Reference lists of primary articles were reviewed for more literature.

Meta-Analysis: Inclusion Criteria and Study Selection

Inclusion criteria are as follows: 1) sufficient data including age, tumor size, tumor site, treatments were provided in a full-length article; 2) study design: prospective or retrospective cohort trials; 3) Outcome measurements: survival rate and corresponding follow up duration. Meanwhile, we excluded studies without enough data for effect sizes calculation or any case reports, review articles, letters, or communications. Two reviewers (SWB, SSC) independently went through the titles and abstracts. A senior reviewer (JJC) would be consulted if any differences exist.

Meta-Analysis: Data Extraction and Quality Assessment

By the Cochrane Collaboration for Systematic Reviews guidelines (18), this process was performed separately by two reviewers (SWB, SSC). Relevant data from the eligible studies were extracted including the 1st author's name, the published year, the number of participants, gender proportion, median age, tumor site, tumor size, tumor grade, tumor presentation, average follow-up time, treatment, and outcome measurements. The methodologic quality of each study was evaluated according to the assessment of the Newcastle–Ottawa scale which comprises three categories, including the selection of the study population. comparability of the groups, and ascertainment of the exposure or outcomes. Each parameter consists of a subcategorized questionnaire based on selection, comparability, and outcomes (19, 20). Two of the authors (SWB, SSC) independently scored the questionnaire for each included study following the user manual of the Newcastle–Ottawa scale.

SEER Database: Selection of Population Data and Outcomes

We chose the SEER 18 database which includes cases recorded between 1973 and 2015 spanning 18 different US geographic areas. The clinical data of patients who were diagnosed with cAS were obtained from the SEER Program. cAS was defined by combining the International Classification of Diseases for Oncology, 3rd edition (ICD-O-3) morphological code 9120/3 and 9170/3, which stands for hemangiosarcoma and lymphangiosarcoma, and topographical codes: C44.0-9. The other variables were included such as age at diagnosis, sex, tumor grade, tumor site, tumor size, SEER historic stage, treatment modalities and survival outcomes. For the SEER historic stages, "local," "regional," and "distant" were used as the End Results Group of National Cancer Institute (NCI).

Statistical Analysis

A single group meta-analysis was performed and results were presented with 95% confidence interval (CI). Studies were then pooled together as appropriate with two-sided $P < 0.05$ considered as statistically significant. The authors calculate the Q-statistic (21) for testing heterogeneity among studies, and $P < 0.05$ was considered as significant too. The authors selected the results with the fixed-effects model if the included studies were homogenous with $P > 0.05$; otherwise, the random-effects model results would be picked on. The I^2 statistic (21) was also calculated to efficiently test for the heterogeneity, with $I^2 < 25\%$, 25%–75%, and $> 75\%$ to represent a low, moderate and high degree of heterogeneity, respectively. We conducted a subgroup analysis to detect the source of heterogeneity furtherly based on the different treatment strategies.

On the other hand, for the SEER database analysis, Kaplan-Meier curves were used to illustrate the overall survival (OS) and cancer-specific survival (CSS) probabilities for the selected patients grouped by different therapies. The univariate and multivariate cox proportional hazards regression models were performed using the log-rank test. Predictors for the multivariate model were the factors identified as statistically significant (P value <0.05) in univariate analysis. Moreover, the authors plotted the trends in the management of patients with cAS with linear regression analysis. All the analysis and plots were generated using R 3.6.2 with packages (22–26): "gemtc," "rjags," "dmetar," "survival," "survminer," and "ggplot2".

RESULTS

Meta-Analysis: Eligible Studies Identification

As shown in **Figure 1**, 445 studies were chosen from databases for further screening. We excluded 66 duplicated articles and 347 other articles because of inappropriate topics (n=254), review articles (n=16), lack of full text (n=5), overlapping author (n=59), and not English (n=13). After assessing articles with full text, 32 studies were selected in total. A large number of studies were short of precise data for a specific treatment arm. In the end, five studies with 276 participants were included for the meta-analysis.

Meta-Analysis: Characteristics of Selected Studies

The clinical characteristics of both selected observational studies and SEER population were summarized in **Table 1**. The detailed characteristics of 32 included studies are shown in **Supplementary Files**. The sample size ranged from 5 to 421 with a median of 44 and 1414 participants in total. Participants of 17 studies were divided into two groups by tumor size. Twenty-eight studies involved information about tumor site and 13 studies involved tumor grade. The majority of studies focused on the efficacy of surgery and RT (n=22).

Meta-Analysis: Summary of Prognosis Results in Eligible Studies

The summary of prognosis parameters: 2-, 3-, 5-, 10-year survival rate, disease-free interval (DFI), mean survival time and 3, 5-year regression free survival (RFS) are shown in **Table 2** severally. The 5-year survival rate in patients receiving surgery was 12.5%–46.9%. In patients treated with RT, the 5-year survival rate was 0%–16.7%. Surgery treatment had the highest 3-year survival rate which was close to that of surgery combined with RT (60.2% and 58.4% respectively). Besides, with the follow-up time extending, the survival rate decreased, especially from 3-year to 5-year: for surgery, from 60.2% to 12.5%–46.9%; for RT, from 33.3% to 0%–16.7%; for surgery and RT, from 58.4% to 0%–33.3%.

Meta-Analysis: Results for Death Rate

Similarly, in **Figure 2**, the treatment of RT and CT had the lowest 5-year death rate followed by the treatment of surgery [risk ratio (RR):0.38, 95% confidential interval (CI) = 0.15–0.65; 0.69, 95% CI = 0.51–0.84; respectively]. However, the small number of patients in RT and CT group should be noted. The heterogeneity was in a moderate degree in the pooled effect ($I^2 = 70\%$, $P < 0.01$) and subgroups of several treatments (**Figure 2**). We also tried to conduct a subgroup analysis to detect the source of heterogeneity furtherly based on other various factors including metastasis condition, age, tumor size, and tumor site, but failed since enrolled articles were lack of appropriate data.

Meta-Analysis: Study Quality of Included Studies

The summary quality assessment of the 32 included studies was illustrated in **Supplementary Files**. We assigned scores of 0–3, 4–6, and 7–9 on the Newcastle-Ottawa scale for the low, moderate and high quality of studies, respectively. The 32 included studies showed the mean quality score was 7 out of 9. In the 5 enrolled studies, three studies reached 8 and two studies were ranked as 7.

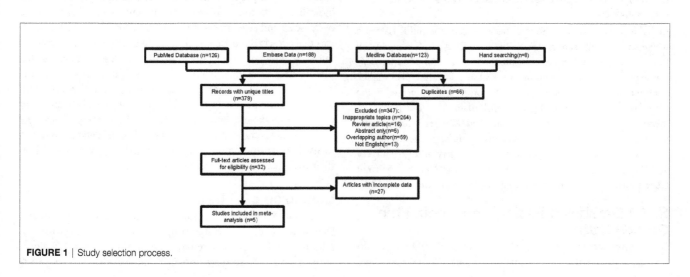

FIGURE 1 | Study selection process.

TABLE 1 | Patient demographics and tumor characteristics for cutaneous angiosarcomas summarized from published literature and SEER database.

	Published literatures	SEER
Sex		
Male	916 (64.8%)	435 (48.4%)
Female	498 (35.2%)	464 (51.6%)
Age		
10–39	72.1 ± 5.15[a]	14 (1.6%)
40–49		31 (3.4%)
50–59		70 (7.8%)
60–69		177 (19.7%)
70–79		280 (31.1%)
80+		327 (36.4%)
Race		
White	–	791 (88.0%)
Black	–	42 (4.6%)
Other	–	49 (5.5%)
Unknown	–	17 (1.9%)
Average follow up (months)[b]	112.9	43.7
Size		
Tumor size ≤5	525 (37.1%)	11 (1.2%)
Tumor size >5	432 (30.6%)	357 (39.7%)
NA/Not reported	457 (32.3%)	531 (59.1%)
Sites		
Scalp/neck/head	721 (51.0%)	345 (39.2%)
Face	367 (26.0%)	211 (21.7%)
Trunk/limb	41 (2.9%)	326 (37.1%)
Unspecific site	152 (10.7%)	17 (1.9%)
Unknown	133 (9.4%)	-
Histologic grade		
Grade I	–	54 (6.0%)
Grade II	–	83 (9.2%)
Grade III	–	138 (15.4%)
Grade IV	–	128 (14.2%)
Unknown	–	496 (55.2%)
SEER historic stage		
Localized	–	437 (51.6%)
Distant	–	291 (34.3%)[c]
Unstaged	–	119 (14.1%)

[a]: Mean ± Standard deviation.
[b]: Mean value of longest follow-up time from each study.
[c]: There are 62 distant and 229 regional patients.
SEER, Surveillance, Epidemiology, and End Results program; NA, not available.

SEER Database: Characteristics of the Population

In **Table 1**, we retrieved 899 cAS patients from the SEER database where 435 patients were male and 464 were female. Interestingly, the ratio of patients with tumor size more than 5 cm versus less than 5cm was exponentially larger than that in published literature data. As for the tumor site, a larger proportion of tumors were documented in the trunk/limb when comparing the SEER data with the published literature data. There are 62 distant and 229 regional patients grouping as distant patients in the following analysis. The number of patients receiving surgery, surgery and RT, surgery and CT, surgery and RT and CT, were 389 (43%), 173 (19%), 61 (7%), and 54 (6%) respectively. There are 108 patients with no treatments recorded (12%).

SEER Database: Factors Influencing the OS and CSS

In the univariate analysis, sites of face (P value < 0.01) and trunk/limb (P value < 0.01) were predictors of both OS and CSS. Ages (P value < 0.01), size (P = 0.03), black race (P value < 0.01), localized stage (P value < 0.01), tumor grades (P value < 0.05) except grade II (P value= 0.54) were all significant predictors of OS. Age (P value < 0.05), sex (P value < 0.01), and SEER historic stage (P value < 0.05) were predictors for CSS (**Supplementary Table 3**). The multivariate models conducted for both OS and CSS included all significant predictors in univariate analysis (**Supplementary Table 4**). We also included the treatment modalities as covariates. All age groups were independently correlated with OS in localized patients. Sites of face and trunk/limb were found to reduce the OS and CSS in localized patients and the OS in metastatic patients when compared with the reference groups (P value < 0.05).

SEER Database: Effectiveness and Trends of Different Treatment Modalities

For a more accurate illustration of the efficacy of different treatment modalities, the multivariate cox regression analysis was performed in which the hazard ratio of OS and CSS were adjusted by the significant factors in the univariate analysis. (Full results were shown in **Supplementary Table 4**). As shown in **Table 3**, the patients were stratified into localized and metastatic groups. Compared with the surgery with RT group, both localized and metastatic patients treated with CT showed significantly worse outcomes in OS and CSS, while the surgery and CT group and surgery and CT and RT group showed significantly worse OS only in localized patients. Particularly, the surgery alone was associated with a higher hazard for OS in metastatic patients compared with the surgery with RT group [hazard ratio (HR): 1.6; 95% CI: (1.05, 2.42); P value: = 0.03]. In **Figure 3**, we plotted the trends of therapies based on the number of patients who received the same therapy each year. Surgery is the most commonly used therapy followed by surgery together with radiotherapy.

DISCUSSION

Given the limited clinical evidence since the rather low incidence of cAS, the discussion for selecting the optimal treatment modality of cAS was in slow progress. Shin et al. (32) conducted a meta-analysis indicating the factors predisposing poor outcomes for angiosarcoma of the scalp and face. In this study, the only treatment-related result was that surgery, compared with no-surgery patients, the 5-year OS rate of angiosarcomas would significantly increase. They also stated the difficulty of comparing different treatment methods since the absence of data. Other studies focusing on the cAS and angiosarcoma patients in SEER database were all short of treatment modalities information (6, 7). To our knowledge, the present study is the first meta-analysis and SEER database research focused on illustrating the prognosis of the cAS patients based on their treatment modalities and extent of the tumor.

Localized cAS Patients

For localized patients, the results from the SEER database suggest that the CT could be inappropriate while the necessity of additional RT to surgery remains uncertain. Because CT alone, surgery and CT, surgery and CT and RT showed worse OS

The Effectiveness of Different Treatment Modalities of Cutaneous Angiosarcoma: Results From Meta-Analysis...

5

TABLE 2 | Summary results of prognosis in included studies.

Therapy type	N	2 year-survival rate (%)	3 year-survival rate (%)	5 year-survival rate (%)	10 year-survival rate (%)	3 year-RFS (%)	5 year-RFS (%)	DFI (month)	Mean survival time (month)	First author
Surgery	7–48		60.2	12.5–46.9	14.3	59.8	25–39.9		12.9	Perez, MC (27); Matsumoto, K (28); Holden, CA (29); Zhang, Y (30)
RT	7–45	29	33.3	0–16.7					10.8	Perez, MC (27); Matsumoto, K (28); Holden, CA (29)
CT	2			0					2	Matsumoto, K (28)
Surgery and RT	3–57	66.7	58.4	0–33.3		27.9	0–27.9	42.8	31.3	Perez, MC (27); Matsumoto, K (28); Holden, CA (29); Zhang, Y (30); Bartelbort, SW (31)
Surgery and CT	8–22			0–14			7		11.9	Matsumoto, K (28); Zhang, Y (30)
Surgery, RT and CT	7–22			13.3–15			0		17.1	Matsumoto, K (28); Zhang, Y (30)
RT and CT	13			61.5					9.3	Matsumoto, K (28)

N, Number of patients enrolled in each study; CT, chemotherapy; RT, radiotherapy; RFS, recurrence-free survival; DFI, disease-free interval.

TABLE 3 | Multivariate cox proportions hazards models for overall survival (OS) and cancer-specific survival (CSS) in SEER patients with cAS.

Treatment modality	Localized						Metastatic					
	OS			CSS			OS			CSS		
	HR	95% CI	P value	HR	95% CI	P value	HR	95% CI	P value	HR	95% CI	P value
Surgery and RT	Ref											
CT	**3.6**	**(1.95,6.62)**	**<0.01**	**3.16**	**(1.17,8.53)**	**0.02**	**4.17**	**(2.05,8.46)**	**<0.01**	**3.53**	**(1.24,10.02)**	**0.02**
None	1.72	(1.01,2.91)	0.05	1.83	(0.83,4.05)	0.13	**4.36**	**(2.3,8.25)**	**<0.01**	**6.78**	**(2.77,16.59)**	**<0.01**
RT	1.62	(0.94,2.77)	0.08	0.9	(0.36,2.24)	0.81	1.61	(0.83,3.11)	0.16	1.37	(0.52,3.62)	0.53
RT+CT	1.61	(0.82,3.15)	0.16	1.17	(0.44,3.13)	0.75	1.11	(0.54,2.25)	0.78	1.82	(0.76,4.33)	0.18
Surgery	0.99	(0.71,1.4)	0.98	0.62	(0.36,1.07)	0.08	**1.6**	**(1.05,2.42)**	**0.03**	1.15	(0.62,2.15)	0.66
Surgery and CT	**2.25**	**(1.19,4.24)**	**0.01**	1.71	(0.57,5.12)	0.34	1.18	(0.67,2.06)	0.56	1.04	(0.46,2.39)	0.92
Surgery, RT and CT	**1.79**	**(1.03,3.13)**	**0.04**	1.89	(0.88,4.04)	0.1	1.3	(0.72,2.33)	0.38	1.87	(0.91,3.86)	0.09

cAS, cutaneous angiosarcoma; OS, overall survival; CSS, cancer-specific survival; CT, chemotherapy; RT, radiotherapy; HR, hazard ratio; CI, confidential interval.
The significant results (P<0.05) were showed in bold.

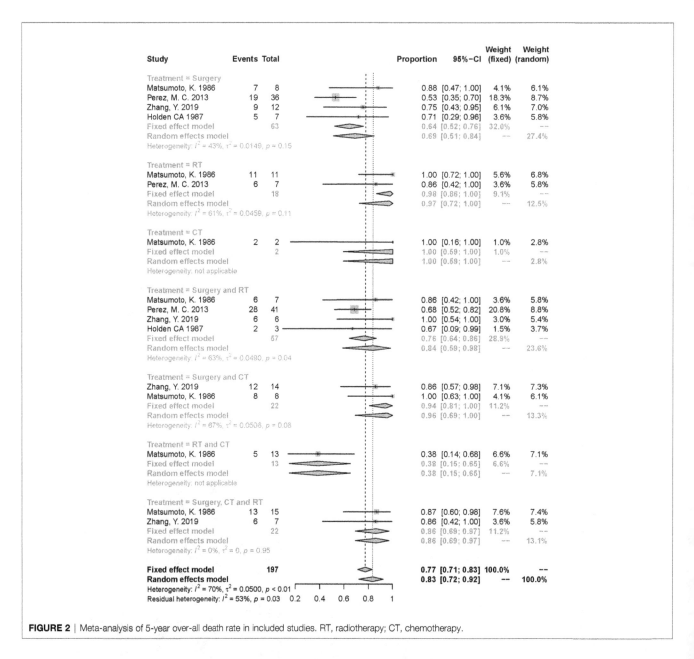

FIGURE 2 | Meta-analysis of 5-year over-all death rate in included studies. RT, radiotherapy; CT, chemotherapy.

results when compared with surgery and RT in the localized patients. The reason could be the intolerance of patients giving a significant proportion of the elderly. What's more, there were no significant results when comparing surgery alone with surgery and RT in the localized patients for both OS and CSS. Several studies (32, 33) have proven that surgery could enhance prognosis in cAS patients with no stratification of patients. Yet, surgery and RT was widely reported for reducing the risk of local recurrence and improving survival rate in localized patients (34, 35). Guadagnolo et al. (36) demonstrated that non-metastatic patients who underwent surgery and RT have statistically greater local control, OS and disease-specific survival compared with those who received surgery or RT alone. Another review (9) stated that surgery followed by RT is the mainstay of the treatment for localized angiosarcoma. Many reasons would

cause this ambiguity. Primarily, the assessment of treatment efficacy should be based on the extent of cAS. Localized cAS patients are prone to receive extensive surgery and with a better prognosis since they are in the early stage of cancer while metastatic patients need more systematic treatment and ended up with a poorer outcome. Thus, any comparison of the treatment regardless of the patients' condition should be treated with caution. Secondly, most studies, including ours, are limited by the retrospective nature. The doses, frequency and time of RT (before or after the surgery) can vary a lot. There was another trial demonstrating the efficacy of chemoradiotherapy followed by maintenance CT in localized patients with large tumors that are hard to control with surgery and RT (37). Further clinical trials or guidelines may focus more on systematically conducting and delicately grouping of patients.

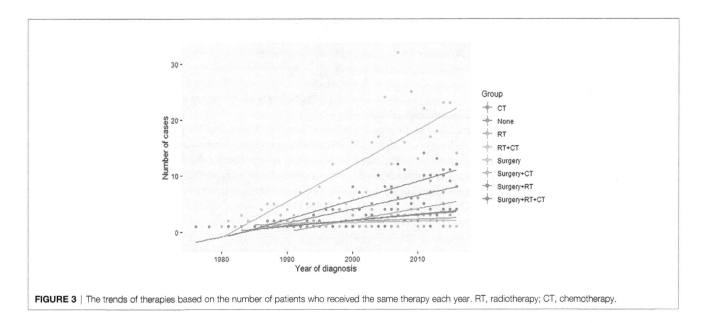

FIGURE 3 | The trends of therapies based on the number of patients who received the same therapy each year. RT, radiotherapy; CT, chemotherapy.

Metastatic cAS Patients

Paclitaxel (taxanes) was recommended as the first-line treatment for metastatic cAS patients in (9), which conflicts with our results: metastatic patients treated with CT alone have worse OS and CSS outcomes than the surgery combined with RT group. This discrepancy could derive from the use of different CT drugs since the quickly evolving process of finding new drugs. Doxorubicin-based drugs have been the preferred choice for advanced soft tissue sarcomas earlier (38, 39), which was replaced by paclitaxel nowadays (9, 38–40). Paclitaxel was rigorously assessed in a phase II trial where 30 metastatic angiosarcoma patients enrolled for a median follow-up of 8 months (40), and the result showed the median time to progression was 4 months and the median overall survival was 8 months. One retrospective study from the same institution including 149 metastatic angiosarcoma patients found there were no statistically significant differences in terms of overall survival between weekly paclitaxel and doxorubicin-based therapy (38).

On the other hand, for metastatic patients, we observed a significantly worse OS outcome receiving surgery alone versus surgery and RT only, which provides evidence for surgery and RT use in metastasis patients except for localized patients. As forementioned, the discussion of the treatment modality for metastatic patients should also consider factors including the patients' tolerance and quality of life and the follow-up duration. Considering the multiple choices of CT drugs, it seems more difficult to reach an agreement. A more systematic treatment modality might be a more reliable choice for metastatic patients based on our findings and current status.

Booming Treatment Options

According to previous results (9, 41), various drugs could be the second-line treatments for advanced cAS including pazopanib (a tyrosine kinase inhibitor), eribulin mesylate (a microtubule-targeting drug), trabectedin (a histone deacetylase inhibitor), bevacizumab (a vascular endothelial growth factor receptor

inhibitor), and propranolol (a beta-blocker). Pazopanib, eribulin mesylate, and trabectedin were firstly published to be effective in treating patients with soft tissue sarcomas (42–44). In later times, a Japanese study showed the potential of pazopanib for the treatment of cAS (45). One prospective clinical study evaluating eribulin mesylate in patients with cAS after taxanes showing a promising response rate (46). Another retrospective study found the 3-month PFS rate was 25% with trabectedin in patients with angiosarcoma (47). Bevacizumab was reported to be effective in treating cAS with a PFS of 6.5 months in a phase II study (48). Notably, propranolol was firstly reported to inhibit the progression of infantile hemangioma (49). Following, several case reports described that the propranolol monotherapy or the combination of propranolol with other chemotherapeutic agents had promising responses in advanced angiosarcoma (50–52).

With the field of cancer immunology growing rapidly, there are also studies linking immune therapy, anti-programmed death ligand-1 (anti-PD-L1), to angiosarcoma treatment. A case report showed a remarkable response in a patient with angiosarcoma with the treatment of anti-PD-L1 (16). Nonetheless, for all the second-line treatments and the immunotherapy, there was not enough evidence to make recommendations for patients with advanced cAS and more prospective studies were needed.

Limitations

Our review has some limitations. Firstly, due to the rarity of cAS and the unclear classification of the treatment modalities, the number of enrolled studies and population is pretty small in the meta-analysis, especially for the CT treatment group. There are also no prospective or randomized studies, which would undermine the quality of our study. Secondly, the detailed baseline information is either absent or ununified in a large number of studies, which prevents the more in-depth analysis. It also contributed to the heterogeneity in pooled results. Additionally, although the retrospective study with the information from SEER was conducted, the treatment details were absent.

CONCLUSION

This study compared the available treatment modalities efficacy of cAS with meta-analysis of observational studies and summarized data from SEER program. The CT could be inappropriate in localized patients. For metastatic patients, the surgery combined RT was recommended compared with surgery alone since its enhanced OS prognosis. Further investigations of long-term and prospective studies are needed for more solid evidence, especially for those newly developed therapies.

AUTHOR CONTRIBUTIONS

Conception and design: YC, JC, and SB. Administrative support: YC and JC. Collection and assembly of data: SB and SC. Data analysis and interpretation: SB, SC, and BW. Article writing: SB, SC, and BW. All authors contributed to the article and approved the submitted version.

REFERENCES

1. Weidema ME, Versleijen-Jonkers YMH, Flucke UE, Desar IME, van der Graaf WTA. Targeting angiosarcomas of the soft tissues: A challenging effort in a heterogeneous and rare disease. *Crit Rev Oncol/Hematol* (2019) 138:120–31. doi: 10.1016/j.critrevonc.2019.04.010

2. Pan Z, An Z, Li Y, Zhou J. Diffuse alveolar hemorrhage due to metastatic angiosarcoma of the lung: A case report. *Oncol Lett* (2015) 10(6):3853–5. doi: 10.3892/ol.2015.3820

3. Cioffi A, Reichert S, Antonescu CR, Maki RG. Angiosarcomas and other sarcomas of endothelial origin. *Hematol/Oncol Clinics North America* (2013) 27(5):975–88. doi: 10.1016/j.hoc.2013.07.005

4. Young RJ, Brown NJ, Reed MW, Hughes D, Woll PJ. Angiosarcoma. *Lancet Oncol* (2010) 11(10):983–91. doi: 10.1016/s1470-2045(10)70023-1

5. Cao J, Wang J, He C, Fang M. Angiosarcoma: a review of diagnosis and current treatment. *Am J Cancer Res* (2019) 9(11):2303–13.

6. Albores-Saavedra J, Schwartz AM, Henson DE, Kostun L, Hart A, Angeles-Albores D, et al. Cutaneous angiosarcoma. Analysis of 434 cases from the Surveillance, Epidemiology, and End Results Program, 1973-2007. *Ann Diagn Pathol* (2011) 15(2):93–7. doi: 10.1016/j.anndiagpath. 2010.07.012

7. Lee KC, Chuang SK, Philipone EM, Peters SM. Characteristics and Prognosis of Primary Head and Neck Angiosarcomas: A Surveillance, Epidemiology, and End Results Program (SEER) Analysis of 1250 Cases. *Head Neck Pathol* (2019) 13(3):378–85. doi: 10.1007/s12105-018-0978-3

8. Florou V, Wilky BA. Current and Future Directions for Angiosarcoma Therapy. *Curr Treat Options Oncol* (2018) 19(3):14. doi: 10.1007/s11864-018-0531-3

9. Ishida Y, Otsuka A, Kabashima K. Cutaneous angiosarcoma: update on biology and latest treatment. *Curr Opin Oncol* (2018) 30(2):107–12. doi: 10.1097/CCO.0000000000000427

10. Choi JH, Ahn KC, Chang H, Minn KW, Jin US, Kim BJ. Surgical Treatment and Prognosis of Angiosarcoma of the Scalp: A Retrospective Analysis of 14 Patients in a Single Institution. *BioMed Res Int* (2015) 2015:321896. doi: 10.1155/2015/321896

11. Oashi K, Namikawa K, Tsutsumida A, Takahashi A, Itami J, Igaki H, et al. Surgery with curative intent is associated with prolonged survival in patients with cutaneous angiosarcoma of the scalp and face -a retrospective study of 38 untreated cases in the Japanese population. *Eur J Surg Oncol* (2018) 44 (6):823–9. doi: 10.1016/j.ejso.2018.02.246

12. Hata M. Radiation Therapy for Angiosarcoma of the Scalp: Total Scalp Irradiation and Local Irradiation. *Anticancer Res* (2018) 38(3):1247–53. doi: 10.21873/anticanres.12346

13. Kajihara I, Kanemaru H, Miyake T, Aoi J, Masuguchi S, Fukushima S, et al. Combination chemotherapy with S-1 and docetaxel for cutaneous angiosarcoma resistant to paclitaxel. *Drug Discovery Ther* (2015) 9(1):75–7. doi: 10.5582/ddt.2015.01005

14. Wada M, Horinaka M, Yasuda S, Masuzawa M, Sakai T, Katoh N. PDK1 is a potential therapeutic target against angiosarcoma cells. *J Dermatol Sci* (2015) 78(1):44–50. doi: 10.1016/j.jdermsci.2015.01.015

15. Florou V, Rosenberg AE, Wieder E, Komanduri KV, Kolonias D, Uduman M, et al. Angiosarcoma patients treated with immune checkpoint inhibitors: a case series of seven patients from a single institution. *J Immunother Cancer* (2019) 7(1):213. doi: 10.1186/s40425-019-0689-7

16. Sindhu S, Gimber LH, Cranmer L, McBride A, Kraft AS. Angiosarcoma treated successfully with anti-PD-1 therapy - a case report. *J Immunother Cancer* (2017) 5(1):58. doi: 10.1186/s40425-017-0263-0

17. Surveillance Epidemiology and End Results Program. (2020). Available at: https://seer.cancer.gov/ (Accessed July 2, 2020).

18. Higgins JPT, Green S. *Cochrane handbook for systematic reviews of interventions*. Chichester (UK: John Wiley & Sons (2008).

19. Stang A. Critical evaluation of the Newcastle-Ottawa scale for the assessment of the quality of nonrandomized studies in meta-analyses. *Eur J Epidemiol* (2010) 25(9):603–5. doi: 10.1007/s10654-010-9491-z

20. Deeks JJ, Dinnes J, D'Amico R, Sowden AJ, Sakarovitch C, Song F, et al. *Evaluating non-randomised intervention studies. Health technology assessment* Vol. 7. Winchester, England: Gray Publishing (2003) p. iii–x, 1-173. doi: 10.3310/hta7270

21. Higgins JP, Thompson SG, Deeks JJ, Altman DG. Measuring inconsistency in meta-analyses. *BMJ (Clin Res ed)* (2003) 327(7414):557–60. doi: 10.1136/bmj.327.7414.557

22. Therneau TM, Grambsch PM. *Modeling Survival Data: Extending the Cox Model*. New York: Springer-Verlag New York (2000). doi: 10.1007/978-1-4757-3294-8

23. Harrer M, Pim C, Toshi AF, David DE. *dmetar: Companion R Package For The Guide "Doing Meta-Analysis in R"*. R package version 0.0. 9000. (2019). Available at: https://bookdown.org/MathiasHarrer/Doing_Meta_Analysis_in_R/.

24. Plummer M. *rjags: Bayesian graphical models using MCMC* Vol. 4. R package version (2016).

25. Wickham H. *ggplot2: Elegant Graphics for Data Analysis*. Springer-Verlag New York (2016).

26. Kassambara A, Kosinski M, Biecek P. survminer: Drawing Survival Curves using 'ggplot2'(2020). Available at: https://CRAN.R-project.org/package=survminer (Accessed July 2, 2020).

27. Perez MC, Padhya TA, Messina JL, Jackson RS, Gonzalez RJ, Bui MM, et al. Cutaneous angiosarcoma: a single-institution experience. *Ann Surg Oncol* (2013) 20(11):3391–7. doi: 10.1245/s10434-013-3083-6

28. Matsumoto K, Inoue K, Fukamizu H. *Prognosis of cutaneous angiosarcoma in Japan: A statistical study of sixty-nine cases* Vol. 8. Verlag GmbH Germany: European Journal of Plastic Surgery (1986) p. 151–8.

29. Holden CA, Spittle MF, Jones EW. Angiosarcoma of the face and scalp, prognosis and treatment. *Cancer* (1987) 59(5):1046–57. doi: 10.1002/1097-0142(19870301)59:5<1046::aid-cncr2820590533>3.0.co;2-6

30. Zhang Y, Yan Y, Zhu M, Chen C, Lu N, Qi F, et al. Clinical outcomes in primary scalp angiosarcoma. *Oncol Lett* (2019) 18(5):5091–6. doi: 10.3892/ol.2019.10886

31. Barttelbort SW, Stahl R, Ariyan S. Cutaneous angiosarcoma of the face and scalp. *Plast Reconstr Surg* (1989) 84(1):55–9. doi: 10.1097/00006534-198907000-00011

32. Shin JY, Roh SG, Lee NH, Yang KM. Predisposing factors for poor prognosis of angiosarcoma of the scalp and face: Systematic review and meta-analysis. *Head Neck* (2017) 39(2):380–6. doi: 10.1002/hed.24554

33. Trofymenko O, Curiel-Lewandrowski C. Surgical treatment associated with improved survival in patients with cutaneous angiosarcoma. *J Eur Acad Dermatol Venereol* (2018) 32(1):e29–31. doi: 10.1111/jdv.14479

34. Fujisawa Y, Yoshino K, Fujimura T, Nakamura Y, Okiyama N, Ishitsuka Y, et al. Cutaneous Angiosarcoma: The Possibility of New Treatment Options Especially for Patients with Large Primary Tumor. *Front Oncol* (2018) 8 (46):46. doi: 10.3389/fonc.2018.00046

35. Wollina U, Koch A, Hansel G, Schönlebe J, Lotti T, Vojvodic A. Cutaneous Angiosarcoma of Head and Neck - A Single-Centre Analysis. *Open Access Maced J Med Sci* (2019) 7(18):2976–8. doi: 10.3889/oamjms.2019.763

36. Guadagnolo BA, Zagars GK, Araujo D, Ravi V, Shellenberger TD, Sturgis EM. Outcomes after definitive treatment for cutaneous angiosarcoma of the face and scalp. *Head Neck* (2011) 33(5):661–7. doi: 10.1002/hed.21513

37. Fujisawa Y, Yoshino K, Kadono T, Miyagawa T, Nakamura Y, Fujimoto M. Chemoradiotherapy with taxane is superior to conventional surgery and radiotherapy in the management of cutaneous angiosarcoma: a multicentre, retrospective study. *Br J Dermatol* (2014) 171(6):1493–500. doi: 10.1111/bjd.13110

38. Penel N, Italiano A, Ray-Coquard I, Chaigneau L, Delcambre C, Robin YM, et al. Metastatic angiosarcomas: doxorubicin-based regimens, weekly paclitaxel and metastasectomy significantly improve the outcome. *Ann Oncol Off J Eur Soc Med Oncol* (2012) 23(2):517–23. doi: 10.1093/annonc/mdr138

39. Italiano A, Cioffi A, Penel N, Levra MG, Delcambre C, Kalbacher E, et al. Comparison of doxorubicin and weekly paclitaxel efficacy in metastatic angiosarcomas. *Cancer* (2012) 118(13):3330–6. doi: 10.1002/cncr.26599

40. Penel N, Bui BN, Bay JO, Cupissol D, Ray-Coquard I, Piperno-Neumann S, et al. Phase II trial of weekly paclitaxel for unresectable angiosarcoma: the ANGIOTAX Study. *J Clin Oncol Off J Am Soc Clin Oncol* (2008) 26(32):5269–74. doi: 10.1200/jco.2008.17.3146

41. Shustef E, Kazlouskaya V, Prieto VG, Ivan D, Aung PP. Cutaneous angiosarcoma: a current update. *J Clin Pathol* (2017) 70(11):917–25. doi: 10.1136/jclinpath-2017-204601

42. van der Graaf WT, Blay JY, Chawla SP, Kim DW, Bui-Nguyen B, Casali PG, et al. Pazopanib for metastatic soft-tissue sarcoma (PALETTE): a randomised,

double-blind, placebo-controlled phase 3 trial. *Lancet (London England)* (2012) 379(9829):1879–86. doi: 10.1016/s0140-6736(12)60651-5

43. Schöffski P, Ray-Coquard IL, Cioffi A, Bui NB, Bauer S, Hartmann JT, et al. Activity of eribulin mesylate in patients with soft-tissue sarcoma: a phase 2 study in four independent histological subtypes. *Lancet Oncol* (2011) 12 (11):1045–52. doi: 10.1016/s1470-2045(11)70230-3

44. Schöffski P, Chawla S, Maki RG, Italiano A, Gelderblom H, Choy E, et al. Eribulin versus dacarbazine in previously treated patients with advanced liposarcoma or leiomyosarcoma: a randomised, open-label, multicentre, phase 3 trial. *Lancet (London England)* (2016) 387(10028):1629–37. doi: 10.1016/s0140-6736(15)01283-0

45. Ogata D, Yanagisawa H, Suzuki K, Oashi K, Yamazaki N, Tsuchida T. Pazopanib treatment slows progression and stabilizes disease in patients with taxane-resistant cutaneous angiosarcoma. *Med Oncol (Northwood London England)* (2016) 33(10):116. doi: 10.1007/s12032-016-0831-z

46. Fujisawa Y, Fujimura T, Matsushita S, Yamamoto Y, Uchi H, Otsuka A, et al. The efficacy of eribulin mesylate for patients with cutaneous angiosarcoma previously treated with taxane: a multi-center, prospective, observational study. *Br J Dermatol* (2020) 20(10):19042. doi: 10.1111/bjd.19042

47. Le Cesne A, Ray-Coquard I, Duffaud F, Chevreau C, Penel N, Bui Nguyen B, et al. Trabectedin in patients with advanced soft tissue sarcoma: a retrospective national analysis of the French Sarcoma Group. *Eur J Cancer (Oxford Engl 1990)* (2015) 51(6):742–50. doi: 10.1016/j.ejca.2015.01.006

48. Agulnik M, Yarber JL, Okuno SH, von Mehren M, Jovanovic BD, Brockstein BE, et al. An open-label, multicenter, phase II study of bevacizumab for the treatment of angiosarcoma and epithelioid hemangioendotheliomas. *Ann Oncol Off J Eur Soc Med Oncol* (2013) 24(1):257–63. doi: 10.1093/annonc/mds237

49. Léauté-Labrèze C, Dumas de la Roque E, Hubiche T, Boralevi F, Thambo JB, Taïeb A. Propranolol for severe hemangiomas of infancy. *New Engl J Med* (2008) 358(24):2649–51. doi: 10.1056/NEJMc0708819

50. Banavali S, Pasquier E, Andre N. Targeted therapy with propranolol and metronomic chemotherapy combination: sustained complete response of a relapsing metastatic angiosarcoma. *Ecancermedicalscience* (2015) 9:499. doi: 10.3332/ecancer.2015.499

51. Chow W, Amaya CN, Rains S, Chow M, Dickerson EB, Bryan BA. Growth Attenuation of Cutaneous Angiosarcoma With Propranolol-Mediated β-Blockade. *JAMA Dermatol* (2015) 151(11):1226–9. doi: 10.1001/jamadermatol.2015.2554

52. Pasquier E, André N, Street J, Chougule A, Rekhi B, Ghosh J, et al. Effective Management of Advanced Angiosarcoma by the Synergistic Combination of Propranolol and Vinblastine-based Metronomic Chemotherapy: A Bench to Bedside Study. *EBioMedicine* (2016) 6:87–95. doi: 10.1016/j.ebiom.2016.02.026

2

Tissue Expression of Carbonic Anhydrase IX Correlates to more Aggressive Phenotype of Basal Cell Carcinoma

Daniela Russo[1†], Silvia Varricchio[1], Gennaro Ilardi[1†], Francesco Martino[1], Rosa Maria Di Crescenzo[1], Sara Pignatiello[1], Massimiliano Scalvenzi[2], Claudia Costa[2], Massimo Mascolo[1], Francesco Merolla[3] and Stefania Staibano[1*]*

[1] Pathology Unit, Department of Advanced Biomedical Sciences, University of Naples "Federico II", Naples, Italy,
[2] Dermatology Unit, Department of Clinical Medicine and Surgery, University of Naples "Federico II", Naples, Italy,
[3] Department of Medicine and Health Sciences "V.Tiberio", University of Molise, Campobasso, Italy

Correspondence:
Francesco Merolla
francesco.merolla@unimol.it
Stefania Staibano
staibano@unina.it

[†]*These authors have contributed equally to this work*

Basal cell carcinoma (BCC) is the most common cancer in the white-skinned population accounting for about 15% of all neoplasms. Its incidence is increasing worldwide, at a rate of about 10% per year. BCC, although infrequently metastasizing, very often causes extensive tissue losses, due to the high propensity toward stromal infiltration, particularly in its dedifferentiated forms, with disfiguring and debilitating results. To date, there still is limited availability of therapeutic treatments alternative to surgery. We evaluated the immunohistochemical expression of the carbonic anhydrase IX (CAIX), one of the main markers of tissue hypoxia, in a set of 85 archived FFPE BCC tissues, including the main subtypes, with different clinical outcomes, to demonstrate a possible relationship between hypoxic phenotype and biological aggressiveness of these neoplasms. Our results showed that the expression level of the CAIX protein contributes to the stratification of BCC in the different risk classes for recurrence. We hypothesize for CAIX a potential therapeutic role as a target therapy in the treatment of more aggressive BCCs, thus providing an alternative to surgical and pharmacological therapy with Hedgehog inhibitors, a promising example of target therapy in BCCs.

Keywords: basal cell carcinoma, carbonic anhydrase IX, IHC, skin cancer, prognosis, risk stratification

INTRODUCTION

Basal cell carcinoma (BCC) is defined by the World Health Organization (WHO) as a locally invasive, slow-growing tumor that originates from the basal layer cells of the epidermis, placed peripherally to the hair bulbs, and that rarely hesitates in metastasis. The main risk associated to BCC are multiple relapses, an event more frequently occurring in case of incomplete excision or multiple primitive tumors, Relapsing BCC can produce, over time, serious anatomic, functional and aesthetic damage, with serious problems of co-morbidity, severely affecting the quality of life (1). Accounting for about 15% of all solid tumors, BCC is the most common malignant neoplasm in the world, with more than 2.8 million new cases diagnosed each year in the

United States of America (2). In the context of non-melanoma skin cancer (NMSC), BCC accounts for about 80% of the cases (3), with a global incidence increase of 3% to 7%/year over last decades (4), BCC represents a serious public health problem. In Italy, the incidence is approximately 100 cases per 100,000 inhabitants (5). These figures could be underestimated because of the diagnostic-therapeutic management for this neoplasia. BCC treatment, in fact, does not usually include hospitalization, and BCC generally does not cause patients' death. BCC develops predominantly in the mature-elderly population (>40 years), prevalently males, with average age at diagnosis of 68 years, in regions of the body chronically exposed to the sun (particularly face and neck, 70% to 85% of cases; 25% to 30% being represented by the nose alone, to follow the trunk and less frequently the limbs). Recently, an epidemiological shift has been reported, with increased incidence in young female population, probably due to the varied habits of exposure of the population (not adequately protected) in the Sun (6). BCC recognizes as the main risk factor exposure to sunlight, especially UVA and UVB ultraviolet rays. Different BCC variants have been described, based on clinical behavior, morphology, growth pattern, architecture, and differentiation (7). Hypoxia is a pathological condition determined by a lack of oxygen in the whole organism (generalized hypoxia) or in one tissue (tissue hypoxia). Hypoxia has emerged as an important feature of tumor microenvironment of neoplasms with more aggressive biological behavior. The uncontrolled growth of tumors is, in fact, accompanied by the induction of insufficient vascularization which results in the formation in most of the malignant solid tumors of heterogeneously distributed hypoxia regions (8, 9). Hypoxia generates a passage to the glycolic metabolism that allows the production of energy in low or absent oxygen conditions and is crucial for the survival of hypoxic cancer cells. Among the molecules most expressed in hypoxia condition are HIF-1 α and carbonic anhydrase IX (CAIX). These molecules are responsible for the process of adapting cells to oxygen deficiency with the formation of new blood vessels, a mechanism that is exploited by tumor tissues to grow and metastasize (10). CAIX belongs to the family of Carbonic Anhydrases (CA), a group of metal zinc-containing enzymes that catalyze the reversible hydration of CO_2 in HCO_3 and H + ions and has recently emerged as the most promising endogenous marker of cellular hypoxia (10, 11). This reaction is fundamental at the level of cells, tissues, and organs in a wide range of biochemical and physiological processes such as acid-base equilibrium, gas exchange, ionic transport, and carbon dioxide fixation. To date, 15 human isoforms of CA have been characterized that differ in catalytic activity, subcellular localization, and tissue distribution (11). Carbonic Anhydrase IX is encoded by a gene located on chromosome 9 and is a transmembrane isoform with a catalytic site in the extracellular portion and has the highest efficiency for the transport of H + between CAs. It consists of a proteoglycan-like domain at the N-terminal end (involved in adhesion and intercellular communication), an extracellular catalytic domain, a trans-membrane hydrophobic portion and a C-terminal cytoplasmic

tail (essential for correct localization on the plasma membrane and proper functioning of the enzyme) (12). It is a tumor-associated protein, as it is expressed in limited quantities in normal tissue, such as the stomach or intestine, and the expression is however limited to the basolateral membrane of epithelial cells endowed with increased proliferative activity, while it is hyper expressed in solid tumor cells linked to a hypoxic phenotype (13). The overexpression of CAIX on the cell membrane of many solid tumors is mediated by the HIF-1 transcription factor and is often associated with poor reactivity to classical radio and chemotherapy. In a recent work, a close association between overexpression of CAIX and the markers of staminality CD44 and Nestin, has been demonstrated in several aggressive and metastasizing neoplasms, with relevance in a series of squamous carcinomas of the tongue (14). This indicates that CAIX action in hypoxic tumors goes beyond intra-tumoral PH control. The clear majority of existing data, in fact, indicates that CAIX has multiple functions in solid tumors, in particular, it plays a key role in encouraging the establishment of chemo-and radio-resistance in the most advanced cases and opens new therapeutic perspectives (14). In the present study, we deepened the role of the Carbonic Anhydrase IX as a possible leading actor and marker of hypoxia in BCC, by evaluating the immunohistochemistry expression of the CAIX protein in a series of archived FFPE BCC tissue samples.

MATERIALS AND METHODS

Patients and Tissue Samples

Formalin-fixed, paraffin-embedded tissue blocks of 85 BCCs, diagnosed and excised with healthy surgical margins from February 2002 to November 2017, were retrieved from the archives of the Pathology Section of the Department of Advanced Biomedical Sciences, "Federico II" University of Naples. Out of 85 cases, 55 males and 30 females, the age at diagnosis ranged between 38 and 88 years (mean age, 67 years). **Table 1** summarizes the histological groups of the study population, together with the associated risk. The clinical data and pathological features of the tumors are reported in **Table 2**. The study design and procedures involving tissue samples collection and handling were performed according to the

TABLE 1 | Study population summary grouped by histological types.

Risk of recurrence	Histotype	Count
Higher risk	Basosquamous carcinoma	14
	Infiltrating BCC	34
	Micronodular BCC	4
	Sclerosing/morphoeic BCC	10
Higher risk, total		62
Lower risk	BCC with adnexal differentiation	2
	Nodular BCC	16
	Superficial BCC	5
Lower risk, total		23
Total		85

Declaration of Helsinki, in agreement with the current Italian law, and to the Institutional Ethical Committee guidelines.

TMAs Construction and Immunohistochemistry

Two pathologists (SS and DR) reviewed the whole routine hematoxylin-eosin (H&E) sections to confirm the original diagnosis and to mark the most representative tumor areas useful for the TMA construction. Tissue cores with a diameter of 3 mm were punched from morphologically representative tissue areas of each "donor" tissue block and brought into one recipient paraffin block using a manual tissue arrayer. The filled recipient blocks were then placed on a metal base mold. The paraffin-embedding was then carried-out, by heating the blocks at 42°C, for 10 min, and flattening their surface by pressing a clean glass slide on them. As a result, four TMAs were built. 4-μm sections were cut from each TMA using an ordinary microtome (15, 16). The first section was stained with H&E to confirm the presence of the tumor and the integrity of tissues. The other section was mounted on a super frost slide (Microm, Walldorf, Germany) for the immunohistochemical evaluation of CAIX. For CAIX IHC assay the sections were deparaffinized routinely in xylene and rehydrated through a series of graded ethanol. CAIX antigen retrieval was performed in EDTA buffer (pH 8) in a hot water bath (94°C) for 20 min and in CITRATE buffer (pH 6) by microwave oven (3 min × 3 times); the backdrop (for blocking non-specific background staining) was removed using the universal blocking serum (Dako Diagnostics, Glostrup, Denmark) for 15 min at room temperature. Endogenous alkaline phosphatase activity was quenched adding Levamisole to buffer AP (Substrate Buffer); the slides were rinsed

with TRIS+Tween20 pH 7.4 buffer and incubated in a humidified chamber with the primary rabbit polyclonal antibody anti-CAIX (sc-25599, Santa Cruz Biotechnology, diluted 1:200 overnight at 4°C). Then used a biotinylated secondary antibody and streptavidin conjugated with alkaline phosphatase. The reaction has been highlighted with the chromogen Fast Red, which showed the presence of antigen that we sought in red (Dako REAL Detection System, Alkaline Phosphatase/RED, Rabbit/Mouse). Again, after a weak nuclear counterstain with hematoxylin, the sections were then mounted with a synthetic medium (Entellan, Merck, Darmstadt, Germany). Positivity for CAIX was visualized as red membranous and cytoplasmic staining. The CAIX expression was defined as high or low depending on whether the percentage of neoplastic cells stained was respectively >/= or <5%.

Statistical Analysis

Correlation between CAIX immunohistochemical expression and BCC clinical-pathologic characteristics was asses through contingency analysis with Fisher exact test. Statistical analysis has been performed using SPSS software (IBM Corp. Released 2013. IBM SPSS Statistics for Windows, Version 22.0. Armonk, NY: IBM Corp.).

RESULTS

Our case series included 85 tumor samples (**Table 2**), out of which, 7 (8%) were not evaluable for CAIX tissue expression due to loss of core integrity. The CAIX protein showed LOW expression score in 35 (45%) out of 78 cases, and a HIGH score in the residual 43 (55%) (**Table 3**). The study population was subdivided, according to the histotype, into two groups: aggressive BCCs (i.e., BCCs with higher risk of recurrence; including basosquamous, morphoeic, infiltrating and micronodular) consisting of 60 cases (60/78, 77%) and the group of ordinary BCCs (i.e., BCCs with lower risk of recurrence; including nodular, superficial, and with adnexal differentiation) consisting of 18 cases (18/78, 23%) (**Table 1**). Among aggressive BCC, 41 out of 60 evaluable cases (68.3%) showed a HIGH CAIX expression score, while in the group of ordinary BCCs only 2 out of 18 cases (11.1%) showed a high score (**Table 4**; **Figure 1A**). **Table 5** shows the distribution of CAIX expression scores per histologic subtypes. The follow-up data for recurrence, detailed per tumor variants, are shown in **Table 6**.

TABLE 2 | Clinical-pathologic characteristics of the study population.

		n	%
Patients	Total	85	100%
Age	Mean	67	
	Range (Min-Max)	38–88	
Sex	Male	55	65%
	Female	30	35%
Tumor site	Area H	46	54%
	Area M	10	12%
	Area L	27	32%
	ND	2	2%
Histologic subtype	BCC with indolent growth	23	27%
	BCC with aggressive growth	62	73%
Follow-up	Recurrence	30	35%
	No recurrence	55	65%
Follow-up time (months)	Mean	39	
	Median	42	
	Min	2	
	Max	153	
Tumor size	>2 cm	25	29%
	<2 cm	59	70%
	N.D.	1	1%

Area H: "mask areas" of face (central face, eyelids, eyebrows, periorbital, nose, lips [cutaneous and vermilion], chin, mandible, preauricular, and postauricular skin/sulci, temple, ear), genitalia, hands, and feet; Area M: cheeks, forehead, scalp, neck, and pretibial; Area L: trunk and extremities; BCC with indolent or ordinary growth: BCC with solid nest, superficial, adenoid, keratotic; BCC with aggressive or aggressive growth: BCC morphoeic, basosquamous, micronodular, dedifferentiated.

TABLE 3 | CAIX IHC tissue expression score frequency distribution in the studied population.

CAIX expression score frequency distribution

CAIX		Frequency	Percentage (Total)	Percentage (Valid)
Valid	Low	35	41%	45%
	High	43	51%	55%
	Tot. Valid	78	92%	100%
Missing		7	8%	
Total		85	100%	

Correlation between CAIX immunohistochemical expression and BCC histotype was assessed through contingency analysis with Fisher exact test, that proved to be statistical significant, with a P value <0.0001. A survival analysis, taking recurrence as endpoint, was carried out and Kaplan-Meier curves are shown in **Figure 1B**: difference between CAIX HIGH and LOW curves is significant as resulted from Log-Rank test (p = 0.05). Taken together our results show that the higher CAIX expression significantly correlates with BCC aggressive behavior. Representative images of CAIX IHC staining in low-risk BCCs are shown in **Figure 2**; representative high-risk BCCs immunostained with anti-CAIX antibody are shown in **Figure 3**.

DISCUSSION

Basal carcinoma (BCC) represents 15% of all neoplasms and constitutes a serious public health problem, being the most common cancer in the white-skinned population. Its incidence is increasing worldwide, with an increase of ≥ 10%/year [Lomas et al. (2)]. BCC is a tumor that, despite its low frequency of distant metastasis, frequently causes extensive tissue losses, due to a marked tendency to stromal infiltration, particularly in its dedifferentiated forms, with disfiguring and debilitating results. The maximum expression of this aggressive behavior is the so-called Ulcus Rodens with destructive consequences for the cartilage and bone tissues. To date, there is still limited availability of alternative therapeutic treatments to surgery.

TABLE 4 | Contingency table of BCC histologic classification by CAIX score.

Contingency Table Classification * CAIX score

		CAIX score		
		High	Low	Total
Classification	Aggressive	41 (68.3%)	19 (31.7%)	60 (100%)
	Ordinary	2 (11.1%)	16(88.9%)	18 (100%)
Total		43(55.1%)	35 (44.9%)	78 (100%)

TABLE 5 | Crosstab of CAIX expression by histologic subtypes.

Histologic type	CAIX score		
	High	Low	Total
Basosquamous carcinoma	9 (64.3%)	5 (35.7%)	14 (100%)
BCC with adnexal differentiation	0	2 (100%)	2(100%)
Infiltrating BCC	22 (66.7%)	11 (33.3%)	33 (100%)
Micronodular BCC	2 (50%)	2 (50%)	4 (100%)
Nodular BCC	1 (8.3%)	11 (91.7%)	12 (100%)
Sclerosing/morphoeic BCC	8 (88.9%)	1 (11.1%)	9 (100%)
Superficial BCC	1 (25%)	3 (75%)	4 (100)

TABLE 6 | Crosstab of recurrence follow-up data by tumor variants.

Histologic type	Follow-Up		
	Not recurrent	Recurrent	Total
Basosquamous carcinoma	10	4	14
BCC with adnexal differentiation	1	1	2
Infiltrating BCC	15	18	33
Micronodular BCC	1	3	4
Nodular BCC	11	1	12
Sclerosing/morphoeic BCC	5	4	9
Superficial BCC	3	1	4
Total	46	32	78

Recently, promising results seem to emerge from the early follow-up of patients treated with molecular anti-Sonic Hedgehog therapy, a pathway associated with the BCC carcinogenesis process. It is compelling to unravel the pathogenetic mechanisms underlying the aggressiveness potential of each BCC subtypes, in order to achieve an effective personalized therapy for these tumors. The need of greater understanding of BCC biology appears even more urgent given that this neoplasia preferentially affects the adult and elderly population and that prevention and early diagnosis are still unattained goals, especially in emerging areas of the World and in Western countries peripheral areas. In recent years, a large body of data has highlighted the importance of the interaction of cancer cells with the tumor microenvironment,

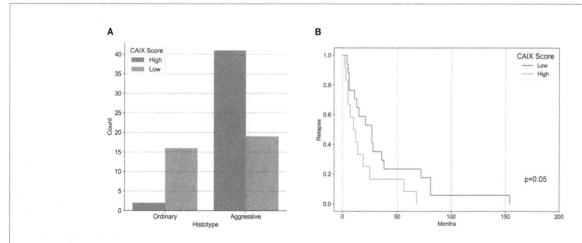

FIGURE 1 | (A) Bar-Graph representation of CAIX immunohistochemical expression in aggressive and ordinary BCC. **(B)** Kaplan-Meier curves of recurrence survival. Difference between CAIX HIGH and CAIX LOW curved proved statistically significant (p = 0.05) as tested by Log-Rank.

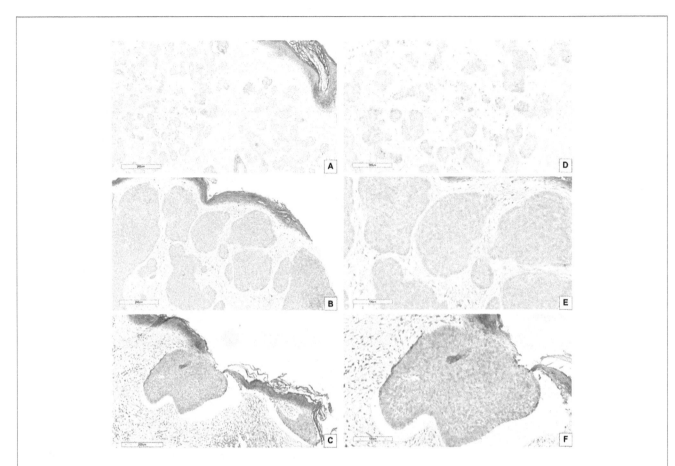

FIGURE 2 | IHC stain with an anti-CAIX antibody in low risk BCC histological variants: **(A–D)** BCC with adnexal differentiation (magnification, 20× and 40×, respectively); **(B–E)** Nodular BCC (magnification, 20× and 40×, respectively); **(C–F)** Superficial BCC (magnification, 20× and 40×, respectively). Scale bars are shown.

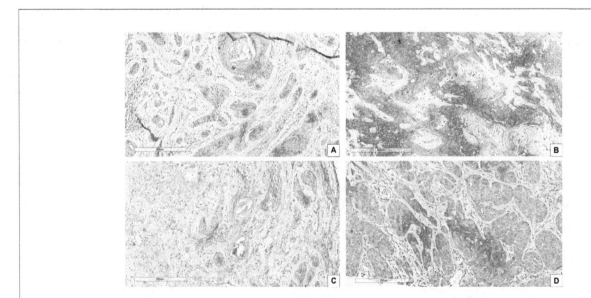

FIGURE 3 | IHC stain with an anti-CAIX antibody in high risk BCC histological variants: **(A)** Infiltrating BCC; **(B)** Morpheaform BCC; **(C)** Micronodular BCC; **(D)** Basosquamous BCC. Scale bars are shown, magnification is 20×.

which provides support for the growth and development of neoplasia. This assumption brought to light new study hypotheses, in order to characterize the heterotypic interaction between the tumor and its microenvironment. Among the alterations of the tumor microenvironment, much attention has been paid, in recent decades, to hypoxia, a pathophysiological feature of locally advanced tumors, resulting from genetic instability, diminished apoptotic potential, and angiogenesis. The hypoxic state also plays an important role in relapsing, metastasis and poor response to treatments, including radiotherapy, chemotherapy and angiogenic treatment. Among the molecules most expressed in hypoxic condition, the carbonic anhydrase IX (CAIX) is considered a marker of hypoxia *in vivo* (17), whose overexpression has been correlated with increased tumor aggression in different types of cancer (18–22). To date, a series of CAIX inhibitors have been synthesized, both in the form of small inhibitory molecules and as monoclonal antibodies, used as antitumor agents in different models of neoplasms (23–31). In a previous work we tested the expression of CAIX in several human solid tumors, extending the CAIX expression information to the expression of the stem cells markers CD44 and nestin in solid cancers, to explore their relationship with the biological behavior of tumors. We found that CAIX is strongly expressed in advanced tumors, including squamous cell invasive cancer of the tongue (14). The role of CAIX as a prognostic biomarker in oral cancer has been recently reviewed by (32), whose systematic review and meta-analysis showed that that immunohistochemical CAIX assessment is a useful OSCC prognostic biomarker. In the present work, the immunohistochemistry expression of the CAIX protein was evaluated in a selected series of patients with BCC divided into two groups based on the histological subtype. The highest levels of protein were found in the aggressive BCC group consisting mainly of morphoeic BCC and Basosquamous BCC. 68.3% of cases showed a high level of expression, and the remaining 31.7% a low level. CAIX expression frequency distribution has been reported in all the histotypes described in our case series, and the statistics of CAIX expression correlation with BCC subtypes have been carried out grouping BCC samples into two categories, aggressive and ordinary one, according to clinical behavior of each subtype, in order to overcome the relative small number of subjects for some subtypes. In the ordinary group, 92% of cases expressed low levels of CAIX and only 8% show a high score. The Fisher Exact Test confirmed that the difference in CAIX immunostain observed between the two BCC groups was statistically significant. The most significant result was obtained by comparing the averages of expression between the aggressive and ordinary groups, and the difference showed a value of $P<0.0001$. In conclusion, these results suggest that the expression levels of the CAIX protein can help to stratify BCCs in different risk classes; moreover, our results let envisage a role for CAIX as a therapeutic target to counteract the most aggressive BCC, providing a viable alternative to the surgical approach, and to the inhibitors of Hedgehog Pathway, a promising tool for target therapy in BCCs, often associated with various degrees of toxicity (muscle spasms, alopecia, dysgeusia, weight loss, fatigue, nausea, decreased appetite and diarrhea) that in the most severe forms (hypovolemic shock, myocardial infarction, meningeal disease, Ischemic stroke) determine the interruption of treatment, with no resolution of the pathology in place.

AUTHOR CONTRIBUTIONS

All authors listed have made a substantial, direct and intellectual contribution to the work, and approved it for publication. All authors contributed to the article and approved the submitted version.

REFERENCES

1. Verkouteren JAC, Ramdas KHR, Wakkee M, Nijsten T. Epidemiology of basal cell carcinoma: scholarly review. *Br J Dermatol* (2017) 177:359–72. doi: 10.1111/bjd.15321
2. Lomas A, Leonardi-Bee J, Bath-Hextall F. A systematic review of worldwide incidence of nonmelanoma skin cancer. *Br J Dermatol* (2012) 166:1069–80. doi: 10.1111/j.1365-2133.2012.10830.x
3. Chinem VP, Miot HA. Epidemiology of basal cell carcinoma. *Anais Brasileiros Dermatol* (2011) 86:292–305. doi: 10.1590/s0365-05962011000200013
4. Leiter U, Keim U, Garbe C. Epidemiology of skin cancer: Update 2019. *Adv Exp Med Biol* (2020) 1268:123–39. doi: 10.1007/978-3-030-46227-7_6
5. AIRTUM Working Group. [Italian cancer figures, report 2011: Survival of cancer patients in Italy]. *Epidemiol E Prevenzione* (2011) 35:1–200.
6. Christenson LJ, Borrowman TA, Vachon CM, Tollefson MM, Otley CC, Weaver AL, et al. Incidence of basal cell and squamous cell carcinomas in a population younger than 40 years. *JAMA* (2005) 294:681–90. doi: 10.1001/jama.294.6.681
7. Elder DE, Massi D, Scolyer RA, Willemze R. *WHO classification of skin tumours*. World Health Organization classification of tumours. 4th. Lyon: International Agency for Research on Cancer (2018).
8. Vaupel P, Mayer A. Hypoxia in cancer: significance and impact on clinical outcome. *Cancer Metastasis Rev* (2007) 26:225–39. doi: 10.1007/s10555-007-9055-1

9. Bache M, Kappler M, Said HM, Staab A, Vordermark D. Detection and specific targeting of hypoxic regions within solid tumors: current preclinical and clinical strategies. *Curr Med Chem* (2008) 15:322–38. doi: 10.2174/092986708783497391
10. Pastorekova S, Gillies RJ. The role of carbonic anhydrase IX in cancer development: links to hypoxia, acidosis, and beyond. *Cancer Metastasis Rev* (2019) 38:65–77. doi: 10.1007/s10555-019-09799-0
11. Pérez-Sayáns M, Supuran CT, Pastorekova S, Suárez-Peñaranda JM, Pilar GD, Barros-Anguiera F, et al. The role of carbonic anhydrase IX in hypoxia control in OSCC. *J Oral Pathol Med: Off Publ Int Assoc Oral Pathologists Am Acad Oral Pathol* (2013) 42:1–8. doi: 10.1111/j.1600-0714.2012.01144.x
12. De Simone G, Supuran CT. Carbonic anhydrase IX: Biochemical and crystallographic characterization of a novel antitumor target. *Biochim Et Biophys Acta* (2010) 1804:404–9. doi: 10.1016/j.bbapap.2009.07.027
13. Breton S. The cellular physiology of carbonic anhydrases. *JOP: J Pancreas* (2001) 2:159–64.
14. Ilardi G, Zambrano N, Merolla F, Siano M, Varricchio S, Vecchione M, et al. Histopathological determinants of tumor resistance: a special look to the immunohistochemical expression of carbonic anhydrase IX in human cancers. *Curr Med Chem* (2014) 21:1569–82. doi: 10.2174/09298673113209990227
15. Mascolo M, Ilardi G, Merolla F, Russo D, Vecchione M, de Rosa G, et al. Tissue microarray-based evaluation of chromatin assembly factor-1 (caf-1)/p60 as tumour prognostic marker. *Int J Mol Sci* (2012) 13:11044–62. doi: 10.3390/ijms130911044

16. Martino F, Varricchio S, Russo D, Merolla F, Ilardi G, Mascolo M, et al. A machine-learning approach for the assessment of the proliferative compartment of solid tumors on hematoxylin-eosin-stained sections. *Cancers* (2020) 12. doi: 10.3390/cancers12051344

17. Swinson DEB, Jones JL, Richardson D, Wykoff C, Turley H, Pastorek J, et al. Carbonic anhydrase IX expression, a novel surrogate marker of tumor hypoxia, is associated with a poor prognosis in non-small-cell lung cancer. *J Clin Oncol: Off J Am Soc Clin Oncol* (2003) 21:473–82. doi: 10.1200/JCO.2003.11.132

18. Hussain SA, Ganesan R, Reynolds G, Gross L, Stevens A, Pastorek J, et al. Hypoxia-regulated carbonic anhydrase IX expression is associated with poor survival in patients with invasive breast cancer. *Br J Cancer* (2007) 96:104–9. doi: 10.1038/sj.bjc.6603530

19. Brennan DC, Daller JA, Lake KD, Cibrik D, Del Castillo D. Thymoglobulin Induction Study Group. Rabbit antithymocyte globulin versus basiliximab in renal transplantation. *New Engl J Med* (2006) 355:1967–77. doi: 10.1056/NEJMoa060068

20. Baniak N, Flood TA, Buchanan M, Dal Cin P, Hirsch MS. Carbonic anhydrase IX (CA9) expression in multiple renal epithelial tumour subtypes. *Histopathology* (2020) 77:659–66. doi: 10.1111/his.14204

21. Jin MS, Lee H, Park IA, Chung YR, Im SA, Lee KH, et al. Overexpression of HIF1α and CAXI predicts poor outcome in early-stage triple negative breast cancer. *Virchows Archiv: Int J Pathol* (2016) 469:183–90. doi: 10.1007/s00428-016-1953-6

22. Lodewijk L, van Diest P, van der Groep P, Ter Hoeve N, Schepers A, Morreau J, et al. Expression of HIF-1α in medullary thyroid cancer identifies a subgroup with poor prognosis. *Oncotarget* (2017) 8:28650–9. doi: 10.18632/oncotarget.15622

23. Supuran CT. Carbonic Anhydrase Inhibition and the Management of Hypoxic Tumors. *Metabolites* (2017) 7. doi: 10.3390/metabo7030048

24. Chafe SC, McDonald PC, Saberi S, Nemirovsky O, Venkateswaran G, Burugu S, et al. Targeting Hypoxia-Induced Carbonic Anhydrase IX Enhances Immune-Checkpoint Blockade Locally and Systemically. *Cancer Immunol Res* (2019) 7:1064–78. doi: 10.1158/2326-6066.CIR-18-0657

25. Lau J, Lin KS, Benard F. Past, Present, and Future: Development of Theranostic Agents Targeting Carbonic Anhydrase IX. *Theranostics* (2017) 7:4322–39. doi: 10.7150/thno.21848

26. Alberti D, Michelotti A, Lanfranco A, Protti N, Altieri S, Deagostino A, et al. In vitro and in vivo BNCT investigations using a carborane containing sulfonamide targeting CAIX epitopes on malignant pleural mesothelioma and breast cancer cells. *Sci Rep* (2020) 10:19274. doi: 10.1038/s41598-020-76370-1

27. Giuntini G, Monaci S, Cau Y, Mori M, Naldini A, Carraro F. Inhibition of Melanoma Cell Migration and Invasion Targeting the Hypoxic Tumor Associated CAXII. *Cancers* (2020) 12. doi: 10.3390/cancers12103018

28. Peppicelli S, Andreucci E, Ruzzolini J, Bianchini F, Nediani C, Supuran CT, et al. The Carbonic Anhydrase IX inhibitor SLC-0111 as emerging agent against the mesenchymal stem cell-derived pro-survival effects on melanoma cells. *J Enzyme Inhibition Med Chem* (2020) 35:1185–93. doi: 10.1080/14756366.2020.1764549

29. Ciccone V, Filippelli A, Angeli A, Supuran CT, Morbidelli L. Pharmacological Inhibition of CA-IX Impairs Tumor Cell Proliferation, Migration and Invasiveness. *Int J Mol Sci* (2020) 21. doi: 10.3390/ijms21082983

30. Aneja B, Queen A, Khan P, Shamsi F, Hussain A, Hasan P, et al. Design, synthesis & biological evaluation of ferulic acid-based small molecule inhibitors against tumor-associated carbonic anhydrase IX. *Bioorg Med Chem* (2020) 28:115424. doi: 10.1016/j.bmc.2020.115424

31. Podolski-Renić A, Dinić J, Stanković T, Jovanović M, Ramović A, Pustenko A, et al. Sulfocoumarins, specific carbonic anhydrase IX and XII inhibitors, interact with cancer multidrug resistant phenotype through pH regulation and reverse P-glycoprotein mediated resistance. *Eur J Pharm Sci: Off J Eur Fed Pharm Sci* (2019) 138:105012. doi: 10.1016/j.ejps.2019.105012

32. Lorenzo-Pouso AI, Gallas-Torreira M, Pérez-Sayáns M, Chamorro-Petronacci CM, Alvarez-Calderon O, Takkouche B, et al. Prognostic value of CAIX expression in oral squamous cell carcinoma: a systematic review and meta-analysis. *J Enzyme Inhibition Med Chem* (2020) 35:1258–66. doi: 10.1080/14756366.2020.1772250

3

Incidence of Skin Cancer in Patients with Chronic Inflammatory Cutaneous Diseases on Targeted Therapies

Salvatore Crisafulli[1†], Lucrezia Bertino[2†], Andrea Fontana[3], Fabrizio Calapai[4], Ylenia Ingrasciotta[1], Massimiliano Berretta[5], Gianluca Trifirò[6] and Claudio Guarneri[1*]

[1] Department of Biomedical and Dental Sciences and Morphofunctional Imaging, University of Messina, Messina, Italy,
[2] Department of Clinical and Experimental Medicine, University of Messina, Messina, Italy, [3] Unit of Biostatistics, Fondazione IRCCS Casa Sollievo della Sofferenza, San Giovanni Rotondo, Italy, [4] Department of Chemical, Biological, Pharmaceutical and Environmental Sciences, University of Messina, Messina, Italy, [5] Department of Clinical and Experimental Medicine, Section of Infectious Diseases, University of Messina, Messina, Italy, [6] Department of Diagnostics and Public Health, University of Verona, Verona, Italy

*Correspondence:
Claudio Guarneri
claudio.guarneri@unime.it

†These authors have contributed equally to this work

Cancer is one of the several comorbidities that have been linked with chronic cutaneous inflammatory diseases namely psoriasis/psoriatic arthritis and hidradenitis suppurativa. Although the chronic inflammatory state, typical of the diseases, may induce pro-tumorigenic effects, the debate whether or not the drugs currently used in clinical practice do in facts increase a patient's risk of malignancy remains largely unsolved. The therapeutic armamentarium has been greatly enhanced at least in the last two decades with the advent of biologics, a heterogeneous group of laboratory-engineered agents with more in the pipeline, and other targeted small molecules. Among the organ systems, skin results as one of the most commonly affected, non-melanoma skin cancers being the main drug-induced manifestations as side effect in course of these treatments. The objective of the study is to systematically review the cutaneous malignancy risk of the newer therapies through an overview of meta-analyses and observational studies on the topic.

Keywords: skin cancer, non-melanoma skin cancer, melanoma, biologics, psoriasis

INTRODUCTION

Psoriasis, psoriatic arthritis and hidradenitis suppurativa are three common inflammatory and immune-mediated skin diseases characterized by increased levels of pro-inflammatory cytokines and chemokines such as tumor necrosis factor (TNF)-α, interleukin (IL)-17 and IL-23 (1–7). Chemical inflammatory mediators involved in the pathogenesis of these diseases may increase the risk of malignancies through the induction of pro-cancerous mutations, adaptive responses, resistance to apoptosis and environmental changes such as the stimulation of angiogenesis (8, 9). A number of observational studies suggested that patients affected by these diseases are at increased risk of developing cancer (10–13). In particular, increased rates of cancer, especially keratinocyte skin cancer and lymphomas were reported in patients with psoriasis or psoriatic arthritis (14). A significantly increased risk of overall cancer was observed also among patients affected by hidradenitis suppurativa in a recently published population-based cohort study (15).

The recent marketing of systemic biological (i.e. the TNF-α inhibitors etanercept, infliximab and adalimumab, the anti-IL-12/23 ustekinumab, the IL-17/IL-17 receptor antagonists secukinumab, ixekizumab and brodalumab and the anti-IL-23 agents tildrakizumab, guselkumab and risankizumab) and chemically synthetized drugs (e.g. apremilast and tofacitinib) as targeted therapies has improved the management of these diseases (16–18). However, since these drugs target molecules that may be relevant to cancer immunosurveillance mechanisms, some concerns were raised about their association with an increased risk of cancer occurrence (19–23). A recent meta-analysis of randomized clinical trials (RCTs) and open-label extension (OLE) studies reported that TNF inhibitors are associated with an increased risk of non-melanoma skin cancers (NMSC) in people with psoriasis. However, the authors of this study found that no real-world evidence was available and acknowledged the significant limitations associated with the study design of the articles included, that make it difficult to extrapolate to real-world practice (24). Evidence on the risk of skin cancer in patients with chronic inflammatory cutaneous diseases on targeted therapies is still sparse controversial. Therefore, the aim of this systematic review and meta-analysis was to assess the risk of cutaneous malignancies in patients with psoriasis, psoriatic arthritis or hidradenitis suppurativa treated with targeted therapies.

METHODS

Search Strategy and Study Selection Criteria

This systematic review and meta-analysis was conducted in accordance with the Preferred Reporting Items for Systematic Reviews and Meta-Analyses (PRISMA) statement, following an *a priori*-established protocol registered on the International Prospective Register of Systematic Reviews (PROSPERO: CRD42020212137). The completed PRISMA checklist is provided in **Supplementary Figure 1**. Two authors (SC, FC) independently searched the bibliographic databases PubMed and EMBASE for literature related to the risk of skin cancer in patients affected by inflammatory cutaneous diseases and treated with targeted therapies. Literature was searched from databases inception until 15th September 2020. The search strategy concerned terms related to inflammatory cutaneous diseases (i.e. psoriasis, psoriatic arthritis and hidradenitis suppurativa), skin

cancers (e.g. squamous cell carcinoma, basal cell carcinoma and melanoma) and targeted therapies (i.e. etanercept, infliximab, adalimumab, ustekinumab, secukinumab, ixekizumab, brodalumab, tildrakizumab, guselkumab, risankizumab, apremilast and tofacitinib). Citations, titles and abstracts were exported into Endnote X9. The detailed literature search strategy for different databases is provided in **Supplementary Table 1**. Original observational studies were included if they (a) included patients affected by psoriasis, psoriatic arthritis or hidradenitis suppurativa; (b) clearly reported a well-defined measure of skin malignancies incidence; (c) included patients treated with biological drugs and/or the small molecules, apremilast and tofacitinib; (d) were written in English. To reduce the risk of publication bias, conference abstracts were also eligible for inclusion. Narrative or systematic reviews, meta-analyses, book chapters, editorials and pooled analyses were not included, but the reference lists in reviews and meta-analyses were screened to potentially identify further studies to include.

After duplicate studies were removed, two authors (SC and FC) individually reviewed titles and abstracts to remove clearly irrelevant articles and, subsequently, full text of the articles that both reviewers considered potentially eligible. Any inconsistencies were resolved at this stage through discussion or the intervention of a third independent assessor (GT or CG).

Data Extraction

For eligible studies, information on the following items was independently collected by the same two authors and stratified by skin cancer type: study authors, year of publication, catchment area, data source, study population, study years, study design and risk estimate. Any disagreements were resolved by consensus with a third author (GT or CG).

Assessment of Risk of Bias and Overall Quality of the Evidence

The risk of bias of the observational studies included in this systematic review was independently assessed by two authors (SC and FC) using the Newcastle-Ottawa quality assessment scale (25). This instrument consists of eight different domains for cohort studies (representativeness of the exposed cohort, selection of the non-exposed cohort, ascertainment of exposure, demonstration that outcome of interest was not present at start of study, comparability of cohorts on the basis of the design or analysis, assessment of outcome, follow-up long enough for outcomes to occur, adequacy of follow up) and case-control studies (adequate case definition, representativeness of the cases, selection of controls, definition of controls, comparability of cases and controls on the basis of the design or analysis, ascertainment of exposure, same method of ascertainment for cases and controls, non-response rate). The included studies were categorized as "low risk of bias" if at least six of the eight domains were judged to be at low risk of bias.

Statistical Analysis

For each included study, skin cancer incidence rates (IR) per 10,000 person-years (PY) were considered as the primary outcome for the meta-analysis. Meta-analysis of IRs was performed assuming that the logarithm of each study-specific rate was normally distributed and the corresponding standard error, used to perform the inverse-variance weighting, was computed from the 95% CI (or p-value) reported in the original IRs. Between-study heterogeneity of the estimates was assessed using the Cochran's Q-test (26) along with its derived measure of inconsistency (I^2), and was considered to be present when Cochran's Q-test p-value was < 0.10 or $I^2 > 40\%$ (27). Estimates were summarized by fixed-effects or random-effects models, according to the absence or the presence of heterogeneity, respectively. It is generally accepted that when there are fewer than ten studies in a meta-analysis, both meta-regression (27) and test for publication bias (28) should not be considered. Both the study specific as well as the pooled epidemiological estimates, were graphically depicted, with their 95% CI, on a forest plot. Analyses were stratified for specific skin cancer types, i.e. NMSCs and melanoma. If a study presented more than one estimate, the most recent one was

used. Two-sided p-values<0.05 were considered for statistical significance. All calculations were carried out using R Foundation for Statistical Computing (version 4.0, package: metafor).

RESULTS

Characteristics of the Studies Included

The original electronic search yielded 1762 (1549 after removing duplicates) papers potentially relevant for this review (**Figure 1**). After removing duplicates, 1549 were initially screened. Of these, 1467 were excluded after the screening of study titles and abstracts. The remaining 82 studies were retrieved for more detailed evaluation and 10 of them met the review inclusion criteria. The main characteristics of the included studies are reported in **Table 1**. Most of the included studies were prospective cohort studies (N= 5; 50.0%) (33–36, 38), three (30.0%) (29, 31, 32) were retrospective cohort studies, one was

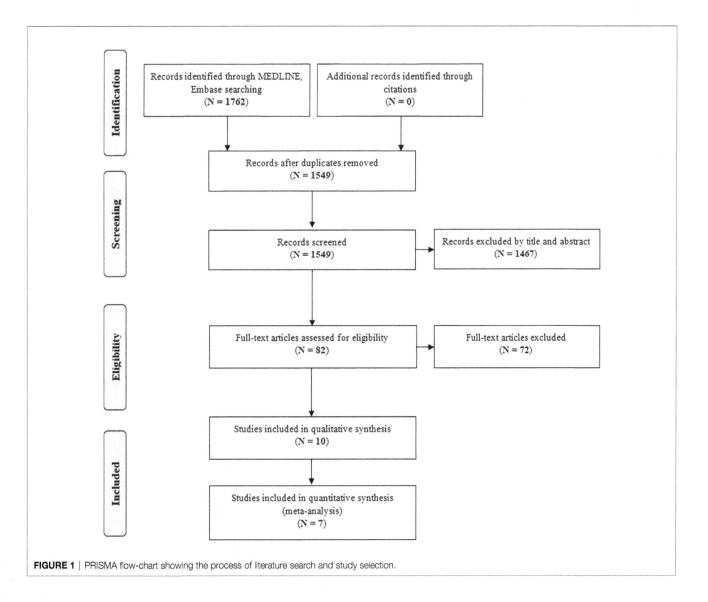

FIGURE 1 | PRISMA flow-chart showing the process of literature search and study selection.

TABLE 1 | Characteristics of the studies included in the systematic review.

Reference	Catchment area	Data source	Study population	Study drugs	Study years	Study design	IR per 10,000 PYs [95%CI]
Non-melanoma skin cancer							
29	California (USA)	Kaiser Permanente Northern California (KPNC)	All KPNC members aged ≥ 18 years, diagnosed with psoriasis between 1998 and 2011 and treated with a systemic antipsoriatic agent	Adalimumab, etanercept, infliximab, ustekinumab	1998-2011	Retrospective cohort study	120 [98-143]
30	USA	US Truven MarketScan database	Patients with moderate to severe PsA, defined by ≥1 inpatient or ≥2 outpatient 696.0 diagnosis codes on 2 unique calendar days	Adalimumab, etanercept, infliximab, apremilast	2010-2015	Clinical trial and real-world data comparison	149.3 [116.5-182.0]
31	United Kingdom	British Society for Rheumatology Biologics Register + National cancer and death registers	All patients diagnosed with PsA starting a TNF-inhibitor and registered in the British Society for Rheumatology Biologics Register	Etanercept, adalimumab, infliximab	2002-2012	Retrospective cohort study	N.A.
32	USA	Market-Scan® database and Medicare	Patients with a diagnosis of psoriasis, with the first outpatient qualifying ICD-9 CM code	Etanercept Adalimumab Infliximab	2005-2009	Retrospective cohort study	185.8 [160.2-211.42]
33	USA, Canada, Germany, France, Czech Republic, Greece, Netherlands, Spain, UK, Austria, Denmark, Ireland, Sweden	ESPRIT Registry	Patients aged ≥ 18 years of age with chronic plaque psoriasis who had been prescribed adalimumab	Adalimumab	2008-2015	Prospective cohort study	62 [52-72]
34	Canada	OBSERVE-5 surveillance registry	Adult patients with moderate to severe psoriasis initiating etanercept	Etanercept	2006-2012	Prospective cohort study	125 [60-240]
34	USA	OBSERVE-5 surveillance registry	Adult patients with moderate to severe psoriasis initiating etanercept	Etanercept	2006-2012	Prospective cohort study	262 [220-310]
35	Germany	The German Psoriasis Registry PsoBest	Adult patients with moderate-to-severe psoriasis at the time point of a new drug to be started	TNF-α inhibitors	2008-2012	Prospective cohort study	38 [12-90]
35	Germany	The German Psoriasis Registry PsoBest	Adult patients with moderate-to-severe psoriasis at the time point of a new drug to be started	Ustekinumab	2008-2012	Prospective cohort study	24 [10-136]
36	The Netherlands	Radboud University Nijmegen Medical Centre pharmacovigilance registry	Patients starting biological treatment for psoriasis in the Dermatology outpatient clinic of the Radboud University Nijmegen Medical Centre	Etanercept, adalimumab, infliximab, ustekinumab	2005-2010	Prospective cohort study	N.A.
Melanoma							
29	California (USA)	Kaiser Permanente Northern California (KPNC)	All KPNC members aged ≥ 18 years old, diagnosed with psoriasis between 1998 and 2011 and treated with a systemic antipsoriatic agent	Adalimumab, etanercept, infliximab, ustekinumab	1998-2011	Retrospective cohort study	8 [3-14]
31	United Kingdom	British Society for Rheumatology Biologics Register + National cancer and death registers	All patients diagnosed with PsA starting a TNF-inhibitor and registered in the British Society for Rheumatology Biologics Register	Etanercept, adalimumab, infliximab	2002-2012	Retrospective cohort study	NA
37	America and Europe	Psoriasis Longitudinal Assessment and Registry (PSOLAR)	Patients aged ≥ 18 years with moderate-to-severe psoriasis who were receiving, or were candidates to receive, systemic therapy	TNF-α inhibitors	2007-2015	Nested case-control study	NA
37	America and Europe	Psoriasis Longitudinal Assessment and Registry (PSOLAR)	Patients aged ≥ 18 years with moderate-to-severe psoriasis who were receiving, or were candidates to receive, systemic therapy	Ustekinumab	2007-2015	Nested case-control study	NA

(Continued)

TABLE 1 | Continued

Reference	Catchment area	Data source	Study population	Study drugs	Study years	Study design	IR per 10,000 PYs [95%CI]
38	USA, Canada, Germany, France, Czech Republic, Greece, Netherlands, Spain, UK, Austria, Denmark, Ireland, Sweden	ESPRIT Registry	Patients aged ≥ 18 years of age with chronic plaque psoriasis who had been prescribed adalimumab	Adalimumab	2008-2013	Prospective cohort study	5 [3-10]
35	Germany	PsoBest Registry	Adult patients with moderate-to-severe psoriasis at the time point of a new drug to be started	Adalimumab, etanercept, infliximab	2008-2012	Prospective cohort study	8 [0-43]

ICD-9 CM: international classification of diseases, 9th revision, clinical modification; IR, incidence rate; NA, not available; PsA, psoriatic arthritis; PYs, person-years; SIR, standardized incidence ratio; TNF, tumor necrosis factor; UK, United Kingdom; USA, United States of America.

a nested case-control study (10.0%) (37) and one was a study comparing clinical trials data and real-world data (10.0%) (30).

All included studies focused on the incidence of skin malignancies in patients treated with TNF-α inhibitors, three of them included also patients treated with ustekinumab (29, 35, 36) and only one study reported NMSC IRs also for apremilast and tofacitinib (30). No observational studies assessing the incidence of skin cancer in patients with inflammatory cutaneous diseases and treated with secukinumab, ixekizumab, brodalumab, tildrakizumab or risankizumab were found. All the included studies used real-world data sources, such as drug or disease registries and claims databases.

Of the 10 studies included in this systematic review, 7 provided data suitable for meta-analysis.

Risk of Bias in Individual Studies

Figure 2 summarizes the risk of bias assessment of individual studies. The overall risk of bias was rated as low for 7 (29, 30, 32–34, 35, 38) of the 10 included studies, while 3 (31, 36, 37) studies

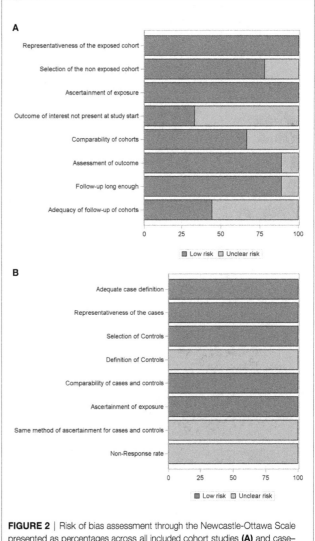

FIGURE 2 | Risk of bias assessment through the Newcastle-Ottawa Scale presented as percentages across all included cohort studies **(A)** and case–control studies **(B)**.

proved to have an unclear risk of bias. Limitations mainly concerned the assessment of the presence or absence of prognostic factors and the adequacy of follow-up.

Targeted Therapies and Skin Cancer Incidence Rates

IRs of NMSC and melanoma reported in the articles included in this systematic review are summarized in **Figure 3**.

Overall, the IR of NMSC in the included studies ranged from 38 (95% CI: 12-90) (35) to 262 (95% CI: 220-310) (34) cases per 10,000 PYs. The pooled IR for the overall risk of NMSC was 124.5 (95% CI 83.4 – 185.8) per 10,000 PYs. A considerable heterogeneity was found among these studies (Cochrane's Q = 173.0; I^2 = 96.5%).

A comparison of the incidence ratio for the overall risk of NMSC in patients exposed to biologics and small molecules versus non-biologic drugs users could be obtained only in two studies (29, 36). In one case (36), the hazard ratio (HR) was 1.42 (95% CI:1.12-1.80), while in the other one the Incidence Rate Ratio (IRR) was 0.74 (95% CI:0.60-0.91) (29).

The IR of melanoma in the included studies ranged from 5 (95% CI: 3-10) (38) to 8 (95% CI: 0-43) (35) cases per 10,000 PYs. The pooled IR for the overall risk of melanoma was 6.1 (95% CI 3.9 – 9.6) per 10,000 PYs. No heterogeneity among studies reporting melanoma IRs was found (Cochrane's Q= 1.0; I^2 = 0.0%). The only study reporting an HR for melanoma between users of biologic drugs and small molecules versus non-biologic users (36) showed no statistically significant difference (HR:1.57, 95% CI: 0.61-4.09).

It was not possible to investigate both the source of heterogeneity and the presence of publication bias, as fewer than ten studies were included in the meta-analysis (28).

DISCUSSION

In recent years, we have witnessed a revolution in the treatment of many skin diseases, ranging from bullous diseases, urticaria, atopic dermatitis, to hidradenitis suppurativa and psoriasis (39). In particular, psoriasis is a chronic cutaneous inflammatory disease affecting an estimated 125 million people worldwide, that is often associated with systemic manifestations such as major adverse cardiovascular event, obesity, inflammatory bowel disease and arthropathic psoriasis (40, 41). The decision to use one therapy over another is significantly influenced by these comorbidities and the severity of the disease. Moreover, a better understanding of the pathogenesis of this systemic disease had led to identification of new therapeutic targets (42). Whereas the older treatment options, such as phototherapy, methotrexate and cyclosporine A, are still effective, biotechnological drugs are substantially improving the therapeutic arsenal. The success of these new therapies lies in their great selectivity of action which allows to obtain, in most cases, a significant therapeutic efficacy in a short time with a reduction in side effects compared to traditional therapies. Through these therapies, even the severest symptoms of psoriasis and psoriatic arthritis can be excellently treated (43, 44). The biological drugs produced so far are

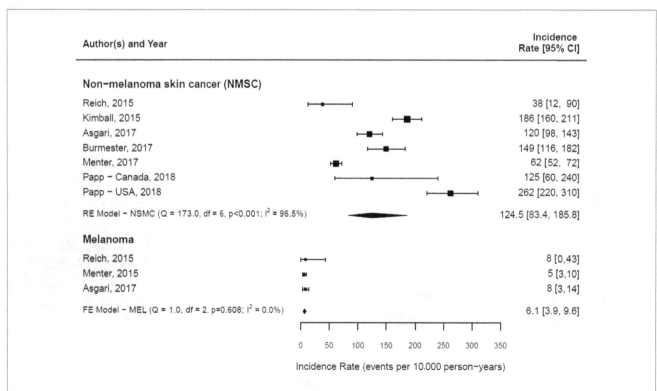

FIGURE 3 | Forest plot of the estimated skin cancer incidence per 10,000 person-years along with 95% confidence intervals, stratified by skin cancer type. RE, Random-Effects model; FE, Fixed Effect model.

monoclonal antibodies and fusion proteins. These products have the enormous advantage of being able to selectively interfere, at various levels and with different modes of action, in the immunological processes that trigger and sustain psoriasis (45). To date they are divided into five classes: TNF-α inhibitors, IL-12/23 inhibitors, IL-17 inhibitors, IL-23 inhibitors and phosphodiesterase type 4 (PDE4) inhibitors (40).

According with the above-mentioned results, our review found no observational studies assessing the incidence of skin cancer in patients with inflammatory cutaneous diseases and treated with biologics targeting selectively IL-17 or IL-23, thus obtaining mainly data on patients under anti-TNF-α therapy and, to a more limited degree, under ustekinumab, apremilast and tofacitinib.

TNF-α inhibitors infliximab, etanercept, adalimumab and certolizumab pegol are the oldest class of currently approved biotechnological drugs for the treatment of both psoriasis and psoriatic arthritis and, limited to adalimumab, of hidradenitis suppurativa. TNF-α exerts several effects. It could promote the progression of cancer (46), but also blocking TNF-α could result in arresting antitumor immune response and in promoting the growth of immunogenic tumors (47–49).

Some of the studies analyzed in this systematic review also included patients receiving ustekinumab, apremilast and tofacitinib (29, 30, 35, 36). Ustekinumab belongs to the class of biologics targeting the IL-12/23 pathway, whereas apremilast is an anti-PDE4 small molecule and tofacitinib a janus kinase inhibitor. The inhibition of these pathways causes a downregulation of the inflammatory response by modulating the expression of TNF-α, IL-23, IL-17 and other inflammatory cytokines, all involved at least in part in the tumorigenesis.

Consequently, whereas these drugs have shown dramatically excellent efficacy, concerns have been raised about the risks related to this class of agents.

Undoubtedly, patients with psoriasis are at an increased risk of cancer. Assessing the baseline risk of cutaneous malignancies in psoriasis patients is challenging due to most studies including both treated and untreated patients, and due to confounding factors like phototherapy and immunosuppressive therapy (50). Moreover NMSC and melanoma are known to arise with increased incidence among patients that have undergone medical radiation procedures or immunosuppressive therapy (51–53), such as those immunosuppressed in an iatrogenic way after a solid organ transplantation (54–56). According to the World Health Organization, age standardized world incidence of melanoma and NMSC are respectively 3,4 and 11 per 100.000 PYs. On the other hand, recent data emerging from literature show that skin cancers have a higher incidence in psoriasis patients than general population with a standardized incidence ratio of 3.37 (95% CI 1.84-5.66) (57). More in detail, Pouplard et al. in a meta-analysis reported a standardized incidence ratio of 5.3 for squamous cell carcinoma (SCC) (95% CI 2.63–10.71) and of 2.00 for basal cell carcinoma (BCC) (95% CI 1.83–2.20), whereas the authors reported a similar risk of melanoma in psoriatic patients compared to the general populations.

When considering the risk of skin cancer in psoriatic patients under treatment, many aspects should be analyzed: predisposing factors, duration and timing of exposure, the cumulative dose, the interaction with other carcinogens and, also, the latency. Despite all these data to be considered, enough evidence confirmed the relation between skin cancer and specific treatment for psoriasis and it has emerged that the risk increases even more respect untreated patients (58).

In particular, oral psoralen and ultraviolet A (PUVA) is associated with an increased risk for skin cancer in a dose dependent fashion: risk of NMSC is greatest with >350 treatments, while melanoma risk is increased with >250 treatments (59, 60). However, the carcinogenic mechanism of PUVA has not been elucidated: it maybe acts in a mutagenic and immunologic way (61). Instead, even if UVB phototherapy may increase photoaging acting with multiple mechanisms (inhibition of DNA synthesis, epidermal keratinocyte hyperproliferation, induction of T-cell apoptosis and of anti-inflammatory cytokines), no increase in skin cancer has been observed, especially with <100 treatments. Only when patients have been treated previously with PUVA and, in a second time, with broadband UVB (>300 treatments), it has been noted a modest increase in SCC (incidence rate ratio 1.37, 95% CI 1.03–1.83) and BCC (incidence rate ratio 1.45, 95% CI 1.07–1.96) (62).

Also systemic non biologic therapies are associated with an increased risk of skin cancers (63), acting primarily as immunosuppressants. Treatment with methotrexate results in higher risk for NMSC, but no association with risk for melanoma was observed (64). In detail, it has been shown that patients in treatment with methotrexate seem to have a doubled risk of SCC compared with people who receive PUVA therapy (65). Cyclosporine is associated with an elevated risk of SCC, which could increase even more in relation to treatment duration (>2 years) and previous therapy (PUVA) (66, 67), as already seen in transplant patients treated with high doses of cyclosporine and for long periods (68–70).

In our systematic review, we also considered studies evaluating the risk of skin cancers in patients with hidradenitis suppurativa in treatment with adalimumab, the only approved biologic agent for moderate-to-severe hidradenitis (71, 72). No articles were found that met the inclusion criteria. Nevertheless, data from literature point to a higher risk of developing NMSC in patients with hidradenitis than general population (15). Compared with psoriatic patients who underwent biologic treatment, patients with hidradenitis start treatment with TNF-α inhibitors after fewer months/years from the diagnosis of the disease and the guidelines do not provide obligatory treatment with first line systemic immunosuppressive drug, such as cyclosporine or methotrexate, before approaching the biologic therapy.

Considering all together the studies included in the metanalysis, the IR emerging from our systematic review shows an incidence of skin cancer in biologic treated patients, 124.5 per 10000 PYs for NMSC and 6.1 per 10000 PYs for melanoma. With regard to NMSC, IRs in literature presented large variability, from 24 in a psoriatic cohort of a German registry to 262 coming from a USA surveillance registry on patients treated with etanercept. The IR has been established on 8 out of 10 studies (**Table 1**). Concerning melanoma, 3 out of 6 studies reported an IR, ranging from 5 to 8 (**Table 1**). As a comparison, these IRs are significantly lower than post-transplant skin cancer IR, that is 1355 per 100.000 PYs for SCC and 125 per 100.000 PYs for melanoma (73).

Our figures substantially agree with those reported in a recent systematic review and metanalysis by Vaengebjerg et al. (14) who reviewed 112 observational studies and more than 2 million persons, thus assessing them for prevalence, incidence and overall risk of cancer in patients with psoriasis and psoriatic arthritis. The reported IR per 1000 PY for overall cancer was 11.75 (95% CI, 8.66-15.31) and 4.35 (95% CI, 3.18-5.70) for keratinocyte cancer, whereas the IR for melanoma was 0.37 per 1000 PYs.

A study by Esse and collaborators was focused on melanoma risk in patients treated with biologics for common inflammatory diseases, such as inflammatory bowel diseases, rheumatoid arthritis and psoriasis (68). In detail, they considered a total of 7 studies, consisting of patients treated with TNF-α inhibitors, one of which regarding patients with psoriasis and, moreover, included in our review (74). According with their findings, the risk of melanoma in biologic-treated patients with IBD and psoriasis compared with their biologic-naïve counterparts receiving conventional systemic therapy showed no statistically significant increases. Esse et al. included in their paper only one study (36) concerning psoriatic patients; this study is currently the only one reporting an HR for melanoma in patients treated with TNF-α inhibitors compared with non-biologic users and shows no significant difference between the two groups.

With regard to NMSC, the paper by Asgari (36) explicitly reported an HR for the same comparison. Our review considered an additional study in which we were able to calculate IRR from the reported data (29). While Asgari et al. (36) reported an increased HR for NMSC in patients treated with TNF-α inhibitors compared with non-biologic users, data coming from the other study (29) showed no statistically significant differences.

The main strengths of our analysis included the use of a well-defined protocol with strict inclusion and exclusion criteria. Complying with the protocol, our search addressed a clearly focused question with standardized data extraction and quality assessment to minimize errors. In addition, the real-world setting of the studies, the inclusion of biologic agents and of patients treated exclusively for common cutaneous inflammatory diseases represent distinctive features of our review and metanalysis.

The main limitation was the small number of eligible studies. The studies were also heterogeneous, which makes comparison difficult. In addition, a major weakness of the analysis was the absence of adjustment for established risk factors for NMSC and melanoma.

Furthermore, in previous studies performed only on patients with PSO it was found that there were no univocal data on the higher or lower incidence of tumors in patients with PSO. In particular, they were studies that analyzed both patients treated with systemic drugs and patients treated with biological drugs (50, 75). In our systematic review and meta-analysis, we considered only patients treated with target therapies suffering from psoriasis, PSA and/or HS.

In common with previous studies, on the other hand, there is the fact that the risk of skin tumors itself cannot be excluded because patients had to undergo immunosuppressive therapy (systemic or not) before being able to carry out treatment with a target therapy.

Another limit that emerges from our systematic review, in common with other articles already present in the literature, is the follow-up time. As demonstrated by many studies, the development and growth times of skin tumors are long and may exceed the observation periods of the clinical trials in the literature.

SUMMARY AND PERSPECTIVES

Although with some limitations, the metanalysis of currently available real-world data seems to suggest that treatment of psoriasis, psoriatic arthritis and/or hidradenitis suppurativa with TNF-α inhibitors, ustekinumab, apremilast or tofacitinib does not increase the risk of NMSC or melanoma compared to "non-biologic" systemic treatments. The cumulative sample size of the studies in literature is certainly conspicuous, but, in the light of the worldwide diffusion and frequency of the aforementioned diseases as well as their multifactorial nature and response to treatment, including undesired effects, further data are desirable.

Additionally, the ending years of the periods analyzed in the available studies range from 2009 to 2015. Similar evaluations of real-world evidence concerning molecules marketed in the last 10-15 years, such as secukinumab, ixekizumab, brodalumab, tildrakizumab or risankizumab, would be of great interest, particularly when considering that these molecules are widely used in current clinical practice. Consequently, to conduct future trials it is necessary to consider the above data and the fact that the number of studies comparing newer molecules and conventional drugs are small. A greater number of new trials will have to be conducted, considering longer follow-up times and, above all, common methods will have to be applied to allow a comparison between the various studies.

In summary, this updated systematic review and meta-analysis seems to suggest that no differences exist between treatment of chronic cutaneous diseases with biotechnological drugs/small molecules and conventional DMARDs in terms of HR/IRR for melanoma, while data on NMSC are more controversial. Nevertheless, periodic dermatologic screening should be ensured for all patients undergoing these therapies.

AUTHOR CONTRIBUTIONS

Conceptualization: CG and SC. Methodology: SC, FC, GT, LB, and CG. Validation: SC, LB, and CG. Resources: SC, AF, FC, GT, YI, LB, MB, and CG. Data curation: SC, AF, FC, YI, GT, MB, and CG. Writing-original draft preparation: SC, LB, and CG. Writing-review and editing: SC, LB, and CG. Supervision: SC, LB, and CG. All authors contributed to the article and approved the submitted version.

ACKNOWLEDGMENTS

We are grateful to Prof. Matthias Augustin, Dr. Christina Sorbe and all the PsoBest Registry team for providing the data of their study (35).

REFERENCES

1. Van Der Zee HH, De Ruiter L, Van Den Broecke DG, Dik WA, Laman JD, Prens EP. Elevated Levels of Tumour Necrosis Factor (TNF)-α, Interleukin (IL)-1β and IL-10 in Hidradenitis Suppurativa Skin: A Rationale for Targeting TNF-α and IL-1β. *Br J Dermatol* (2011) 164:1292–8. doi: 10.1111/j.1365-2133.2011.10254.x

2. Kelly G, Hughes R, McGarry T, Van Den Born M, Adamzik K, Fitzgerald R, et al. Dysregulated Cytokine Expression in Lesional and Nonlesional Skin in Hidradenitis Suppurativa. *Br J Dermatol* (2015) 173:1431–9. doi: 10.1111/bjd.14075

3. Menon B, Gullick NJ, Walter GJ, Rajasekhar M, Garrood T, Evans HG, et al. Interleukin-17+CD8+ T Cells Are Enriched in the Joints of Patients With Psoriatic Arthritis and Correlate With Disease Activity and Joint Damage Progression. *Arthritis Rheumatol* (2014) 66:1272–81. doi: 10.1002/art.38376

4. Nickoloff BJ, Qin JZ, Nestle FO. Immunopathogenesis of Psoriasis. *Clin Rev Allergy Immunol* (2007) 33:45–56. doi: 10.1007/s12016-007-0039-2

5. Sabat R, Philipp S, Höflich C, Kreutzer S, Wallace E, Asadullah K, et al. Immunopathogenesis of Psoriasis. *Exp Dermatol* (2007) 16:779–98. doi: 10.1111/j.1600-0625.2007.00629.x

6. Gisondi P, Talamonti M, Chiricozzi A, Piaserico S, Amerio P, Balato A, et al. Treat-to-Target Approach for the Management of Patients With Moderate-to-Severe Plaque Psoriasis: Consensus Recommendations. *Dermatol Ther (Heidelb)* (2021) 11:235–52. doi: 10.1007/s13555-020-00475-8

7. Ceccarelli M, Venanzi Rullo E, Vaccaro M, Facciolà A, d'Aleo F, Paolucci IA, et al. HIV-Associated Psoriasis: Epidemiology, Pathogenesis, and Management. *Dermatol Ther* (2019) 32(2):e12806. doi: 10.1111/dth.12806

8. Shacter E, Weitzman SA. Chronic Inflammation and Cancer. *Oncology (Williston Park)* (2002) 16(2):217–26. doi: 10.1201/b12696-15

9. Tchernev G, Guarneri C, Bevelacqua V, Wollina U. Carcinoma Cuniculatum in Course of Etanercept: Blocking Autoimmunity But Propagation of Carcinogenesis? *Int J Immunopathol Pharmacol* (2014) 27:261–6. doi: 10.1177/039463201402700213

10. Lapins J, Ye W, Nyrén O, Emtestam L. Incidence of Cancer Among Patients With Hidradenitis Suppurativa. *Arch Dermatol* (2001) 137:730–4. doi: 10-1001/pubs.Arch Dermatol.-ISSN-0003-987x-137-6-dst00132

11. Rastogi S, Patel KR, Singam V, Ali Y, Gao J, Amin A, et al. Vulvar Cancer Association With Groin Hidradenitis Suppurativa: A Large, Urban, Midwestern US Patient Population Study. *J Am Acad Dermatol* (2019) 80:80–10. doi: 10.1016/j.jaad.2018.10.008

12. Lee JH, Kim HJ, Han KD, Kim HN, Park YM, Lee JY, et al. Cancer Risk in 892 089 Patients With Psoriasis in Korea: A Nationwide Population-Based Cohort Study. *J Dermatol* (2019) 46:95–102. doi: 10.1111/1346-8138.14698

13. Malaponte G, Signorelli SS, Bevelacqua V, Polesel J, Taborelli M, Guarneri C, et al. Increased Levels of NF-κb-Dependent Markers in Cancer-Associated Deep Venous Thrombosis. *PloS One* (2015) 10(7):e0132496. doi: 10.1371/journal.pone.0132496

14. Vaengebjerg S, Skov L, Egeberg A, Loft ND. Prevalence, Incidence, and Risk of Cancer in Patients With Psoriasis and Psoriatic Arthritis: A Systematic Review and Meta-Analysis. *JAMA Dermatol* (2020) 156:421–9. doi: 10.1001/jamadermatol.2020.0024

15. Jung JM, Lee KH, Kim YJ, Chang SE, Lee MW, Choi JH, et al. Assessment of Overall and Specific Cancer Risks in Patients With Hidradenitis Suppurativa. *JAMA Dermatol* (2020) 156:844–53. doi: 10.1001/jamadermatol.2020.1422

16. Di Lernia V, Neri I, Pintoton PC, Di Nuzzo S, Stingeni L, Guarneri C, et al. T Reatment Patterns With Systemic Antipsoriatic Agents in Childhood Psoriasis: An Italian Database Analysis. *G Ital di Dermatologia e Venereol* (2017) 152:327–32. doi: 10.23736/S0392-0488.16.05287-X

17. Marcianò I, Randazzo MP, Panagia P, Intelisano R, Sgroi C, Ientile V, et al. Real-World Use of Biological Drugs in Patients With Psoriasis/Psoriatic Arthritis: A Retrospective, Population-Based Study of Years 2010-2014 From Southern Italy. *G Ital Dermatol Venereol* (2020) 155:441–51. doi: 10.23736/S0392-0488.18.05753-X

18. Skarmoutsou E, Bevelacqua V, D'Amico F, Russo A, Spandidos DA, Scalisi A, et al. FOXP3 Expression is Modulated by TGF-β1/NOTCH1 Pathway in Human Melanoma. *Int J Mol Med* (2018) 42:392–404. doi: 10.3892/ijmm.2018.3618

19. Bilal J, Berlinberg A, Bin RI, Faridi W, Bhattacharjee S, Ortega G, et al. Risk of Infections and Cancer in Patients With Rheumatologic Diseases Receiving Interleukin Inhibitors: A Systematic Review and Meta-Analysis. *JAMA Netw Open* (2019) 2:e1913102. doi: 10.1001/jamanetworkopen.2019.13102

20. Khazaei Z, Ghorat F, Jarrahi AM, Adineh HA, Sohrabivafa M, Goodarzi E. Global Incidence and Mortality of Skin Cancer by Histological Subtype and its Relationship With the Human Development Index (HDI); an Ecology Study in 2018. *WCRJ* (2019) 6:e1265. doi: 10.32113/wcrj_20194_1265

21. Askling J, Fahrbach K, Nordstrom B, Ross S, Schmid CH, Symmons D. Cancer Risk With Tumor Necrosis Factor Alpha (TNF) Inhibitors: Meta-analysis of Randomized Controlled Trials of Adalimumab, Etanercept, and Infliximab Using Patient Level Data. *Pharmacoepidemiol Drug Saf* (2011) 20:119–30. doi: 10.1002/pds.2046

22. Mariette X, Matucci-Cerinic M, Pavelka K, Taylor P, Van Vollenhoven R, Heatley R, et al. Malignancies Associated With Tumour Necrosis Factor Inhibitors in Registries and Prospective Observational Studies: A Systematic Review and Meta-Analysis. *Ann Rheum Dis* (2011) 70:1895–904. doi: 10.1136/ard.2010.149419

23. Moran GW, Lim AWK, Bailey JL, Dubeau MF, Leung Y, Devlin SM, et al. Review Article: Dermatological Complications of Immunosuppressive and Anti-TNF Therapy in Inflammatory Bowel Disease. *Aliment Pharmacol Ther* (2013) 38:1002–24. doi: 10.1111/apt.12491

24. Peleva E, Exton LS, Kelley K, Kleyn CE, Mason KJ, Smith CH. Risk of Cancer in Patients With Psoriasis on Biological Therapies: A Systematic Review. *Br J Dermatol* (2018) 178:103–13. doi: 10.1111/bjd.15830

25. Sidwell K. Lucian A Selection. Ed. and Trm.D. Macleod. Warminster: Aris and Phillips, 1991. Pp. Iv + 316. £35.00 (Bound), £12.50 (Paper). *J Hell Stud* (1993) 113:198–9. doi: 10.2307/632432

26. Higgins JPT, Thompson SG, Deeks JJ, Altman DG. Measuring Inconsistency in Meta-Analyses. *Br Med J* (2003) 327:557–60. doi: 10.1136/bmj.327.7414.557

27. Higgins J, Green S. Cochrane Handbook for Systematic Reviews of Interventions, *version 5.1*. Cochrane Collab (2011).

28. Sterne JAC, Sutton AJ, Ioannidis JPA, Terrin N, Jones DR, Lau J, et al. Recommendations for Examining and Interpreting Funnel Plot Asymmetry in Meta-Analyses of Randomised Controlled Trials. *BMJ* (2011) 343:d4002. doi: 10.1136/bmj.d4002

29. Asgari MM, Ray GT, Geier JL, Quesenberry CP. Malignancy Rates in a Large Cohort of Patients With Systemically Treated Psoriasis in a Managed Care Population. *J Am Acad Dermatol* (2017) 76:632–8. doi: 10.1016/j.jaad.2016.10.006

30. Burmester GR, Curtis JR, Yun H, FitzGerald O, Winthrop KL, Azevedo VF, et al. An Integrated Analysis of the Safety of Tofacitinib in Psoriatic Arthritis Across Phase III and Long-Term Extension Studies With Comparison to Real-World Observational Data. *Drug Saf* (2020) 43:379–92. doi: 10.1007/s40264-020-00904-9

31. Fagerli KM, Kearsley-Fleet L, Mercer LK, Watson K, Packham J, Symmons DPM, et al. Malignancy and Mortality Rates in Patients With Severe Psoriatic Arthritis Requiring Tumour-Necrosis Factor Alpha Inhibition: Results From the British Society for Rheumatology Biologics Register. *Rheumatol (United Kingdom)* (2019) 58:80–5. doi: 10.1093/rheumatology/key241

32. Kimball AB, Schenfeld J, Accortt NA, Anthony MS, Rothman KJ, Pariser D. Cohort Study of Malignancies and Hospitalized Infectious Events in Treated and Untreated Patients With Psoriasis and a General Population in the United States. *Br J Dermatol* (2015) 173:1183–90. doi: 10.1111/bjd.14068

33. Menter A, Thaçi D, Wu JJ, Abramovits W, Kerdel F, Arikan D, et al. Long-Term Safety and Effectiveness of Adalimumab for Moderate to Severe Psoriasis: Results From 7-Year Interim Analysis of the ESPRIT Registry. *Dermatol Ther (Heidelb)* (2017) 7:365–81. doi: 10.1007/s13555-017-0198-x

34. Papp KA, Bourcier M, Poulin Y, Lynde CW, Gilbert M, Poulin-Costello M, et al. Observe-5: Comparison of Etanercept-Treated Psoriasis Patients From Canada and the United States. *J Cutan Med Surg* (2018) 22:297–303. doi: 10.1177/1203475418755998

35. Reich K, Mrowietz U, Radtke MA, Thaci D, Rustenbach SJ, Spehr C, et al. Drug Safety of Systemic Treatments for Psoriasis: Results From The German Psoriasis Registry Psobest. *Arch Dermatol Res* (2015) 307:875–83. doi: 10.1007/s00403-015-1593-8

36. Van Lümig PPM, Driessen RJB, Berends MAM, Boezeman JBM, Van De Kerkhof PCM, De Jong EMGJ. Safety of Treatment With Biologics for Psoriasis in Daily Practice: 5-Year Data. *J Eur Acad Dermatol Venereol* (2012) 26:283–91. doi: 10.1111/j.1468-3083.2011.04044.x

37. Fiorentino D, Ho V, Lebwohl MG, Leite L, Hopkins L, Galindo C, et al. Risk of Malignancy With Systemic Psoriasis Treatment in the Psoriasis Longitudinal Assessment Registry. *J Am Acad Dermatol* (2017) 77:845–54. doi: 10.1016/j.jaad.2017.07.013

38. Menter A, Thaçi D, Papp KA, Wu JJ, Bereswill M, Teixeira HD, et al. Five-Year Analysis From the ESPRIT 10-Year Postmarketing Surveillance Registry of Adalimumab Treatment for Moderate to Severe Psoriasis A Portion of the Data in This Manuscript Was Presented in at the Fall European Academy of Dermatology and Venereology 2. *J Am Acad Dermatol* (2015) 73:410–9. doi: 10.1016/j.jaad.2015.06.038

39. Yiqiu Y, Ravn Jørgensen AH, Thomsen SF. Biologics for Chronic Inflammatory Skin Diseases: An Update for the Clinician. *J Dermatolog Treat* (2020) 31:108–30. doi: 10.1080/09546634.2019.1589643

40. Armstrong AW, Read C. Pathophysiology, Clinical Presentation, and Treatment of Psoriasis: A Review. *JAMA - J Am Med Assoc* (2020) 323:1945–60. doi: 10.1001/jama.2020.4006

41. Dattilo G, Borgia F, Guarneri C, Casale M, Bitto R, Morabito C, et al. Cardiovascular Risk in Psoriasis: Current State of the Art. *Curr Vasc Pharmacol* (2017) 17:85–91. doi: 10.2174/1570161115666171116163816

42. Kaushik SB, Lebwohl MG. Psoriasis: Which Therapy for Which Patient: Psoriasis Comorbidities and Preferred Systemic Agents. *J Am Acad Dermatol* (2019) 80:27–40. doi: 10.1016/j.jaad.2018.06.057

43. Kamata M, Tada Y. Efficacy and Safety of Biologics for Psoriasis and Psoriatic Arthritis and Their Impact on Comorbidities: A Literature Review. *Int J Mol Sci* (2020) 21:1690. doi: 10.3390/ijms21051690

44. Ceccarelli M, Venanzi Rullo E, Berretta M, Cacopardo B, Pellicanò GF, Nunnari G, et al. New Generation Biologics for the Treatment of Psoriasis and Psoriatic Arthritis. State of the Art and Considerations About the Risk of Infection. *Dermatol Ther* (2021) 34(1):e14660. doi: 10.1111/dth.14660

45. Di Lernia V, Guarneri C, Stingeni L, Gisondi P, Bonamonte D, Calzavara Pinton PG, et al. Effectiveness of Etanercept in Children With Plaque Psoriasis in Real Practice: A One-Year Multicenter Retrospective Study. *J Dermatolog Treat* (2018) 29:217–9. doi: 10.1080/09546634.2017.1364692

46. Balkwill F. Tnf-α in Promotion and Progression of Cancer. *Cancer Metastasis Rev* (2006) 25:409–16. doi: 10.1007/s10555-006-9005-3

47. Larmonier N, Cathelin D, Larmonier C, Nicolas A, Merino D, Janikashvili N, et al. The Inhibition of TNF-α Anti-Tumoral Properties by Blocking Antibodies Promotes Tumor Growth in a Rat Model. *Exp Cell Res* (2007) 313:2345–55. doi: 10.1016/j.yexcr.2007.03.027

48. Facciolà A, Venanzi Rullo E, Ceccarelli M, D'Andrea F, Coco M, Micali C, et al. Malignant Melanoma in HIV: Epidemiology, Pathogenesis, and Management. *Dermatol Ther* (2020) 33(1):e13180. doi: 10.1111/dth.13180

49. Berretta M, Martellotta F, Francia RD, Spina M, Vaccher E, Balestreri L, et al. Clinical Presentation and Outcome of Non-AIDS Defining Cancers, in HIV-Infected Patients in the ART-Era: The Italian Cooperative Group on AIDS and Tumors Activity. *Eur Rev Med Pharmacol Sci* (2015) 19:3619–34.

50. Geller S, Xu H, Lebwohl M, Nardone B, Lacouture ME, Kheterpal M. Malignancy Risk and Recurrence With Psoriasis and Its Treatments: A Concise Update. *Am J Clin Dermatol* (2018) 19:363–75. doi: 10.1007/s40257-017-0337-2

51. Berge LAM, Andreassen BK, Stenehjem JS, Heir T, Karlstad Ø, Juzeniene A, et al. Use of Immunomodulating Drugs and Risk of Cutaneous Melanoma: A Nationwide Nested Case-Control Study. *Clin Epidemiol* (2020) 12:1389–401. doi: 10.2147/CLEP.S269446

52. Maiorino A, De Simone C, Perino F, Caldarola G, Peris K. Melanoma and non-Melanoma Skin Cancer in Psoriatic Patients Treated With High-Dose Phototherapy. *J Dermatolog Treat* (2016) 27:443–7. doi: 10.3109/09546634.2015.1133882

53. IAS S. Beneficial Role of Vitamin D in Common Cancers: Is the Evidence Compelling Enough? *WCRJ* (2020) 7:e1574. doi: 10.32113/wcrj_20205_1574

54. Collins L, Asfour L, Stephany M, Lear JT, Stasko T. Management of Non-Melanoma Skin Cancer in Transplant Recipients. *Clin Oncol* (2019) 31:779–88. doi: 10.1016/j.clon.2019.08.005

55. Guarneri C, Bevelacqua V, Polesel J, Falzone L, Cannavo PS, Spandidos DA, et al. Nf-κb Inhibition Is Associated With OPN/MMP-9 Downregulation in Cutaneous Melanoma. *Oncol Rep* (2017) 37:737–46. doi: 10.3892/or.2017.5362

56. Goodarzi E, Khazaei Z, Moayed L, Adineh HA, Sohrabivafa M, Darvishi I. Dsl. Epidemiology and Population Attributable Fraction of Melanoma to Ultraviolet Radiation in Asia: An Ecological Study. *Wcrj* (2018) 5:1–8. doi: 10.32113/wcrj_20189_1114

57. Polachek A, Muntyanu A, Lee KA, Ye JY, Chandran V, Cook RJ, et al. Malignancy in Psoriatic Disease: Results From Prospective Longitudinal Cohorts. *Semin Arthritis Rheum* (2021) 51:144–9. doi: 10.1016/j.semarthrit.2020.12.008

58. Naldi L. Malignancy Concerns With Psoriasis Treatments Using Phototherapy, Methotrexate, Cyclosporin, and Biologics: Facts and Controversies. *Clin Dermatol* (2010) 28:88–92. doi: 10.1016/j.clindermatol.2009.03.003

59. Stern RS. The Risk of Squamous Cell and Basal Cell Cancer Associated With Psoralen and Ultraviolet A Therapy: A 30-Year Prospective Study. *J Am Acad Dermatol* (2012) 66:553–62. doi: 10.1016/j.jaad.2011.04.004

60. Stern RS, Nichols KT, Väkevä LH. Malignant Melanoma in Patients Treated for Psoriasis With Methoxsalen (Psoralen) and Ultraviolet A Radiation (PUVA). *N Engl J Med* (1997) 336:1041–5. doi: 10.1056/nejm199704103361501

61. Morison WL, Baughman RD, Day RM, Forbes PD, Hoenigsmann H, Krueger GG, et al. Consensus Workshop on the Toxic Effects of Long-Term PUVA Therapy. *Arch Dermatol* (1998) 134:595–8. doi: 10.1001/archderm.134.5.595

62. Lee E, Koo J, Berger T. UVB Phototherapy and Skin Cancer Risk: A Review of the Literature. *Int J Dermatol* (2005) 44:355–60. doi: 10.1111/j.1365-4632.2004.02186.x

63. Balak DMW, Gerdes S, Parodi A, Salgado-Boquete L. Long-Term Safety of Oral Systemic Therapies for Psoriasis: A Comprehensive Review of the Literature. *Dermatol Ther (Heidelb)* (2020) 10:589–613. doi: 10.1007/s13555-020-00409-4

64. Polesie S, Gillstedt M, Paoli J, Osmancevic A. Methotrexate Treatment for Patients With Psoriasis and Risk of Cutaneous Melanoma: A Nested Case-Control Study. *Br J Dermatol* (2020) 183:684–91. doi: 10.1111/bjd.18887

65. Stern RS, Laird N. The Carcinogenic Risk of Treatments for Severe Psoriasis. *Cancer* (1994) 73:2759–64. doi: 10.1002/1097-0142(19940601)73:11<2759::AID-CNCR2820731118>3.0.CO;2-C

66. Paul CF, Ho VC, McGeown C, Christophers E, Schmidtmann B, Guillaume JC, et al. Risk of Malignancies in Psoriasis Patients Treated With Cyclosporine: A 5 Y Cohort Study. *J Invest Dermatol* (2003) 120:211–6. doi: 10.1046/j.1523-1747.2003.12040.x

67. Di Lernia V, Stingeni L, Boccaletti V, Calzavara Pinton PG, Guarneri C, Belloni Fortina A, et al. Effectiveness and Safety of Cyclosporine in Pediatric Plaque Psoriasis: A Multicentric Retrospective Analysis. *J Dermatolog Treat* (2016) 27:395–8. doi: 10.3109/09546634.2015.1120852

68. Zafar SY, Howell DN, Gockerman JP. Malignancy After Solid Organ Transplantation: An Overview. *Oncologist* (2008) 13:769–78. doi: 10.1634/theoncologist.2007-0251

69. Malaponte G, Hafsi S, Polesel J, Castellano G, Spessotto P, Guarneri C, et al. Tumor Microenvironment in Diffuse Large B-Cell Lymphoma: Matrixmetalloproteinases Activation is Mediated by Osteopontin Overexpression. *Biochim Biophys Acta - Mol Cell Res* (2016) 1863:483–9. doi: 10.1016/j.bbamcr.2015.09.018

70. D'Aniello C, Perri F, Scarpati GDV, Pepa CD, Pisconti S, Montesarchio V, et al. Melanoma Adjuvant Treatment: Current Insight and Clinical Features. *Curr Cancer Drug Targets* (2017) 18:442–56. doi: 10.2174/1568009617666170208163714

71. Flood KS, Porter ML, Kimball AB. Biologic Treatment for Hidradenitis Suppurativa. *Am J Clin Dermatol* (2019) 20:625–38. doi: 10.1007/s40257-019-00439-5

72. Giuffrida R, Cannavò SP, Coppola M, Guarneri C. Novel Therapeutic Approaches and Targets for the Treatment of Hidradenitis Suppurativa. *Curr Pharm Biotechnol* (2020) 22:59–72. doi: 10.2174/1389201021666200505100556

73. Garrett GL, Blanc PD, Boscardin J, Lloyd AA, Ahmed RL, Anthony T, et al. Incidence of and Risk Factors for Skin Cancer in Organ Transplant Recipients in the United States. *JAMA Dermatol* (2017) 153:296–303. doi: 10.1001/jamadermatol.2016.4920

4

Interference of COVID-19 Vaccination with PET/CT Leads to Unnecessary Additional Imaging in a Patient with Metastatic Cutaneous Melanoma

Rafał Czepczyński[1,2]*, Jolanta Szczurek[1,2], Jacek Mackiewicz[3] and Marek Ruchała[1]

[1] *Department of Endocrinology, Metabolism and Internal Diseases, Poznan University of Medical Sciences, Poznań, Poland,* [2] *Department of Nuclear Medicine, Affidea, Poznań, Poland,* [3] *Department of Medical and Experimental Oncology, Poznan University of Medical Sciences, Poznań, Poland*

Correspondence:
Rafał Czepczyński
czepczynski@ump.edu.pl

The COVID-19 pandemic has widely influenced oncological imaging mainly by presenting unexpected pulmonary and mediastinal lesions. The ongoing global program of vaccination has led to incidental diagnosis of axillary lymphadenopathy. We present a case of increased accumulation of ^{18}F-FDG in an axillary lymph node in a PET/CT scan performed in a 43-year-old female patient with metastatic melanoma. The scan was performed 4 days after the AZD1222 vaccination. The occurrence of lymphadenopathy was verified with another PET/CT scan scheduled one month later. This case report presents a possible misinterpretation of PET/CT images caused by the recent COVID-19 vaccination. To avoid distress of the patient and unnecessary oncological diagnostics to verify the findings, we recommend avoiding scheduling PET/CT shortly after vaccination.

Keywords: malignant melanoma, PET/CT, COVID-19, vaccination, metastases

INTRODUCTION

Positron emission tomography with computed tomography (PET/CT) using ^{18}F-fluoro-deoxyglucose (^{18}F-FDG) is a valuable tool used to monitor treatment of melanoma, especially its metastatic forms subjected to immunotherapy (1). In stage III cutaneous melanoma, sensitivity in detecting distant metastases during follow-up ranges between 82 and 100%, and the specificity ranges between 45 and 100% (2). With regard to lymph node metastases, PET/CT shows sensitivity of 91% for nodes >10 mm and 69% for smaller nodes (with a similar specificity of 71%) (3). The inflammatory reaction of the lymph nodes is one of the main causes of the false positive PET/CT findings in oncological patients. A non-specific nodal ^{18}F-FDG uptake may lead to a false diagnosis of metastases and to the initiation of an unnecessary treatment.

The widespread COVID-19 vaccination has raised a lot of questions with regard to its potential complications and side-effects. Many patients experience local pain in the injection site; some of them suffer from generalized inflammatory reactions, including fever and fatigue (4). As it has been recently shown, local inflammatory reaction in the lymphatic system may have potential implications for imaging. The vaccine-induced lymphadenopathy may also pose a challenge in the PET/CT interpretation (5). In this paper, we report a patient with stage IV melanoma who had a PET/CT performed incidentally few days after COVID-19 vaccination that resulted in a false positive finding in an axillary lymph node.

CASE PRESENTATION

A 43-year-old female with the diagnosis of metastatic melanoma treated with nivolumab was reported for a ^{18}F-FDG PET/CT scan to exclude disease progression shortly after COVID-19 vaccination.

The timeline of the history of the patient is presented in **Figure 1**. She was diagnosed of a primary cutaneous melanoma of the right thigh in June 2015. The patient was previously healthy, with no history of other malignancies, surgery, or medication. There was no personal or family history of melanoma. The lesion was removed, and the final diagnosis was: cutaneous melanoma, *BRAF* wild-type, pT2aN0M0. In January 2019, a recurrence of the disease in form of the subcutaneous and brain metastases was diagnosed with the use of CT. A single cerebral metastasis was confirmed by MRI. After two weeks, nivolumab treatment was initiated, with a dose of 480 mg every 4 weeks. After the first dose of nivolumab, the cyberknife radiotherapy of the brain metastasis was performed. After two months of systemic treatment, all subcutaneous metastases disappeared; however six new brain metastases were detected in another MRI. All these new lesions were subsequently treated with cyberknife. The patient continued the nivolumab therapy beyond progression. Thereafter, during nivolumab treatment, she developed a further disease progression in the brain (04.2019, 05.2019, 01.2020, 12.2020). With each progression, one or two new brain metastases were found in the MRI. These lesions did not exceed 1 cm and were asymptomatic. After each occurrence, the cerebral metastases

were treated with cyberknife. All extracerebral metastases were still in regression until December 2020 when some metabolically active lymph nodes in the right iliac region were detected in a PET/CT scan (PET1). In January 2021, a robot-assisted right iliac lymphadenectomy was performed, and the metastatic character of the iliac lymph nodes was histologically confirmed.

In February 2021, the patient underwent AZD1222 COVID-19 vaccination (first dose injected into her left arm). Four days later, another PET/CT was performed to exclude new extracerebral metastases (PET2). No sign of melanoma recurrence was found in the iliac lymph nodes or central nervous system. However, a metabolically active lymph node in the left axillary region was noted (**Figure 2**). The lymph node had the dimension of 9 × 7 mm, and the maximal standardized uptake value was 5.2. Additionally, an area of increased ^{18}F-FDG accumulation was found in the left deltoid muscle that corresponded to the site of the recent vaccination. An inflammatory reaction to the injection was suspected to be responsible for the ^{18}F-FDG accumulation in the axillary lymph node. However, in order to rule out a melanoma metastasis in the axillary lymph node, a follow-up PET/CT (PET3) was recommended 28 days later (March 2021, 32 days after vaccination). This scan did not present any ^{18}F-FDG accumulation in the reported lymph node. The diameter of the node did not change. No other finding was reported, except for a focus of slightly increased ^{18}F-FDG accumulation (diameter of 10 mm) in the right cerebellar lobe that had not been present in the PET2 scan. Fortunately, the subsequent MRI did not confirm any lesion in the cerebellum and did not show any other intracranial recurrence. However, further MRI monitoring of the central nervous system has been recommended.

To date (June, 2021), the patient does not present any active metastases (NED—no evidence of disease). Moreover, her performance status remains WHO 0 from the initial diagnosis until now. The treatment beyond disease progression was beneficial to the patient. In addition, at each disease progression, the patient was offered a second line treatment

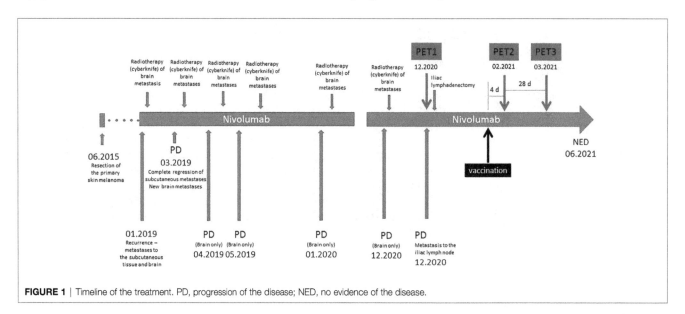

FIGURE 1 | Timeline of the treatment. PD, progression of the disease; NED, no evidence of the disease.

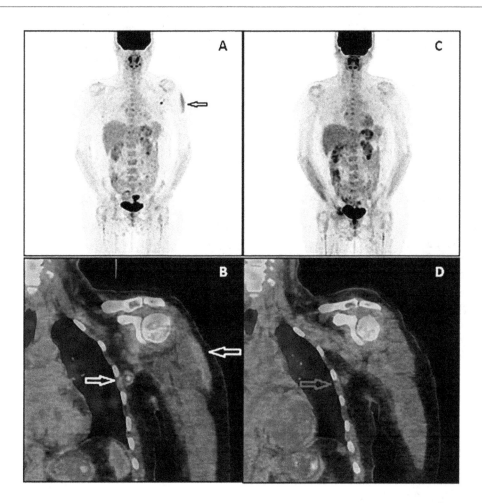

FIGURE 2 | PET/CT image performed 4 days after vaccination **(A, B)**. The multiple-intensity projection image **(A)** showing increased ^{18}F-FDG uptake in the left deltoid muscle (black arrow) and in the left axillary region. Fused coronal image **(B)** showing the uptake in the muscle (white arrow) and in the axillary lymph node (yellow arrow). PET/CT image performed 32 days after vaccination **(C, D)**. Both the muscular uptake and nodal uptake have disappeared. The referred axillary lymph node (red arrow) shows similar morphology but no ^{18}F-FDG accumulation.

with ipilimumab, to which the patient did not consent due to its high toxicity and low efficacy (6). The patient was informed that there was insufficient evidence for the treatment with nivolumab beyond confirmed progression (7). Due to the fact that the patient did not consent to the ipilimumab treatment, as well as to the lack of a clinical trial, the continuation of nivolumab therapy was the only reasonable treatment option. In conclusion, the continued treatment beyond progression was decided due to the low tumor burden, the motivation of the patient and good performance status and, the lack of other treatment options.

The patient gave consent for the publication of her case.

DISCUSSION

PET/CT is an established imaging modality used in oncology on an every-day basis. It is well-known that foci of non-oncological pathology can accumulate ^{18}F-FDG similarly to the malignant tumors, nodal and distant metastases. The examples of such

benign, metabolically active lesions include pulmonary tuberculosis, benign thyroid nodules, diverticulitis, *etc.* (8–10). Also, reactive lymph nodes can present as metabolically active, mimicking nodal metastases (11). Common situations like that include cervical lymphadenopathy after infection of the upper respiratory tract or tonsillitis, mediastinal lymphadenopathy in case of pneumonia or sarcoidosis, and inguinal lymph node metabolic stimulation due to a lower extremity injury. Careful anamnesis prior to the scan, not excluding apparently irrelevant conditions, like tooth pain or transient fever, may prevent a misinterpretation of the images.

In the every-day practice of a PET/CT department, the occurrence of vaccination-induced lymphadenopathy is a new phenomenon. Several authors have already reported the unexpected findings of increased ^{18}F-FDG accumulation in the axillary lymph nodes (5, 12–14). It may cause serious doubts regarding the character of lymphadenopathy in cases of melanoma and other malignancies with an aggressive dissemination pattern. The presented patient had a history of lymph node metastases in the inguinal region that was obviously correlated with the primary location in the ipsilateral lower extremity. However, the metastatic behavior of melanoma can be unpredictable, and a metastasis in the contralateral axillary fossa could not be excluded, especially when knowing that the progression of the disease with new brain metastases during systemic treatment had occurred several times. The coexistence of all these risk factors has led to the recommendation of an early follow-up scan (PET3). Although the axillary metastasis has been excluded by the negative PET/CT, an increased caution of the reporting physician, who was aware of the history of the patient, led to another false positive finding—the cerebellar focus suspected of being another recurrence in the central nervous system. The reporting attention of the physician to possible intracranial foci was alerted because of the well-known low sensitivity of ^{18}F-FDG PET/CT in the detection of brain metastases due to the physiological radionuclide uptake in the gray matter. The rapid application of MR has led to the exclusion of relapse.

Worldwide COVID-19 vaccination is an unprecedented program of the medical interventions performed on an enormous global population in a relatively short time (4). What is more, commonly, the intramuscular vaccine injection is performed twice in each subject. Also oncological patients, referred to a PET/CT scan as a part of their routine management, are independently vaccinated and the schedules of the vaccination and imaging are not always coordinated, as they are being organized by separate institutions. This may lead to a situation of equivocal PET/CT findings as presented in this case report.

Interestingly, the sign of elevated ^{18}F-FDG accumulation does not occur in all vaccinated patients. In a recent study by Schroeder et al., the ^{18}F-FDG-positive axillary lymph nodes were found in four out of 54 patients subjected to COVID-19 vaccination performed at the median time of 10–13 days earlier (15). This observation may cause even more uncertainty of the PET/CT image interpretation. Recently, authors from Israel have reported a much higher incidence of the vaccination-related axillary lymphadenopathy: 36.4% after the first vaccine dose

and as much as 53.9% after the booster dose (16). It must be emphasized, however, that these results refer to the mRNA vaccine (Pfizer BNT162b2), not the viral vector vaccine, as in the presented case. If the vaccination and the PET/CT are to be performed in a short interval, we recommend to schedule the PET/CT before the COVID-19 vaccination. This may not always be feasible, especially if the patient undergoes an oncological treatment with a strict protocol. In such a situation, a delayed PET/CT scan would be a preferable solution. Considering the optimal time of PET/CT after vaccination, no firm data are available. From our experience, a great majority of patients who present the sign of increased axillary ^{18}F-FDG accumulation received their vaccine in the recent 10 days. In rare cases, however, we have seen this sign even more than 4 weeks after the injection and this observation is supported by other authors (5). It is noteworthy that a prolonged nodal hypermetabolism is more likely to be found after the booster dose of a mRNA vaccine (16). Therefore, we recommend performing the PET/CT imaging *ca.* 4 weeks after the vaccination if the treatment protocol allows that. In any case, the physician responsible for reporting the PET/CT scan must be aware of the vaccination date.

CONCLUSION

This case report presents possible misinterpretation of PET/CT images caused by a recent COVID-19 vaccination. To avoid distress of the patient and unnecessary oncological diagnostics to verify the findings, we recommend avoiding scheduling PET/CT shortly after vaccination.

AUTHOR CONTRIBUTIONS

RC wrote the manuscript. JS performed image acquisition and prepared images. JM prepared clinical data and the time-line and reviewed the manuscript. MR reviewed the manuscript. All authors contributed to the article and approved the submitted version.

REFERENCES

1. Ayati N, Sadeghi R, Kiamanesh Z, Lee ST, Zakavi SR, Scott AM. The Value of 18F-FDG PET/CT for Predicting or Monitoring Immunotherapy Response in Patients With Metastatic Melanoma: A Systematic Review and Meta-Analysis. *Eur J Nucl Med Mol Imaging* (2021) 48:428–48. doi: 10.1007/s00259-020-04967-9

2. Bisschop C, de Heer EC, Brouwers AH, Hospers GAP, Jalving M. Rational Use of 18F-FDG PET/CT in Patients With Advanced Cutaneous Melanoma: A Systematic Review. *Crit Rev Oncol Hematol* (2020) 153:103044. doi: 10.1016/j.critrevonc.2020.103044

3. Cha J, Kim S, Wang J, Yun M, Cho A. Evaluation of 18F-FDG PET/CT Parameters for Detection of Lymph Node Metastasis in Cutaneous Melanoma. *Nucl Med Mol Imaging* (2018) 52(1):39–45. doi: 10.1007/s13139-017-0495-4

4. Baden LR, El Sahly HM, Essink B, Kotloff J, Frey S, Novak R, et al. Efficacy and Safety of the mTNA-1273 SARS-CoV-2 Vaccine. *N Engl J Med* (2021) 384:403–16. doi: 10.1056/NEJMoa2035389

5. McIntosh LJ, Bankier AA, Vijayaraghavan GR, Licho R, Rosen MP. COVID-19 Vaccination-Related Uptake on FDG PET/CT: An Emerging Dilemma and Suggestions for Management. *Am J Roentgenol* (2021). doi: 10.2214/AJR.21.25728

6. Long GV, Robert C, Blank CU, Ribas A, Mortiel R, Schachter J, et al. (2016). Outcomes in Patients Treated With Ipilimumab After Pembrolizumab in KEYNOTE-006. In: *Society of Melanoma Research 2016 Congress*. Boston, MA, USA (2016).

7. Da Silva IP, Ahmed T, Reijers ILM, Weppler AM, Warner AB, Patrinely JR, et al. Ipilimumab Alone or Ipilimumab Plus Anti-PD-1 Therapy in Patients With Metastatic Melanoma Resistant to Anti-PD-(L)1 Monotherapy: A Multicentre, Retrospective, Cohort Study. *Lancet Oncol* (2021) 22(6):836–47. doi: 10.1016/S1470-2045(21)00097-8

8. Hu Y, Zhao X, Zhang J, Han J, Dai M. Value of 18 F-FDG PET/CT Radiomic Features to Distinguish Solitary Lung Adenocarcinoma From Tuberculosis. *Eur J Nucl Med Mol Imaging* (2021) 48(1):231–40. doi: 10.1007/s00259-020-04924-6

9. Stangierski A, Woliński K, Czepczyński R, Czarnywojtek A, Łodyga M, Wyszomirska A, et al. The Usefulness of Standardized Uptake Value in

Differentiation Between Benign and Malignant Thyroid Lesions Detected Incidentally in 18F-FDG PET/CT Examination. *PloS One* (2014) 9(10): e109612. doi: 10.1371/journal.pone.0109612

10. Shen YY, Kao CH, Yeh LH, Chou YH, Liang JA, Hsieh TC. Vanishing Spot on Dual-Time-Point FDG PET/CT: Colonic Diverticulitis. *Clin Nucl Med* (2010) 35(7):529–31. doi: 10.1097/RLU.0b013e3181e06067

11. Karunanithi S, Kumar G, Sharma P, Bal C, Kumar R. Potential Role of (18)F-2-Fluoro-2-Deoxy-Glucose Positron Emission Tomography/Computed Tomography Imaging in Patients Presenting With Generalized Lymphadenopathy. *Indian J Nucl Med* (2015) 30(1):31–8. doi: 10.4103/0972-3919.147532

12. Nawwar AA, Searle J, Singh R, Lyburn ID. Oxford-AstraZeneca COVID-19 Vaccination Induced Lymphadenopathy on [18F]Choline PET/CT - Not Only an FDG Finding. *Eur J Nucl Med Mol Imaging* (2021) 4:1–2. doi: 10.1007/s00259-021-05279-2

13. Avner M, Orevi M, Caplan N, Popovtzer A, Lotem M, Cohen JE. COVID-19 Vaccine as a Cause for Unilateral Lymphadenopathy Detected by 18F-FDG PET/CT in a Patient Affected by Melanoma. *Eur J Nucl Med Mol Imaging* (2021) 6:1–2. doi: 10.1007/s00259-021-05278-3

14. Ulaner GA, Giuliano P. 18f-FDG-Avid Lymph Nodes After COVID-19 Vaccination of 18F-FDG PET/CT. *Clin Nucl Med* (2021) 46(5):433–4. doi: 10.1097/RLU.0000000000003633

15. Schroeder DG, Jang S, Johnson DR, Takahashi H, Navin PJ, Broski SM, et al. Frequency and Characteristics of Nodal and Deltoid FDG and 11C-Choline Uptake on PET Imaging Performed After COVID-19 Vaccination. *Am J Roentgenol* (2021). doi: 10.2214/AJR.21.25928

16. Cohen D, Krauthammer SH, Wolf I, Even-Sapir E. Hypermetabolic Lymphadenopathy Following Administration of BNT162b2 mRNA Covide-19 vaccineL Incidence Assessed by [^{18}F]FDG PET-CT and Relevance to Study Interpretation. *Eur J Nucl Med Mol Imaging* (2021) 48:1854–63. doi: 10.1007/s00259-021-05314-2

Sonidegib for the Treatment of Advanced Basal Cell Carcinoma

Gabriella Brancaccio[1], Federico Pea[2,3], Elvira Moscarella[1] and Giuseppe Argenziano[1]*

[1] Dermatology Unit, University of Campania "Luigi Vanvitelli", Naples, Italy, [2] Department of Medicine, University of Udine, Udine, Italy, [3] Institute of Clinical Pharmacology, Azienda Ospedaliero-Universitaria Santa Maria Della Misericordia, Azienda Sanitaria Universitaria Friuli Centrale, Udine, Italy

*Correspondence:
Gabriella Brancaccio
gabri.brancaccio@gmail.com

Basal cell carcinoma (BCC) accounts for almost 80% of skin cancers, and its healthcare workload burden is substantial within dermatology departments. Although most BCCs are small, well-defined tumors amenable of surgery or conservative procedures, in a small proportion of patients, BCCs can progress to an advanced stage including locally advanced BCC. The goal of the clinician in the treatment of BCC should be the right therapeutic approach at diagnosis, and different guidelines propose treatment strategies in order to prevent relapses or disease progression. In case of unresectable and untreatable BCC with radiotherapy, the first-choice medical therapy is Hedgehog-GLI (HH) pathway inhibitors. Sonidegib was approved by the U.S. Food and Drug Administration (FDA) and European Medicines Agency (EMA) as a first-line treatment for adult patients with locally advanced BCC, becoming the second HH pathway inhibitor receiving approval after vismodegib. In this review, data on pharmacology, safety, tolerability, and efficacy of sonidegib are summarized and compared to those of vismodegib. Lastly, indications on the management of advanced basal cell carcinoma based on author's clinical experience are provided.

Keywords: basal cell carcinoma, advanced basal cell carcinoma, hedgehog inhibitors, sonidegib, skin cancer

INTRODUCTION

Basal cell carcinoma (BCC) accounts for almost 80% of skin cancers, and its oncogenesis rely on the interplay between constitutional predisposition (genotypic and phenotypic characteristics) and subsequent exposure to environmental risk factors, with ultraviolet radiation exposure as the principal one (1).

Actual BCC tumor burden is much greater in the population than it is apparent from normal incidence rates. Many reasons make the true BCC incidence difficult to calculate as 1) routine recording of BCC is often not performed by cancer registries; 2) in clinical practice not all the BCCs are histologically confirmed and 3) when recorded, often only the first histologically confirmed BCC per patient is taken into account. These factors translate into a complete absence of BCC rates in the most accounted statistical datasets (2), where it is even excluded from the group of non-melanoma skin cancer. However, the healthcare workload burden and cost of BCC are substantial within dermatology departments (3), and it is even much higher considering the subset of advanced BCC which accounts for the highest morbidity due to cosmetic disfigurement and functional morbidity.

Although most BCCs are small or intermediate-size, well-defined tumors amenable of surgery or conservative procedures, in a small proportion of patients, BCCs can progress to an advanced stage including metastatic BCC (mBCC) or locally advanced BCC (laBCC) (4). Advanced BCC is an entity not yet clearly defined as there is a lack of consensus on the diagnostic criteria which are hardly objectified. Usually, advanced BCCs are extended tumors characterized by destructive growth after multiple relapse, often located on the head and neck areas that have become difficult to treat through standard surgery and radiotherapy. In order to distinguish between BCCs that may progress to mBCC or laBCC, an innovative classification in easy-to-treat and difficult-to-treat BCCs has been recently proposed. It takes into account size, location, definition of borders, previous treatments, and related recurrences and even some patient's characteristics as comorbidities interfering with surgery or

reluctance to proposed treatments (5). The distinction between easy- and difficult-to-treat BCC may have practical implication considering the wide availability of therapeutic option for the first group of tumors and the need of an immediate resolutive treatment for the latter one (**Table 1**, **Figure 1**). Different guidelines (5, 6) propose treatment strategies in order to identify the better care pathway and, thus, prevent relapses or persistence of the tumor. The multidisciplinary approach is the mainstay of management of difficult-to-treat BCCs, that should be managed in a tertiary care center (referral center).

Surgery should be always considered as primary therapeutic option, even after neoadjuvant approaches. Mohs surgery should be performed in case of large, high-risk tumors located on the face, in case of surgery after a previous relapse, or in case of BCCs arising on a previous irradiated area, scars or areas of chronic inflammation. However, despite very high cure rate, Mohs

TABLE 1 | Recommended therapeutic approach to easy-to-treat and difficult-to-treat BCCs (5).

	Treatment	Type of recommendation	Grade of recommendation–Level of evidence
Easy-to-treat BCC	Surgery	Highly effective in any type of BCC	A-3
	5% Imiquimod (sBCC)	Effective in sBCC	A-2
		Potential role in nBCC	B-2
	5% 5-Fluoruracil	Effective in sBCC	A-2
	Curettage + electrodedissication and cryoterapy	Potential role in low-risk BCC on the trunk and extremities	B-3
	PDT with MAL or ALA	Effective in sBCC and thin nBCC	A-1
Difficult-to-treat BCC	Surgery	Evaluation of suitability by multidisciplinary team	Expert opinion
	Radiotherapy	Role in elderly patients and patients not candidates for surgery (any BCC)	A-1
	HH inhibitors	To be offered in laBCC and mBCC	B-3

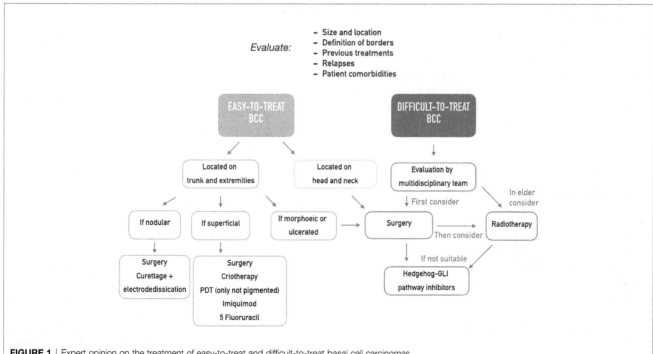

FIGURE 1 | Expert opinion on the treatment of easy-to-treat and difficult-to-treat basal cell carcinomas.

surgery is a costly, time-consuming procedure that requires specialized training and has very little spread in some countries.

Radiotherapy should be taken into account as second-line treatment in elderly patients (>60 years old) suffering from a BCC not amenable of surgery. Radiotherapy is also an option in adjuvant setting in case of positive margins after primary excision. However, due to concerns with long-term sequelae as well as adverse events with intermediate onset, indication to radiotherapy may be questioned by the multidisciplinary team.

Once evolved to laBCC or mBCC, the most appropriate therapeutic option is the target therapy through Hedgehog inhibitors.

HEDGEHOG-GLI PATHWAY AND ITS INHIBITORS

Hedgehog-GLI (HH) signaling plays a major role during the development and is involved in cell proliferation and differentiation (7, 8). The HH pathway is normally silenced in most adult tissues, and it was shown that it may be aberrantly activated in the pathogenesis of various types of tumors (9). This may promote the subsequent activation of transcription factors of the Glioma-associated oncogene (GLI) family, which may favor tumor proliferation (9). Smoothened (SMO) is the main transducer of HH signaling, and in the last few years, it has emerged as a promising therapeutic target for anticancer therapy. Natural and synthetic antagonists have been developed for SMO, and many have undergone clinical trials with varying degrees of success. SMO inhibition was first characterized through binding studies of cyclopamine, a natural steroidal alkaloid derived from *Veratrum californicum*. Derivatives of cyclopamine have been developed with the aim of increasing specificity and pharmacological potency while limiting side effects (10). The first HH pathway inhibitor to be approved by the FDA and EMA was vismodegib, a second-generation cyclopamine derivative. Later, sonidegib was approved by the FDA and EMA as a first-line treatment for adult patients with locally advanced BCC, becoming the second HH pathway inhibitor receiving approval (10). A new SMO inhibitor is also in development for topical administration in patients affected by Gorlin syndrome (11).

SONIDEGIB FOR THE TREATMENT OF ADVANCED BASAL CELL CARCINOMA

Sonidegib is an oral small molecule that acts as a selective antagonist of the SMO receptor, a G protein-coupled receptor-like structure that is fundamental for the correct action of the HH signaling pathway (12).

Sonidegib exhibited dose- and exposure-dependent inhibition of the expression of the GLI homolog 1 in tumor and normal skin biopsies (13) and is currently indicated for the treatment of adults with advanced basal cell carcinomas at the daily dosage of 200 mg (12).

PHARMACOKINETIC PROFILE

Sonidegib pharmacokinetics (PK) was studied in patients with cancer after a single dose ranging between 100 mg and 3000 mg (13). Under fasting condition, absorption resulted quite rapidly with a time to peak concentration (T_{max}) of 2–4 h. Oral bioavailability (F_{OS}) was quite low under fasted state as it was estimated to be around 6–7% after a single 800 mg dose in healthy volunteers (14). F_{OS} increased by 7.8-fold when in the presence of high-fat meal with an almost proportional increase in drug exposure of 7.4-fold in terms of area under the plasma concentration–time curve (AUC) from zero to infinity (15). For this reason, it is recommended that sonidegib is taken under fasting conditions, at least 1–2 h before meal (15).

One of the most interesting pharmacokinetic properties of sonidegib is represented by the wide distribution within tissues (14). A population pharmacokinetic analysis carried out among 351 patients who received sonidegib at a dose ranging between 100 mg and 3,000 mg showed that the volume of distribution (Vd) was of 9,170 L (15). This may explain why sonidegib may either achieve skin concentration sixfold higher than in plasma (15) or effectively cross the blood brain barrier (16). Sonidegib is bound for >97% to plasma protein in a concentration independent mode (15–17).

Sonidegib has a very long-elimination half-life of around 28 days (16, 18). This means that steady-state is reached after more or less 4 months from starting daily dosing treatment (16, 18), with an estimated accumulation of around 19-fold (13, 15). Sonidegib undergoes metabolism mainly *via* oxidation and hydrolysis by the 3A4 isoform of the cytochrome (CYP) P450 (15, 19). All of the metabolites are several-folds less pharmacologically active than the parent compound. Sonidegib is the main circulating moiety in plasma (36%), and both the parent compound and its metabolites are eliminated by the feces (overall 93% of the administered dose) (14).

Overall, the PK profile of sonidegib is quite different from that of the other SMO antagonist vismodegib (**Table 2**). Both drugs are very highly bound to plasma proteins (>97%), but the binding is concentration-independent for sonidegib (16, 17) and concentration-dependent for vismodegib (21, 22). The Vd is much higher for sonidegib than for vismodegib, accordingly to a major grade of lipophilicity. This may reflect in extensive accumulation of sonidegib within tissues, as documented by the finding of concentrations sixfold higher in the skin compared with plasma (15). Conversely, the distribution of vismodegib is mainly limited to the plasma and to the extracellular spaces (23). Theoretically, these differences in the distribution pattern might translate into potential differences in the pharmacodynamic profile of efficacy and toxicity of these two SMO inhibitors (20). Another relevant PK difference is related to the elimination half-life, which is three to fourfold longer for sonidegib (28–30 days) (16, 18) compared with vismodegib (4–12 days) (23, 24). This means that the time needed to achieve steady concentrations during continued treatment (namely the steady-state) is of around 3–4 months for sonidegib (16, 18) and of around 7–21 days for vismodegib (23, 24). The differences in

TABLE 2 | Comparative PK characteristic and efficacy of sonidegib and vismodegib.

PK	Sonidegib 200 mg daily	Vismodegib 150 mg daily
Plasma protein binding	>97% (concentration-independent) (8, 9),	>99% (concentration-dependent) (12, 13),
Vd (L)	9166 (7, 8),	16.4–26.6 (14)
$t_{1/2}$ (days)	28–30 (8, 10),	4–12 (14, 16),
Time to steady-state (days)	90–120 (8, 10),	17–21 (14, 16),
Efficacy	Central review RECIST-like 18-month follow-up (BOLT trial) (20)	Central review RECIST 21-month follow-up (Erivance trial) (20)
Overall response rate n (%); 95% CI	40 (60.6); 47.8–72.4	30 (47.6); 35.5–60.6
Complete response n (%)	14 (21.2%)	14 (22.2%)
Partial response n (%)	26 (39.4%)	16 (25.4%)
Stable disease n (%)	20 (30.3%)	22 (34.9%)
Progressive disease n (%)	1 (1.5%)	8 (12.7%)
Unknown n (%)	5 (7.6%)	3 (4.8%)

RECIST, Response Evaluation Criteria in Solid Tumors. Adapted by Dummer et al. J Eur Acad Dermatol Venereol. 2020.

time to steady state between the two HH inhibitors do not seem to correlate with the time to response, as the median time to response was 3.9 months for sonidegib in BOLT and 5.6 months for vismodegib in ERIVANCE trial (20).

Drug–Drug Interactions

Sonidegib is a substrate of CYP3A4 and it is expected that its pharmacokinetic profile may be altered by modulators of the activity of this metabolizing enzyme (15, 19). Thus, the recommendation on the EMA product label is to avoid co-administration with strong CYP 3A4 inhibitors or to reduce sonidegib dose to 200 mg every other day during co-treatment with strong CYP 3A4 inhibitors in order not to exceed a twofold increase in sonidegib exposure (15, 19). Similarly, co-treatment with strong CYP 3A4 inducers should be avoided (15, 19). However, if co-treatment with inducers is needed, sonidegib dose may be increased to 400–800 mg in order to prevent >80% reduction in sonidegib exposure (15, 19). Concomitant treatment with strong CYP inducers should be avoided in the case of vismodegib as well. The product label does not provide any advice on dose adjustment if co-administration is necessary [Erivedge EMA label].

Pharmacokinetic Profile in Special Patient Populations

The pharmacokinetic behavior of sonidegib was evaluated also in special patient populations. The effect of mild to severe hepatic impairment on the pharmacokinetics of sonidegib was assessed in a phase 1 multicenter, open label, parallel-group study (25) concluding that in patients with any grade of hepatic impairment dose adjustments are unnecessary.

Sonidegib has not been studied in a dedicated pharmacokinetic study in patients with renal impairment. Based on the available data, sonidegib elimination *via* the kidney is negligible. A population pharmacokinetic analysis found that mild or moderate renal impairment did not have a significant effect on the apparent clearance of sonidegib, suggesting that dose adjustment is not necessary in patients with renal impairment. No efficacy and safety data are available in patients with severe renal impairment [Odomzo EMA label].

Additionally, safety and efficacy data in patients aged 65 years and older do not suggest that a dosage adjustment is required in these patients [Odomzo EMA label].

A population pharmacokinetic analysis of sonidegib was carried out among healthy volunteers and patients with advanced solid tumors (18). Covariate analysis showed that age, weight, gender, ethnicity, mild hepatic impairment, mild and moderate renal impairment did not affect sonidegib pharmacokinetics. This means that no sonidegib dose adjustment is indicated in relation to these conditions. Conversely, clinically relevant effects on sonidegib F_{OS} were induced by high-fat meal (fivefold increase), and by co-administration of proton pump inhibitors (30% decrease). In regard to the former effect, it is recommended that sonidegib is assumed under fasted condition for avoiding unpredictable overexposure (15). In regard to the latter effect, a phase 1 study carried out among 42 healthy volunteers showed that co-administration of esomeprazole (40 mg 5-days pretreatment plus combination on day 6) with a single 200 mg dose of sonidegib resulted in a modest reduction of sonidegib absorption under fasted conditions (decreased sonidegib AUC by 32-38%) (26).

TOLERABILITY AND SAFETY

The safety and the tolerability of sonidegib was assessed in the double-blind, phase 2 pivotal trial (BOLT) in which patients with locally advanced or metastatic basal cell carcinoma were randomized to receive 200 or 800 mg oral sonidegib daily (27).

A comprehensive analysis assessed whether an exposure–response relationship would exist for effectiveness and safety of sonidegib among patients with advanced solid tumors (28). For the exposure–efficacy analysis, data from 190 patients receiving sonidegib at 200 or 800 mg daily were included. Logistic regression analysis showed no relationship between sonidegib exposure in terms of trough level (C_{min}) resulting from 200 or 800 mg doses at week 5 and the objective response rate in terms of complete and/or partial response. Exposure–safety analysis was carried out among 336 patients receiving dosages ranging from 100 to 3,000 mg once daily and 250 to 750 mg twice daily. The findings showed that increased exposure was associated with a greater risk of grades 3–4 creatine kinase (CK) elevation, and that the risk was lower in females *vs.* males. Consistently, it is recommended that CK level is monitored periodically throughout the duration of treatment with sonidegib (29).

A pooled analysis of the change in the QT interval was carried out for assessing the eventual prolongation QT caused by sonidegib. Data coming from four patient studies (n = 341) were merged with those coming from four healthy volunteer studies (n = 204) (30). Overall, data showed that sonidegib did not cause QTc prolongation as ΔQTc were always <5 ms both for the 200 and 800 mg dose.

With regard to tolerability, the most frequent adverse events (AEs) resulted in muscle spasms, alopecia, and dysgeusia, mostly of grade 1–2 (17). The most common grade 3–4 AEs occurring in ≥2% of patients receiving the 200 mg daily dose were fatigue, weight decrease, and muscle spasms. Even if data from the two pivotal studies are not directly comparable, sonidegib resulted in being associated with the same AEs of vismodegib but with an approximately 10% lower incidence (4). AEs reported with sonidegib were also slightly less severe and with a slightly longer median time to onset (4). Specifically, the median time to onset of the most frequent AEs with vismodegib 150 mg and sonidegib 200 mg, namely muscle spasms, alopecia and dysgeusia, were 1.89 vs 2.07 months, 3.38 vs 5.55 months and 1.48 vs 3.71 months, respectively.

EFFICACY

The phase 2 trial (BOLT) that led to the approval in both US and Europe compared sonidegib at a dosage of 200 and 800 mg in patients affected by laBCC (n = 194) and mBCC (n = 36). As sonidegib 200 mg demonstrated a better benefit-risk profile than sonidegib 800 mg, we will focus only on the former, which is the approved dose in the setting of laBCC (15).

Primary endpoint of the BOLT trial was overall response rate (ORR) by central review, while secondary endpoints were ORR by investigator review, duration of response (DOR), progression free survival (PFS), overall survival (OS), time to response, safety and quality of life (QoL). Noteworthy, assessment of laBCC in BOLT trial was performed using the BCC-modified RECIST criteria (mRECIST) (27). BCC-mRECIST is a multimodal assessment method integrating magnetic resonance imaging per RECISTv1.1, standard and annotated color photography per WHO guidelines, and histology in multiple biopsy specimens surveying the lesion area. Overall, these criteria for assessing partial and complete response, as well as progression disease, are more stringent compared to the RECISTv1.1 criteria used in vismodegib studies (4). mRECIST is more likely to detect minimal signs of disease and disease progression, thus classifying a given treatment response as partial, whereas the same response may be considered as complete using RECIST. Similarly, mRECIST is more likely to detect signs of slight disease progression that may be classified as stable disease (SD) under RECIST (20). This aspect is crucial when comparing efficacy data from sonidegib and vismodegib trial analyses (17, 27, 31, 32) (**Table 2**). Despite similar baseline patient characteristics, endpoints, and role of central and investigator review, the difference in assessment criteria makes a head-to-head comparison of the two drugs difficult. However, in the 30-month analysis of the BOLT study, a pre-planned analysis adjusted the outcomes from BOLT with RECIST-like criteria. As underlined in a recent expert opinion paper, the most correct match is between adjusted ORR of sonidegib and ORR of vismodegib at the closest follow-up time points across the studies with central review (20). At 21-month follow-up, vismodegib ORR was 47.6%, with 22.2% complete response (CR) and 25.4% partial response (PR). At 18-month follow-up, adjusted ORR of sonidegib was 60.6% with 21.2% CR and 39.4% PR. Adjusting efficacy data using RECIST criteria make just a slight increase in sonidegib overall response rate (ORR) (from 56.1 to 60.6%) while the number of CR increases significantly at the expense of PR. The rate of progressive disease (PD) is higher for vismodegib than for sonidegib (12.7 and 1.5%, respectively) (20), and this data is consistent with reports of acquired resistance during treatment with vismodegib (4). However, it is likely that the responsible genomic mutations affecting SMO confer resistance to different SMO inhibitors. Further studies are needed to find the right therapeutic strategy in constitutionally or acquired resistant laBCC, through drug associations or different molecules. Lastly, the centrally reviewed median duration of response (mDOR) and median progression free survival (mPFS) with sonidegib at 30 months were longer than vismodegib at 21 months (17, 31). The longest (39 months) follow-up report of vismodegib includes only investigator reviewed data, therefore is not appropriate for a comparison (32). However, the investigator reviewed mDOR results are longer with vismodegib.

CLINICAL IMPLICATIONS AND CONCLUSIONS

The goal of the clinician in the treatment of BCC should be the right therapeutic approach at diagnosis, thus preventing the evolution into laBCC or mBCC. Many treatments are available depending on the clinical features of the primitive lesion and on patient characteristics (**Table 1**), and the distinction into easy-to-treat and difficult-to-treat BCCs may be helpful in the clinical practice (**Figure 1**). Easy-to-treat BCCs may be properly managed by the territorial health care or in the private practice, while difficult-to-treat BCCs should be referred to a secondary/tertiary care center in order to be evaluated by a multidisciplinary team. Obviously, the experience of each center differs from one country to another and in the same country and may influence the therapeutic decision, but general recommendations should be followed (5).

For the treatment of difficult-to-treat BCCs, surgery should be the first therapeutic option, but it should be carefully planned, and appropriate imaging to determine the extent of the tumor should be performed when perineural involvement or bone invasion is suspected. When available, Mohs surgery should be preferred. Radiotherapy is an alternative option in elderly patient affected by BCCs not amenable of surgery or in patients who are not candidates to surgery; it is devoted to elderly people because the potential risk of very-long-term trophic disorders is not well addressed (5).

In case of unresectable and untreatable BCC with radiotherapy (laBCC), the first-choice medical therapy is HH pathway inhibitors. Chemotherapy showed a low response rate and a short duration of response in few reports, so it can be considered a last-line treatment, while studies on the efficacy of immunotherapy in BCC are currently ongoing (5).

To date, the choice between the two HH inhibitors available, vismodegib and sonidegib, is based on expert opinion and indirect comparison, as a head-to-head trial is not available. However, a subset of patients who could benefit more from one drug than another has not been clearly identified. Vismodegib, being the first approved HH inhibitor, has been used for longer time and real-world data are available. Although no laboratory tests are required by label (except for pregnancy test), we routinely perform a metabolic panel every 1–2 months, depending on patient comorbidities, with special attention to liver and kidney functionality and creatinine kinase levels. We experienced the efficacy of vismodegib in many laBCC patients, with both complete and partial responses, but also some disease progressions after the onset of resistance, as reported in literature. The main pitfall is the adherence to a long, otherwise chronic, treatment due to the onset of adverse events and their impact on quality of life. The most reported and least tolerated side effect seems to be muscle spasms; it occurs relatively early during the treatment and implementation through magnesium or levocarnitine shows a mild effectiveness in few cases. Dysgeusia and alopecia are of later onset but equally impairing AEs. To overcome this issue, different preventive and management strategies have been proposed, mainly drug holydays. However, since no dose adjustments are present in the vismodegib data sheet, any individual modifications that may be introduced are off-label.

Sonidegib is the latest HH inhibitor to be approved; thus its real-life experience is being built. However, both trial results and clinical experience confirm a similar efficacy profile to vismodegib. Comparing the adjusted results of BOLT trial at 18-month follow-up to the results of ERIVANCE trial at 21-month follow-up points out slightly higher ORR and PR, similar CR and SD, and a lower PD for sonidegib (20). Like vismodegib, also sonidegib is not contraindicated in any specific patient subset, but monitoring of CK levels is indicated. We usually prescribe the same laboratory tests for vismodegib. With regard to tolerability, sonidegib shares the same class-dependent AEs of vismodegib; however, they seem to be less frequent and with a slightly longer time to onset, probably due to a different pharmacokinetic profile. The availability of an alternative administration schedule included in the label (200 mg every other day) is very helpful in managing the entity of specific AEs, such as high CK levels, and thus the rate of treatment discontinuation may be lowered.

To understand which patient could benefit from vismodegib or sonidegib, real-world data on the latter drug are needed. Only one case report described the experience of a laBCC successfully treated with sonidegib with complete response and with no side effects (33). A case series collecting experience in our center is under review. However, making any definitive directives for the choice between the two HHi is premature. Besides real-world data on sonidegib use, a head-to-head trial should be designed in order to produce more reliable comparative data. Also, intermittent trials, sequential trials, or cross-over trials of the two HH inhibitors in laBCC patients who discontinued treatment due to AEs may demonstrate the impact of the pharmacokinetic profile differences and improve the awareness of the clinician on the use of HH inhibitors.

AUTHOR CONTRIBUTIONS

All the authors contributed equally to this work. All authors contributed to the article and approved the submitted version.

REFERENCES

1. Verkouteren JAC, Ramdas KHR, Wakkee M, Nijsten T. Epidemiology of basal cell carcinoma: scholarly review. *Br J Dermatol* (2017) 177(2):359–72. doi: 10.1111/bjd.15321

2. Bray F, Ferlay J, Soerjomataram I, Siegel RL, Torre LA, Jemal A. Global cancer statistics 2018: GLOBOCAN estimates of incidence and mortality worldwide for 36 cancers in 185 countries. *CA Cancer J Clin Nov* (2018) 68(6):394–424. doi: 10.3322/caac.21492

3. Venables ZC, Nijsten T, Wong KF, Autier P, Broggio J, Deas A, et al. Epidemiology of basal and cutaneous squamous cell carcinoma in the U.K. 2013-15: a cohort study. *Br J Dermatol* (2019) 181(3):474–82. doi: 10.1111/bjd.17873

4. Migden MR, Chang ALS, Dirix L, Stratigos AJ, Lear JT. Emerging trends in the treatment of advanced basal cell carcinoma. *Cancer Treat Rev* (2018) 64:1–10. doi: 10.1016/j.ctrv.2017.12.009

5. Peris K, Fargnoli MC, Garbe C, Kaufmann R, Bastholt L, Seguin NB, et al. European Dermatology Forum (EDF), the European Association of Dermato-Oncology (EADO) and the European Organization for Research and Treatment of Cancer (EORTC). Diagnosis and treatment of basal cell carcinoma: European consensus-based interdisciplinary guidelines. *Eur J Cancer* (2019) 118:10–34. doi: 10.1016/j.ejca.2019.06.003

6. National Comprehensive Cancer Network. NCCN clinical practice guidelines in oncology: basal cell skin cancer. (2020). Version 1. Available at: https://www.nccn.org/professionals/physician_gls/pdf/nmsc.pdf.

7. Ingham PW, Nakano Y, Seger C. Mechanisms and functions of Hedgehog signalling across the metazoa. *Nat Rev Genet* (2011) 12(6):393–406. doi: 10.1038/nrg2984

8. Choudhry Z, Rikani AA, Choudhry AM, Tariq S, Zakaria F, Asghar MW, et al. Sonic hedgehog signalling pathway: a complex network. *Ann Neurosci* (2014) 21(1):28–31. doi: 10.5214/ans.0972.7531.210109

9. Carpenter RL, Lo HW. Hedgehog pathway and GLI1 isoforms in human cancer. *Discovery Med* (2012) 13(69):105–13.

10. Pietrobono S, Stecca B. Targeting the Oncoprotein Smoothened by Small Molecules: Focus on Novel Acylguanidine Derivatives as Potent Smoothened Inhibitors. *Cells* (2018) 7(12):272. doi: 10.3390/cells7120272

11. National Cancer Institute. Trial of patidegib gel 2%, 4%, and vehicle to decrese the number of surgically eligible basal cell carcinomas in Gorlin syndrome

patients. Available at: https://clinicaltrials.gov/ct2/show/NCT02762084 (Accessed 20 Apr 2020).

12. Burness CB. Sonidegib: First Global Approval. *Drugs* (2015) 75(13):1559–66. doi: 10.1007/s40265-015-0458-y

13. Rodon J, Tawbi HA, Thomas AL, Stoller RG, Turtschi CP, Baselga J, et al. multicenter, open-label, first-in-human, dose-escalation study of the oral smoothened inhibitor Sonidegib (LDE225) in patients with advanced solid tumors. *Clin Cancer Res* (2014) 20(7):1900–9. doi: 10.1158/1078-0432.CCR-13-1710

14. Zollinger M, Lozac'h F, Hurh E, Emotte C, Bauly H, Swart P. Absorption, distribution, metabolism, and excretion (ADME) of (1)(4)C-sonidegib (LDE225) in healthy volunteers. *Cancer Chemother Pharmacol* (2014) 74 (1):63–75. doi: 10.1007/s00280-014-2468-y

15. *Odomzo EMA Summary of product characteristics.* Available at: https://www.ema.europa.eu/en/documents/product-information/odomzo-epar-product-information_en.pdf, checked on 19 March 2020.

16. Pan S, Wu X, Jiang J, Gao W, Wan Y, Cheng D, et al. Discovery of NVP-LDE225, a Potent and Selective Smoothened Antagonist. *ACS Med Chem Lett* (2010) 1(3):130–4. doi: 10.1021/ml1000307

17. Lear JT, Migden MR, Lewis KD, Chang ALS, Guminski A, Gutzmer R, et al. Long-term efficacy and safety of sonidegib in patients with locally advanced and metastatic basal cell carcinoma: 30-month analysis of the randomized phase 2 BOLT study. *J Eur Acad Dermatol Venereol* (2018) 32(3):372–81. doi: 10.1111/jdv.14542

18. Goel V, Hurh E, Stein A, Nedelman J, Zhou J, Chiparus O, et al. Population pharmacokinetics of sonidegib (LDE225), an oral inhibitor of hedgehog pathway signaling, in healthy subjects and in patients with advanced solid tumors. *Cancer Chemother Pharmacol* (2016) 77(4):745–55. doi: 10.1007/s00280-016-2982-1

19. Einolf HJ, Zhou J, Won C, Wang L, Rebello S. A Physiologically-Based Pharmacokinetic Modeling Approach To Predict Drug-Drug Interactions of Sonidegib (LDE225) with Perpetrators of CYP3A in Cancer Patients. *Drug Metab Dispos* (2017) 45(4):361–74. doi: 10.1124/dmd.116.073585

20. Dummer R, Ascierto PA, Basset-Seguin N, Dreno B, Garbe C, Gutzmer R, et al. Sonidegib and vismodegib in the treatment of patients with locally advanced basal cell carcinoma: a joint expert opinion. *J Eur Acad Dermatol Venereol* (2020). doi: 10.1111/jdv.16230

21. Graham RA, Lum BL, Cheeti S, Jin JY, Jorga K, Von Hoff DD, et al. Pharmacokinetics of hedgehog pathway inhibitor vismodegib (GDC-0449) in patients with locally advanced or metastatic solid tumors: the role of alpha-1-acid glycoprotein binding. *Clin Cancer Res* (2011) 17(8):2512–20. doi: 10.1158/1078-0432.CCR-10-2736

22. Lorusso PM, Jimeno A, Dy G, Adjei A, Berlin J, Leichman L, et al. Pharmacokinetic dose-scheduling study of hedgehog pathway inhibitor vismodegib (GDC-0449) in patients with locally advanced or metastatic solid tumors. *Clin Cancer Res* (2011) 17(17):5774–82. doi: 10.1158/1078-0432.CCR-11-0972

23. Graham RA, Hop CE, Borin MT, Lum BL, Colburn D, Chang I, et al. Single and multiple dose intravenous and oral pharmacokinetics of the hedgehog pathway inhibitor vismodegib in healthy female subjects. *Br J Clin Pharmacol* (2012) 74(5):788–96. doi: 10.1111/j.1365-2125.2012.04281.x

24. Lu T, Wang B, Gao Y, Dresser M, Graham RA, Jin JY. Semi-Mechanism-Based Population Pharmacokinetic Modeling of the Hedgehog Pathway Inhibitor Vismodegib. *CPT Pharmacometr Syst Pharmacol* (2015) 4 (11):680–9. doi: 10.1002/psp4.12039

25. Horsmans Y, Zhou J, Liudmila M, Golor G, Shibolet O, Quinlan M, et al. Effects of Mild to Severe Hepatic Impairment on the Pharmacokinetics of Sonidegib: A Multicenter, Open-Label, Parallel-Group Study. *Clin Pharmacokinet* (2018) 57(3):345–54. doi: 10.1007/s40262-017-0560-2

26. Zhou J, Quinlan M, Glenn K, Boss H, Picard F, Castro H, et al. Effect of esomeprazole, a proton pump inhibitor on the pharmacokinetics of sonidegib in healthy volunteers. *Br J Clin Pharmacol* (2016) 82(4):1022–9. doi: 10.1111/bcp.13038

27. Migden MR, Guminski A, Gutzmer R, Dirix L, Lewis KD, Combemale P, et al. Treatment with two different doses of sonidegib in patients with locally advanced or metastatic basal cell carcinoma (BOLT): a multicentre, randomised, double-blind phase 2 trial. *Lancet Oncol* (2015) 16(6):716–28. doi: 10.1016/S1470-2045(15)70100-2

28. Zhou J, Quinlan M, Hurh E, Sellami D. Exposure-Response Analysis of Sonidegib (LDE225), an Oral Inhibitor of the Hedgehog Signaling Pathway, for Effectiveness and Safety in Patients With Advanced Solid Tumors. *J Clin Pharmacol* (2016) 56(11):1406–15. doi: 10.1002/jcph.749

29. Carpenter RL, Ray H. Safety and Tolerability of Sonic Hedgehog Pathway Inhibitors in Cancer. *Drug Saf* (2019) 42(2):263–79. doi: 10.1007/s40264-018-0777-5

30. Quinlan M, Zhou J, Hurh E, Sellami D. Exposure-QT analysis for sonidegib (LDE225), an oral inhibitor of the hedgehog signaling pathway, for measures of the QT prolongation potential in healthy subjects and in patients with advanced solid tumors. *Eur J Clin Pharmacol* (2016) 72(12):1427–32. doi: 10.1007/s00228-016-2128-8

31. Sekulic A, Migden MR, Lewis K, Hainsworth JD, Solomon JA, Yoo S, et al. Pivotal ERIVANCE basal cell carcinoma (BCC) study: 12-month update of efficacy and safety of vismodegib in advanced BCC. *J Am AcadDermatol* (2015) 72(6):1021–6. doi: 10.1016/j.jaad.2015.03.021

32. Sekulic A, Migden MR, Basset-Seguin N, Garbe C, Gesierich A, Lao CD, et al. Long-term safety and efficacy of vismodegib in patients with advanced basal cell carcinoma: final update of the pivotal ERIVANCE BCC study. *BMC Cancer* (2017) 17(1):332. doi: 10.1186/s12885-017-3286-5

33. Villani A, Fabbrocini G, Costa C, Scalvenzi M. Complete remission of an advanced basal cell carcinoma after only 3-month treatment with sonidegib: Report of a case and drug management during COVID-19 pandemic. *Dermatol Ther* (2020) 1:e14200. doi: 10.1111/dth.14200

6

Mucosal Invasion, but not Incomplete Excision, has Negative Impact on Long-Term Survival in Patients with Extramammary Paget's Disease

Hiroki Hashimoto[*], Yumiko Kaku-Ito, Masutaka Furue and Takamichi Ito

Department of Dermatology, Graduate School of Medical Sciences, Kyushu University, Fukuoka, Japan

*Correspondence:
Hiroki Hashimoto
h-hashi@dermatol.med.kyushu-u.ac.jp

Background: Extramammary Paget's disease (EMPD) sometimes spreads from the skin to mucosal areas, and curative surgical excision of these areas is challenging. The aim of this study is to analyze the impact of mucosal involvement and surgical treatment on the survival of patients with EMPD.

Methods: We conducted a retrospective review of 217 patients with EMPD. We also assessed the associations between tumor involvement in boundary areas (anal canal, external urethral meatus, vaginal introitus), prognostic factors, and survival in 198 patients treated with curative surgery.

Results: Of 217 patients, 75 (34.6%) had mucosal boundary area involvement. Lesions in these areas were associated with frequent lymphovascular invasion ($p = 0.042$), lymph node metastasis ($p = 0.0002$), incomplete excision ($p < 0.0001$), and locoregional recurrence ($p < 0.0001$). Boundary area involvement was an independent prognostic factor associated with disease-specific survival, per multivariate analysis (HR: 11.87, $p = 0.027$). Incomplete excision was not significantly correlated with disease-specific survival (HR: 1.05, $p = 0.96$).

Conclusion: Boundary area tumor involvement was a major risk factor for incomplete excision, local recurrence, and poor survival outcomes. However, incomplete removal of primary tumors was not significantly associated with poor prognosis. A less invasive surgical approach for preserving anogenital and urinary functions may be acceptable as the first-line treatment for resectable EMPD.

Keywords: extramammary Paget's disease, mucosal invasion, surgery, prognostic factor, invasive surgery, radical surgery

INTRODUCTION

Extramammary Paget's disease (EMPD) is a rare neoplastic condition (1). It commonly affects areas rich in apocrine sweat glands, including the vulva, perineal area, perianal area, scrotal area, and penile skin (1, 2). EMPD typically affects Caucasian females and Asian males older than 60 years (3–7). Most EMPD tumors are restricted to the epidermis as *in situ* lesions, and they are associated with good prognosis because of their slow-growing nature (1, 8). However, approximately 15–40% of EMPD lesions display dermal invasion, which is known as invasive EMPD, and this increases the risk of lymph node and distant metastasis (2, 4). Management is notoriously complicated, and the recurrence rate is high (15–61%) despite aggressive surgeries (9–12).

Several prognostic factors regarding primary tumors have been reported, including tumor thickness (13, 14), level of tumor invasion (15–18), lymphovascular invasion (8, 17, 19), and perianal location (13, 20–22). Ohara et al. (8) recently conducted a multicenter analysis of 301 invasive EMPD cases, and they proposed a new tumor, node, and metastasis (TNM) classification and staging system in which the T category was determined based on tumor thickness and lymphovascular invasion. The Japanese Skin Cancer Society is currently proposing the use of this EMPD-specific TNM classification and staging system. However, the classification is still tentative.

EMPD lesions sometimes spread from the skin to mucosal areas *via* boundary areas (anal canal, external urethral meatus, vaginal introitus) and deep toward internal organs (rectum, uterus, urinary bladder). Curative surgical excision of lesions in boundary areas is challenging since radical excision impairs organ functions and requires additional functional reconstruction (colostomy, etc.). To preserve organ function, surgical margins are determined at specific sites (e.g., dentate line) regardless of tumor spread, but it can be difficult to maintain sufficient surgical margins at these sites. Perianal lesions indicate poor prognosis partly due to difficult total excision (20). A recent report suggested frequent incomplete excision in cases of EMPD with mucosal involvement (23). However, the prognostic impact of mucosal involvement has not been elucidated.

In this study, we reviewed the data of 217 EMPD patients in our institution over a 23-year period. We showed that lesions involving boundary areas were associated with high risk for poor survival outcomes, regardless of whether complete surgical removal was achieved, and that incomplete excision of EMPD did not affect patient outcomes. We also aimed to verify the newly proposed EMPD-specific TNM staging system (8).

MATERIALS AND METHODS

Patients

This retrospective review was conducted according to the guidelines of the Declaration of Helsinki. This study was

Abbreviations: EMPD, extramammary Paget's disease; TNM, tumor, node, and metastasis; DSS, disease-specific survival; SLNB, sentinel lymph node biopsy; CLND, completion lymph node dissection.

approved by the Ethics Committee of Kyushu University Hospital (30–363; November 27, 2018). We retrieved the data of 217 patients with primary EMPD lesions. These patients were treated at the Department of Dermatology of Kyushu University in Fukuoka, Japan, between January 1997 and October 2020. At least three experienced dermatopathologists confirmed the diagnosis. Patients with secondary EMPD, which involved direct invasion from visceral organs, were carefully excluded.

The following data on all patients were retrieved from our prospectively maintained databank and then analyzed: demographic data (sex, age at initial presentation), clinical data (tumor site, primary lesion size), and histopathological data obtained *via* hematoxylin and eosin staining (tumor thickness [measured to the second decimal place, as per the latest melanoma classification guidelines of the American Joint Committee on Cancer] (24), lymphovascular invasion). For patients with two or more primary lesions, we recorded the greatest tumor thickness and the total tumor size. Tumor thickness was measured from the total excised specimen. For cases without total excision, tumor thickness was calculated from biopsy specimens. In situ lesions on biopsy were further confirmed by clinical findings (lack of erosions, ulcerations, formation of nodules). Involvement of mucosal boundary areas (anal canal, external urethral meatus, vaginal introitus) was recorded from clinicopathological data. Lymph node metastasis was primarily determined by histopathology. Patients who had lymphadenopathy detected by physical examination or imaging studies (ultrasonography, computed tomography [CT], and/or positron emission tomography with computed tomography [PET/CT]) were also considered to have metastasis. The N category was defined according to the classification system proposed by Ohara et al. (8): N0, no lymph node metastasis; N1, metastasis involving one lymph node; and N2, metastasis involving two or more lymph nodes. Distant metastasis was determined by using imaging studies (ultrasonography, chest X-ray, CT, and/or PET/CT). Lymph node metastasis beyond the regional lymphatic basin was also classified as distant metastasis. For the M category, M0 indicated no distant metastasis, and M1 indicated distant metastasis (8).

Mucosal Boundary Area Involvement and Surgical Outcomes

Next, the data of patients treated with curative surgery were collected. Patients were divided into two groups, that is, with or without involvement of mucosal boundary areas, as involvement of these areas influences surgical strategies. In addition to the data mentioned above, we compared data pertaining to surgical treatments and outcomes, including surgical margin, margin status after surgery (complete or incomplete excision), local recurrence, and new regional lymph node metastasis after initial treatment, between these two groups. Complete excision was defined as complete removal of the primary tumor with histopathologically negative margins and complete dissection of regional lymph nodes (if lymph node metastases were present). Patients with distant metastases at surgery were excluded when comparing surgical outcomes. Reconstruction of skin/mucosal defects was performed by using simple sutures, skin grafting, or musculocutaneous flaps, as appropriate.

Follow-Up

The patients were monitored by physical examination every 3–6 months and imaging studies (ultrasonography, chest X-ray, and/or CT). Survival data, including time of locoregional and distant recurrence, survival length, and cause of death, were recorded. The median follow-up period was 61.4 months (range: 2.0–264.7 months). By the last follow-up, 164 patients were alive, 20 died of EMPD, and 33 died of other causes.

Statistical Analysis

All statistical analyses were performed by using JMP version 14.2 (SAS Institute, Cary, NC, USA). The χ^2 test or Fisher's exact test and Mann-Whitney U test were used for analysis of categorical variables and continuous variables, respectively. We used the Kaplan-Meier method to evaluate disease-specific survival (DSS), and we compared survival curves by using the log-rank test. DSS was calculated from the date of the first histological examination to the date of death due to EMPD or the last follow-up prior to October 31, 2020. Data on patients who did not die were censored on October 31, 2020. Data on patients who died of other causes were censored at the time of death. The associations between clinical and histopathological factors and DSS were determined by using a multivariate Cox proportional hazards regression model. Probability values less than 0.05 were regarded as statistically significant.

RESULTS

Clinicopathological Data of the Study Cohort

The demographic and clinical data of the 217 patients with primary EMPD are shown in **Table 1**. All patients were Japanese, with a mean age of 72.9 years (range: 34–95 years). There were 130 male patients (59.9%) and 87 female patients (40.1%). Tumors were predominantly localized in the genital area (83.9%), followed by the perianal area (4.1%), then the axillary area (2.3%). Multiple lesions or tumors spreading over two areas were seen in 21 patients (9.7%). There were 95 patients (44.4%) with small primary lesions (< 25 cm^2) and 119 (55.6%) with large lesions (≥ 25 cm^2). A total of 109 patients (50.2%) had tumors in situ. Tumor thickness was stratified as ≤ 1 mm, 1–4 mm, or > 4 mm for invasive tumors. There were 38 patients (17.5%) with tumors ≤ 1 mm, 45 (20.7%) with tumors 1–4 mm, and 19 (8.8%) with tumors > 4 mm. Lymphovascular invasion was observed in 14 patients (6.5%); lymphovascular invasion was not evident in 203 patients (93.5%). A total of 75 patients (34.6%) exhibited boundary area involvement. Regional lymph node metastasis was found in 27 patients (12.4%). Seven patients (3.2%) had one metastatic lymph node, and 20 (9.2%) had two or more. Distant metastasis was observed in six patients (2.8%). Data on primary lesion size and tumor thickness were unavailable for three and six patients, respectively.

TABLE 1 | Demographics and clinical data of all 217 patients.

Parameter	n (%)
Sex	
Male	130 (59.9)
Female	87 (40.1)
Age (years)	
Mean ± SD	72.9 ± 10.0
Median (range)	73 (34-95)
Tumor site	
Genital area only	182 (83.9)
Perianal area only	9 (4.1)
Axillary area only	5 (2.3)
Genital + perianal areas	13 (6.0)
Genital + axillary areas	5 (2.3)
Other areas	3 (1.4)
Primary lesion size (cm^2)	
<25	95 (44.4)
≥25	119 (55.6)
Unknown	3 (0.4)
Tumor thickness (mm)	
In situ	109 (50.2)
≤1	38 (17.5)
1-4	45 (20.7)
>4	19 (8.8)
Unknown	6 (2.8)
Lymphovascular invasion	
Present	14 (6.5)
Absent	203 (93.5)
Boundary area involvement	
Present	75 (34.6)
Absent	142 (65.4)
Metastasis	
Regional lymph node metastasis	
N0	190 (87.6)
N1	7 (3.2)
N2	20 (9.2)
Distant metastasis	
M0	211 (97.2)
M1	6 (2.8)

SD, standard deviation.

Treatment, Locoregional Recurrence, and Distant Metastasis

A total of 204 patients (94.0%) underwent surgical excision for primary lesions. Of these patients, 200 underwent curative excision with wide margins (0.5–5.0 cm), typically after mapping biopsy, and four underwent palliative surgery. Surgical margins were positive in 46 of these 204 patients (22.5%). Additional excision was performed in seven of these 46 patients. A total of 13 patients (6.0%) with disseminated metastasis or complications or who were unable to give consent for surgical excision received the following alternative treatments, alone or in combination: topical imiquimod cream (n = 3), topical 5-fluorouracil ointment (n = 3), cryotherapy (n = 2), photodynamic therapy (n = 1), radiation therapy (n = 5), or systemic chemotherapy (n = 4). Only two patients received palliative care as the primary treatment. There were 33 patients without lymphadenopathy who underwent sentinel lymph node biopsy (SLNB); eight of them (24.2%) were positive. There were 19 patients with lymphadenopathy who underwent swollen lymph node biopsy; nine of them (47.4%) had confirmed metastasis. Completion lymph node dissection (CLND) was performed in 18 patients (8.3%). Systemic chemotherapy/ targeted therapy was performed in six patients (2.8%). Radiation therapy was performed in seven patients (3.2%). A summary of the initial treatments is available in **Supplementary Table 1**.

Of 200 patients who underwent curative excision with wide margins, 13 patients had local recurrence during the follow-up period. They underwent wide surgical excision (n = 9), radiation therapy (n = 2), or treatment with topical imiquimod cream (n = 2). The details of the 13 patients with local recurrence are shown in **Supplementary Table 2**. Regional lymph node metastasis or distant metastasis (distant lymph node, lung, liver, brain, or bone metastasis) occurred for the first time in 18 patients during the follow-up period, and 13 of these patients underwent CLND, systemic chemotherapy/targeted therapy, or radiation therapy (alone or in combination).

Stage Classification and Disease-Specific Survival: Corroboration of the Newly Proposed TNM Staging System

Most patients were stage 0 (T0N0M0) (n = 109, 50.2%), followed by stage I (T1N0M0) (n = 70, 32.3%), stage II (T2N0M0) (n = 9, 4.1%), stage IIIa (TanyN1M0) (n = 7, 3.2%), stage IIIb (TanyN2M0) (n = 16, 7.4%), and stage IV (TanyNanyM1) (n = 6, 2.8%). The 5-year DSS of each stage was 100.0%, 97.4%, 42.9%, 80.0%, 23.3%, and 0.0%, respectively. The prognosis between stages I and II, classified by tumor thickness of invasive EMPD without remote regional lymph node or

distant metastasis, showed a significant difference ($p < 0.0001$). All patients with distant metastasis (stage IV) died within 5 years, and the survival rate was significantly different from that of all other stages (0 vs. IV, $p < 0.0001$; I vs. IV, $p < 0.0001$; II vs. IV, $p = 0.0027$; IIIa vs. IV, $p = 0.0003$; IIIb vs. IV, $p < 0.0001$). No significant difference was found between stages IIIa and IIIb, classified by the number of lymph node metastases ($p = 0.066$). There were significant differences in survival between stages I and IIIa ($p = 0.034$) and stages I and IIIb ($p < 0.0001$). The survival rate of stages II was opposite that of patients in stage IIIa, although there was no significant difference ($p = 0.47$). The Kaplan-Meier DSS curves of patients stratified by TNM stage are shown in **Figure 1**.

Characteristics of Patients Treated With Curative Surgery

Next, the data of 198 patients treated with curative surgery were analyzed to assess the associations between mucosal boundary area involvement and prognostic factors. Patients with distant metastasis (stage IV) were excluded from this analysis. There were 65 patients (32.8%) with boundary area involvement and 133 (67.2%) without.

The demographic and clinicopathological data of each group are listed in **Table 2**. Patients with involvement of boundary areas were mostly female ($p < 0.0001$), and the location was most frequently the perianal area ($p = 0.0018$). Tumor size showed no significant difference between the two groups ($p = 0.29$). Histopathologically, patients with boundary area involvement

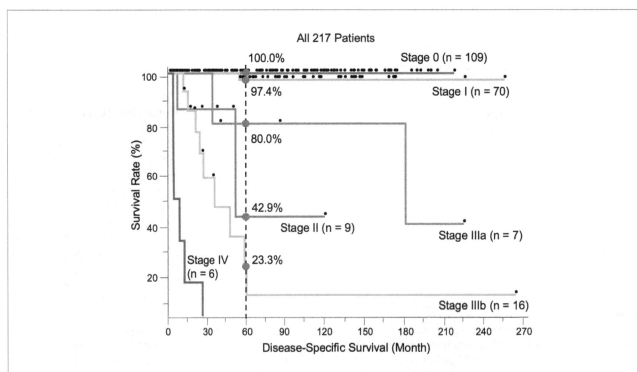

FIGURE 1 | Kaplan-Meier disease-specific survival curves of all 217 patients stratified by TNM stage. The 5-year survival was 100.0% (Stage 0, n = 109), 97.4% (I, n = 70), 42.9% (II, n = 9), 80.0% (IIIa, n = 7), 23.3% (IIIb, n = 16), and 0.0% (IV, n = 6). The log-rank test showed the results of survival as follows: 0 vs I, p = 0.17; I vs II, p < 0.0001; I vs IIIa, p = 0.034; I vs IIIb, p < 0.0001; II vs IIIa, p = 0.47; II vs IIIb, p = 0.24; IIIa vs IIIb, p = 0.066; 0 vs. IV, p < 0.0001; I vs. IV, p < 0.0001; II vs. IV, p = 0.0027; IIIa vs. IV, p = 0.0003; IIIb vs. IV, p < 0.0001.

TABLE 2 | Demographics and clinical data of the 198 patients treated with curative surgery.

Parameter	Involvement of mucosal boundary areas		P-value*
	Present (n = 65)	Absent (n = 133)	
Sex			
Male	16 (24.6%)	105 (78.9%)	**<0.0001**
Female	49 (75.4%)	28 (21.1%)	
Age (year)			
Mean ± SD	69.7 ± 10.3	73.5 ± 9.12	**0.0091**
Tumor site			
Perianal area	12 (18.5%)	5 (3.8%)	**0.0018**
Other areas	53 (81.5%)	128 (96.2%)	
Primary lesion size (cm²)			
<25	26 (40.0%)	64 (48.1%)	0.29
≥25	39 (60.0%)	69 (51.9%)	
Tumor thickness (mm)			
In situ	30 (46.2%)	72 (54.1%)	0.12†
≤4	26 (40.0%)	54 (40.6%)	
>4	9 (13.8%)	7 (5.3%)	
Lymphovascular invasion			
Present	7 (10.8%)	4 (3.0%)	**0.042**
Absent	58 (89.2%)	129 (97.0%)	
Regional LN metastasis			
Present	13 (20.0%)	4 (3.0%)	**0.0002**
Absent	52 (80.0%)	129 (97.0%)	
Number of regional LN metastases			
1	4 (30.8%)	3 (75.0%)	0.25
2 or more	9 (69.2%)	1 (25.0%)	
TNM stage			
0	30 (46.2%)	72 (54.1%)	**0.0014**
I	20 (30.8%)	50 (37.6%)	
II	2 (3.1%)	7 (5.3%)	
IIIa	4 (6.2%)	3 (2.3%)	
IIIb	9 (13.9%)	1 (0.8%)	
Local recurrence			
Present	12 (18.5%)	0 (0.0%)	**<0.0001**
Absent	53 (71.5%)	133 (100.0%)	
Follow-up period (month)			
Mean ± SD	82.8 ± 64.0	83.7 ± 57.4	0.73
Median (range)	58.2 (7.2–256.5)	78.9 (2.0–264.7)	

Significant values are shown in boldface.
*Mann-Whitney U tests were used for continuous variables, and χ^2 or Fisher's exact tests were used for categorical variables.
†In situ vs. ≤ 4 mm, p = 0.65; in situ vs. > 4 mm, p = 0.040; ≤ 4 mm vs. > 4 mm, p = 0.077.
SD, standard deviation; LN, lymph node; TNM, tumor, node, metastasis.

tended to have thicker tumors in invasive EMPD (*in situ* vs. ≤ 4 mm, $p = 0.65$; *in situ* vs. > 4 mm, $p = 0.040$; ≤ 4 mm vs. > 4 mm, $p = 0.077$). Lymphovascular invasion was more frequently observed in patients with involvement of boundary areas ($p = 0.042$). Patients with boundary area involvement had more advanced primary tumors. The rate of regional lymph node metastasis in patients with boundary area involvement was statistically higher than in patients without boundary area involvement ($p = 0.0002$). In each group, patients were classified in accordance with the TNM staging system. Patients with involvement of boundary areas tended to be classified with advanced TNM stages.

Twelve patients had local recurrence during the follow-up period, and all of them had involvement of boundary areas. They underwent wide surgical excision (n = 9), radiation therapy (n = 1), or treatment with topical imiquimod cream (n = 2). The details of the patients with local recurrence are shown in **Supplementary Table 2**.

Initial Treatment of Patients Treated With Curative Surgery: Boundary Area Involvement as a Risk Factor for Incomplete Excision

The initial treatment patterns of these 198 patients, who were divided into two groups based on boundary area involvement, are summarized in **Table 3**.

For primary tumor excision, the distance of the surgical margin showed no significant difference in the two groups (mean: 1.56 cm vs. 1.72 cm, $p = 0.18$). Surgical margins were positive in 42 of the 198 patients (21.2%). The positive site was predominantly at the mucosal side (n = 30), followed by the skin side (n = 8), and then both the mucosal and skin sides (n = 4). The positive surgical margin rate was significantly higher in patients with boundary area involvement than in patients without boundary area involvement ($p < 0.0001$). Additional excision was performed in seven of the 42 patients with positive surgical margins (six patients with additional mucosal excision and one with additional skin excision), and all seven of these patients were confirmed to have negative surgical margins. Only three patients underwent colostomy or urinary diversion. There was no significant difference in the rate of SLNB performed ($p = 0.41$). However, the rate of metastasis in SLNB cases was significantly different between the two groups ($p = 0.0048$). The rate of metastasis in lymphadenopathy cases was not significantly different between the two groups ($p = 0.12$). CLND was performed in 13 patients with boundary area involvement and four patients without boundary area involvement ($p = 0.0002$). Curative excision was completed in 37 patients with boundary area involvement (56.9%) and 126 patients without boundary area involvement (94.7%) ($p < 0.0001$). All incomplete excisions were for primary tumors. There were no patients with incomplete removal of regional lymph nodes. Five patients among 35 patients with incomplete excision (14.3%) experienced local recurrence (**Supplementary Table 2**).

Factors Associated With Disease-Specific Survival of Patients Treated With Curative Surgery: Negative Impact of Boundary Area Involvement on Long-Term Survival

We evaluated the possible clinical and histopathological factors associated with DSS in the 198 patients treated with curative surgery by using a multivariate Cox proportional hazards regression model. The following factors were included as explanatory variables: sex, age, tumor site, tumor thickness, boundary area involvement, complete excision, and regional lymph node metastasis. The results are listed in **Table 4**. Univariate analysis results revealed that tumor thickness > 4 mm, boundary area involvement, and regional lymph node metastasis were statistically significant factors for poor survival. Multivariate analysis results showed that tumor thickness > 4 mm (HR: 7.23, $p = 0.0037$), boundary area involvement

TABLE 3 | Initial treatment of the 198 patients treated with curative surgery.

Treatment		Involvement of boundary areas		P-value*
		Present (n = 65)	Absent (n = 133)	
For primary lesions	Surgical margin (cm)			
	Mean ± SD	1.56 ± 0.84	1.72 ± 0.84	0.18
	Surgical margin status			
	Positive	34 (52.3%)	8 (6.0%)	**<0.0001**
	Negative	31 (47.7%)	125 (94.0%)	
	Additional excision			
	Done	6 (17.7%)	1 (12.5%)	1.00
	Not done	28 (82.3%)	7 (87.5%)	
For regional LNs	SLNB			
	Done	8 (12.3%)	24 (18.1%)	0.41
	Not done	57 (87.7%)	109 (81.9%)	
	SLNB			
	LN metastasis present	5 (62.5%)	2 (8.3%)	**0.0048**
	No LN metastasis	3 (37.5%)	22 (91.7%)	
	Biopsy of lymphadenopathy			
	Done	8 (12.3%)	8 (6.0%)	0.16
	Not done	57 (87.7%)	125 (94.0%)	
	Biopsy of lymphadenopathy			
	LN metastasis present	5 (62.5%)	1 (12.5%)	0.12
	No LN metastasis	3 (37.5%)	7 (87.5%)	
	CLND			
	Done	13 (20.0%)	4 (3.0%)	**0.0002**
	Not done	52 (80.0%)	129 (97.0%)	
Overall	Complete excision†			
	Complete	37 (56.9%)	126 (94.7%)	**<0.0001**
	Incomplete	28 (43.1%)	7 (5.3%)	
Adjuvant therapy	Chemotherapy	0 (0.0%)	1 (0.75%)	1.00
	Radiation therapy	1 (0.75%)	0 (0.0%)	1.00

Significant values are shown in boldface.
*Mann-Whitney U tests were used for continuous variables, and Fisher's exact tests were used for categorical variables.
†Complete excision was defined as complete removal of the primary tumor with histopathologically negative margins and complete dissection of regional lymph nodes (if lymph node metastases were present).
SD, standard deviation; LN, lymph node; SLNB, sentinel lymph node biopsy; CLND, completion lymph node dissection.

(HR: 11.87, p = 0.027), and regional lymph node metastasis (HR: 27.91, p = 0.031) were also statistically independent factors associated with DSS. Incomplete excision was not significantly correlated with survival (HR: 1.05, p = 0.96). The Kaplan-Meier curves of patients stratified by boundary area involvement and achievement of complete excision are shown in **Figures 2**, **3**.

As an additional analysis, these possible prognostic factors were evaluated in the 65 patients with boundary area involvement by using a multivariate analysis for DSS. The results revealed that incomplete excision was not significantly correlated with survival (HR: 3.11, p = 0.34). The detailed data are available in **Supplementary Table 3**.

DISCUSSION

Complete surgical tumor removal is the treatment of choice for resectable EMPD. Due to the slow-growing nature of this kind of tumor, nearly 90% of the patients at our hospital show no lymph node or distant metastasis. Treatment strategies for primary lesions are therefore key for curing this disease in these patients. EMPD lesions are most likely to arise in the anogenital area, sometimes extending toward visceral organs *via* boundary areas (anal canal, external urethral meatus, vaginal introitus). When tumors involve these boundary areas, surgeons are forced to choose whether radical surgical excision with extensive reconstruction should be performed or whether less invasive surgery should be performed to preserve defecation and urination functions. This choice is challenging, as most EMPD patients are elderly, and radical surgery impairs patients' quality of life. The latter choice is often chosen in our institute after deep discussion with patients and their families, unless the tumors are invasive (with nodule formation, etc.) in boundary areas. Reconstruction of skin/mucosal defects is typically accomplished by using simple sutures or split-skin grafting. One of the aims of this study was to evaluate the reasonability of this kind of surgery. We retrospectively summarized 23 years of experience treating 217 patients with EMPD and assessed their outcomes. This is one of the largest studies conducted at a single institute, and we identified several important findings.

We showed for the first time that patients with EMPD lesions in boundary areas had significantly shortened DSS compared to other patients (p < 0.0001, **Figure 2**). This was corroborated by the results of multivariate analyses, which were adjusted by some known prognostic factors (HR: 11.87, 95% CI: 1.32–106.73, p = 0.027). Representative prognostic factors of primary tumors

TABLE 4 | Multivariate Cox proportional hazard analyses for disease-specific survival.

Variable	Univariate analysis			Multivariate analysis		
	HR	95% CI	P-value	HR	95% CI	P-value
Sex, male	1.78	0.47-6.72	0.39	0.26	0.012-5.42	0.38
Age (year)†	1.01	0.92-1.05	0.49	1.05	0.97-1.14	0.24
Perianal lesion	1.11	0.14-8.72	0.92	1.53	0.13-16.90	0.73
Tumor thickness > 4 mm	30.56	8.73-109.94	**<0.0001**	7.23	1.13-46.19	**0.037**
Boundary area involvement	21.13	2.70-165.60	**0.0037**	11.87	1.32-106.73	**0.027**
Incomplete excision	0.94	0.20-4.38	0.94	1.05	0.16-6.74	0.96
Regional LN metastasis	36.60	9.51-140.92	**<0.0001**	27.91	1.35-576.63	**0.031**

Significant values are shown in boldface.
†Continuous variable.
HR, hazard ratio; CI, confidence interval; LN, lymph node.

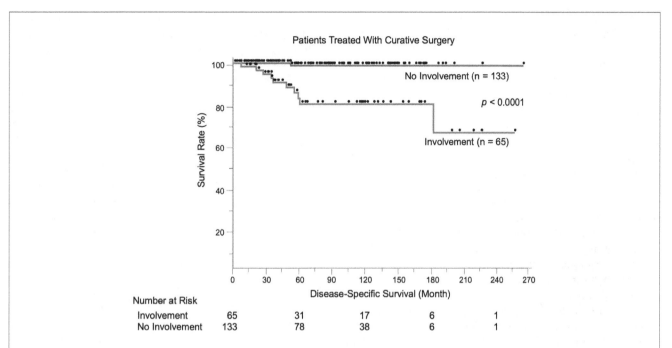

FIGURE 2 | Kaplan-Meier disease-specific survival curves of the 198 patients treated with curative surgery stratified by boundary area involvement. Patients with EMPD lesions in boundary areas had significantly shortened their survival ($p < 0.0001$). The number at risk is also shown.

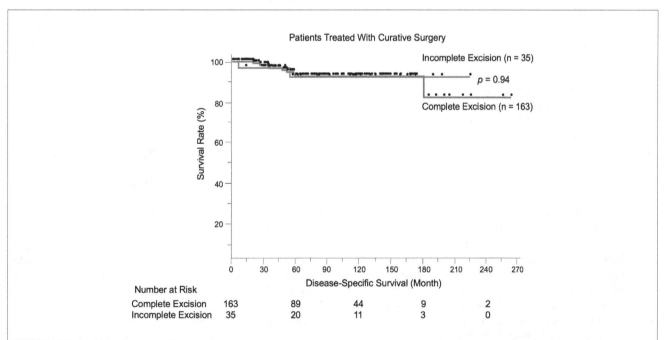

FIGURE 3 | Kaplan-Meier disease-specific survival curves of the 198 patients treated with curative surgery stratified by achievement of complete excision. Incomplete excision was not correlated with worse survival compared to complete excision ($p = 0.94$). The number at risk is also shown.

include nodule formation (14, 25), tumor thickness (8, 13, 14), level of tumor invasion (15–18), lymphovascular invasion (8, 17, 19), perianal location (13, 20–22), and vaginal location (26). Human epidermal growth factor receptor 2/neu (27–29) and nectin cell adhesion molecule 4 (30) expression are other factors associated with tumor recurrence and DSS, respectively. We previously evaluated the efficacy of mapping biopsy and surgical treatment of EMPD, and we found a high tumor-positive rate of surgical margins in EMPD lesions with mucosal boundary area involvement (19/36, 52.8%) (23). This high positive rate may be due to difficulty both in delineating tumor borders and in setting sufficient surgical margins in these areas. In the current study, the positive rate was similar to our previous one (34/65, 52.3%). Some factors were associated with the presence of boundary area involvement. Female patients more frequently had boundary and perianal lesions compared to male patients (data not shown) since female anogenital areas are close to boundary areas. Other factors included thicker tumors, the presence of lymphovascular invasion, and lymph node metastasis, suggesting that advanced EMPD lesions are likely to extend to boundary areas. In this study, 12 patients experienced local recurrence of primary lesions, and all had boundary lesions.

Of note, among the 198 patients treated with curative surgery, incomplete excision of primary tumors was not correlated with worse DSS compared to complete removal ($p = 0.94$). Similarly, when analyzing the patients with boundary area involvement (n = 65), incomplete excision was not a poor prognostic factor ($p = 0.34$ per Cox multivariate analysis). Furthermore, only five patients among 35 patients with incomplete excision (14.3%) experienced local recurrence. Most of the patients with the disease were elderly (mean age: 72.9 years), and among the 53 patients who died during the follow-up period, EMPD was the direct cause only in 20 patients (37.7%); the other 33 patients (62.3%) died of other causes. These results raise an important question: is it always necessary to pursue negative margins in primary EMPD? Previous studies have reported no correlation between positive surgical margins and local recurrence in vulvar EMPD (9–11, 31, 32). Nasioudis et al. (6) conducted a large database study and reported that the presence of positive surgical margins was not associated with overall survival. Correlations between surgical margins and patient survival have been controversial, and the current study offered new insights into this issue. Furthermore, some radical surgical procedures (proctectomy, urethrectomy, total cystectomy) are accompanied by simultaneous creation of colostomy and urinary diversions, which can lead to troublesome complications (33–36). Formijne Jonkers et al. (37) reported that 82% of patients who underwent creation of an intestinal stoma experienced one or more stoma-related complications within 1 year. Radical surgeries with creation of colostomy or urinary diversions deteriorate patients' organ functions, as well as patients' quality of life (33, 38–40). In our cohort, only three of 75 patients (4.0%) with boundary area involvement underwent colostomy or urinary diversion. Whereas lesions in boundary areas had increased risks of incomplete excision and local recurrence, these lesions were also associated with advanced tumor status (thicker tumors, frequent lymphovascular invasion, and lymph node metastasis). Most localized EMPD lesions were unaggressive, with high 5-year survival rates (100% in stage 0 and 97.4% in stage I). Collectively, the less invasive approach we performed (preserving anorectal and urinary functions) may be a reasonable treatment choice for patients with EMPD.

Another interesting finding was that patient survival in this study fit well with the newly proposed TNM staging system (8). Although TNM staging is crucial in cancer treatment, no widely accepted staging system specific for EMPD has been established due to the rarity of the disease. In this study, we classified patients in accordance with the newly proposed, EMPD-specific TNM staging system (8) and assessed its validity. The T category (classified by tumor thickness and lymphovascular invasion), N category (classified by lymph node metastasis), and M category (classified by distant metastasis) were significantly associated with worse survival, and their survival curves were consistent with previous reports. Interestingly, the survival of patients in stage II (localized invasive tumors) was worse than that of patients in stage IIIa (one regional lymph node metastasis), although the difference did not reach statistical significance ($p = 0.47$). These inverse survival results were also observed in the original report of the TNM staging system for EMPD (8). The exact mechanisms of this inversion is still unclear but this is also noted in malignant melanoma (41, 42). EMPD and melanoma exhibit a similar invasion process (first arising in the epidermis, horizontally spreading, and later invading vertically into the dermis with the destruction of basal membrane). One possible explanation is the hematogenous metastasis, however, more data is required to test this hypothesis.

CONCLUSION

We retrospectively reviewed 23 years of data of 217 patients with EMPD. Most patients (n = 198, 91.2%) were candidates for curative surgery. Tumor involvement in boundary areas was a major risk factor for incomplete excision, local recurrence, and poor survival outcomes. However, incomplete removal of primary tumors was not significantly associated with poor prognosis. A less invasive surgical approach for preserving anogenital and urinary functions may be acceptable as the first-line treatment for resectable EMPD.

AUTHOR CONTRIBUTIONS

HH, TI, and YK-I participated in manuscript preparation. TI designed the methodology. HH participated in data analysis and figure preparation. HH and YK-I collected the detailed information of the patients. TI and MF reviewed and revised the manuscript. All authors contributed to the article and approved the submitted version.

ACKNOWLEDGMENTS

The authors thank all patients for their participation, as well as the members of our laboratory for their helpful advice.

REFERENCES

1. Kanitakis J. Mammary and extramammary Paget's disease. *J Eur Acad Dermatol Venereol* (2007) 21:581–90. doi: 10.1111/j.1468-3083.2007.02154.x

2. Shepherd V, Davidson EJ, Davies-Humphreys J. Extramammary Paget's disease. *BJOG* (2005) 112:273–9. doi: 10.1111/j.1471-0528.2004.00438.x

3. Simonds RM, Segal RJ, Sharma A. Extramammary Paget's disease: a review of the literature. *Int J Dermatol* (2019) 58:871–9. doi: 10.1111/ijd.14328

4. Ito T, Kaku-Ito Y, Furue M. The diagnosis and management of extramammary Paget's disease. *Expert Rev Anticancer Ther* (2018) 18:543–53. doi: 10.1080/14737140.2018.1457955

5. Funaro D, Krasny M, Lam C, Desy D, Sauthier P, Bouard D. Extramammary Paget disease: epidemiology and association to cancer in a Quebec-based population. *J Low Genit Tract Dis* (2013) 17:167–74. doi: 10.1097/LGT.0b013e31825f4b4f

6. Nasioudis D, Bhadra M, Ko EM. Extramammary Paget disease of the vulva: management and prognosis. *Gynecol Oncol* (2020) 157:146–50. doi: 10.1016/j.ygyno.2019.11.009

7. Morris CR, Hurst EA. Extramammary Paget's disease: a review of the literature – Part I: history, epidemiology, pathogenesis, presentation, histopathology, and diagnostic work-up. *Dermatol Surg* (2020) 46:151–8. doi: 10.1097/DSS.0000000000002064

8. Ohara K, Fujisawa Y, Yoshino K, Kiyohara Y, Kadono T, Murata Y, et al. A proposal for a TNM staging system for extramammary Paget disease: retrospective analysis of 301 patients with invasive primary tumors. *J Dermatol Sci* (2016) 83:234–9. doi: 10.1016/j.jdermsci.2016.06.004

9. Cai Y, Sheng W, Xiang L, Wu X, Yang H. Primary extramammary Paget's disease of the vulva: the clinicopathological features and treatment outcomes in a series of 43 patients. *Gynecol Oncol* (2013) 129:412–6. doi: 10.1016/j.ygyno.2013.02.029

10. Black D, Tornos C, Soslow RA, Awtrey CS, Barakat RR, Chi DS. The outcomes of patients with positive margins after excision for intraepithelial Paget's disease of the vulva. *Gynecol Oncol* (2007) 104:547–50. doi: 10.1016/j.ygyno.2006.09.017

11. Nitecki R, Davis M, Watkins JC, Wu YE, Vitonis AF, Muto MG, et al. Extramammary Paget disease of the vulva: a case series examining treatment, recurrence, and malignant transformation. *Int J Gynecol Cancer* (2018) 28:632–8. doi: 10.1097/IGC.0000000000001189

12. Delport ES. Extramammary Paget's disease of the vulva: an annotated review of the current literature. *Australas J Dermatol* (2013) 54:9–21. doi: 10.1111/j.1440-0960.2012.00898.x

13. Shiomi T, Noguchi T, Nakayama H, Yoshida Y, Yamamoto O, Hayashi N, et al. Clinicopathological study of invasive extramammary Paget's disease: subgroup comparison according to invasion depth. *J Eur Acad Dermatol Venereol* (2013) 27:589–92. doi: 10.1111/j.1468-3083.2012.04489.x

14. Ito T, Kaku Y, Nagae K, Nakano-Nakamura M, Nakahara T, Oda Y, et al. Tumor thickness as a prognostic factor in extramammary Paget's disease. *J Dermatol* (2015) 42:269–75. doi: 10.1111/1346-8138.12764

15. Tsutsuimida A, Yamamoto Y, Minakawa H, Yoshida T, Kokubu I, Sugihara T. Indications for lymph node dissection in the treatment of extramammary Paget's disease. *Dermatol Surg* (2003) 29:21–4. doi: 10.1046/j.1524-4725.2003.29001.x

16. Hatta N, Yamada M, Hirano T, Fujimoto A, Morita R. Extramammary Paget's disease: treatment, prognostic factors and outcome in 76 patients. *Br J Dermatol* (2008) 158:313–8. doi: 10.1111/j.1365-2133.2007.08314.x

17. Dai B, Kong YY, Chang K, Qu YY, Ye DW, Zhang SL, et al. Primary invasive carcinoma associated with penoscrotal extramammary Paget's disease: a clinicopathological analysis of 56 cases. *BJU Int* (2015) 115:153–60. doi: 10.1111/bju.12776

18. Van der Linden M, Oonk MHM, van Doorn HC, Bulten J, van Dorst EBL, Fons G, et al. Vulvar Paget disease: a national retrospective cohort study. *J Am Acad Dermatol* (2018) 81:956–62. doi: 10.1016/j.jaad.2018.11.016

19. Yoshino K, Yamazaki N, Yamamoto A, Namikawa K, Abe M, Yoshida H. On the TNM classification of extramammary Paget's disease. *Jpn J Dermatol* (2006) 116:1313–8.

20. Herrel LA, Weiss AD, Goodman M, Johnson TV, Osunkoya AO, Delman KA, et al. Extramammary Paget's disease in males: survival outcomes in 495 patients. *Ann Surg Oncol* (2015) 22:1625–30. doi: 10.1245/s10434-014-4139-y

21. Weng S, Zhu N, Li D, Chen Y, Tan Y, Chen J, et al. Clinical characteristics, treatment, and prognostic factors of patients with primary extramammary Paget's disease (EMPD): a retrospective analysis of 44 patients from a single center and an analysis of data from the Surveillance, Epidemiology, and End Results (SEER) database. *Front Oncol* (2020) 10:1114:1114. doi: 10.3389/fonc.2020.01114

22. Karam A, Dorigo O. Treatment outcomes in a large cohort of patients with invasive extramammary Paget's disease. *Gynecol Oncol* (2012) 125:346–51. doi: 10.1016/j.ygyno.2012.01.032

23. Kaku-Ito Y, Ito T, Tsuji G, Nakahara T, Hagihara A, Furue M, et al. Evaluation of mapping biopsies for extramammary Paget disease: a retrospective study. *J Am Acad Dermatol* (2018) 78:1171–7. doi: 10.1016/j.jaad.2017.12.040

24. Gershenwald JE, Scolyer RA. Melanoma staging: American Joint Committee on Cancer (AJCC) 8th edition and beyond. *Ann Surg Oncol* (2018) 25:2105–10. doi: 10.1245/s10434-018-6513-7

25. Ito Y, Igawa S, Ohishi Y, Uehara J, Yamamoto AI, Iizuka H. Prognostic indicators in 35 patients with extramammary Paget's disease. *Dermatol Surg* (2012) 38:1938–44. doi: 10.1111/j.1524-4725.2012.02584.x

26. Yao H, Xie M, Fu S, Guo J, Peng Y, Cai Z, et al. Survival analysis of patients with invasive extramammary Paget disease: implications of anatomic sites. *BMC Cancer* (2018) 18:403. doi: 10.1186/s12885-018-4257-1

27. Kang Z, Zhang Q, Zhang Q, Li X, Hu T, Xu X, et al. Clinical and pathological characteristics of extramammary Paget's disease: report of 246 Chinese male patients. *Int J Clin Exp Pathol* (2015) 8:13233–40.

28. Fukuda K, Funakoshi T. Metastatic extramammary Paget's disease: pathogenesis and novel therapeutic approach. *Front Oncol* (2018) 8:38:38. doi: 10.3389/fonc.2018.00038

29. Hu J, Ge W, Mao S, Ding Q, Hu M, Jiang H, et al. First-time versus recurrent penoscrotal extramammary Paget's disease: clinicopathological characteristics and risk factors in 164 Chinese male patients. *Indian J Dermatol Venereol Leprol* (2020) 86:134–40. doi: 10.4103/ijdvl.IJDVL_382_18

30. Murata M, Ito T, Tanaka Y, Kaku-Ito Y, Furue M. NECTIN4 expression in extramammary Paget's disease: implication of a new therapeutic target. *Int J Mol Sci* (2020) 21:5891. doi: 10.3390/ijms21165891

31. Parker LP, Parker JR, Bodurka-Bevers D, Deavers M, Bevers MW, Shen-Gunther J, et al. Paget's disease of the vulva: pathology, pattern of involvement, and prognosis. *Gynecol Oncol* (2000) 77:183–9. doi: 10.1006/gyno.2000.5741

32. Sopracordevole F, Di Giuseppe J, De Piero G, Canzonieri V, Buttignol M, Giorda G, et al. Surgical treatment of Paget disease of the vulva: prognostic significance of stromal invasion and surgical margin status. *J Low Genit Tract Dis* (2016) 20:184–8. doi: 10.1097/LGT.0000000000000191

33. Nastro P, Knowles CH, McGrath A, Heyman B, Porrett TR, Lunniss PJ. Complications of intestinal stomas. *Br J Surg* (2010) 97:1885–9. doi: 10.1002/bjs.7259

34. Hemelrijck M, Thorstenson A, Smith P, Adolfsson J, Akre O. Risk of in-hospital complications after radical cystectomy for urinary bladder carcinoma: population-based follow-up study of 7608 patients. *BJU Int* (2013) 112:1113–20. doi: 10.1111/bju.12239

35. Steinhagen E, Colwell J, Cannon LM. Intestinal stomas–postoperative stoma care and peristomal skin complications. *Clin Colon Rectal Surg* (2017) 30:184–92. doi: 10.1055/s-0037-1598159

36. Morris CR, Hurst EA. Extramammary Paget's disease: a review of the literature Part II: treatment and prognosis. *Dermatol Surg* (2020) 46:305–11. doi: 10.1097/DSS.0000000000002240

37. Formijne Jonkers HA, Draaisma WA, Roskott AM, van Overbeeke AJ, Broeders IA, Consten EC. Early complications after stoma formation: a prospective cohort study in 100 patients with 1-year follow-up. *Int J Color Dis* (2012) 27:1095–9. doi: 10.1007/s00384-012-1413-y

38. Nasvall P, Dahlstrand U, Lowenmark T, Rutegård J, Gunnarsson U, Strigård K. Quality of life in patients with a permanent stoma after rectal cancer surgery. *Qual Life Res* (2017) 26:55–64. doi: 10.1007/s11136-016-1367-6

39. Kretschmer A, Grimm T, Buchner A, Stief CG, Karl A. Prognostic features for quality of life after radical cystectomy and orthotopic neobladder. *Int Braz J Urol* (2016) 42:1109–20. doi: 10.1590/s1677-5538.ibju.2015.0491

40. Gunther V, Malchow B, Schubert M, Andresen L, Jochens A, Jonat W, et al. Impact of radical operative treatment on the quality of life in women with vulvar cancer - a retrospective study. *Eur J Surg Oncol* (2014) 40:875–82. doi: 10.1016/j.ejso.2014.03.027

41. Kim CC, Najita JS, Tan S, Varada S, Tong LX, Lee HD, et al. Factors associated with worse outcome for patients with AJCC stage IIC relative to stage IIIA melanoma. *J Clin Oncol* (2015) 33:9078–8. doi: 10.1200/jco.2015.33.15_suppl.9078

42. Yushak M, Mehnert J, Luke J, Poklepovic A. Approaches to high-risk resected stage II and III melanoma. *Am Soc Clin Oncol Annu Meeting* (2019) 39:e207–11. doi: 10.1200/EDBK_239283

7

Usefulness of High-Frequency Ultrasonography in the Diagnosis of Melanoma

Maria Paola Belfiore[1], Alfonso Reginelli[1*], Anna Russo[1], Gaetano Maria Russo[1],
Maria Paola Rocco[1], Elvira Moscarella[2], Marilina Ferrante[1], Antonello Sica[1],
Roberto Grassi[1,3] and Salvatore Cappabianca[1]

[1] Department of Precision Medicine, University of Campania Luigi Vanvitelli, Naples, Italy, [2] Dermatology Unit, University of Campania Luigi Vanvitelli, Naples, Italy, [3] Italian Society of Medical Radiology (SIRM) Foundation, Milan, Italy

*Correspondence:
Alfonso Reginelli
alfonsoreginelli@hotmail.com

High-frequency equipment is characterized by ultrasound probes with frequencies of over 10 MHz. At higher frequencies, the wavelength decreases, which determines a lower penetration of the ultrasound beam so as to offer a better evaluation of the surface structures. This explains the growing interest in ultrasound in dermatology. This review examines the state of the art of high-frequency ultrasound (HFUS) in the assessment of skin cancer to ensure the high clinical approach and provide the best standard of evidence on which to base clinical and policy decisions.

Keywords: Melanoma, high frequency ultrasound, oncology research and diseases, MDT, Dermatology

INTRODUCTION

Cutaneous melanoma (CM) has a high incidence rate, even among young people; it has steadily increased over the last several decades (1, 2). Moreover this incidence is 1.5 times higher in males (3). However, this data is related to the age of onset; it has been seen that melanoma affects young women and older men. The main risky factors implicated in melanoma development are exposure to ultraviolet (UV) for their genotoxic effect, the number of melanocytic nevi, familiar history, and genetic susceptibility (3). It has been noted that patients with a previous history of melanoma have a 1% to 8% risk of developing other primary melanomas (4). These numbers highlight the health and socio-economic implications of this skin cancer. Melanoma is related to a poor prognosis in the general population. The main important prognostic factors for survival are the Breslow's index and the presence of ulceration. In the eighth edition, the AJCC melanoma expert panel described the impact of the tumor thickness subcategorizing T1 melanomas (5). The main prognostic factors for survival are still primary tumor (Breslow) thickness and ulceration. They are also useful to define T-category strata in cutaneous melanoma. As in prior editions, also in the eighth edition, tumor thickness has to be measured to the nearest 0.1 mm, not 0.01 mm. In this edition, melanoma thickness threshold of 1.0, 2.0, and 4.0 mm continues to define the T category. Consequently, those tumors that measure from 0.95 to 1.04 would be rounded to 1.0 mm. While in the seventh edition, a subset of these melanomas measuring 1.01 to 1.04 would have been staged as T2 (a: w/o ulceration, b: with ulceration). The clinical implication, if any, of this small group of patients who are mentioned in the eighth edition, has not yet been formally explored. Previous studies have detected a clinically significant treshold in the region of 0.7 to 0.8 mm in patients with T1 melanoma. In the eighth edition AJCC the analysis of the T1 melanoma patient cohort, multivariable analysis of factors that predict melanoma-specific survival (MSS) [i.e. tumor thickness, ulceration, mitotic rate as a dichotomous variable (<1 mitosis/mm^2 vs ≥1 mitosis/mm^2)] revealed that tumor thickness dichotomized as < 0.8 mm and 0.8 to 1.0 mm and ulceration could predict MSS more efficiently than mitotic rate (as a dichotomous variable).

The subcategorization of T1 melanomas (0.8 threshold) is important for the role of Sentinel Lymph nodes biopsy(SNLB) considering that SLN metastases are very infrequent (< 5%) in patients whose melanoma is < 0.8 mm in thickness and nonulcerated (i.e., AJCC eighth edition T1a) but it occurs in approximately 5% to 12% of patients with primary melanomas 0.8 to 1.0 mm in thickness. The SLN biopsy can be performed in the patients with a primary tumor thickness 0.8–1.0 mm and also in patients with thinner ulcerated tumors (i.e., all patients with AJCC eighth edition T1b melanomas). The SLN biopsy had to be performed for patients with T2 and thicker melanomas, and when performed in patients with a T1 melanoma, the status of the SLN was used (5).

The thickness of the melanoma also determines an increased risk of lymph node involvement. Patients with melanoma spread to the nearby lymph nodes have a survival rates at 5 years of 65% (6). For all patients with primary melanoma with Breslow's index > 0.8 mm is indicated the Sentinel lymph nodes. This procedure allows the detection of metastatic involvement of the lymph nodes and the detection of nodal disease with no clinical or radiographic evidence. The outcome of SNLB may change future therapeutic management, including the choice of performing a complete lymph nodes dissection, or an adjuvant therapy, but also set up different program of clinical and imaging follow-up. For whole-body staging are used advanced imaging techniques, such as computed tomography (CT), magnetic resonance (MR), and positron emission tomography-CT (PET-CT) (7). There is no single consensus regarding surveillance imaging in melanoma patients, in fact, according to National Comprehensive Cancer Network (NCCN), the CT or PET scan is recommended every 3 to 12 months for patients with stage IIB-IV asymptomatic melanoma. While, The European Society of Medical Oncology recommends only physical examination

every three months (8). However, ultrasound is the first diagnostic approach used to monitor regional lymph node basins for recurrence. It has been demonstrated that ultrasound has the highest sensitivity and specificity, 96% and 99% respectively, for lymph node surveillance (9–11), as well as for the evaluation of nodal disease. Thanks to the use of high-frequency probes, it has proved useful for the determination of ultrasound Breslow index, which means evaluating the depth of tumor invasion (**Figure 1**). Moreover, Color Doppler is an additional tool that can improve diagnostic accuracy through the identification of intra-tumor vessels and characterizations of their distributions (12) (**Figure 2**).

High accurate pre-treatment evaluation of the melanoma is useful tool for taking a correct therapeutic approach and improving the survival rate and follow-up (13).

The HFUS, and even more the ultra-HFUS, provide important information, previously obtained only thanks to biopsy samples.

Further information can be obtained thanks to the use of strain elastography (SE). This technique estimates the tissues elasticity according to assumption that tissues affected by tumor invasion are less deformable than normal tissues (14). An evaluation is then achieved by comparing the elasticity of the target lesion with the surrounding tissues. The data obtained on the relative stiffness is converted into a color-coded image that overlaps the two-dimensional images (15–17) (**Figure 3**).

This review examines the state of the art of HFUS in the assessment of melanoma to ensure the best clinical evaluation for the correct therapeutic strategies.

METHODS

Using the Medline, Embase, and ISI web of Science (Science Citation Index Expanded) databases, we searched different articles with these keywords: "melanoma", "melanoma ultrasound", "skin cancer melanoma diagnosis" (18).

The reference lists of all retrieved studies were used as additional sources of pertinent documents (18). We evaluated the title and abstract of these selected articles. If the abstract was eligible, the article was downloaded and read by two of the authors

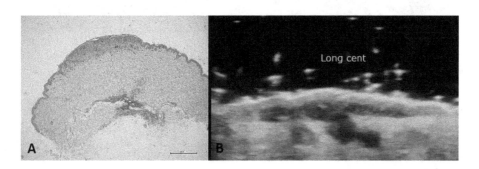

FIGURE 1 | Histological specimen **(A)** and ultrasound examination **(B)** in case of cutaneous melanoma. High-frequency probes are useful for the determination of the ultrasound Breslow index, which means evaluating the depth of tumor invasion.

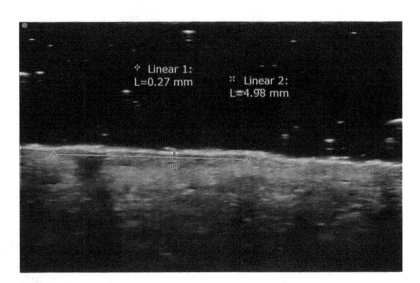

FIGURE 2 | High-frequency transducers allow the determination of ultrasound Breslow index, which means evaluating the depth of tumor invasion. This example shows skin melanoma considered with HFUS (70 MHz).

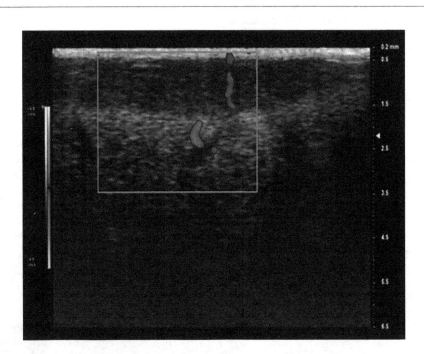

FIGURE 3 | Doppler is an additional tool that can identify intra-tumor vessels and characterize their distribution, improving diagnostic accuracy. On Color Doppler examination, it is possible to see a hypoechoic lesion with an increased vascular signal.

(MB and AR). We included human observational studies published from 1997 to 2020. These studies reported melanoma thickness with ultrasound (US). Furthermore, the ability to identify with HFUS the skip lesions and lymph nodes using 95% confidence intervals or other measures of statistical uncertainty. The studies included in the meta-analysis consider different epidemiological data. Many of these studies relied on specific reference incidence rates based on gender, age, and provided a relative standardized incidence ratio as risky measures (**Table 1**).

We excluded case reports, editorials, non-independent studies, and cohort or case-control studies.

Between two articles with overlapping numbers of melanoma cases, we chose the study with the highest number of total patients (18) (**Figure 4**).

TABLE 1 | List of the main studies related to the use of the HFUS in melanoma.

Author	Year	Frequency Probes	Results
Lassau et al.	1997	20 MHz	Proved that in 12 cases of melanoma the difference between histologic and US measurement was ≤ 0.2 mm.
Harland et al.	2000	20 MHz	US is a non-invasive aid for evaluating the acoustic differences between common pigmented lesions.
Clement et al.	2001	20 MHz	US is useful for differential diagnosis of skin lesions.
Bessoud et al.	2003	20 MHz	Sonographic and histologic measurement of melanoma thickness are strongly related, and US coupled with Color Doppler is a simple and useful tool for pigmented skin lesions management.
Pellacani et al.	2003	20 MHz	US measurements were slightly overestimated compared to the histological size but US has a strength correlation with melanoma thickness.
Rallan et al.	2007	20 MHz	Demonstration of quantitative differences between benign and malign skin lesions.
Gambichler et al.	2007	20 MHz	US measurements were slightly overestimated compared to the histological size but US has a strength correlation with melanoma thickness.
Machet et al.	2009	20 MHz	US measurements were slightly overestimated compared to the histological size but US has a strength correlation with melanoma thickness.
Kaikaris et al.	2011	14 MHz	They found a low US correlation between the Breslow index for thin melanomas (1-2 mm) and a significant correlation for thicker melanomas (> 2 mm).
Solivetti et al.	2014	18MHz or 22MHz (in case of very small and superficial lesions)	All of 52 lesions (in-transit metastases) were detected with HFUS.
Botar et al.	2015	40 MHz	There is not substantial difference between Breslow index and US thickness.
Reginelli et al.	2019	50-70 MHz	There is a favorable agreement between HFUS and Breslow thickness in 7 lesions examined.

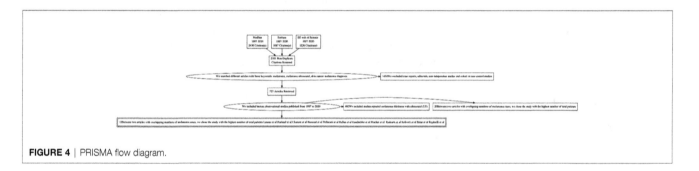

FIGURE 4 | PRISMA flow diagram.

DATA EXTRACTION

Only one co-author (MB) pulled the data into a predefined database.

The following information was considered valid for the analysis: study's year, country, type of melanoma, number of patients, the average age, gender, and lastly, median person years accumulated by patients (18).

DISCUSSION

The application of new imaging techniques has also changed the staging work-up of patients with cutaneous melanoma. Chest and abdominal computed tomography (CT) scanning should be restricted to patients with high-risk melanoma (stage IIIA with a macroscopic lymph node, IIIB, IIIC) and used to evaluate the potential metastatic sites. Magnetic resonance imaging (MRI) of the brain is used in patients with stage IV, optional in stage III and not used in patients with stage I and II disease. The diagnosis of metastases is evaluated by Positron emission tomography (PET)/CT. This technique complements conventional CT/MRI imaging

in the staging of patients who have solitary or oligometastatic disease where surgical resection is most relevant. The lesions suspected of cutaneous melanoma are subjected to dermoscopic examination and if dermatologist deems it necessary, evaluated with excisional biopsy. The histological examination allows to decide whether to perform a further surgical excision and an SNLB; after a correct melanoma staging to decide the subsequent treatment (19, 20). Therefore after the excision of the lesion and histologic evaluation it is mandatory to perform a correct staging to decide whether a further surgical excision should be performed. Ultrasonography is widely used in medicine (21–23). In recent years, US and especially HFUS have become popular among dermatologists. Skin US offers essential information for the diagnosis, therapeutical management, and follow-up of tumoral and non-tumoral cutaneous pathology. It seems that HFUS examination may be useful in pre-operative evaluation of CM, and it may correlate with histology (24). Modern HFUS equipment allows highly accurate visualization of the skin layers and appendages up to histological details (25–28). Probes ranged from 15 to 22 MHz allowed visualization of the epidermis and dermis, including adjacent tissues 1 to 2 cm deep from the basal dermal layer (16).

Moreover ultra-HFUS has ultrasound frequencies higher than 30 MHz, which allow to obtain submillimeter resolution of superficial anatomical structures (29).

The image quality is influenced by the resolution, the key element in measuring the thickness and depth of skin changes (30). The typical ultrasound image of healthy skin is composed of three elements: epidermis, also known as epidermal echo, dermis and subcutaneous tissue (30).

HFUS cannot detect pigments such as melanin but allows a non-invasive evaluation of the primary tumor. It is already able to calculate a Breslow index in a large number of patients with CM (1).

Many literature studies provide US information on primary skin melanoma lesions (30–32). The first US evaluations were performed with 14 MHz probes. The 20-MHz probe was used in five studies, it has an axial resolution that goes from 50 to 80 μm and lateral resolutions to 100 μm in Bessoud et al., 2003, Clement et al., 2001, Lassau et al., 1997 and Rallan et al., 2007 at 300 μm in Harland et al., 2000 (12, 33–36).

As far as these studies are concerned, it remains unclear how the authors obtained the resolution values. Some parameters such as dynamic signal range and signal-to-noise ratio were not reported in the studies, and more often the diagnostic information provided on the lesions appeared to be poorly detailed (37).

Bessoud et al., 2003 evaluated with HFUS 130 pigmented lesions and added a Color Doppler study in 107 lesions. Ultrasound features were linked with anatomo-pathological specimen. Of these lesions: 57% invasive melanoma, 29% benign nevi, 4% basal cell carcinoma (BCC), 4% seborrheic keratosis and other benign lesions (32, 34).

Lassau et al., 1997 evaluated 70 skin lesions, clinically suspected of CM (35) and of BCC (32). HFUS and color Doppler were performed for each lesion, only eight lesions of these were not visualized and therefore excluded. Of these lesions 19 (27%) were invasive melanoma, 31 (44%) BCC, one neurosarcoma, and 12 (17%)were benign nevi (3 of the seven lesions not visualized on HFUS were melanomas) (12). In both studies, the sensitivity of the combined characteristics of HFUS was 100% with a specificity of 33% (95% CI 20% to 48%) in Bessoud et al, 2003 (130 lesions; 65 melanomas) and 73% (95% CI 57% to 85%) in Lassau et al., 1997 (62 lesions; 19 melanomas) (the lower limits of the 95% CIs for sensitivity were 94% and 82%, respectively).

Lassau et al., 1997 determined a specificity of 8% (95% CI 0% to 36%) on 32 lesions, 19 of which were melanomas. Both studies have not visualized five melanomas in the US (38).

Lassau et al., 1997 who evaluated the hypoechoic, homogeneous, well-defined and vascularized lesions, saw that there is no difference in the sensitivity and specificity achieved using HFUS alone for the discrimination of invasive melanoma (n = 19) from all other included lesions (n = 44) (39).

The HFUS and Doppler features can be combined according to both Bessoud et al., 2003 and Lassau et al., 1997, sensitivities were 34% (95% CI 22% to 47%; n = 65 melanomas) and 16% (95% CI 3% to 40%; n = 19 melanomas) with 100% specificity (95% CI 92% to 100%) respectively for both studies (n = 45 and n = 44).

Harland et al., 2000 and Rallan et al., 2007 reported quantitative assessments of the US image evaluating the acoustic differences between common pigmented lesions.

Both studies included only melanoma, melanoma in situ, benign naevi, or seborrheic keratosis (n = 19, 6, 15, 29 in Harland et al., 2000; and n =14, 11, 38, 24 in Rallan et al., 2007).

Harland et al., 2000 compared melanoma and seborrheic keratosis (benign naevi excluded) (35, 36).

Rallan et al., 2007's work on a prototype 3D HFUS C-scan with "reflex transmission" imaging found significant differences in the mean values between melanoma and seborrheic keratosis and between melanoma and benign naevi (39).

Kaikaris et al., 2011 described the use of HFUS (14 MHz) and the association between US and morphological findings in measuring melanoma thickness.

They found a low US correlation between the Breslow index for thin melanomas (1–2 mm) and a significant correlation for thicker melanomas (> 2 mm). Measurements made with ultra-HFUS (20 MHz) were found to be well correlated with the depth of thick melanomas but were not accurate enough for thinner melanomas.

Evidence suggests that HFUS (20 MHz) may be the best tool for the estimations of tumor volume more than 2D-US (40). The first significant US reports of melanoma were performed using fixed HF probes ranging from 20 to 100 MHz.

Solivetti et al., 2014, define the HFUS as a useful technique for the detection of melanoma in-transit metastases (41). This study was performed on 600 patients with melanoma (thickness> 1 mm) resulted negative to objective examination at clinical follow-up; the US detected in-transit metastases in 63 patients with a total of 95 lesions (41). All these lesions have not reported false positive or false negative (41).

Botar et al., 2015 document the positive correlation between the Breslow index with the involvement of the lymph nodes and risk of distant metastasis. This study performed the characterization of the lesion with elastography but used the 40-MHz probe for the semiquantitative analysis. The information obtained with HFUS showed a good correlation between sonometry and histometry (r = 0.88), with an average difference of 0.39 mm (relative difference 28%) (35, 42). Tumors with a thickness between 0.55 and 0.95 mm were found to be incorrectly classified according to histology in 34%, and tumors with a thickness between 1.30 and 1.70 mm were classified incorrectly in 50% of cases. These last results are due to the low penetration of ultrasound with fixed frequency equipment (about 6 mm at 20 MHz, 3 mm at 75 MHz, and 1 mm at 100 MHz).

On the other hand, probes with variable frequency from 10 to 15 MHz and multi-channeled color Doppler evaluation allow differentiating melanomas measuring < o > 1 mm in thickness (43). This evaluation is essential in choosing to perform an SNL biopsy, which is indicated in melanomas measuring more than 1 mm in thickness (42).

Gambichler et al., found an almost similar relationship to histology, with a correlation coefficient of 0.99 with both 20- and 100-MHz transducers (44).The use of 100 MHz was more accurate than the 20 MHz. They included only lesions ≤ 1 mm thick, limiting the evaluation of lesions> 1 mm thick. Machet et al., Gambichler et al., and Pellacani et al., found that the US measurements were slightly overestimated compared to the histological size but concluded that US has a strength correlation with melanoma thickness (10, 45, 46).

For the first time, Reginelli et al., described the HFUS analysis of the CM using probes ranged from 50 to 70 MHz. In this study 14 CM have been analyzed. They present oval aspects and a fusiform shape, inhomogeneous, hypoechoic, smooth edges, and variable vascularization (1, 47, 48).

After several studies on small animals, the first HFUS for clinical use could be introduced for clinical use. The availability to use HF between 50 and 70 MHz is much higher than the conventional US systems, providing a resolution up to 30 microns and a penetration of about 15 mm (1). They considered the US performed with HF probes more accurate because the result corresponds to *in vivo* tissue without dehydration or fixation. The thickness obtained from US evaluation was compared to that obtained on the biopsy piece, and a favorable agreement was seen with the Breslow thickness (39, 49–51).

CONCLUSIONS

The application of ultrasound to dermatology is becoming more and more frequent. The ultrasound examination offers significant advantages and being it minimally invasive it is easily repeatable. In particular, the use of equipment with high-frequency probes provides important information, especially in the pre-operative, thus allowing a broader diagnostic-therapeutic evaluation, as well as later follow-up.

AUTHOR CONTRIBUTIONS

All the authors contributed equally to this work. All authors contributed to the article and approved the submitted version.

REFERENCES

1. Reginelli A, Belfiore MP, Russo A, Turriziani F, Moscarella E, Troiani T, et al. A Preliminary Study for Quantitative Assessment With HFUS (High-Frequency Ultrasound) of Nodular Skin Melanoma Breslow Thickness in Adults Before Surgery: Interdisciplinary Team Experience. *Curr Radiopharm* (2020) 13:48–55. doi: 10.2174/1874471012666191007121626

2. Scally CP, Wong SL. Intensity of Follow-Up After Melanoma Surgery. *Ann Surg Oncol* (2014) 21:752–7. doi: 10.1245/s10434-013-3295-9

3. Rastrelli M, Tropea S, Rossi CR, Alaibac M. Melanoma: Epidemiology, Risk Factors, Pathogenesis, Diagnosis and Classification. *In Vivo* (2014) 28:1005–11.

4. Bradford PT, Freedman DM, Goldstein AM, Tucker MA. Increased Risk of Second Primary Cancers After a Diagnosis of Melanoma. *Arch Dermatol* (2010) 146:265–72. doi: 10.1001/archdermatol.2010.2

5. Keung EZ, Gershenwald JE. The Eighth Edition American Joint Committee on Cancer (AJCC) Melanoma Staging System: Implications for Melanoma Treatment and Care. *Expert Rev Anticancer Ther* (2018) 18:775–84. doi: 10.1080/14737140.2018.1489246

6. Melanoma Statistics. Available at: https://www.cancer.net/cancer-types/melanoma/statistics.

7. Balch CM, Gershenwald JE, Soong S-J, Thompson JF, Atkins MB, Byrd DR, et al. Final Version of 2009 AJCC Melanoma Staging and Classification. *J Clin Oncol Off J Am Soc Clin Oncol* (2009) 27:6199–206. doi: 10.1200/JCO.2009.23.4799

8. Howard MD. Melanoma Radiological Surveillance: A Review of Current Evidence and Clinical Challenges. *Yale J Biol Med* (2020) 93:207–13.

9. Bafounta M-L, Beauchet A, Chagnon S, Saiag P. Ultrasonography or Palpation for Detection of Melanoma Nodal Invasion: A Meta-Analysis. *Lancet Oncol* (2004) 5:673–80. doi: 10.1016/S1470-2045(04)01609-2

10. Machet L, Belot V, Naouri M, Boka M, Mourtada Y, Giraudeau B, et al. Preoperative Measurement of Thickness of Cutaneous Melanoma Using High-Resolution 20 MHz Ultrasound Imaging: A Monocenter Prospective Study and Systematic Review of the Literature. *Ultrasound Med Biol* (2009) 35:1411–20. doi: 10.1016/j.ultrasmedbio.2009.03.018

11. Voit C, Mayer T, Kron M, Schoengen A, Sterry W, Weber L, et al. Efficacy of Ultrasound B-scan Compared With Physical Examination in Follow-Up of Melanoma Patients. *Cancer* (2001) 91:2409–16. doi: 10.1002/1097-0142(20010615)91:12<2409::AID-CNCR1275>3.0.CO;2-S

12. Lassau N, Spatz A, Avril MF, Tardivon A, Margulis A, Mamelle G, et al. Value of High-Frequency US for Preoperative Assessment of Skin Tumors. *Radiographics* (1997) 17:1559–65. doi: 10.1148/radiographics.17.6.9397463

13. Di Grezia G, Somma F, Serra N, Reginelli A, Cappabianca S, Grassi R, et al. Reducing Costs of Breast Examination: Ultrasound Performance and Inter-Observer Variability of Expert Radiologists Versus Residents. *Cancer Invest* (2016) 34:355–60. doi: 10.1080/07357907.2016.1201097

14. Sica A, Vitiello P, Caccavale S, Sagnelli C, Calogero A, Doraro CA, et al. Primary Cutaneous Dlbcl Non-GCB Type: Challenges of a Rare Case. *Open Med (Warsaw Poland)* (2020) 15:119–25. doi: 10.1515/med-2020-0018

15. Alexander H, Miller DL. Determining Skin Thickness With Pulsed Ultra Sound. *J Invest Dermatol* (1979) 72:17–9. doi: 10.1111/1523-1747.ep12530104

16. Bard RL. High-Frequency Ultrasound Examination in the Diagnosis of Skin Cancer. *Dermatol Clin* (2017) 35:505–11. doi: 10.1016/j.det.2017.06.011

17. Botar Jid C, Bolboacă SD, Cosgarea R, Şenilă S, Rogojan L, Lenghel M, et al. Doppler Ultrasound and Strain Elastography in the Assessment of Cutaneous Melanoma: Preliminary Results. *Med Ultrason* (2015) 17:509–14. doi: 10.11152/mu.2013.2066.174.dus

18. Caini S, Boniol M, Botteri E, Tosti G, Bazolli B, Russell-Edu W, et al. The Risk of Developing a Second Primary Cancer in Melanoma Patients: A Comprehensive Review of the Literature and Meta-Analysis. *J Dermatol Sci* (2014) 75:3–9. doi: 10.1016/j.jdermsci.2014.02.007

19. Morton DL, Cochran AJ, Thompson JF. The Rationale for Sentinel-Node Biopsy in Primary Melanoma. *Nat Clin Pract Oncol* (2008) 5:510–1. doi: 10.1038/ncponc1205

20. Sondak VK, Gibney GT. Indications and Options for Systemic Therapy in Melanoma. *Surg Clin North Am* (2014) 94:1049–58, viii. doi: 10.1016/j.suc.2014.07.007

21. Badea R, Crişan M, Lupşor M, Fodor L. Diagnosis and Characterization of Cutaneous Tumors Using Combined Ultrasonographic Procedures (Conventional and High Resolution Ultrasonography). *Med Ultrason* (2010) 12:317–22.

22. Botar-Jid CM, Cosgarea R, Bolboacă SD, Şenilă SC, Lenghel LM, Rogojan L, et al. Assessment of Cutaneous Melanoma by Use of Very- High-Frequency Ultrasound and Real-Time Elastography. *AJR Am J Roentgenol* (2016) 206:699–704. doi: 10.2214/AJR.15.15182

23. Fernández Canedo I, de Troya Martín M ,F únez Liébana R, Rivas Ruiz F, Blanco Eguren G, Blázquez Sánchez N. Preoperative 15-MHz Ultrasound Assessment of Tumor Thickness in Malignant Melanoma. *Actas Dermosifiliogr* (2013) 104:227–31. doi: 10.1016/j.ad.2012.06.007

24. Heibel HD, Hooey L, Cockerell CJ. A Review of Noninvasive Techniques for Skin Cancer Detection in Dermatology. *Am J Clin Dermatol* (2020) 21:513–24. doi: 10.1007/s40257-020-00517-z

25. Samimi M, Perrinaud A, Naouri M, Maruani A, Perrodeau E, Vaillant L, et al. High-Resolution Ultrasonography Assists the Differential Diagnosis of Blue

Naevi and Cutaneous Metastases of Melanoma. *Br J Dermatol* (2010) 163:550–6. doi: 10.1111/j.1365-2133.2010.09903.x

26. Solivetti FM, Di Luca Sidozzi A, Pirozzi G, Coscarella G, Brigida R, Eibenshutz L. Sonographic Evaluation of Clinically Occult in-Transit and Satellite Metastases From Cutaneous Malignant Melanoma. *Radiol Med* (2006) 111:702–8. doi: 10.1007/s11547-006-0067-7

27. Berritto D, Iacobellis F, Rossi C, Reginelli A, Cappabianca S, Grassi R. Ultra High-Frequency Ultrasound: New Capabilities for Nail Anatomy Exploration. *J Dermatol* (2017) 44:43–6. doi: 10.1111/1346-8138.13495

28. Mlosek RK, Malinowska S. Ultrasound Image of the Skin, Apparatus and Imaging Basics. *J Ultrason* (2013) 13:212–21. doi: 10.15557/JoU.2013.0021

29. Izzetti R, Oranges T, Janowska A, Gabriele M, Graziani F, Romanelli M. The Application of Ultra-High-Frequency Ultrasound in Dermatology and Wound Management. *Int J Low Extrem Wounds* (2020) 19:334–40. doi: 10.1177/1534734620972815

30. Piłat P, Borzęcki A, Jazienicki M, Krasowska D. Skin Melanoma Imaging Using Ultrasonography: A Literature Review. *Postep Dermatol i Alergol* (2018) 35:238–42. doi: 10.5114/ada.2018.76211

31. Bezugly A. High Frequency Ultrasound Study of Skin Tumors in Dermatological and Aesthetic Practice. *Med Ultrason* (2015) 17:541–4. doi: 10.11152/mu.2013.2066.174.hfy

32. Farberg AS, Rigel DS. Non-Invasive Technologies for the Diagnosis and Management of Skin Cancer. *Dermatol Clin* (2017) 35:i. doi: 10.1016/s0733-8635(17)30099-2

33. Clément A, Hoeffel C, Fayet P, Benkanoun S, Sahut D'izarn J, Oudjit A. Value of High Frequency (20mhZ) and Doppler Ultrasound in the Diagnosis of Pigmented Cutaneous Tumors. *J Radiol* (2001) 82(5):563–71.

34. Bessoud B, Lassau N, Koscielny S, Longvert C, Avril M-F, Duvillard P, et al. High-Frequency Sonography and Color Doppler in the Management of Pigmented Skin Lesions. *Ultrasound Med Biol* (2003) 29:875–9. doi: 10.1016/s0301-5629(03)00035-8

35. Rallan D, Bush NL, Bamber JC, Harland CC. Quantitative Discrimination of Pigmented Lesions Using Three-Dimensional High-Resolution Ultrasound Reflex Transmission Imaging. *J Invest Dermatol* (2007) 127:189–95. doi: 10.1038/sj.jid.5700554

36. Harland CC, Kale SG, Jackson P, Mortimer PS, Bamber JC. Differentiation of Common Benign Pigmented Skin Lesions From Melanoma by High-Resolution Ultrasound. *Br J Dermatol* (2000) 143:281–9. doi: 10.1046/j.1365-2133.2000.03652.x

37. Klebanov N, Gunasekera NS, Lin WM, Hawryluk EB, Miller DM, Reddy BY, et al. Clinical Spectrum of Cutaneous Melanoma Morphology. *J Am Acad Dermatol* (2019) 80:178–88. doi: 10.1016/j.jaad.2018.08.028

38. Jones OT, Ranmuthu CKI, Hall PN, Funston G, Walter FM. Recognising Skin Cancer in Primary Care. *Adv Ther* (2020) 37:603–16. doi: 10.1007/s12325-019-01130-1

39. Dinnes J, Bamber J, Chuchu N, Bayliss SE, Takwoingi Y, Davenport C, et al. High-Frequency Ultrasound for Diagnosing Skin Cancer in Adults. *Cochrane Database Syst Rev* (2018) 12:CD013188. doi: 10.1002/14651858.CD013188

40. Kaikaris V, Samsanavičius D, Maslauskas K, Rimdeika R, Valiukevičienė S, Makštienė J, et al. Measurement of Melanoma Thickness–Comparison of Two Methods: Ultrasound Versus Morphology. *J Plast Reconstr Aesthet Surg* (2011) 64:796–802. doi: 10.1016/j.bjps.2010.10.008

41. Solivetti FM, Desiderio F, Guerrisi A, Bonadies A, Maini CL, Filippo S, et al. HF Ultrasound vs PET-CT and Telethermography in the Diagnosis of in-Transit Metastases From Melanoma:a Prospective Study and Review of the Literature. *J Exp Clin Cancer Res* (2014) 33:1–7. doi: 10.1186/s13046-014-0096-3

42. Wortsman X. Sonography of the Primary Cutaneous Melanoma: A Review. *Radiol Res Pract* (2012) 2012:1–6. doi: 10.1155/2012/814396

43. Wortsman X. Ultrasound in Dermatology: Why, How, and When? *Semin Ultrasound CT MRI* (2013) 34:177–95. doi: 10.1053/j.sult.2012.10.001

44. DiGiacinto D, Bagley J, Goldsbury AM. The Value of Sonography in the Assessment of Skin Cancers and Their Metastases. *J Diagn Med Sonogr* (2016) 32:140–6. doi: 10.1177/8756479316643959

45. Gambichler T, Moussa G, Bahrenberg K, Vogt M, Ermert H, Weyhe D, et al. Preoperative Ultrasonic Assessment of Thin Melanocytic Skin Lesions Using a 100-MHz Ultrasound Transducer: A Comparative Study. *Dermatol Surg* (2007) 33:818–24. doi: 10.1111/j.1524-4725.2007.33175.x

46. Pellacani G, Seidenari S. Preoperative Melanoma Thickness Determination by 20-MHZ Sonography and Digital Videomicroscopy in Combination. *Arch Dermatol* (2003) 139:293–8. doi: 10.1001/archderm.139.3.293

47. Guevara M, Rodríguez-Barranco M, Puigdemont M, Minicozzi P, Yanguas-Bayona I, Porras-Povedano M, et al. Disparities in the Management of Cutaneous Malignant Melanoma. A Population-Based High-Resolution Study. *Eur J Cancer Care (Engl)* (2019) 28:e13043. doi: 10.1111/ecc.13043

48. Narayanamurthy V, Padmapriya P, Noorasafrin A, Pooja B, Hema K, Firus Khan AY, et al. Skin Cancer Detection Using non-Invasive Techniques. *RSC Adv* (2018) 8:28095–130. doi: 10.1039/c8ra04164d

49. Hambardzumyan M, Hayrapetyan A. Ultrasound Analytic Criteria for Diagnosing Cutaneous Malignant Melanoma. *Madridge J Dermatol Res* (2018) 3:33–7. doi: 10.18689/mjdr-1000108

50. Vidal CI, Armbrect EA, Andea AA, Bohlke AK, Comfere NI, Hughes SR, et al. Appropriate Use Criteria in Dermatopathology: Initial Recommendations From the American Society of Dermatopathology. *J Cutan Pathol* (2018) 45:563–80. doi: 10.1111/cup.13142

51. Svoboda RM, Prado G, Mirsky RS, Rigel DS. Assessment of Clinician Accuracy for Diagnosing Melanoma on the Basis of Electrical Impedance Spectroscopy Score Plus Morphology Versus Lesion Morphology Alone. *J Am Acad Dermatol* (2019) 80:285–7. doi: 10.1016/j.jaad.2018.08.048

8

Non-Melanoma Skin Cancer in People Living with HIV: From Epidemiology to Clinical Management

Emmanuele Venanzi Rullo[1], Maria Grazia Maimone[1], Francesco Fiorica[2],
Manuela Ceccarelli[1,3], Claudio Guarneri[4], Massimiliano Berretta[1*] and Giuseppe Nunnari[1]

[1] Unit of Infectious Disease, Department of Clinical and Experimental Medicine, University of Messina, Messina, Italy,
[2] Department of Radiation Oncology and Nuclear Medicine, State Hospital "Mater Salutis" Azienda Unità Locale Socio
Sanitaria (AULSS) 9, Legnago, Italy, [3] Unit of Infectious Disease, Department of Clinical and Experimental Medicine, University
of Catania, Catania, Italy, [4] Unit of Dermatology, Department of Biomedical and Dental Sciences and Morphofunctional
Imaging, University of Messina, Messina, Italy

*Correspondence:
Massimiliano Berretta
massimiliano.berretta@unime.it

Skin cancers represent the most common human tumors with a worldwide increasing incidence. They can be divided into melanoma and non-melanoma skin cancers (NMSCs). NMSCs include mainly squamous cell (SCC) and basal cell carcinoma (BCC) with the latest representing the 80% of the diagnosed NMSCs. The pathogenesis of NMSCs is clearly multifactorial. A growing body of literature underlies a crucial correlation between skin cancer, chronic inflammation and immunodeficiency. Intensity and duration of immunodeficiency plays an important role. In immunocompromised patients the incidence of more malignant forms or the development of multiple tumors seems to be higher than among immunocompetent patients. With regards to people living with HIV (PLWH), since the advent of combined antiretroviral therapy (cART), the incidence of non-AIDS-defining cancers (NADCs), such as NMSCs, have been increasing and now these neoplasms represent a leading cause of illness in this particular population. PLWH with NMSCs tend to be younger, to have a higher risk of local recurrence and to have an overall poorer outcome. NMSCs show an indolent clinical course if diagnosed and treated in an early stage. BCC rarely metastasizes, while SCC presents a 4% annual incidence of metastasis. Nevertheless, metastatic forms lead to poor patient outcome. NMSCs are often treated with full thickness treatments (surgical excision, Mohs micro-graphic surgery and radiotherapy) or superficial ablative techniques (such as cryotherapy, electrodesiccation and curettage). Advances in genetic landscape understanding of NMSCs have favored the establishment of novel therapeutic strategies. Concerning the therapeutic evaluation of PLWH, it's mandatory to evaluate the risk of interactions between cART and other treatments, particularly antiblastic chemotherapy, targeted therapy and immunotherapy. Development of further treatment options for NMSCs in PLWH seems needed. We reviewed the literature after searching for clinical trials, case series, clinical cases and available databases in Embase and Pubmed. We review the incidence of NMSCs among PLWH, focusing our attention on any differences in clinicopathological features of BCC and SCC between PLWH and HIV negative persons, as well as on any differences in efficacy and safety of treatments and response to immunomodulators and finally on any differences in rates of metastatic disease and outcomes.

Keywords: human immunodeficiency virus, non-melanoma skin cancer, basal cell cancer, squamous cell cancer, immunedeficiency, review (article)

INTRODUCTION

The natural history of HIV has been significantly modified by the advent of combined antiretroviral therapy (cART) that has prolonged life expectancy and reduced mortality and morbidity of people living with HIV (PLWH). Even if highly active, cART cannot cure HIV and so it is a lifelong therapy because of a hidden, even though active, reservoir (1, 2) that is able to escape the treatment. Over the past twenty years, many important factors, as increased age of PLWH and (3) coinfection with oncogenic viruses have promoted the emergence of other malignant neoplasms that collectively are classified as non-AIDS-defining cancers (NADCs) and that, over the years, overtook the incidence of AIDS-defining cancers in PLWH (4–14).

Non-melanoma skin cancers (NMSCs) include primarily basal cell (BCC) and squamous cell carcinoma (SCC). They represent the most frequent malignant neoplasms in the white population, with a worldwide increasing incidence (15). NMSCs develop from epidermal cells and their incidence increases in older age. The pathogenesis is multifactorial: chronic sun exposure is the main environmental risk factor. Other risk factors include increased longevity, genetic mutations, immunodeficiency, concurrent disease and dedicated therapy (i.e., psoriasis) (16). In immunocompromised patients, such as HIV positive patients, the incidence of more malignant form or the development of multiple tumors seems to be higher than among immunocompetent people. In PLWH these malignancies are often more aggressive compared with the general population and they need multidisciplinary assistance (17–26).

The purpose of this review is to describe the incidence of NMSCs among PLWH, focusing on any difference in clinicopathologic features of BCC and SCC between PLWH and HIV negative persons, as well as on any difference in efficacy and safety of treatments and response to immunomodulators, and finally any differences in rates of metastatic disease and outcomes.

MATERIALS AND METHODS

A systematic search of the EMBASE and Medline databases was performed to identify potentially relevant papers reporting original research on NMSCs in PLWH. This research was performed from inception to 3 March 2021, and it was restricted to humans. Clinical trials, prospective and retrospective studies, case series, case control studies and metanalysis concerning the topic of NMSCs in PLWH published in English, Spanish and Italian with available abstracts, were selected if they addressed one or more of the following topics: BCC, SCC, basal cell carcinoma, squamous cell carcinoma, HIV. The following search strings were used: "BCC OR basal cell carcinoma AND HIV", "SCC OR squamous cell carcinoma AND HIV". Reviews, expert opinions, book chapters and articles lacking original data were excluded. The title and abstract of all articles retrieved were check by two reviews (EVR and MGM) who selected relevant articles for full text evaluation according to predetermined criteria. Discrepancies were resulted by a third reviewer (MB). Studies were compared by title and abstracts to eliminate duplicates. A Preferred Reporting Items for Systematic Reviews and Meta-Analyses (PRISMA) flow diagram (Downloaded 03 March 2021, http://prisma-statement.org/PRISMAStatement/FlowDiagram.aspx.) was set to illustrate the review process (**Supplementary Materials**). We summarized the review according to PRISMA guidelines, represented below).

EPIDEMIOLOGICAL PROFILE OF NMSCs

Non-melanoma skin cancers (NMSCs) are the most frequent neoplasms in Caucasians and their incidence is increasing worldwide, with 80% diagnosed as BCC followed by SCC being both more common than melanomas (27). They are much common in white population than in skin color people. Their incidence results 18-20 times higher than that of melanoma (28). Epidemiologic studies highlight that the worldwide incidence varies widely. In fact, BCC has higher incidence in equatorial latitudes and lower in polar latitudes. Australia is the country with highest incidence of BCC, followed by the US and Europe, although the real incidence is globally underestimated (29). In Australia the rate for BCC is more than 1,000 per 100,000 person-years (2,448/100.000), followed by Europe (91 in women and 129 in men per 100,000 person-years) and the US (450 per 100,000 person-years). Cutaneous SCC is the most common skin cancer, behind BCC, and it represents approximately 20 percent of NMSCs (30). Its incidence increases more quickly with age than BCC. In PLWH cancer is becoming a growing problem representing now the first cause of death. It is clear that cancer risk is higher in PLWH in comparison with the general population (31), less clear are the reasons behind it. The advent of cART has improved the morbidity and mortality of PLWH, prolonging their life expectancy (32). A large body of literature has highlighted that HIV infection is associated to an increased risk of several different type of cancers besides NMSCs, such as lung cancer, cancer of the colon and rectum, Hodgkin disease, hepato-cellular carcinoma, head and neck SCC (HNSCC), conjunctival SCC and anogenital SCC (10, 17, 19, 20, 33, 34). BCC in PLWH show a 1.8-fold increased risk in comparison with HIV negative people (35), but it could be better in patients that have a good control of the infection. The occurrence of multiple BCC in PLWH without additional risk factors is uncommon. In HIV positive patients BCC is essentially more frequent than SCC (36) and ratios around 4:1 of BCC versus SCC have been found, similar to the general population (4:1) (33). In a retrospective cohort that studied 36821 HIV negative and 6560 HIV positive patients it has been shown an increased risk for BCC among PLWH. In fact, in this Californian cohort, the risk of developing a BCC was about twice as likely in non-Hispanic white PLWH than in the same HIV negative population. So that, it has been denoted that patients with HIV showed a meaningful tendency to develop BCC as HIV negative persons (37). Regarding HNSCCs, they are a heterogeneous group of cancers occurring in various anatomic sites, including scalp, oral cavity, lips, oropharynx, nasopharynx and larynx.

Focus on SCC of the Scalp

SCC of the scalp represents approximately 16% of scalp cancers (38), with a mean age of 65 years at diagnosis. It has a positive correlation with advanced age.

Known risk factors for developing SCC of the scalp are older age, history of ionizing radiation chronic scarring, androgenetic alopecia, ultraviolet light exposure, actinic damage.

Immunosuppression is a crucial risk factor for all SCCs (39) that represent the most common cancer in immunosuppressed patients, with greater potential for tumor growth, cell differentiation, and aggressiveness. Furthermore, SCC may show a higher risk of metastatic disease and death in immunocompromised patients compared with immunocompetent individuals (40).

A retrospective study showed that twenty out of fifty-tree immunocompromised patients affected by cutaneous SCC of the scalp had bone invasion, that is associated with poor prognosis (41).

The aggressive behavior of SCC on the scalp in immunosuppressed patients has been described by Lang et al. (42). It is recommendable to manage scalp tumors aggressively and appropriately because they are associated with important morbidity and mortality. So that, it is essential to monitor for bone invasion, recurrence, perineural invasion and metastasis. A better knowledge of the mechanisms of recurrency could be helpful to prevent morbidity and mortality in this specific group of patients. Concerning the clinical presentation of SCC of the scalp in HIV positive patients, Ferreira CP et al. have described a case report of a sixty years-old male, white, and HIV positive in use of zidovudine, lamivudine and efavirenz, presenting tumor located in scalp, progressing with rapid growth for one year. The histopathological examination revealed a diagnosis of well differentiated SCC. Immuno-virological profile revealed CD4: 62 cells/mm³; CD8: 1,654 cells/mm³; viral load: 91,000 copies. CT brain scan revealed cerebral foci of calcification in the suprasellar

region as well as in basal ganglia on the left, with a diameter of 15 mm and invasion to the skull along the interparietal suture. The patient had subsequent pneumonia that was the final cause of death. Fortunately, SCC is often diagnosed before the invasion to the skull because of its slow progression. Rarely, SCC can extend to the brain and invade, in late stages, the skull and the dura mater. When this event occurs, patients may present neurological symptoms (43). Because of the anatomical profile of the scalp region, margin excision is not always possible. Preoperative imaging is essential to define the proper extent of invasion and choose the correct treatment strategy. The treatment of SCC in advanced stages is challenging starting from the multidisciplinary surgical approach needed for a proper excision. Further studied are required for advanced disease.

RISK FACTORS AND PATHOGENESIS

Among immunocompetent light-skin color people, the development of NMSCs is favored mainly by chronic sun exposure and increasing age. There are important phenotypic characteristics, such as fair skin type, light-colored eyes, red hair, northern European origin and childhood freckling (44) that influence vulnerability to solar radiation. The frequency and intensity of sun exposure are also important.

Other environmental risk factors that contribute an increased risk for NMSCs include older age, family history of skin cancer, immunodeficiency (45), previous radiotherapy, long-term immunosuppressive treatment, genetic syndromes and chronic, mostly occupational, exposure to arsenic (46).Moreover, several observational studies have documented a correlation between use of photosensitizing molecules and increased risk for BCC (47).

The Genetic Landscape of NMSCs

Mutations of numerous tumor suppressor genes and proto-oncogenes play a key role as drivers in BCC formation (48). In almost 90% of cases, mutations that activate the Hedgehog pathway (HH) play an established role in the development of BCC (48), while SCC is characterized by a high neoantigen burden (37). In about 50% of BCC cases, TP53 tumor-suppressor gene mutations are caused by UV radiation. TP53 encodes the P53 protein involved in maintain genomic stability by regulating the cell cycle, inducing apoptosis and activating DNA repair. Furthermore, mutations identified in PTCH1 and TP53 are so-called UV signature mutations, because in most cases they are consistent with ultraviolet radiation-induced mutagenesis.

Among genetic syndromes that may increase the risk for the development of BCC, we should keep on mind Gorlin-Goltz syndrome, also called Nevoid BCC syndrome, an autosomal dominant disease with multiple lesions of the skin, pits of the palm and developmental defects (49).

Moreover, oculocutaneous albinisms and xeroderma pigmentosum, which are known as genetic diseases with deficiencies of the protective mechanisms against UVR, are characterized by multiple and early BCCs (50).

Concerning the genetic landscape of SCC, multiple studies have shown that genes altered by UVR exposition are TP53, CDKN2A, NOTCH1, NOTCH2 and p16 suppressor gene. Moreover, mutations in DNA repair pathways include missense mutations in ATR, PIK3CA, ERRB4 and NF1 (51). In addition, association between SCC and genetic syndromes as oculocutaneous albinism, xeroderma pigmentosum, Fanconi anemia, epidermolysis bullosa and Lynch syndrome has been found (52).

A Brief Focus on Possible Links Between the Innate Immune System and NMSCs

A large body of studies highlights that innate immunity play a key role in NMSCs development and progression. Their role has attracted increasing attention recently. As well known, the innate immune system cells can recognize numerous exogenous ligands, such as infectious agents, through various mechanisms. The most important genetic pathway networks involve a crucial group of receptors, called toll-like receptors (TLRs) (53). They are a family of ten transmembrane glycoproteins that directly recognize a wide spectrum of pathogen-associated molecular patterns (PAMPs) and damage-associated molecular patterns (DAMPs), against which they activate the innate immune response and initiate the adaptive immune response (54).

TLRs play a crucial role in the activation of innate immunity, promoting cancer progression; therefore, their activation induces genes that encode for numerous inflammatory cytokines, such as tumor necrosis factor-α (TNF-α), INF-1, IL-6, IL-1, granulocyte-colony stimulating factor and different chemokines, including CCL2 and CXCL10 (54, 55).

It has been observed that some TLRs are involved in the pathogenesis of numerous inflammatory and autoimmune skin disorders. Particularly, there is evidence that Imiquimod, a synthetic agonist of TLR-7, presents high efficacy for treatment of superficial BCC, with a cure rate ranging from 43-94% (56).

The high efficacy of this TLR-7 agonist against superficial BCC, suggests a possible role of this receptor in the pathogenesis of BCC. As a possible consequence, polymorphisms of this receptor could change host immune responses, determining a different susceptibility to BCC and others cancers and autoimmune diseases (57).

A recent case control study performed by Russo et al. (58) highlights the possible association between the susceptibility to BCC and a functional single-nucleotide polymorphism within the promoter of TLR-7 gene (SNP rs 179008/Gln11Leu).

Further genetic research of this receptor and its ligands are needed to improve the knowledge of the pathogenesis of BCC and other UV-related skin cancers.

An increasing body of evidence shows that BCC is an immunogenic tumor (59). Several immune-related markers have been implicated in BCC pathogenesis. IL-23/Th17 related cytokines, as 17, 23, 22, play a significant role in cutaneous inflammatory diseases, but their involvement in skin carcinogenesis is controversial and is poorly investigated in BCC. A recent study of Pellegrini C et al. has highlighted the role of INF-γ in BCC pathogenesis, supporting the involvement of IL-23/Th 17 related cytokines. Particularly, it has observed that BCC is characterized by higher levels of IFN-γ, IL-17, IL-22 and IL-23. Their expression could be correlated to the severity of the inflammatory infiltrate.

Concerning cSCCs, as well known, they are characterized by high mutational burden and cellular heterogeneity (60).

The role of immunosuppression in cSCC risk is supported by higher incidence among recipients of solid organ transplants and PLWH (37, 61), suggesting that this tumor type has enhanced many elements of innate immune response compared to normal skin. The immune system plays complex roles over the entire process of cancer initiation, promotion and progression.

Presentation of tumor antigens to CD8+ cytotoxic T cells and CD4+ helper T cells by HLA class I and class II molecules, respectively, is a key component of this process. The immune response is modulated by human leukocyte antigens (HLAs), which are encoded by a cluster of highly polymorphic genes located on chromosome 6. At the same time, inflammation can facilitate cell transformation by providing pro-tumorigenic cytokines and growth factors to tumor cells and forming an immune suppressive microenvironment within the tumor, which ultimately lead to immune escape and clinical manifestation of the tumors (62). A growing body of literature shows that variation in the expression pattern of these proteins, involved in the presentation of tumor antigens to T lymphocytes, has been implicated in multiple cancers by influencing host defenses against tumorigenesis. The exact mechanisms underlying these associations need to be elucidated. The strongest association between amino acid changes and cSCC risk was found for codon 26 of HLA-DRB1. However, the true functional impact of the phenylalanine to leucine change remains to be elucidated. The identification of specific amino acid changes in the HLA class II genes, if confirmed, helps provide mechanistic clues to the relationship between HLA-mediated immune response and cSCC tumorigenesis. Future studies that examine the mechanism underlying the association between HLA class II and cSCC risk need to be performed. The immune system impacts cSCC susceptibility and pathogenesis, as evidenced by the substantially higher incidence of cSCC in immunocompromised patients. Furthermore, susceptibility to the effects of UVR is known to be genetically determined (63). Variations in immunological makeup of human hosts may influence their ability to recruit immune responses needed to prevent cSCC development. Particular HLA genetic variants are associated with cSCC in immunocompetent and immunosuppressed patients, with more evidence for class I HLA-cSCC associations in immunosuppressed patients than in immunocompetent patients. Class I HLA could play a more important role in cSCC in immunosuppressed patients because HPV may be a co-factor in tumorigenesis- class I HLA proteins present intracellular peptide antigens, including viral proteins degraded into peptides. Further researches of tumor antigens involved in cSCC pathogenesis are needed, to better understand cSCC pathogenesis from an immunological point of view, and try to provide an effective prevention and treatment of cSCC (64).

Skin Cancer, Chronic Inflammation, and Immunodeficiency: A Mènage A Tròis

Cutaneous manifestations often may reveal themselves important clinical clues of many diseases in general, including neoplastic skin diseases, that brings the patient to the physician.

The cutaneous immune system is usually linked to defense against pathogens and external agents; it can also promote the neoplastic process and tumor progression through inflammation.

As known, inflammation plays a key role in oncogenesis (**Figure 1**). Different kinds of cancers arise from infections or chronic inflammation that represent the main promoters of chronic activation of immune system. This prolonged immune activation triggers various stages of carcinogenesis.

As known, immunodepression HIV-related determines an increased risk of tumors (65).

Moreover, HIV shows a tropism for cells of the human immune system, such as macrophages, dendritic cells and T-lymphocytes. HIV infection, through different processes, leads to the reduction of CD4 T-cells to a critical level. Below this level, cell-mediated immunity is lost, and this event allows the rise of opportunistic infections and AIDS development.

Regarding the mechanisms by which HIV virus induced lytic activities, Pope et al. (66) suggested that direct contact between CD4 T cells and HIV pulsed dendritic antigen-presenting cells triggers replication of the virus, leading to a death to both cell types. Furthermore, delayed-type hypersensitivity tests usually have been used as monitors for the progression of the infection, because of the compromise of cutaneous immune system is crucial (67). When CD4 and antigen-presenting cells count decrease meaningfully, skin becomes susceptible to numerous opportunistic infections and neoplastic diseases. In addition, HIV virus seems to activate proto-oncogenes (68), cause alterations in cell cycle regulation and inhibit tumor suppressor genes including p53 (69). Moreover, HIV could determine microsatellite gene instability and genetic alterations, promoting formation of different cancers, including NMSCs (70) (**Figure 2**).

Finally, HIV infection may booster pro-angiogenesis signaling that could lead to endothelial abnormalities. These alterations could promote tumor growth and metastasis (71).

Cutaneous malignancies are the majority of cancers among HIV positive patients (72) and NMSCs are now the most frequent cutaneous malignancies among PLWH. The main risk factors for NMSCs are similar to HIV negative people. Accumulate worldwide studies have shown that NMSCs are usually more aggressive in immunocompromised patients, as evidenced by an increased risk of metastatic disease and mortality in comparison with immunocompetent individuals (73). Frequent opportunistic infections represent also important risk factors for NMSCs (74).

In a study by BURGI et al. (72), cART therapy was associated with lower rates of NMSCs, whereas the standardized incidence ratio (SIR) for NMSCs was reported not to be decreased in the post-cART era among patients recorded in the Swiss cohort study (36). Moreover, a study by Silverberg et al. has suggested that the cART use is associated with decreased risk. Generally, PLWH with BCC and SCC tend to be younger, to have an increased rate of recurrence and they seem to have an overall poorer outcome (75). They often present with more advanced stages of the disease, with a greater degree of infiltrative disease and poorer outcomes (76). In PLWH possible etiologies of NMSCs include the HIV virus, coinfection with oncogenic viruses, such us hepatitis B virus (HBV) (77), hepatitis C virus (HCV) (78), human papilloma virus (HPV) and Epstein Barr virus (EBV) (79), cART agents and tobacco exposure. HPV skin infections are common but the exact correlation between HPV infection and the developing of cutaneous SCC remains still less clear (80). Multiple studies have reported indirect evidence supporting an etiologic relationship (81).

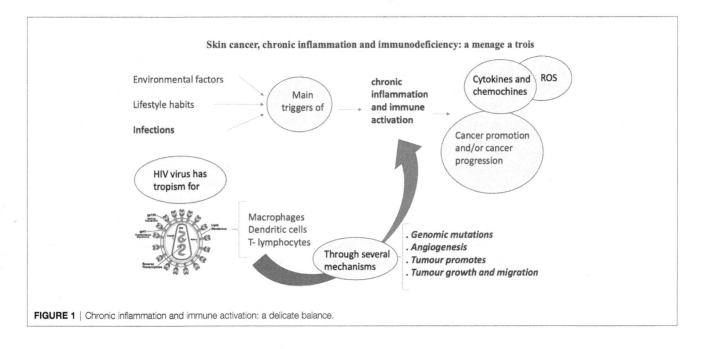

FIGURE 1 | Chronic inflammation and immune activation: a delicate balance.

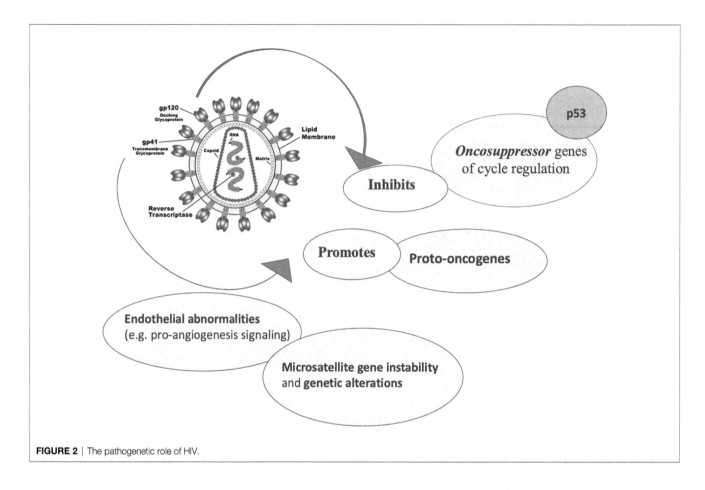

FIGURE 2 | The pathogenetic role of HIV.

Exploring the Link Between Viral-Immunologic Profile of HIV Positive Patients and Risk of NMSCs

Current knowledge of the correlation between viral-immunologic profile of HIV positive patients and NMSCs is evolving. A peculiar correlation between decreased immune-surveillance and carcinogenic virus co-infections might favor oncogenesis, increasing the risk of developing tumors in these subjects (see **Figure 3**).

CD4 cell count is one of the main investigations in the clinical evaluation and management of HIV-infected patients and the skin is richly endowed with these cells. Immunocompetent and PLWH seemed to share the same genetic and environmental factors that lead to the formation of NMSC. Immunosuppression can increase risk to develop NMSCs, mostly SCC (82). An increased rate of neoplasms could be likely to explained by the progressive decline and dysfunction of T cells associated with HIV infection.

HIV infection causes reduced activation of both CD4 and CD8 cells and an increased synthesis of TH2 cytokine subsets. This event leads to cell-mediated immunity deficiency and accumulation of genetic mutations. HIV produces specific proteins, such as nef and tat, that alter MHC signaling and chemokine production (83).

How HIV infection could be the cause of oncogenesis it is complicated to demonstrate, especially because it seems not to be correlated with the overall immune status (CD4 counts and viral load) (84). A meta-analysis of Grulich et al. (85) have showed that immune deficiency caused an increased risk of cancer. HIV positive patients, with CD4 counts <200/microL and high viral loads > 10,000 copies/mL, have a twofold increased risk of developing a primary SCC. The association between level of immunodeficiency and risk of NMSCs is less clear, with a correlation with only SCC having been observed (37). Recently, it has been demonstrated an increased rate of NMSCs among PLWH (37). In 2017, Asgari et al. reported that non-Hispanic white PLWH had a greater risk of developing a new subsequent SCC and that this risk is correlated with lower CD4 counts and higher viral loads. The study failed to demonstrate the same for BCC. In PLWH a 15% increased risk of NMSC has been demonstrated. In particular, the possibility of a subsequent NMSC seemed to be correlated with profound immune-compromission (CD4 <200) (86).

These findings suggest that HIV-related immunodeficiency can determine an increased risk of NMSC overall and SCC in particular. In addition, the HIV viral load, often influenced by antiretroviral therapy adherence, was associated with subsequent primary SCC (hazard ratio of 2.28 with a VL above 10,000 copies/mL) but not for BCC (86). However, this study presents some limitations. The confidence intervals surrounding their HRs are not wide, suggesting that their findings were sufficiently powered. PLWH, especially those with poor immune control,

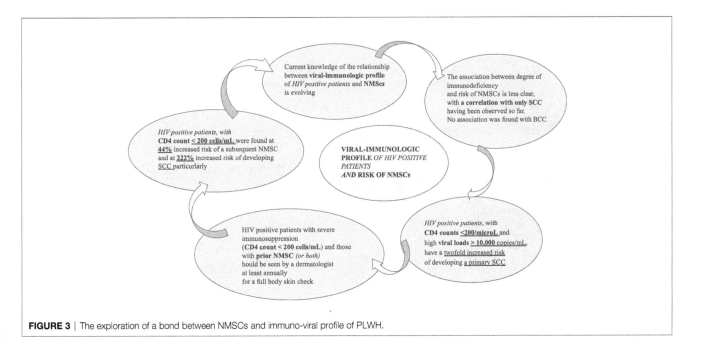

FIGURE 3 | The exploration of a bond between NMSCs and immuno-viral profile of PLWH.

could potentially benefit from targeted monitoring for SCC. In these cases, Sarah J Coates et al. recommended that patients with prior NMSC should undergo a careful dermatologic evaluation at least every year (87).

CLINICAL PRESENTATION AND DIAGNOSIS

BCC derives from the deepest cell layer of the epidermis, the basal layer of keratinocytes. Its clinical presentation is notably heterogeneous. It usually appears as a waxy, translucent, or pearly lesion that often shows a central ulceration and a raised pale border. Telangiectasias are frequent and they often bleed. Moreover, they lead to friability and poor healing. The lesion can appear atrophic and the borders can be indistinct (88). Approximately, in 9 cases out of 10, BCC arises on the head and in 7 cases out of 10 on the trunk and extremities (89). Although BCC shows minimal metastatic potential (<0,1%), local tissue effects can be destructive and disfiguring (88). Diagnosis is primarily histologically. The main histologic patterns are: nodular, superficial, morpheaform/infiltrative, basosquamous, micronodular and pigmented. Morpheaform/ infiltrative, micronodular and basosquamous are considered more "aggressive growth" subtypes of BCC. Moreover, some lesions present a mixed histology.

SCC arises from atypical proliferation of keratinizing cells of the epidermis or its appendages. It often develops from actinic keratosis and Bowen's disease (SCC *in situ*) which are considered precancerous lesions. It can also grow *de novo* or on irradiated skin regions, or on chronic inflammatory skin disorders. In contrast to BCC which rarely metastasizes, SCC can metastasize initially to regional lymph-nodes and subsequently

to distant regions (90). Typical clinical aspect of SCC is a raised pink papule or plaque, sometimes with scaling or an ulcerated center. The borders often are irregular and bleed easily. During the first years of follow-up, it seems to be less frequent that AKs turns into invasive SCC. When SCC arises from actinic keratosis, it appears scaly, but it tends to grow thicker, and a pink macular area develops into an erythematous raised base. Because SCC may seem quite similar to actinic keratosis, only skin biopsy accurately identifies significant cytologic atypia and invasion of SCC (89). Clinical appearance of SCC is extremely heterogeneous, and it depends also on the anatomical region and subtype. The diagnosis of SCC is primarily histologically. In all clinically suspicious lesions, a skin incisional biopsy or excision, need for a histologic confirmation, should be performed initially, depending on the size of the cancer and treatment approach (see **Figure 4**). It is possible to perform an incisional (punch or shave biopsy) or an excisional biopsy of the whole lesion. Moreover, in rare cases of uncertain diagnosis, immunohistochemical markers of differentiation, such as cytokeratin or molecular biological markers can be applied (50).

Generally, PLWH with SCC and BCC present identically to immunocompetent individuals (91). BCC generally appears on the trunk, while SCC on the head and neck regions. Superficial type BCC is the most typical clinical and histologic presentation, which tends to be multiple, involving the trunk. Generally, in PLWH malignant cancers show a more aggressive phenotype and poorer survival rates in comparison with immunocompetent persons. NADCs show often earlier age at onset, higher tumor degree, more aggressive clinical course and/or more advanced stage at presentation, highlighting the need for prompt and aggressive treatment. More aggressive clinical course has been correlated with multiple factors, such as anatomic site, size at onset, growth rate, histologic features and recurrence after treatment (92). A substantial body of evidence on metastatic

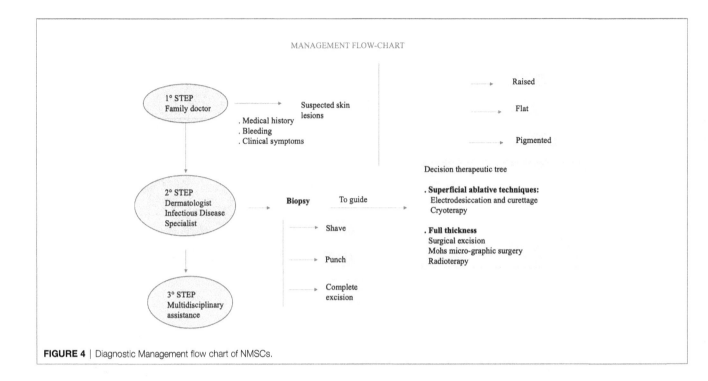

FIGURE 4 | Diagnostic Management flow chart of NMSCs.

SCC highlights that head and neck are primary sites; particularly the temporal and zygomatic regions seem to have a clear tendency for metastasis, maybe because of rich and direct lymphatic drain-age to the parotid gland (93).

Nguyen et all. have demonstrated that PLWH can develop rapidly growing SCC at a young age, with a high risk of local recurrence and metastasis. Management of high-risk SCC should be aggressive and not palliative in PLWH (92). However, cART has certain improved the life quality of PLWH and their outcome that appears more similar as in the general population. Several worldwide studies have highlight that in PLWH, NMSCs are usually characterized by a more aggressive clinical course, higher cancer grade, advanced stages at cancer diagnosis and shorter survival compared with HIV negative individuals (74). SCC seem to be more dangerous in the context of HIV disease. R. N. Motta et al. have described the case of a 59-year-old male patient with advanced HIV infection who presented with a highly aggressive SCC lesion scalp area with destruction of the underlying parietal bone and fulminant clinical progression (94).

Nguyen et al. (92) have described ten cases of aggressive SCC. They recorded 41 different SCC lesions: 75% in head and neck, 7% in the trunk and 8% in extremities.

based on rapid growth rate, a diameter of over 1.5 cm, a history of recurrence and/or evidence of metastasis. A total of 41 SCC lesions were recorded from 10 patients. The head and neck were the most frequently involved regions (31 lesions), followed by the trunk (7 lesions) and extremities (1 lesion). The article stated that those patients initially treated with radiation therapy and surgery combined as well as those treated with radical neck dissection had the best outcomes (92). This paper suggests that high-risk SCC should be treated aggressively and not palliatively in patients infected with HIV.

FROM PREVENTION TO THERAPY

Skin cancer can be avoided by following simple prevention rules (95). Primary prevention is of utmost importance. In particular, sun exposure should be reduced and totally avoided when at its peak during the day, and intensive tanning discouraged. Secondary prevention should be aimed to reduce morbidity and mortality, mainly through early detection of skin cancer, as close clinical evaluation of the arms, face and upper chest can uncover many lesions. In PLWH it is vital a careful evaluation with early biopsy of suspicious lesions. Precancerous lesions should be undergone an early diagnosis to prevent the development of invasive SCC. When cycle of therapy is concluded, patients should undergo a regular follow-up with evaluation of local recurrence or nodal metastasis, particularly for SCC. Other important prevention strategies include smoking cessation and prevention and/or treatment of oncogenic viruses' coinfections, such as HPV, HBV, HCV (13, 26). HPV plays an important etiologic role in genital SCC, so that the quadrivalent HPV vaccination has been strongly suggested (96). Generally, cancer therapy is chosen on the basis of location of primary disease, extension and spread and host comorbidities. Moreover, it depends on histology, lesion aspect, size and location, as well as patient compliance. BCC and SCC should be primarily treated with complete surgical excision (97) (see **Figure 5**).

Management of BCC remains primarily surgical (98), as in immunocompetent people. Management of SCC is influenced by clinical presentation (i.e., palpable lymph nodes) and histopathologic features. Generally, a full skin examination should be performed in all patients, followed by lymph node examination and by surgical and medical management involving a team of experts. It is important to extend the excision at least

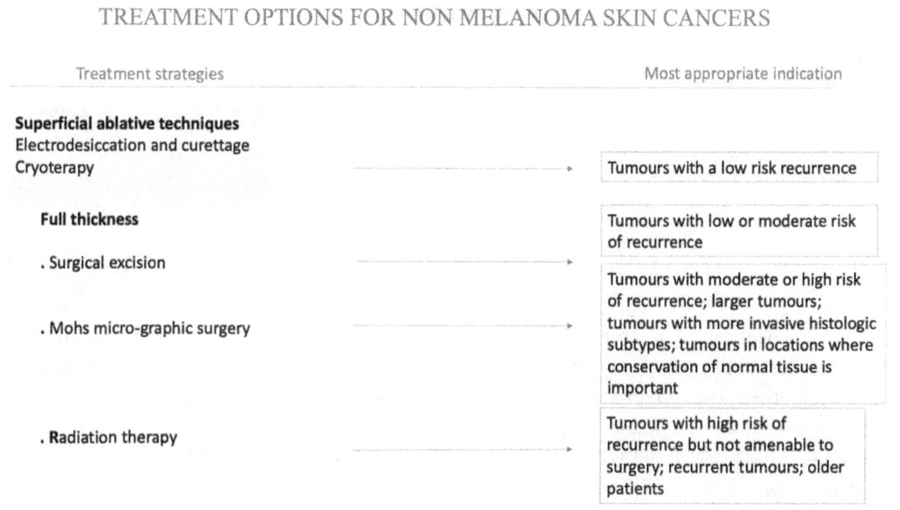

FIGURE 5 | Treatment options for NMSCs.

6 mm from the margins independently from the site whenever it is possible (98). Standard treatment should be applied to all PLWH with a newly diagnosed NMSCs (99); however, when combining cART with chemotherapy, potential drug-drug interactions and overlapping toxicities such as nausea and diarrhea, myelosuppression, neuropathies may occur (99). In case of overlapping toxicity occurs, it is recommendable to change cART or the chemotherapy agent rather than stopping the antiretroviral therapy or decreasing the dosage of chemotherapy (99). Many studies suggested that outcomes can be similar in PLWH with a good control of their infection and HIV negative people (100). However, PLWH with advanced disease show a poor tolerance of therapy and they more likely have worse outcomes compared with HIV negative individuals (101). In immunocompromised individual oral retinoids could be effective to reduce cancer load and to partially prevent the occurrence of new lesions. Unfortunately oral retinoids are teratogenic and that represent a limitation in their use (102). Morbidity and mortality of aggressive SCC in PLWH depend on the control of the disease in the early stages (92). People with higher risk cancers should receive loco regional adjunctive radiotherapy or chemotherapy or both and sentinel node procedures. These recommendations apply regardless of CD4 counts. There is no evidence that BCC in PLWH need more aggressive therapy. For example, Wilkins et al. recommend the use of the same treatment protocols for treatment of BCC even if there is no evidence for imiquimod for BCC in PLWH (91). Among factors influencing prognosis, any kind of immunocompromised patient present more rapid growth, an higher risk of local recurrence and metastasis, even 10 times higher (82). Intensity and duration of immunodeficiency plays a great role (103). Immunocompromised patients should be followed-up closely, at least twice a year (50). PLWH can die of a metastatic SCC, so the treatment of SCC in PLWH should never be less aggressive or prompt than the treatment of HIV

negative individuals. Concerning metastatic SCC, it is important to keep in mind that late treatment of high-risk SCC could lead to metastatic diseases especially in immunocompromised people. Moreover, perineural invasion is clearly linked to recurrence and higher risk of metastasis. Generally, the most chosen surgical option in these high-risk cases is Mohs surgery. But the presence of perineural invasion requires additional adjuvant therapy (104). Similarly, high-risk SCC in HIV infected patients should be treated initially by ablative therapy with histologic control and, if necessary, adjuvant therapy. A retrospective study of Nguyen has illustrated the potential for rapid growth of SCC in HIV infected people. An initial less aggressive therapeutical approach in PLWH is linked to higher rates of recurrence, metastasis and death. For this reason PLWH with SCC should receive a combination of surgery and radiotherapy or of surgery and radical neck dissection (92). NMSCs are a striking example of immunodeficiency-related neoplasm, and they offer further opportunities for therapeutic and pathogenetic insights. In fact, multiple clinical phenomena highlight the close correlation between immunity and skin cancers.

The main therapeutic techniques, superficial ablative and full thickness, for NMSCs will be broadly reviewed above (see **Table 1**).

Surgical Excision
Surgery is the treatment of choice. Depending on the affected area, it can be followed by plastic reconstruction. Moreover, histological examination of the excised tissues allows diagnosis, prognosis and treatment tailoring.

In SCC, surgical excision is immediately followed by histopathological examination of excision margins, which allows to confirm the cancer type and assess the absence of cancer cells from the resection margins. Another procedure to obtain the same result is micrographically controlled surgery

TABLE 1 | Classification of BCC according to risk for recurrence (105, 106).

LOW RISK	INTERMEDIATE RISK	HIGH RISK
Superficial primary BCC	Superficial recurrent BCC	Clinical forms: Morpheaform or ill-defined
Nodular primary BCC when:	Nodular primary BCC when:	Nodular primary BCC when:
<1 cm in intermediate risk area	<1 cm in high-risk area	>1 cm in high-risk area
<2 cm in low-risk area	>1 cm in intermediate risk area	
	>2 cm in low-risk area	
Pinkus tumor BCC		Histological forms:
		Aggressive
		Recurrent forms

(MCS). For low-risk NMSCs limited to dermis, traditional excision preferred (89). Aesthetically, excision offers better results than ablative techniques. Moreover, it offers the advantage of obtaining specimens for histologic examination. With surgery, cure rates are higher than 90%. It is neither recommended, nor cost-effective, storing frozen sections of tumor margins of every suspected NMSC. MMS is applied for recurrent tumors, tumors in high-risk areas, tumors ≥ 2 cm, recurrent tumors, tumors which margins are not clear and tumors in cosmetically sensitive areas (107). Wide removals should be done when margins are smaller than the recommended safety margins due to the tissue shrinkage, while re-excision should be done for operable cases in the event of positive margins (108). In the context of high-risk SCC, usefulness of a sentinel lymph node biopsy is still not clear (109). In fact, SCC does not invade deeper tissues as quickly as cutaneous malignant melanoma. The reason consists in absence of lymphatic drainage in superficial dermis and epidermis. Therefore, SCC is less likely to spread *via* lymphatics. There are still no guidelines about how to approach regional nodal disease in patients with SCC. Moreover, available directions are based on studies concerning head and neck mucosal SCC (110). Patients affected by metastases from SCC spread to lymph nodes should be treated surgically, as well as patients with melanoma or Merkel cell carcinoma. When surgery is not indicated, e.g., for patient-related factors, a nonsurgical approach by a multidisciplinary group should be evaluated.

Radiotherapy

Radiotherapy (RT) may be applied in an adjuvant setting, after surgical resection, in patients with high-risk features. A host factors as immunosuppression is considered by the American Joint Committee of Cancer (AJCC) as a risk for having a poorer outcome when diagnosed with NMSC. Obviously, the presence of other risk factors such as location, particularly ears and lips, poor differentiation and perineural invasion (PNI) can worsen outcomes. American Society for Radiation Oncology (ASTRO) guidelines recommends postoperative radiotherapy (PORT) in the setting of chronic immunosuppression (111).

Bimodality therapy (surgery and PORT) is used in the context of immune suppression, especially with head and neck cutaneous SCC. As a matter of fact, it frequently presents a lower outcome than immunocompetent patients, with a significantly lower progression-free survival at 2 years ($p = 0.002$) (112). When necessary, adjuvant RT should not be delayed. It is

demonstrated that exceeding a time of 6 weeks after the excision may worsen the prognosis (113). Irradiation volume must consider cancer location and risk factors, such as PNI, lymphatic and vascular invasion, to decide whether to include the first lymph node. The results of phase III TROG 05.01 trial (114) suggest no benefit in overall survival, disease free survival and locoregional relapse with the addition of weekly carboplatin to RT as adjuvant therapy.

RT is recommended as the only treatment modality in patients with NMSCs who cannot benefit from surgical resection. In fact, NMSCs can obtain an optimal local control because they are radio responsive carcinomas. Marconi et al. (115), using definitive RT, demonstrated that BCC had a 5- and 10-year local control of 96% and 94%, while for SCC 5- and 10-year control were 92% and 87%, respectively. It is important to keep in mind that in case of underlying genetic syndromes RT is discouraged because of higher radio-sensitivity in patients affected by Li-Fraumeni or Gorlin syndrome, ataxia telangiectasia. Furthermore, connective tissue disorders represent a contraindication to treatment whenever not under control (111).

Cryotherapy

Cryotherapy represents a therapeutic option for BCC, although tissue destruction is not perfectly targeted. It is based on two consecutive 30-second freeze-thaw cycles and is particularly effective on facial lesions, with a 95% cure rate (116).

Electrodesiccation and Curettage

Generally, these therapeutic options are considered only when assessing low-risk lesions. These techniques have a worse cosmetic yield than surgical excision, often ending in a round, hypopigmented and possibly hypertrophic scar (89). National Comprehensive cancer Network (NCCN) guidelines reported that curettage and electrodessication may be considered for small and low-risk primary SCC (117).

Chemotherapy

Systemic chemotherapy has a meaningful role in the management of local advanced and/or metastatic NMSC. Aggressive management with polychemotherapy should be considered for difficult to treat cases. Usually, mono-chemotherapy should be considered as a first-line treatment (50). Metastatic SCCs are notably difficult to treat, representing a challenge for clinicians. Platinum based chemotherapeutic agents, such as cisplatin or carboplatin, can be considered for local advanced and metastatic SCCs not amenable for surgical excision or radiotherapy. Other chemotherapeutic drugs, such as cyclophosphamide, bleomycin, doxorubicin, methotrexate and 5-FU, may also be used alone or in combination (118). However, guidelines for the use of classic chemotherapy in NMSC are based on low-level evidence, as the trials had several limitations, such as lack of randomization and heterogeneous patient populations. Recently, it has been highlighted that patients with stage I and II lip SCC can be successfully treated with monotherapy *via* superficial temporal artery administration of bleomycin, in order to obtain a cure in 70.8% of patients (119). Currently, chemotherapy is recommended in NCCN guidelines in a combination with radiotherapy, especially in localized, high-risk SCCs for patients who cannot undergo surgery (117). Before the advent of molecular target therapies, metastatic BCC had been treated with various conventional chemotherapeutic agents. However, metastatic BCC is rare, and the available literature about the effectiveness of these treatments is mostly episodic. In a short review collecting twelve elsewhere published cases treated with platinum, five showed complete response and four showed partial response (120).

Immunotherapy and Target Therapy of NMSCs: New Promising Neoadjuvant Therapy

Given actual evidence, targeted therapy and immunotherapy represent the frontiers in neoadjuvant therapy of NMSCs, being much more selective than traditional chemotherapy. Emerging clinical data (see **Table 2**) show that immunotherapy, particularly checkpoint inhibition, is a useful therapy option for advanced cSCC, while targeted therapy with sonic hedgehog pathway inhibitors results an effective treatment option for locally advanced or multiple BCC (121). The role of immune system has been linked to the occurrence of NMSCs by epidemiologic evidence that led to several studies about the immunology of NMSCs (122). These studies demonstrated the elevated number

of neoantigens expressed by NMSCs' cells that could represent the right target for a successful immune therapy. These kinds of observations have led to ongoing clinical trials based on novel immunotherapies of NMSCs as a neoadjuvant approach (123). By definition, a neoadjuvant approach aims to reduce the size of the tumor, before the subsequent potentially curative techniques. Immunotherapy acts by inhibiting immune checkpoints, eventually improving the activity of the immune system against the tumoral cells and reducing regulatory T cell-mediated immunosuppression. Unfortunately, these new treatment options appear quite expensive; moreover, immunotherapy can cause important and irreversible adverse effects (121). A thorough knowledge of SCC carcinogenesis is needed to develop new treatment approaches. The main immune checkpoints include CTLA-4, PD-1 and PD-L1, while sonic hedgehog pathway inhibitors include Vismodegib and Sonidegib, that we briefly describe above.

Anti-Programmed Cell Death Receptor-1 Immune Checkpoint Inhibitor
Cemiplimab
It is indicated for advanced or metastatic SCC in patients who are not amenable for surgery or radiotherapy. The phase I/II study (EMPOWER-CSCC-1) of patients with locally advanced or metastatic SCC has been the first trial that led to drug approval, producing a response rate of 47% in a cohort of 59 patients (124). Recently, this study led to the U.S. Food and Drug Administration approval of cemiplimab for locally advanced or metastatic SCC on September 28, 2018. The phase II clinical study of Cemiplimab in patients with advanced cutaneous SCC is ongoing and it is currently recruiting participants. (NCT02760498).

Another study (NCT03969004) is currently recruiting participants to study cemiplimab use in the adjuvant setting after surgery and radiation in patients with high risk of recurrence. Numerous ongoing clinical trials are studying the use of cemiplimab in patients with advanced BCC with a progression of disease while on Hedgehog pathway inhibitor therapy (125). Between them, the study (NCT03132636) is

TABLE 2 | Immune Checkpoint inhibitors.

Stage of disease	SCC	BCC
I	Nivolumab ± Ipilimumab(II)	N/A
II	Nivolumab ± Ipilimumab (II)	N/A
	Cemiplimab (II)	
III	Nivolumab ± Ipilimumab (II)	N/A
	Cemiplimab (II)	
IVA	Nivolumab ± Ipilimumab (II)	Nivolumab ± Ipilimumab (II)
	Avelumab (II)	
	Cemiplimab (II)	
	Pembrolizumab (II)	
IVB	Nivolumab (II)	Nivolumab ± Ipilimumab (II)
	Avelumab (II)	
	Cemiplimab (II)	
	Pembrolizumab (II)	

Immune Checkpoint inhibitors currently under investigation for the treatment of squamous cell carcinoma and basal cell carcinoma. Between brackets the phase of the study. SCC, squamous cell carcinoma; BCC, basal cell carcinoma; N/A, not applicable. Data extracted from https://clinicaltrials.gov/.

active, not recruiting. Another ongoing clinical trial is studying CTLA-4/PD-1 combinations, such as ipilimumab/nivolumab for treatment of advanced BCC. This study (NCT03521830) is currently recruiting participants with locally advanced or metastatic BCC.

Pembrolizumab

There are currently ongoing studies that are investigating the treatment of recurrent or metastatic cSCC (126). Between them, (NCT02964559) is an active study, not recruiting participants. It is also being evaluated in advanced SCC (NCT03284424), an active study, not recruiting for treatment of recurrent or metastatic cSCC.

Nivolumab

It is also being evaluated in advanced SCC: (NCT04204837) is an active study, not recruiting.

Anti-Programmed Cell Death Ligand-1

Avelumab

Several ongoing studies for advanced SCC are investigating avelumab with or without cetuximab (121). The study (NCT03944941) is currently open to enrollment. Another study, (NCT03737721) is currently recruiting participants with unresectable SCC treated with avelumab and radical radiotherapy. This study is called UNSCARRed study.

Atezolizumab

The study (NCT03108131) studies how cobimetinib/atezolizumab association works in treating participants with rare tumors that have spread to other places in the body (advanced) or that does not respond to treatment (refractory). This study is currently recruiting participants. Cobimetinib may block some of the enzymes involved in cell growth. So that, immunotherapy with monoclonal antibodies, such as atezolizumab, could interfere with the capability of tumor cells to grow and spread.

Cosibelimab

Cosibelimab is a fully human monoclonal antibody of IgG1 subtype that directly blocks its interactions with the Programmed Death-1 (PD-1) and B7.1 receptors (121). The study (NCT03212404), based on cosibelimab/atezolizumab association, is currently recruiting participants. The aim of this study is to assess the safety, tolerability and efficacy of CK-301 when administered intravenously as a single agent to subjects with recurrent or metastatic cancers.

Anti-Cytotoxic T-Lymphocyte-Associated Protein 4 Immune Checkpoint Inhibition

Ipilimumab

Emerging data showing ipilimumab use in SCC are limited to case reports. A patient with metastatic cSCC had a durable remission of both malignancies. Concerning BCC, there is an ongoing study regarding locally-advanced unresectable or metastatic BCC which investigates ipilimumab in association with nivolumab in one of the arms (NCT03521830) (127). This study is currently open to enrollment.

Hedgehog Pathway Inhibitors: Vismodegib and Sonidegib

Genetic and molecular studies have highlighted genetic mutations in the hedgehog signaling pathway characterize almost all BCCs. These alterations result in excessive activation leading to uncontrolled proliferation of basal cells. In addition, they determine loss of function of patched homologue 1 (PTCH1). PTCH1 blocks the signaling activity of smoothened homologue (SMO), a seven-transmembrane protein.

Vismodegib and sonidegib are two anti-tumor drugs targeting the HH pathway, called hedgehog pathway inhibitors (HPIs). Currently, there are no recommendations about when to prefer one molecule rather than the other. Moreover, these molecules have similar efficacy and tolerability, although they differ under a pharmacokinetic aspect (128). As a matter of fact, both are metabolized through cytochrome P450. Vismodegib is prevalently metabolized by CYP2C9, while sonidegib passes through CY3A4. Therefore, CYP3A4 inhibitors increases the blood concentration of sonidegib. Among them, ritonavir e saquinavir, two antiretroviral drugs. Whenever it is not possible to avoid the simultaneous use of sonidegib and strong inhibitors of CYP3A4, a dose reduction to sonidegib 200 mg every second day is recommended (129). Muscle spasms, alopecia, dysgeusia and weight loss are the most frequent side effects described in the literature. Of interest, many cases of SCC have been observed in patients treated with vismodegib for BCC therapy or single agent (BRAF) inhibitors, such as vemurafenib, for melanoma therapy (130).

All the current conventional treatments and ongoing trials are summarized in **Table 3**. Further studies are required to better understand the correct management of the drug, alternative dosing regimens and differences with the other HPIs.

Target Therapy in PLWH

Immunotherapy has paved new paths for treatment of HIV-related cancers and, thanks to monoclonal antibodies and immunomodulatory drugs, have shown to be effective in HIV-related cancers. In particular, the effectiveness of checkpoint inhibitors targeting the PD-1/PD-L1 pathway in the treatment of many malignancies in PLWH it has been suggested by recent data, hopefully stronger evidence on this matter will follow with the inclusion of PLWH in immune-oncology studies. Recently, ASCO and the Food and Drug Association (FDA) have provided guidance to include PLWH in clinical trials on neoplastic diseases.

A recent FDA-approved sonic hedgehog (SHH) signaling pathway inhibitor, Vismodegib, can be used to treat locally advanced, metastatic and recurrent BCCs that are inoperable and cannot be treated with radiotherapy, showing promising results (131). Although this molecule seems to be a safe option for those patients that cannot undergo surgery for advanced and metastatic BCC, in high-risk patients the optimal treatment protocol is unknown. The safety of Vismodegib in PLWH and its interactions with cART are not well known. Recently, Scalvenzi et al. have described a case-report of a HIV positive patient with an inoperable ulcerative BCC of the ear.

TABLE 3 | Conventional and New promising neoadjuvant therapies.

CONVENTIONAL THERAPY	
SURGICAL EXCISION	Generally adopted as **first step** for most NMSCs and it is considered a **potentially curative treatment**
RADIOTHERAPY	Effective non-surgical option and used in the **definitive, adjuvant and palliative settings**
CRYOTHERAPY	Reserved only for **low-risk lesions**
ELECTRODESICCATION AND CURETTAGE	Reserved only for **low-risk lesions**
CHEMIOTHERAPY	Topic mono-chemotherapy, e.g. with **5-fluorouracil** or **Imiquimod**, can be considered for **superficial lesions**
NEW PROMISING NEOADJUVANT THERAPY	
TARGETED THERAPY	Targeted therapy with sonic hedgehog pathway inhibitors is very effective in **locally advanced or**
-Sonic hedgehog pathway inhibitors: Vismodegib and Sonidegib	**multiple BCC.**
IMMUNOTHERAPY	Immunotherapy with immune checkpoint inhibitors appears to be promising for **advanced cutaneous**
- Anti-programmed cell death receptor-1 checkpoint inhibitor **(Anti PD-1)**	**SCC.** Several **ongoing clinical trials** are investigating their use. **Cemiplimab** is the only checkpoint inhibitor approved for locally advanced or metastatic cSCC.
- Anti-cytotoxic T-lymphocyte-associated protein 4 immune checkpoint inhibition **(Anti CTLA-4)**	
- Anti-programmed cell death ligand-1 **(Anti PD-L1)**	

Conventional and New promising neoadjuvant therapies. SCC, squamous cell carcinoma; cSCC, cutaneous squamous cell carcinoma; BCC, basal cell carcinoma.

After a specialistic evaluation also of the immune status (high CD4 T cell count) the patient started oral Vismodegib 150 mg daily. In about 6 months of therapy the patient obtained a complete resolution, after which Vismodegib was discontinued. The article reports good tolerance and no interactions between Vismodegib and the previous cART (132). Reports on SHH inhibitors in immunocompromised patients witch locally advanced or metastasizing BCC are rare (133). Effectual use of Vismodegib and the lack of drug to drug interaction with cART (tenofovir/emtricitabine/rilpivirine) has been described in a single case (132). Recently, Hoffmann V. et al. have described a successful case of treatment with Sonidegib in a patient on cART. However, it's mandatory to evaluate the risk of interactions between cART and antiblastic chemotherapy, target therapy and immunotherapy (134). In fact, it is true that the new antiretroviral drugs (135) are less toxic but they still have long-term side effects that need to be careful evaluated (136).

CONCLUSIONS AND FUTURE PERSPECTIVES

PLWH have an elevated propensity to develop cancers compared to the general population. It has been clearly shown that in this population immunosuppression and concomitant infection with oncogenic viruses play an important role. NMSCs are the most frequent cause of cutaneous malignancy in PLWH, and they represent a new oncologic challenge due increasing age of HIV-infected patients. In this paper, we tried to review the incidence of NMSCs among PLWH, any different clinical presentations of squamous cell and basal cell carcinoma between PLWH and HIV negative persons and any differences in efficacy and safety of treatments and response to immunomodulators (see **Table 4**). According to several authors ratios of BCC and SCC are similar between PLWH and HIV negative persons (4:1) (140), with BCC essentially more frequent than SCC. PLWH with NMSCs tend to

be younger, to have a higher risk of local recurrence and to have an overall poorer outcome. The main risk factors for NMSCs are similar to HIV negative individuals. Superficial BCC is the most frequent variant and is more often found on the trunk and in multiple lesions. SCC tends to be more aggressive in HIV infected people and it presents at significantly younger age, with higher risk of local recurrence and metastasis (141). The treatment of SCC in people with HIV should be at least aggressive as the treatment in HIV seronegative individuals. There is no strong evidence of how the depth of the immune compromision (CD4 counts) directly influence the risk of NMSCs, and this evidence supports mainly the risk of SCC rather than BCC. It is mandatory to suggest to PLWH a proper screening of all precancerous lesions besides a careful prevention with sun avoidance and use of sunscreen. Notably, there is a lack of official recommendation and guidelines on these subjects. Recently, Vismodegib and Sonidegib, two hedgehog signaling pathway inhibitors, have been approved to treat unresectable BCCs that are not amenable for surgery and radiotherapy. It is difficult to compare the efficacy of Sonidegib and Vismodegib due to the absence of trials designed to prove it and also because the first is only approved for locally advanced BCC while the last is also used for metastasizing BCC (128). It is time to answer to this lack of knowledge with appropriate trials that study the role of targeted therapy for BCC, in PLWH that result to be inoperable. The effectiveness of checkpoint inhibitors targeting the PD-1/PD-L1 pathway in the treatment of many malignancies in PLWH it has been suggested by recent data, hopefully stronger evidence on this matter will follow. In order to improve knowledge, PLWH must be included in immune-oncology studies. In conclusion, the treatment of advanced NMSC represents still an important challenge for clinician, mainly because of the lack of high-quality evidence and randomized trials. Further studies are required to focus on the

TABLE 4 | Synoptic picture with differences between PLWH and immunocompetent.

	GENERAL POPULATION	HIV POSITIVE PATIENTS
RATIOS BCC/SCC	4:1 (30)	4:1 (33)
MORE FREQUENT SUBTYPE OF BCC	Nodular (75)	Superficial (137)
PREVALENCE M/W	Slight male predilection (after age of 45 years) (138)	Increased risk of NMSC in both male and female patients (139)
AGE AT DIAGNOSIS	60 -70 years	Tendency to earlier age (~ 45 years) (83)
RISK FACTORS FOR DEVELOPMENT OF NMSCs	Chronic sun-exposure, fair phenotypic features, family history, older age, genetic mutations	The same as for general population plus immunodeficiency and coinfection with oncogenic viruses (83)
ANATOMIC DISTRIBUTION	Sun-exposed areas (more frequent on head and neck regions)	Trunk and extremities (generally lesions are multiple) (83)
CLINICAL COURSE	Usually indolent; nevertheless, metastatic forms lead to poor patient outcome	Generally more aggressive compared to the general population (83)
RISK METASTATIC DISEASE	Generally BCC shows minimal metastatic potential (88); SCC has a 4% annual incidence of metastatic disease (90)	Higher compared to the general population (83)
TREATMENT	**Full thickness Treatment** (93) Surgical excision Mohs micro-graphic surgery Radiotherapy **Superficial ablative techniques** **Targeted Therapy**	The same as standard of care for general population. However, it's mandatory to evaluate the risk of drug interactions (between cART and other treatments) (134)

best therapeutic approaches to NMSCs and mostly on the impact of cancer screening interventions among HIV-infected patients, in order to improve cancer diagnosis at an earlier stage. Further studies are needed to learn and apply pathogenetic insights to obtain new therapeutic options and correlate the degree of HIV-related immunodeficiency with disease outcome.

AUTHOR CONTRIBUTIONS

ER, MB, and GN designed the study. ER, MM, MB, and MC performed the screening of articles following the inclusion criteria. ER, MM, and FF wrote the article. CG, MB, and GN supervised the part of diagnosis and treatment. All authors contributed to the article and approved the submitted version.

REFERENCES

1. Venanzi Rullo E, Cannon L, Pinzone MR, Ceccarelli M, Nunnari G, O'Doherty U. Genetic Evidence That Naive T Cells Can Contribute Significantly to the Human Immunodeficiency Virus Intact Reservoir: Time to Re-Evaluate Their Role. *Clin Infect Dis* (2019) 69:2236–7. doi: 10.1093/cid/ciz378
2. Venanzi Rullo E, Pinzone MR, Cannon L, Weissman S, Ceccarelli M, Zurakowski R, et al. Persistence of an Intact HIV Reservoir in Phenotypically Naive T Cells. *JCI Insight* (2020) 5:105. doi: 10.1172/jci.insight.133157
3. Atteritano M, Mirarchi L, Venanzi Rullo E, Santoro D, Iaria C, Catalano A, et al. Vitamin D Status and the Relationship With Bone Fragility Fractures in HIV-Infected Patients: A Case Control Study. *Int J Mol Sci* (2018) 19 (1):119. doi: 10.3390/ijms19010119
4. Facciolà A, Venanzi Rullo E, Ceccarelli M, D'Andrea F, Coco M, Micali C, et al. Malignant Melanoma in HIV: Epidemiology, Pathogenesis, and Management. *Dermatol Ther* (2019) 33(1):e13180. doi: 10.1111/dth.13180
5. Facciolà A, Venanzi Rullo E, Ceccarelli M, D'Aleo F, Visalli G, Pinzone MR, et al. Hodgkin's Lymphoma in People Living With HIV: Epidemiology and Clinical Management. *World Cancer Res J* (2019) 6:e1295. doi: 10.32113/wcrj_20195_1295
6. D'Andrea F, Pellicanò GF, Venanzi Rullo E, Nunnari G, Ceccarelli M. Cervical Cancer in Women Living With HIV: A Review of the Literature. *World Cancer Res J* (2019) 6:1–6. doi: 10.32113/wcrj_20193_1224
7. D'Andrea F, Ceccarelli M, Facciolà A, Nunnari G, Pellicanò GF. Breast Cancer in Women Living With HIV. *Eur Rev Med Pharmacol Sci* (2019) 23:1158–64. doi: 10.26355/eurrev_201902_17007
8. Facciolà A, Ceccarelli M, Venanzi Rullo E, D'Aleo F, Condorelli F, Visalli G, et al. Prostate Cancer in HIV-Positive Patients- a Review of the Literature. *World Cancer Res J* (2018) 5:e1136. doi: 10.32113/wcrj_20189_1136
9. Visalli G, Facciolà A, D'Aleo F, Pinzone MR, Condorelli F, Picerno I, et al. HPV and Urinary Bladder Carcinoma: A Review of the Literature. *World Cancer Res J* (2018) 5:e1038. doi: 10.32113/wcrj_20183_1038
10. D'Aleo F, Cama BAV, Paolucci IA, Venanzi Rullo E, Condorelli F, Facciolà A, et al. New and Old Assumptions on Lung Cancer in People Living With HIV. *World Cancer Res J* (2018) 5:e1036. doi: 10.32113/wcrj_20183_1036
11. Ceccarelli M, Venanzi Rullo E, Facciolà A, Madeddu G, Cacopardo B, Taibi R, et al. Head and Neck Squamous Cell Carcinoma and Its Correlation With Human Papillomavirus in People Living With HIV: A Systematic Review. *Oncotarget* (2018) 9:17171–80. doi: 10.18632/oncotarget.24660
12. Ceccarelli M, Condorelli F, Venanzi Rullo E, Pellicanò GF. Improving Access and Adherence to Screening Tests for Cancers: A New, Though Old, Challenge in the HIV Epidemics. *World Cancer Res J* (2018) 5:e1030. doi: 10.1093/cid/ciu773
13. D'Andrea F, Ceccarelli M, Venanzi Rullo E, Facciolà A, D'Aleo F, Cacopardo B, et al. Cancer Screening in Hiv-Infected Patients: Early Diagnosis in a High-Risk Population. *World Cancer Res J* (2018) 5:e1130. doi: 10.32113/wcrj_20189_1130

14. D'Aleo F, Ceccarelli M, Facciolà A, Condorelli F, Pinzone MR, Cacopardo B, et al. HIV and Colorectal Cancer. New Insights and Review of the Literature. *World Cancer Res J* (2018) 5:e1122. doi: 10.32113/wcrj_20189_1122

15. Khazaei Z, Ghorat F, Jarrahi AM, Adineh A, Sohrabivafa M, Goodarzi E. Global Incidence and Mortality of Skin Cancer by Histological Subtype and Its Relationship With the Human Development Index (HDI) - An Ecology Study in 2018. *World Cancer Res J* (2019) 6:1–14. doi: 10.4103/AIHB.AIHB_2_19

16. Ceccarelli M, Venanzi Rullo E, Vaccaro M, Facciolà A, D'Aleo F, Paolucci IA, et al. HIV-Associated Psoriasis: Epidemiology, Pathogenesis, and Management. *Dermatol Ther* (2018) 32(2):e12806. doi: 10.1111/dth.12806

17. Berretta M, Martellotta F, Di Francia R, Spina M, Vaccher E, Balestreri L, et al. Clinical Presentation and Outcome of Non-AIDS Defining Cancers, in HIV-Infected Patients in the ART-Era: The Italian Cooperative Group on AIDS and Tumors Activity. *Eur Rev Med Pharmacol Sci* (2015) 19:3619–34.

18. La Ferla L, Pinzone MR, Nunnari G, Martellotta F, Lleshi A, Tirelli U, et al. Kaposi's Sarcoma in HIV-Positive Patients: The State of Art in the HAART-Era. *Eur Rev Med Pharmacol Sci* (2013) 17:2354–65.

19. Martellotta F, Berretta M, Cacopardo B, Fisichella R, Schioppa O, Zanghì A, et al. Clinical Presentation and Outcome of Squamous Cell Carcinoma of the Anus in HIV-Infected Patients in the HAART-Era: A GICAT Experience. *Eur Rev Med Pharmacol Sci* (2012) 16:1283–91.

20. Berretta M, Garlassi E, Cacopardo B, Cappellani A, Guaraldi G, Cocchi S, et al. Hepatocellular Carcinoma in HIV-Infected Patients: Check Early, Treat Hard. *Oncologist* (2011) 16:1258–69. doi: 10.1634/theoncologist.2010-0400

21. Simonelli C, Tedeschi R, Gloghini A, Talamini R, Bortolin MT, Berretta M, et al. Plasma HHV-8 Viral Load in HHV-8-Related Lymphoproliferative Disorders Associated With HIV Infection. *J Med Virol* (2009) 81:888–96. doi: 10.1002/jmv.21349

22. Zanet E, Berretta M, Benedetto FD, Talamini R, Ballarin R, Nunnari G, et al. Pancreatic Cancer in HIV-Positive Patients. *Pancreas* (2012) 41:1331–5. doi: 10.1097/MPA.0b013e31824a0e40

23. Ceccarelli M, Venanzi Rullo E, Marino MA, D'Aleo F, Pellicanò GF, D'Andrea F, et al. Non-AIDS Defining Cancers: A Comprehensive Update on Diagnosis and Management. *Eur Rev Med Pharmacol Sci* (2020) 24:3849–75. doi: 10.26355/eurrev_202004_20852

24. Ceccarelli M, Facciolà A, Taibi R, Pellicanò GF, Nunnari G, Venanzi Rullo E. The Treatment of Kaposi's Sarcoma: Present and Future Options, A Review of the Literature. *Eur Rev Med Pharmacol Sci* (2019) 23:7488–97. doi: 10.26355/eurrev_201909_18860

25. Guarneri C, Tchernev G, Bevelacqua V, Lotti T, Nunnari G. The Unwelcome Trio: HIV Plus Cutaneous and Visceral Leishmaniasis. *Dermatol Ther* (2016) 29:88–91. doi: 10.1111/dth.12303

26. D'Aleo F, Ceccarelli M, Venanzi Rullo E, Pellicanò GF, Nunnari G. Anal Cancer in People Living With HIV: The Importance of the Screening and of Early Diagnosis. *World Cancer Res J* (2019) 6:1–9. doi: 10.32113/wcrj_20196_1319

27. Leiter U, Eigentler T, Garbe C. Epidemiology of Skin Cancer. In: *Advances in Experimental Medicine and Biology*. New York, NY: Springer (2014). p. 120–40. doi: 10.1007/978-1-4939-0437-2_7

28. Eide MJ, Krajenta R, Johnson D, Long JJ, Jacobsen G, Asgari MM, et al. Identification of Patients With Nonmelanoma Skin Cancer Using Health Maintenance Organization Claims Data. *Am J Epidemiol* (2010) 171:123–8. doi: 10.1093/aje/kwp352

29. Bray F, Ferlay J, Soerjomataram I, Siegel RL, Torre LA, Jemal A. Global Cancer Statistics 2018: GLOBOCAN Estimates of Incidence and Mortality Worldwide for 36 Cancers in 185 Countries. *CA Cancer J Clin* (2018) 68:394–424. doi: 10.3322/caac.21492

30. Kaira PS, Han J, Schmults CD. Cutaneous Squamous Cell Carcinoma: Estimated Incidence of Disease, Nodal Metastasis, and Deaths From Disease in the United States. *J Am Acad Dermatol* (2012) 2013) 68:957–66. doi: 10.1016/j.jaad.2012.11.037

31. Engels EA, Pfeiffer RM, Goedert JJ, Virgo P, McNeel TS, Scoppa SM, et al. Trends in Cancer Risk Among People With AIDS in the United States 1980-2002. *AIDS* (2006) 20:1645–54. doi: 10.1097/01.aids.0000238411.75324.59

32. Palella FJ, Delaney KM, Moorman AC, Loveless MO, Fuhrer J, Satten GA, et al. Declining Morbidity and Mortality Among Patients With Advanced Human Immunodeficiency Virus Infection. *N Engl J Med* (1998) 338:853–60. doi: 10.1056/NEJM199803263381301

33. Chang AY, Doiron P, Maurer T. Cutaneous Malignancies in HIV. *Curr Opin HIV AIDS* (2017) 12:57–62. doi: 10.1097/COH.0000000000000338

34. Nunnari G, Berretta M, Pinzone MR, Di Rosa M, Berretta S, Cunsolo G, et al. Hepatocellular Carcinoma in HIV Positive Patients. *Eur Rev Med Pharmacol Sci* (2012) 16:1257–70.

35. Omland SH, Ahlström MG, Gerstoft J, Pedersen G, Mohey R, Pedersen C, et al. Risk of Skin Cancer in Patients With HIV: a Danish Nationwide Cohort Study. *J Am Acad Dermatol* (2018) 79:689–95. doi: 10.1016/j.jaad.2018.03.024

36. Clifford GM, Polesel J, Rickenbach Mon behalf of the Swiss HIV Cohort Study, , Dal Maso L, Keiser O, et al. Cancer Risk in the Swiss HIV Cohort Study: Associations With Immunodeficiency, Smoking, and Highly Active Antiretroviral Therapy. *JNCI J Natl Cancer Inst* (2005) 97:425–32. doi: 10.1093/jnci/dji072

37. Silverberg MJ, Leyden W, Warton EM, Quesenberry CP, Engels EA, Asgari MM. HIV Infection Status, Immunodeficiency, and the Incidence of Non-Melanoma Skin Cancer. *J Natl Cancer Inst* (2013) 105:350–60. doi: 10.1093/jnci/djs529

38. Chiu CS, Lin CY, Kuo TT, Kuan YZ, Chen MJ, Ho HC, et al. Malignant Cutaneous Tumors of the Scalp: A Study of Demographic Characteristics and Histologic Distributions of 398 Taiwanese Patients. *J Am Acad Dermatol* (2007) 56:448–52. doi: 10.1016/j.jaad.2006.08.060

39. Fahradyan A, Howell AC, Wolfswinkel EM, Tsuha M, Sheth P, Wong AK. Updates on the Management of Non-Melanoma Skin Cancer (NMSC). *Healthcare (Basel)* (2017) 5:82. doi: 10.3390/healthcare5040082

40. Harwood CA, Toland AE, Proby CM, Euvrard S, Hofbauer GFL, Tommasino M, et al. The Pathogenesis of Cutaneous Squamous Cell Carcinoma in Organ Transplant Recipients. *Br J Dermatol* (2017) 177:1217–24. doi: 10.1111/bjd.15956

41. Jambusaria-Pahlajani A, Kanetsky PA, Karia PS, Hwang W-T, Gelfand JM, Whalen FM, et al. Evaluation of AJCC Tumor Staging for Cutaneous Squamous Cell Carcinoma and a Proposed Alternative Tumor Staging System. *JAMA Dermatol* (2013) 149:402–10. doi: 10.1001/jamadermatol.2013.2456

42. Lang PG, Braun MA, Kwatra R. Aggressive Squamous Carcinomas of the Scalp. *Dermatol Surg* (2006) 32:1163–70. doi: 10.1111/j.1524-4725.2006.32258.x

43. Gupta SK, Sandhir RK, Jaiswal AK, Kumar S. Marjolin's Ulcer of the Scalp Invading Calvarial Bone, Dura and Brain. *J Clin Neurosci* (2005) 12:693–5. doi: 10.1016/j.jocn.2004.08.030

44. Zanetti R, Rosso S, Martinez C, Navarro C, Schraub S, SanchoGarnier H, et al. The Multicentre South European Study "Helios".1. Skin Characteristics and Sunburns in Basal Cell and Squamous Cell Carcinomas of the Skin. *Br J Cancer* (1996) 73:1440–6. doi: 10.1038/bjc.1996.274

45. Saladi RN, Persaud AN. The Causes of Skin Cancer: a Comprehensive Review. *Drugs Today (Barc)* (2005) 41:37–53. doi: 10.1358/dot.2005.41.1.875777

46. Karagas MR, Nelson HH, Zens MS, Linet M, Stukel TA, Spencer S, et al. Squamous Cell and Basal Cell Carcinoma of the Skin in Relation to Radiation Therapy and Potential Modification of Risk by Sun Exposure. *Epidemiology* (2007) 18:776–84. doi: 10.1097/EDE.0b013e3181567ebe

47. Kaae J, Boyd HA, Hansen AV, Wulf HC, Wohlfahrt J, Melbye M. Photosensitizing Medication Use and Risk of Skin Cancer. *Cancer Epidemiol Biomarkers Prev* (2010) 19:2942–9. doi: 10.1158/1055-9965.EPI-10-0652

48. Pellegrini C, Maturo MG, Di Nardo L, Ciciarelli V, Gutiérrez García-Rodrigo C, Fargnoli MC. Understanding the Molecular Genetics of Basal Cell Carcinoma. *Int J Mol Sci* (2017) 18(11):2485. doi: 10.3390/ijms18112485

49. Bresler SC, Padwa BL, Granter SR. Nevoid Basal Cell Carcinoma Syndrome (Gorlin Syndrome). *Head Neck Pathol* (2016) 10:119–24. doi: 10.1007/s12105-016-0706-9

50. Stratigos A, Garbe C, Lebbe C, Malvehy J, del Marmol V, Pehamberger H, et al. Diagnosis and Treatment of Invasive Squamous Cell Carcinoma of the Skin: European Consensus-Based Interdisciplinary Guideline. *Eur J Cancer* (2015) 51:1989–2007. doi: 10.1016/j.ejca.2015.06.110

51. Ventura A, Pellegrini C, Cardelli L, Rocco T, Ciciarelli V, Peris K, et al. Telomeres and Telomerase in Cutaneous Squamous Cell Carcinoma. *Int J Mol Sci* (2019) 20(6):1333. doi: 10.3390/ijms20061333

52. Martincorena I, Roshan A, Gerstung M, Ellis P, Van Loo P, McLaren S, et al. High Burden and Pervasive Positive Selection of Somatic Mutations in Normal Human Skin. *Science* (2015) 348:880–6. doi: 10.1126/science.aaa6806

53. Muehleisen B, Jiang SB, Gladsjo JA, Gerber M, Hata T, Gallo RL. Distinct Innate Immune Gene Expression Profiles in Non-Melanoma Skin Cancer of Immunocompetent and Immunosuppressed Patients. *PloS One* (2012) 7: e40754. doi: 10.1371/journal.pone.0040754

54. Akira S, Hemmi H. Recognition of Pathogen-Associated Molecular Patterns by TLR Family. *Immunol Lett* (2003) 85:85–95. doi: 10.1016/s0165-2478(02) 00228-6

55. Eiró N, Ovies C, Fernandez-Garcia B, Álvarez-Cuesta CC, González L, González LO, et al. Expression of TLR3, 4, 7 and 9 in Cutaneous Malignant Melanoma: Relationship With Clinicopathological Characteristics and Prognosis. *Arch Dermatol Res* (2013) 305:59–67. doi: 10.1007/s00403-012-1300-y

56. Gupta AK, Cherman AM, Tyring SK. Viral and Nonviral Uses of Imiquimod: A Review. *J Cutan Med Surg* (2004) 8:338–52. doi: 10.1007/s10227-005-0023-5

57. Kutikhin AG. Association of Polymorphisms in TLR Genes and in Genes of the Toll-Like Receptor Signaling Pathway With Cancer Risk. *Hum Immunol* (2011) 72:1095–116. doi: 10.1016/j.humimm.2011.07.307

58. Russo I, Cona C, Saponeri A, Bassetto F, Baldo V, Alaibac M. Association Between Toll-Like Receptor 7 Gln11leu Single-Nucleotide Polymorphism and Basal Cell Carcinoma. *BioMed Rep* (2016) 4:459–62. doi: 10.3892/br.2016.597

59. Malaponte G, Hafsi S, Polesel J, Castellano G, Spessotto P, Guarneri C, et al. Tumor Microenvironment in Diffuse Large B-Cell Lymphoma: Matrixmetalloproteinases Activation Is Mediated by Osteopontin Overexpression. *Biochim Biophys Acta* (2016) 1863:483–9. doi: 10.1016/j.bbamcr.2015.09.018

60. Dotto GP, Rustgi AK. Squamous Cell Cancers: A Unified Perspective on Biology and Genetics. *Cancer Cell* (2016) 29:622–37. doi: 10.1016/j.ccell.2016.04.004

61. Euvrard S, Kanitakis J, Claudy A. Skin Cancers After Organ Transplantation. *N Engl J Med* (2003) 348:1681–91. doi: 10.1056/NEJMra022137

62. Vinay DS, Ryan EP, Pawelec G, Talib WH, Stagg J, Elkord E, et al. Immune Evasion in Cancer: Mechanistic Basis and Therapeutic Strategies. *Semin Cancer Biol* (2015) 35 Suppl:S185–98. doi: 10.1016/j.semcancer.2015.03.004

63. Lindström LS, Yip B, Lichtenstein P, Pawitan Y, Czene K. Etiology of Familial Aggregation in Melanoma and Squamous Cell Carcinoma of the Skin. *Cancer Epidemiol Biomarkers Prev* (2007) 16:1639–43. doi: 10.1158/1055-9965.EPI-07-0047

64. Al-Rohil RN, Tarasen AJ, Carlson JA, Wang K, Johnson A, Yelensky R, et al. Evaluation of 122 Advanced-Stage Cutaneous Squamous Cell Carcinomas by Comprehensive Genomic Profiling Opens the Door for New Routes to Targeted Therapies. *Cancer* (2016) 122:249–57. doi: 10.1002/cncr.29738

65. Hernandez-Ramirez RU, Shiels MS, Dubrow R, Engels EA. Cancer Risk in HIV-Infected People in the USA From 1996 to 2012: A Population-Based, Registry-Linkage Study. *Lancet HIV* (2017) 4:E495–504. doi: 10.1016/S2352-3018(17)30125-X

66. Pope M, Betjes M, Romani N, Hirmand H, Cameron P, Hoffman L, et al. Conjugates of Dendritic Cells and Memory T-Lymphocytes From Skin Facilitate Productive Infection With HIV-1. *Cell* (1994) 78:389–98. doi: 10.1016/0092-8674(94)90418-9

67. Gordin FM, Hartigan PM, Klimas NG, Zollapazner SB, Simberkoff MS, Hamilton JD. Delayed-Type Hypersensitivity Skin-Tests Are an Independent Predictor of Human-Immunodeficiency-Virus Disease Progression. *J Infect Dis* (1994) 169:893–7. doi: 10.1093/infdis/169.4.893

68. Guo H-G, Pati S, Sadowska M, Charurat M, Reitz M. Tumorigenesis by Human Herpesvirus 8 vGPCR Is Accelerated by Human Immunodeficiency Virus Type 1 Tat. *J Virol* (2004) 78:9336–42. doi: 10.1128/JVI.78.17.9336-9342.2004

69. Li CJ, Wang C, Friedman DJ, Pardee AB. Reciprocal Modulations Between P53 and Tat of Human Immunodeficiency Virus Type 1. *Proc Natl Acad Sci* (1995) 92:5461–4. doi: 10.1073/pnas.92.12.5461

70. Wistuba II, Behrens C, Milchgrub S, Virmani AK, Jagirdar J, Thomas B, et al. Comparison of Molecular Changes in Lung Cancers in HIV-Positive and HIV-Indeterminate Subjects. *JAMA* (1998) 279:1554–9. doi: 10.1001/jama.279.19.1554

71. Corallini A, Campioni D, Rossi C, Albini A, Possati L, Rusnati M, et al. Promotion of Tumour Metastases and Induction of Angiogenesis by Native HIV-1 Tat Protein From BK Virus/Tat Transgenic Mice. *AIDS* (1996) 10:701–10. doi: 10.1097/00002030-199606001-00003

72. Burgi A, Brodine S, Wegner S, Milazzo M, Wallace MR, Spooner K, et al. Incidence and Risk Factors for the Occurrence of Non-AIDS-Defining Cancers Among Human Immunodeficiency Virus-Infected Individuals. *Cancer* (2005) 104:1505–11. doi: 10.1002/cncr.21334

73. Tedeschi R, Caggiari L, Silins I, Kallings I, Andersson-Ellstrom A, De Paoli P, et al. Seropositivity to Human Herpesvirus 8 in Relation to Sexual History and Risk of Sexually Transmitted Infections Among Women. *Int J Cancer* (2000) 87:232–5. doi: 10.1002/1097-0215(20000715)87:2<232::AID-IJC13>3.0.CO;2-T

74. Berretta M, Cinelli R, Martellotta F, Spina M, Vaccher E, Tirelli U. Therapeutic Approaches to AIDS-Related Malignancies. *Oncogene* (2003) 22:6646–59. doi: 10.1038/sj.onc.1206771

75. Di Stefani A, Chimenti S. Basal Cell Carcinoma: Clinical and Pathological Features. *G Ital Dermatol Venereol* (2015) 150:385–91.

76. Puoti M, Bruno R, Soriano V, Donato F, Gaeta GB, Quinzan GP, et al. Hepatocellular Carcinoma in HIV-Infected Patients: Epidemiological Features, Clinical Presentation and Outcome. *AIDS* (2004) 18:2285–93. doi: 10.1097/00002030-200411190-00009

77. D'Andrea F, Venanzi Rullo E, Marino A, Moscatt V, Celesia BM, Cacopardo B, et al. Hepatitis B Virus Infection and Hepatocellular Carcinoma in PLWH: Epidemiology, Pathogenesis and Treatment. *World Cancer Res J* (2020) 7:e1537. doi: 10.32113/wcrj_20203_1537

78. D'Aleo F, Ceccarelli M, Facciolà A, Di Rosa M, Pinzone MR, Condorelli F, et al. Hepatitis C-Related Hepatocellular Carcinoma: Diagnostic and Therapeutic Management in HIV-Patients. *Eur Rev Med Pharmacol Sci* (2017) 21:5859–67. doi: 10.26355/eurrev_201712_14035

79. D'Andrea F, Venanzi Rullo E, Facciolà A, Di Rosa M, Condorelli F, Marino A, et al. Epstein Barr Virus Related Cancer in People Living With HIV: A Review of the Literature. *World Cancer Res J* (2020) 7:e1512. doi: 10.32113/wcrj_20203_1512

80. Arron ST, Ruby JG, Dybbro E, Ganem D, Derisi JL. Transcriptome Sequencing Demonstrates That Human Papillomavirus Is Not Active in Cutaneous Squamous Cell Carcinoma. *J Invest Dermatol* (2011) 131:1745–53. doi: 10.1038/jid.2011.91

81. Wang J, Aldabagh B, Yu J, Arron ST. Role of Human Papillomavirus in Cutaneous Squamous Cell Carcinoma: A Meta-Analysis. *J Am Acad Dermatol* (2014) 70:621–9. doi: 10.1016/j.jaad.2014.01.857

82. Euvrard S, Kanitakis J, Claudy A. Skin Cancers After Organ Transplantation - Reply. *N Engl J Med* (2003) 349:613–4. doi: 10.1056/NEJM200308073490618

83. Wilkins K, Turner R, Dolev JC, LeBoit PE, Berger TG, Maurer TA. Cutaneous Malignancy and Human Immunodeficiency Virus Disease. *J Am Acad Dermatol* (2006) 54:189–206. doi: 10.1016/j.jaad.2004.11.060

84. Crum-Cianflone N, Hullsiek KH, Satter E, Marconi V, Weintrob A, Ganesan A, et al. Cutaneous Malignancies Among HIV-Infected Persons. *Arch Intern Med* (2009) 169:1130–8. doi: 10.1001/archinternmed.2009.104

85. Grulich AE, van Leeuwen MT, Falster MO, Vajdic CM. Incidence of Cancers in People With HIV/AIDS Compared With Immunosuppressed Transplant Recipients: A Meta-Analysis. *Lancet* (2007) 370:59–67. doi: 10.1016/S0140-6736(07)61050-2

86. Asgari MM, Ray GT, Quesenberry CP, Katz KA, Silverberg MJ. Association of Multiple Primary Skin Cancers With Human Immunodeficiency Virus Infection, CD4 Count, and Viral Load. *JAMA Dermatol* (2017) 153:892–6. doi: 10.1001/jamadermatol.2017.1716

87. Coates SJ, Leslie KS. What's New in HIV Dermatology? *F1000Res* (2019) 8: F1000. doi: 10.12688/f1000research.16182.1

88. Stulberg DL, Crandell B, Fawcett RS. Diagnosis and Treatment of Basal Cell and Squamous Cell Carcinomas. *Am Fam Phys* (2004) 70:1481–8.

89. Netscher DT, Leong M, Orengo I, Yang D, Berg C, Krishnan B. Cutaneous Malignancies: Melanoma and Nonmelanoma Types. *Plast Reconstruct Surg* (2011) 127:37e–56e. doi: 10.1097/PRS.0b013e318206352b

90. Toll A, Margalef P, Masferrer E, Ferrándiz-Pulido C, Gimeno J, Pujol RM, et al. Active Nuclear IKK Correlates With Metastatic Risk in Cutaneous Squamous Cell Carcinoma. *Arch Dermatol Res* (2015) 307:721–9. doi: 10.1007/s00403-015-1579-6

91. Wilkins K, Dolev JC, Turner R, LeBoit PE, Berger TG, Maurer TA. Approach to the Treatment of Cutaneous Malignancy in HIV-Infected Patients. *Dermatol Ther* (2005) 18:77–86. doi: 10.1111/j.1529-8019.2005.05003.x

92. Nguyen P, Vin-Christian K, Ming ME, Berger T. Aggressive Squamous Cell Carcinomas in Persons Infected With the Human Immunodeficiency Virus. *Arch Dermatol* (2002) 138:758–63. doi: 10.1001/archderm.138.6.758

93. Otley CC. Immunosuppression and Skin Cancer - Pathogenetic Insights, Therapeutic Challenges, and Opportunities for Innovation. *Arch Dermatol* (2002) 138:827–8. doi: 10.1001/archderm.138.6.827

94. Neves-Motta R, De Almeida Ferry FR, Basílio-De-Oliveira CA, De Souza Carvalho R, Martins CJ, Eyer-Silva WA, et al. Highly Aggressive Squamous Cell Carcinoma in an HIV-Infected Patient. *Rev Soc Bras Med Trop* (2004) 37:496–8. doi: 10.1590/S0037-86822004000600013

95. Olson AL, Gaffney CA, Starr P, Dietrich AJ. The Impact of an Appearance-Based Educational Intervention on Adolescent Intention to Use Sunscreen. *Health Educ Res* (2008) 23:763–9. doi: 10.1093/her/cym005

96. Reusser NM, Downing C, Guidry J, Tyring SK. HPV Carcinomas in Immunocompromised Patients. *J Clin Med* (2015) 4:260–81. doi: 10.3390/jcm4020260

97. Alam M, Armstrong A, Baum C, Bordeaux JS, Brown M, Busam KJ, et al. Guidelines of Care for the Management of Cutaneous Squamous Cell Carcinoma. *J Am Acad Dermatol* (2018) 78:560–78. doi: 10.1016/j.jaad.2017.10.007

98. Bejar C, Basset-Seguin N, Faure F, Fieschi C, Frances C, Guenne C, et al. French ENT Society (SFORL) Guidelines for the Management of Immunodeficient Patients With Head and Neck Cancer of Cutaneous Origin. *Eur Ann Otorhinolaryngol Head Neck Dis* (2014) 131:121–9. doi: 10.1016/j.anorl.2014.02.002

99. Deeken JF, Tjen-A-Looi A, Rudek MA, Okuliar C, Young M, Little RF, et al. The Rising Challenge of Non-AIDS-Defining Cancers in HIV-Infected Patients. *Clin Infect Dis* (2012) 55:1228–35. doi: 10.1093/cid/cis613

100. Blazy A, Hennequin C, Gornet J-M, Furco A, Gérard L, Lémann M, et al. Anal Carcinomas in HIV-Positive Patients: High-Dose Chemoradiotherapy Is Feasible in the Era of Highly Active Antiretroviral Therapy. *Dis Colon Rectum* (2005) 48:1176–81. doi: 10.1007/s10350-004-0910-7

101. Biggar RJ, Kirby KA, Atkinson T, McNeel TS, Engels E, Grp ACMS. Cancer Risk in Elderly Persons With HIV/AIDS. *JAIDS J Acquir Immune Defic Syndr* (2004) 36:861–8. doi: 10.1097/00126334-200407010-00014

102. Hofbauer GF, Anliker M, Arnold A, Binet I, Hunger R, Kempf W, et al. Swiss Clinical Practice Guidelines for Skin Cancer in Organ Transplant Recipients. *Swiss Med Wkly* (2009) 139(29–30):407–15. doi: 10.5167/uzh-25639

103. Euvrard S, Kanitakis J, Pouteilnoble C, Dureau G, Touraine J, Faure M, et al. Comparative Epidemiologic-Study of Premalignant and Malignant Epithelial Cutaneous Lesions Developing After Kidney and Heart-Transplantation. *J Am Acad Dermatol* (1995) 33:222–9. doi: 10.1016/0190-9622(95)90239-2

104. Hochman M, Lang P. Skin Cancer of the Head and Neck. *Med Clin North Am* (1999) 83:261–. doi: 10.1016/s0025-7125(05)70101-2

105. Trakatelli M, Morton C, Nagore E, Ulrich C, Del Marmol V, Peris K, et al. Update of the European Guidelines for Basal Cell Carcinoma Management. *Eur J Dermatol* (2014) 24(3):312–29. doi: 10.1684/ejd.2014.2271

106. Dandurand T, Petit P, Martel P, Guillot B. Management of Basal Cell Carcinoma in Adults Clinical Practice Guidelines. *Eur J Dermatol* (2006) 16(4):394–401.

107. Rowe DE. Comparison of Treatment Modalities for Basal Cell Carcinoma. *Clin Dermatol* (1995) 13:617–20. doi: 10.1016/0738-081x(95)00067-p

108. Stratigos AJ, Garbe C, Dessinioti C, Lebbe C, Bataille V, Bastholt L, et al. European Interdisciplinary Guideline on Invasive Squamous Cell Carcinoma of the Skin: Part 2. Treatment. *Eur J Cancer* (2020) 128:83–102. doi: 10.1016/j.ejca.2020.01.008

109. Reschly MJ, Messina JL, Zaulyanov LL, Cruse W, Fenske NA. Utility of Sentinel Lymphadenectomy in the Management of Patients With High-Risk Cutaneous Squamous Cell Carcinoma. *Dermatol Surg* (2003) 29:135–40. doi: 10.1046/j.1524-4725.2003.29035.x

110. Veness MJ, Morgan GJ, Palme CE, Gebski V. Surgery and Adjuvant Radiotherapy in Patients With Cutaneous Head and Neck Squamous Cell Carcinoma Metastatic to Lymph Nodes: Combined Treatment Should be Considered Best Practice. *Laryngoscope* (2005) 115:870–5. doi: 10.1097/01.MLG.0000158349.64337.ED

111. Likhacheva A, Awan M, Barker CA, Bhatnagar A, Bradfield L, Brady MS, et al. Definitive and Postoperative Radiation Therapy for Basal and Squamous Cell Cancers of the Skin: Executive Summary of an American Society for Radiation Oncology Clinical Practice Guideline. *Pract Radiat Oncol* (2020) 10:8–20. doi: 10.1016/j.prro.2019.10.014

112. Manyam BV, Garsa AA, Chin R-I, Reddy CA, Gastman B, Thorstad W, et al. A Multi-Institutional Comparison of Outcomes of Immunosuppressed and Immunocompetent Patients Treated With Surgery and Radiation Therapy for Cutaneous Squamous Cell Carcinoma of the Head and Neck. *Cancer* (2017) 123:2054–60. doi: 10.1002/cncr.30601

113. Babington S, Veness MJ, Cakir B, Gebski VJ, Morgan GJ. Squamous Cell Carcinoma of the Lip: Is There a Role for Adjuvant Radiotherapy in Improving Local Control Following Incomplete or Inadequate Excision? *ANZ J Surg* (2003) 73:621–5. doi: 10.1046/j.1445-2197.2003.t01-1-02710.x

114. Porceddu SV, Bressel M, Poulsen MG, Stoneley A, Veness MJ, Kenny LM, et al. Postoperative Concurrent Chemoradiotherapy Versus Postoperative Radiotherapy in High-Risk Cutaneous Squamous Cell Carcinoma of the Head and Neck: The Randomized Phase III TROG 05.01 Trial. *J Clin Oncol* (2018) 36:1275–83. doi: 10.1200/JCO.2017.77.0941

115. Grossi Marconi D, da Costa Resende B, Rauber E, de Cassia Soares P, Fernandes JM, Mehta N, et al. Head and Neck Non-Melanoma Skin Cancer Treated By Superficial X-Ray Therapy: An Analysis of 1021 Cases. *PloS One* (2016) 11:e0156544. doi: 10.1371/journal.pone.0156544

116. Mallon E, Dawber R. Cryosurgery in the Treatment of Basal Cell Carcinoma - Assessment of One and Two Freeze-Thaw Cycle Schedules. *Dermatol Surg* (1996) 22:854–8. doi: 10.1111/j.1524-4725.1996.tb00588.x

117. Miller SJ. The National Comprehensive Cancer Network (NCCN) Guidelines of Care for Nonmelanoma Skin Cancers. *Dermatol Surg* (2000) 26:289–92. doi: 10.1111/j.1524-4725.2000.00005.x

118. Amaral T, Garbe C. Non-Melanoma Skin Cancer: New and Future Synthetic Drug Treatments. *Expert Opin Pharmacother* (2017) 18:689–99. doi: 10.1080/14656566.2017.1316372

119. Cheraghi N, Cognetta AJ, Goldberg D. Radiation Therapy in Dermatology: Non-Melanoma Skin Cancer. *J Drugs Dermatol* (2017) 16:464–9.

120. Carneiro B, Watkin W, Mehta U, Brockstein B. Metastatic Basal Cell Carcinoma: Complete Response to Chemotherapy and Associated Pure Red Cell Aplasia. *Cancer Invest* (2006) 24:396–400. doi: 10.1080/07357900600705474

121. Zelin E, Zalaudek I, Agozzino M, Dianzani C, Dri A, Di Meo N, et al. Neoadjuvant Therapy for Non-Melanoma Skin Cancer: Updated Therapeutic Approaches for Basal, Squamous, and Merkel Cell Carcinoma. *Curr Treat Options Oncol* (2021) 22:35. doi: 10.1007/s11864-021-00826-3

122. Yanik EL, Pfeiffer RM, Freedman DM, Weinstock MA, Cahoon EK, Arron ST, et al. Spectrum of Immune-Related Conditions Associated With Risk of Keratinocyte Cancers Among Elderly Adults in the United States. *Cancer Epidemiol Biomarkers Prev* (2017) 26:998–1007. doi: 10.1158/1055-9965.EPI-17-0003

123. Hall ET, Fernandez-Lopez E, Silk AW, Dummer R, Bhatia S. Immunologic Characteristics of Nonmelanoma Skin Cancers: Implications for Immunotherapy. *Am Soc Clin Oncol Educ Book* (2020) 40:1–10. doi: 10.1200/EDBK_278953

124. Migden MR, Rischin D, Schmults CD, Guminski A, Hauschild A, Lewis KD, et al. PD-1 Blockade With Cemiplimab in Advanced Cutaneous Squamous-Cell Carcinoma. *N Engl J Med* (2018) 379:341–51. doi: 10.1056/NEJMoa1805131

125. Falchook GS, Leidner R, Stankevich E, Piening B, Bifulco C, Lowy I, et al. Responses of Metastatic Basal Cell and Cutaneous Squamous Cell Carcinomas to Anti-PD1 Monoclonal Antibody REGN2810. *J Immunother Cancer* (2016) 4:70. doi: 10.1186/s40425-016-0176-3

126. Chang ALS, Tran DC, Cannon JGD, Li S, Jeng M, Patel R, et al. Pembrolizumab for Advanced Basal Cell Carcinoma: An Investigator-Initiated, Proof-of-Concept Study. *J Am Acad Dermatol* (2019) 80:564–6. doi: 10.1016/j.jaad.2018.08.017

127. Mohan SV, Kuo KY, Chang ALS. Incidental Regression of an Advanced Basal Cell Carcinoma After Ipilimumab Exposure for Metastatic Melanoma. *JAAD Case Rep* (2016) 2:13–5. doi: 10.1016/j.jdcr.2015.11.007

128. Dummer R, Ascierto PA, Basset-Seguin N, Dréno B, Garbe C, Gutzmer R, et al. Sonidegib and Vismodegib in the Treatment of Patients With Locally Advanced Basal Cell Carcinoma: A Joint Expert Opinion. *J Eur Acad Dermatol Venereol* (2020) 34:1944–56. doi: 10.1111/jdv.16230

129. Hoffmann V, Husak R, Maiwirth F, Sasama B, Zahn A, Guski S, et al. Sonidegib in a Patient With Multiple Basal Cell Carcinomas and HIV Infection. *J Dtsch Dermatol Ges* (2021) 19(4):592–4. doi: 10.1111/ddg.14355

130. Peng L, Wang Y, Hong Y, Ye X, Shi P, Zhang J, et al. Incidence and Relative Risk of Cutaneous Squamous Cell Carcinoma With Single-Agent BRAF Inhibitor and Dual BRAF/MEK Inhibitors in Cancer Patients: A Meta-Analysis. *Oncotarget* (2017) 8:83280–91. doi: 10.18632/oncotarget.21059

131. Sekulic A, Migden MR, Oro AE, Dirix L, Lewis KD, Hainsworth JD, et al. Efficacy and Safety of Vismodegib in Advanced Basal-Cell Carcinoma. *N Engl J Med* (2012) 366:2171–9. doi: 10.1056/NEJMoa1113713

132. Scalvenzi M, Villani A, Mazzella C, Cappello M, Salvatores GDF, Costa C. Vismodegib Treatment in a HIV Positive Patient on Antiretroviral Therapy. *Indian J Dermatol Venereol Leprol* (2018) 84:758–60. doi: 10.4103/ijdvl.IJDVL_92_18

133. Tran AQ, Patete CL, Blessing NW, Rong AJ, Garcia AL, Dubovy S, et al. Orbito-Scleral-Sinus Invasion of Basal Cell Carcinoma in an Immunocompromised Patient on Vismodegib. *Orbit* (2021) 40:155–8. doi: 10.1080/01676830.2020.1753783

134. Berretta M, Caraglia M, Martellotta F, Zappavigna S, Lombardi A, Fierro C, et al. Drug-Drug Interactions Based on Pharmacogenetic Profile between Highly Active Antiretroviral Therapy and Antiblastic Chemotherapy in Cancer Patients with HIV Infection. *Front Pharmacol* (2016) 7:71. doi: 10.3389/fphar.2016.00071

135. Venanzi Rullo E, Ceccarelli M, Condorelli F, Facciolà A, Visalli G, D'Aleo F, et al. Investigational Drugs in HIV: Pros and Cons of Entry and Fusion Inhibitors (Review). *Mol Med Rep* (2019) 19(3):1987–95. doi: 10.3892/mmr.2019.9840

136. Pinzone MR, Ceccarelli M, Venanzi Rullo E, Maresca M, Bruno R, Condorelli F, et al. Circulating Angiopoietin-Like Protein 2 Levels Are Associated With Decreased Renal Function in HIV+ Subjects on cART: A Potential Marker of Kidney Disease. *BioMed Rep* (2019) 10:140–4. doi: 10.3892/br.2019.1183

137. Cullen R, Hasbún P, Campos-Villenas M. Carcinoma Basocelular Superficial. *Med Clin* (2017) 149:140. doi: 10.1016/j.medcli.2016.10.017

138. Apalla Z, Calzavara-Pinton P, Lallas A, Argenziano G, Kyrgidis A, Crotti S, et al. Histopathological Study of Perilesional Skin in Patients Diagnosed With Nonmelanoma Skin Cancer. *Clin Exp Dermatol* (2016) 41:21–5. doi: 10.1111/ced.12713

139. Zhao H, Shu G, Wang S. The Risk of Non-Melanoma Skin Cancer in HIV-Infected Patients: New Data and Meta-Analysis. *Int J STD AIDS* (2016) 27:568–75. doi: 10.1177/0956462415586316

140. Garlassi E, Harding V, Weir J, Francis N, Nelson M, Newsom-Davis T, et al. Nonmelanoma Skin Cancers Among HIV-Infected Persons in the HAART Era. *J Acquir Immune Defic Syndr* (2012) 60:e63–5. doi: 10.1097/QAI.0b013e318251b004

141. Berretta M, Lleshi A, Zanet E, Bearz A, Simonelli C, Fisichella R, et al. Bevacizumab Plus Irinotecan-, Fluorouracil-, and Leucovorin-Based Chemotherapy With Concomitant HAART in an HIV-Positive Patient With Metastatic Colorectal Cancer. *Onkologie* (2008) 31:394–7. doi: 10.1159/000132360

Research Interest and Public Interest in Melanoma: A Bibliometric and Google Trends Analysis

Hanlin Zhang[†‡], Yuanzhuo Wang[†‡], Qingyue Zheng[†], Keyun Tang[†], Rouyu Fang[†], Yuchen Wang[†] and Qiuning Sun[*†]

Department of Dermatology, Peking Union Medical College Hospital, Chinese Academy of Medical Sciences, Peking Union Medical College, Beijing, China

*Correspondence:
Qiuning Sun
doctorjenny1@163.com

†ORCID:
Hanlin Zhang
orcid.org/0000-0001-5065-4086
Yuanzhuo Wang
orcid.org/0000-0002-1940-9741
Qingyue Zheng
orcid.org/0000-0003-4503-3423
Keyun Tang
orcid.org/0000-0002-5128-2648
Rouyu Fang
orcid.org/0000-0002-9224-8163
Yuchen Wang
orcid.org/0000-0002-1507-0701
Qiuning Sun
orcid.org/0000-0002-1912-341X

‡These authors have contributed
equally to this work and share first
authorship

Introduction: Melanoma is a severe skin cancer that metastasizes quickly. Bibliometric analysis can quantify hotspots of research interest. Google Trends can provide information to address public concerns.

Methods: The top 15 most frequently cited articles on melanoma each year from 2015 to 2019, according to annual citations, were retrieved from the Web of Science database. Original articles, reviews, and research letters were included in this research. For the Google Trends analysis, the topic "Melanoma" was selected as the keyword. Online search data from 2004 to 2019 were collected. Four countries (New Zealand, Australia, the United States and the United Kingdom) were selected for seasonal analysis. Annual trends in relative search volume and seasonal variation were analyzed, and the top related topics and rising related topics were also selected and analyzed.

Results: The top 15 most frequently cited articles each year were all original articles that focused on immunotherapy (n=8), omics (n=5), and the microbiome (n=2). The average relative search volume remained relatively stable across the years. The seasonal variation analysis revealed that the peak appeared in summer, and the valley appeared in winter. The diseases associated with or manifestations of melanoma, treatment options, risk factors, diagnostic tools, and prognosis were the topics in which the public was most interested. Most of the topics revealed by bibliometric and Google Trends analyses were consistent, with the exception of issues related to the molecular biology of melanoma.

Conclusion: This study revealed the trends in research interest and public interest in melanoma, which may pave the way for further research.

Keywords: melanoma, bibliometric analysis, Google Trends, research interest, public interest

INTRODUCTION

Melanoma is a severe skin cancer that metastasizes quickly. Cutaneous melanoma causes 55,000 deaths each year, and once the disease spreads, it rapidly becomes life-threatening (1). Cases of cutaneous melanoma account for approximately 1.7% of all newly diagnosed cases of primary malignant cancers (1). The incidence and mortality rate of melanoma vary around the world. Fair-skinned populations are particularly prone to melanoma, and the incidence of melanoma is the highest in New Zealand and Australia (2). Exposure to ultraviolet radiation, number of atypical moles, and genetic background are common risk factors for melanoma (3).

Bibliometric analysis is a method used to quantify hot topics and research interest in the research community (4–6). Bibliometric analysis can provide physicians and investigators with crucial messages in a specific field. A thorough bibliometric analysis of the most frequently cited articles may facilitate an understanding of disciplinary development and future directions of a research field (7, 8). Google Trends is a commonly used tool for addressing online health issues. Infodemiological methods using Google Trends can estimate the epidemiological characteristics, explore the public interest, and monitor the dynamic variations in infectious diseases (9). Previously, some studies demonstrated positive correlations between the online search frequency of "melanoma" and that of its risk factors (10–12). However, McDonald and Bloom reported negative results on the association between the search index and the incidence of melanoma (13, 14).

Compared to bibliometric analysis, which provides information on research interest, Google Trends analysis provides information on public interest. Physicians and investigators should know not only the hotspots of scientific research on melanoma but also the issues of interest for the general public. This study aimed to update the topics of research interest and public interest in melanoma using bibliometric and Google Trends analyses and compare the similarities and differences, which may pave the way for further research.

METHODS

Bibliometric Analysis

We analyzed the top 15 most frequently cited articles on melanoma each year from 2015 to 2019 according to the bibliometric analysis method. These publications were retrieved from the Web of Science in descending order according to their numbers of annual citations. Two researchers (H. Zhang and Y. Wang) independently screened the abstracts and reached a consensus on the qualifying papers. Articles focusing on multiple diseases, conference articles, patents, comments, or case reports were all excluded. Original articles, reviews, and research letters were all included in this research.

Search Tool and Keyword Selection

Online search data were collected from Google Trends. Google Trends provided an index, namely, the relative search volume (RSV), to facilitate comparisons between terms, times, and locations. The RSV was restricted to a range from 0 to 100. An RSV of 100 represented the highest search count in a given period (weeks, months, or years), and the search counts were proportionally assigned lower numbers in other periods. For example, an RSV of 50 indicates that half as many searches were performed in the selected period compared to the searches

indicated by an RSV of 100 (15). An RSV of 0 did not necessarily indicate 0 searches but may represent an extremely low search count compared to other periods (16). Google Trends also automatically adjusted the RSV based on population sizes to allow a comparison between populated areas and underpopulated areas (17).

The keywords were selected under the instruction of a previous guideline (18). Words or short phrases that were specific and not prone to be confused with other words or short phrases were preferable. Google Trends provided two types of query modes. One mode was the "Terms," which could be combined for exhaustive search, but the results would only be shown in the given language. The other type was "Topics," which were defined as groups of terms that shared the same concept in any language. This mode also included related searches in non-English speaking countries and might contain the most associated information (16). The mesh words of PubMed only provided "melanomas" for possible synonyms or homonyms of "melanoma" and allowed us to compare the two types of query modes by inputting different patterns of keywords, including "melanoma" alone as a term or topic, "melanomas" alone as a term, and "melanoma + melanomas" as a combination of terms in Google Trends. Both tests yielded similar fluctuations and patterns, but the topic "melanoma" produced the highest RSV. Therefore, the topic "Melanoma" was selected as the keyword in this study.

Data Query

The "Health" category was chosen to exclude unrelated information. The time range was set from January 2004 to December 2019. On 1 September 2020, the RSV data were exported to Microsoft Excel 2019. Four English-speaking countries with high RSVs were selected for seasonal variation analysis. Two countries (the United Kingdom and the United States) were located in the Northern Hemisphere, and the other two countries (Australia and New Zealand) were located in the Southern Hemisphere.

Google Trends Analysis

Topics related to the search term were also extracted from Google Trends to analyze the public interest. Google Trends provided two types of related topics: "Top related topics" and "Rising related topics." "Top related topics" are defined as the most frequently searched topics within the chosen category, time, or country. "Rising related topics" are topics with high RSV growth and are presented as a percentage of fold changes. We queried the "Top related topics" and "Rising related topics" each year from 2014 to 2019 globally to analyze the variation in the public interest over time. The results were manually examined by two searchers (H. Zhang and Y. Wang) to exclude irrelevant information.

Statistical Analysis

R software (v 3.6.2) was used for statistical analysis and plotting graphs. A diagram was plotted using the "plot" function in R to observe the trend in the annual average RSV. A cosinor model was applied for seasonal analysis according to Barnett's research

(19). Boxplots of the seasonal variation for different countries were plotted by the "season" package in R. A p-value < 0.05 was considered statistically significant.

Ethical Requirements

This study did not involve animal experiments or clinical trials. Thus, permission from the ethical committee was not needed.

RESULTS

Bibliometric Analysis

Table 1 shows the 15 top articles on melanoma with the most annual citations from 2015 to 2019. Seven articles were published in 2015, three were published in 2016, three were published in 2017, and two were published in 2018 (20–34). The annual number of citations of these articles ranged from 167.0 to 485.0, with a median of 212.6 (170.8, 283.5). Seven of the articles were published in the *New England Journal of Medicine*, followed by *Science* (n = 4), *Cell* (n = 2), *Nature* (n = 1), and *Lancet Oncology* (n=1). All of the articles were original articles. These articles were

then classified into three different research focuses: immunotherapy (n = 8), omics (n = 5), and microbiome (n = 2).

Annual trends and seasonal variation in Google Trends

The annual trends for the RSV of melanoma in Google Trends are shown in **Figure 1A**. The maximum value appeared in June 2005, and the minimum value was observed in December 2012. The average RSV remained relatively stable across the years. The seasonal variation curve fit with the "cosinor" model for the RSV is shown in **Figure 1B** (p-value < 0.05). The analysis revealed that the peak RSV of melanoma occurred in summer (January for Australia and New Zealand and June for the United States and the United Kingdom) and the valley occurred in winter (July for Australia and New Zealand and December for the United States and the United Kingdom).

Related Topics

Topics related to melanoma from 2004 to 2019 are summarized in **Table 2**. Regarding the top related topics, "Skin" was the most related (RSV = 100), followed by "Skin cancer" (RSV = 70),

---

TABLE 1 | List of the top 15 most frequently cited articles on melanoma from 2015 to 2019.

Title	Year of publication	Article type	Research focus	Journal of publication	Total citations	Annual citations	Rank by annual citations
Nivolumab in Previously Untreated Melanoma without BRAF Mutation	2015	Original article	Immunotherapy	New England Journal of Medicine	2910	485	1
Pembrolizumab versus Ipilimumab in Advanced Melanoma	2015	Original article	Immunotherapy	New England Journal of Medicine	2783	463.83	2
Gut Microbiome Modulates Response to Anti-PD-1 Immunotherapy in Melanoma Patients	2018	Original article	Microbiome	Science	888	296	3
Overall Survival with Combined Nivolumab and Ipilimumab in Advanced Melanoma	2017	Original article	Immunotherapy	New England Journal of Medicine	1134	283.5	4
Nivolumab and Ipilimumab versus Ipilimumab in Untreated Melanoma	2015	Original article	Immunotherapy	New England Journal of Medicine	1618	269.67	5
Nivolumab versus Chemotherapy in Patients with Advanced Melanoma Who Progressed after Anti-CTLA-4 Treatment (CheckMate 037): a Randomised, Controlled, Open-label, Phase 3 trial	2015	Original article	Immunotherapy	Lancet Oncology	1474	245.67	6
Improved Overall Survival in Melanoma with Combined Dabrafenib and Trametinib	2015	Original article	Immunotherapy	New England Journal of Medicine	1277	212.83	7
Mutations Associated with Acquired Resistance to PD-1 Blockade in Melanoma	2016	Original article	Omics	New England Journal of Medicine	1063	212.6	8
An Immunogenic Personal Neoantigen Vaccine for Patients with Melanoma	2017	Original article	Immunotherapy	Nature	752	188	9
The Commensal Microbiome is Associated with Anti-PD-1 Efficacy in Metastatic Melanoma Patients	2018	Original article	Microbiome	Science	558	186	10
Genomic Classification of Cutaneous Melanoma	2015	Original article	Omics	Cell	1110	185	11
Genomic and Transcriptomic Features of Response to Anti-PD-1 Therapy in Metastatic Melanoma	2016	Original article	Omics	Cell	854	170.8	12
Adjuvant Nivolumab versus Ipilimumab in Resected Stage III or IV Melanoma	2017	Original article	Immunotherapy	New England Journal of Medicine	679	169.75	13
Genomic Correlates of Response to CTLA-4 Blockade in Metastatic Melanoma	2015	Original article	Omics	Science	1005	167.5	14
Dissecting the Multicellular Ecosystem of Metastatic Melanoma by Single-cell RNA-seq	2016	Original article	Omics	Science	835	167	15

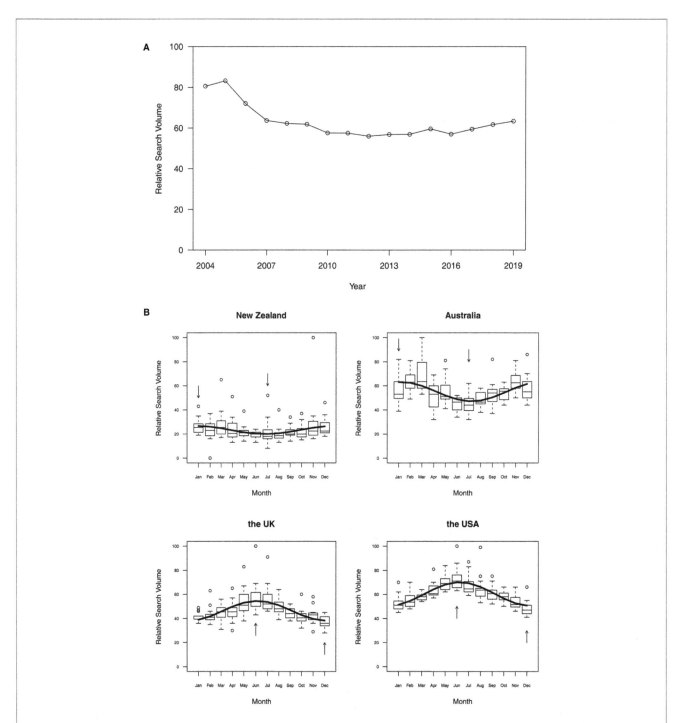

FIGURE 1 | Annual trends **(A)** and seasonal variation **(B)** of the relative search volume on melanoma. a. Annual trends from 2004 to 2019. **(B)** Seasonal variation in New Zealand, Australia, the United Kingdom, and the United States. **(A)** The lines represent the overall trend of RSV variation, and the circles represent the data points of the 12-month average RSV for each year. **(B)** The seasonal analysis was conducted and fit by the cosinor model with a p-value < 0.05. The arrows indicate the extreme value of the 16-year average RSV. (Box: interquartile range (IQR). The horizontal line inside each box: median. Whisker: maximum and minimum within median ± 1.5 × IQR. Circle: outlier outside 1.5 IQR.)

"Metastasis" (RSV = 34), "Melanocytic nevus" (RSV = 32), "Nevus" (RSV = 25), "Basal-cell carcinoma" (RSV = 16), "Prognosis" (RSV = 11), "Squamous cell carcinoma" (RSV = 10), and others. Melanoma mostly originates from the skin and represents a crucial kind of metastatic skin cancer that has a poor prognosis and is difficult to distinguish from benign melanocytic nevus or other metastatic lesions, including basal cell carcinoma and squamous cell carcinoma. Regarding the rising related topics, pathological genes and monoclonal antibodies, including "BRAF," "Ipilimumab," "Nivolumab," "Pembrolizumab," and "Vemurafenib," exhibited an

TABLE 2 | Top related and rising related topics on melanoma from 2004 to 2019.

Top related topics	Relative search volume	Rising related topics	Fold changes
Skin	100	BRAF	Breakout*
Skin cancer	70	Ipilimumab	Breakout*
Metastasis	34	Nivolumab	Breakout*
Melanocytic nevus	32	Pembrolizumab	Breakout*
Nevus	25	Vemurafenib	Breakout*
Basal-cell carcinoma	16	Squamous cell carcinoma	500%
Prognosis	11	Cancer staging	500%
Squamous cell carcinoma	10	Basal-cell carcinoma	400%
Survival rate	8	Melanocytic nevus	350%
Carcinoma	7	Nevus	250%
Malignancy	7	Skin	250%
Cancer staging	7	Carcinoma	200%
Melanin	7	Skin cancer	190%
BRAF	5	Metastasis	170%
Ipilimumab	3	Malignancy	150%
Nivolumab	3	Prognosis	120%
Pembrolizumab	2	Survival rate	110%
Vemurafenib	2		

*Breakout means an increase of over 5000%.

TABLE 3 | Annual topics related to melanoma from 2004 to 2019.

Year	Top related topics	Relative search volume	Rising related topics	Fold Changes
2004	Skin	100	Basal-cell carcinoma	Breakout*
	Skin cancer	73	Melanin	Breakout*
	Metastasis	28	Prognosis	Breakout*
2005	Skin	100	Birthmark	Breakout*
	Skin cancer	79	Kaposi's sarcoma	Breakout*
	Metastasis	30	Lymphadenectomy	Breakout*
2006	Skin	100	Melanosis	Breakout*
	Skin cancer	84	Dacarbazine	160%
	Melanocytic nevus	30	American Joint Committee on Cancer	160%
2007	Skin	100	American Joint Committee on Cancer	Breakout*
	Skin cancer	80	Dermatoscopy	Breakout*
	Metastasis	34	Freckle	250%
2008	Skin	100	Sarcoma	200%
	Skin cancer	71	Immunotherapy	180%
	Metastasis	30	Survival rate	90%
2009	Skin	100	BRAF	300%
	Skin cancer	70	Sun tanning	130%
	Metastasis	37	Dermatoscopy	120%
2010	Skin	100	Ipilimumab	400%
	Skin cancer	74	Freckle	200%
	Metastasis	33	BRAF	180%
2011	Skin	100	Melancholia	Breakout*
	Skin cancer	74	Vemurafenib	170%
	Metastasis	35	Lentigo	90%
2012	Skin	100	Mohs surgery	120%
	Skin cancer	68	Melanosis	60%
	Metastasis	36	Liver spot	60%
2013	Skin	100	Programmed cell death protein 1	300%
	Skin cancer	70	Dermatoscopy	60%
	Metastasis	34	Cell culture	60%
2014	Skin	100	Pembrolizumab	350%
	Skin cancer	70	Nivolumab	180%
	Metastasis	35	Immunotherapy	120%
2015	Skin	100	Bob Marley	150%
	Skin cancer	81	Nivolumab	150%
	Metastasis	34	Pembrolizumab	120%
2016	Skin	100	Immunotherapy	70%
	Skin cancer	75	Liver spot	50%
	Metastasis	35	Dermatoscopy	50%
2017	Skin	100	American Joint Committee on Cancer	100%
	Skin cancer	62	Melasma	90%
	Melanocytic nevus	32	Exeresis	70%
2018	Skin	100	Subungual hematoma	50%
	Skin cancer	66	Relapse	50%
	Metastasis	33	Eye neoplasm	50%
2019	Skin	100	Vulvar cancer	90%
	Skin cancer	62	Stadion	40%
	Metastasis	28	Dysplastic nevus	40%

*Breakout means an increase of over 5000%.

increase over 5,000%, followed by associated diseases, including the topics "Squamous cell carcinoma" (n = 500%), "Basal-cell carcinoma" (n = 400%), "Melanocytic nevus" (n = 350%), and "Nevus" (n = 250%). Prognosis factors, including "Cancer staging" (n = 500%), "Metastasis" (n = 170%), "Malignancy" (n = 150%) and "Survival rate" (n = 110%), also attracted attention.

Annual Related Topics

The annual related topics are also compared in **Table 3** to identify the trends of the public interest over time. The top related topics each year were consistent with the above results. "Skin," "Skin cancer," "Metastasis," and "Melanocytic nevus" were the only four top related topics during the 16-year interval that had nearly stable ranks, which reflected the search habits of the population. In contrast, 36 rising related topics during this period were identified and showed different emphases across the years. To facilitate comprehension, we summarized the frequency of occurrence and then classified them into several subgroups.

The diseases associated with or manifestations of melanoma appeared most frequently (17/48, 35.4%), including the terms "Freckle," "Liver spot," and "Melanosis" (2/48, 4.2%), followed by "Basal-cell carcinoma," "Birthmark," "Dysplastic nevus," "Eye neoplasm," "Kaposi's sarcoma," "Lentigo," "Melancholia," "Melasma," "Sarcoma," "Subungual hematoma," and "Vulvar cancer" (1/48, 2.1%). Treatment options (13/48, 27.1%) included "Immunotherapy" (3/48, 6.3%), "Nivolumab," "Pembrolizumab" (2/48, 4.2%), "Dacarbazine," "Exeresis," "Ipilimumab," "Lymphadenectomy," "Mohs surgery," and "Vemurafenib" (1/ 48, 2.1%). Risk factors (5/48, 10.4%), such as the terms "BRAF" (2/48, 4.2%), "Programmed cell death protein 1," "Sun tanning," and "Melanin" (1/48, 2.1%), also attracted attention. Diagnostic tools (5/48, 10.4%) and prognosis (3/48, 6.3%) of melanoma, such as "Dermatoscopy" (4/48, 8.3%), "Cell culture," "Relapse,"

"Prognosis," and "Survival rate" (1/48, 2.1%), also accounted for small portions of the annual rising related topics. Other topics (5/ 48, 10.4%) included the "American Joint Committee on Cancer" (3/48, 6.3%); and "Bob Marley" (1/48, 2.1%), who was a celebrity who died of melanoma; and "Stadion" (1/48, 2.1%), which had little relationship with melanoma.

DISCUSSION

This study updated the topics of research interest and public interest related to melanoma and provided physicians and investigators with a detailed description of the hot issues in which scientists and the public are interested. Google Trends data are a powerful tool to monitor and evaluate public interest in melanoma. The combination of Google Trends and bibliometric analysis may allow researchers to better anticipate research interests to serve melanoma patients.

Using bibliometric analysis, we determined the 15 most frequently cited articles on melanoma with the high numbers of annual citations published from 2015 to 2019. Using annual citations instead of the total citations as bibliometric parameters for ranking yielded benefits because this ranking included newly published articles that can provide emerging insights in the analysis (35). Our analysis indicated that the majority of these articles were published in the *New England Journal of Medicine*, followed by *Science, Cell, Nature,* and *Lancet Oncology*, which could be attributed to the high quality of these journals or the inherent bias with which researchers tend to select high impact factor journals for citations (36, 37). All the publications were original articles, reflecting the substantial demand of the community for revolutionary innovation and discoveries related to melanoma. The average numbers of citations of these most frequently cited articles were dramatically higher than those of other bibliometric analysis studies, such as those on rosacea (8), oral lichen planus (38), or psoriatic arthritis (38). This phenomenon reflects a high degree of research interest regarding melanoma. In addition, the articles were all classic with more than 400 citations, even for the articles published in 2018, showing the impact of the literature (8, 39).

Eight of the 15 annual most frequently cited articles were about immunotherapies, such as anti-PD1 therapies (33), nivolumab, or ipilimumab treatment (25), and nivolumab treatment in patients without BRAF mutations (27). The molecular mechanisms and the star genes that the immunotherapeutic drugs targeted, including the "Programmed cell death protein 1" (PD-1) and "B-Raf proto-oncogene" (BRAF), generated research interest (40–42). PD-1 is an immune checkpoint molecule expressed on tumor cells that inhibits CD8+ T cells and induces adaptive immune inhibition (43). PD-1 inhibitors, including "Nivolumab" and "Pembrolizumab," have been demonstrated to show clinical activities in melanoma (44). BRAF mutations were found in approximately 60% of melanomas (45), and the inhibitors "Vemurafenib" and "Dabrafenib" were proven to be efficient in melanoma patients with the mutation (46, 47).

Furthermore, researchers might focus on other topics to provide new insights into melanoma that the public might not know. Examples include omics analysis and microbiome analysis. Genomic studies have identified activating driver mutations that stimulate the development of targeted therapies for patients (48). The overall mutational load, neoantigen load, and expression of cytolytic markers in the immune microenvironment were significantly associated with clinical benefits (29). In addition, the commensal microbiome might

have a mechanistic impact on antitumor immunity in melanoma patients (23). The results suggested that patients with a favorable gut microbiome might express enhanced systemic and antitumor immunity (21).

Google Trends was particularly helpful in monitoring health information-seeking behavior and analyzing public interest. The results showed that the global average RSV for melanoma was relatively stable across the years, illustrating the continued attention given by the public to melanoma (49). Regarding seasonal analysis, in Australia and New Zealand, the peak RSV appeared in January (summer). During that time, the incidence of melanoma is predominantly high in those countries (50), and previous research has demonstrated the correlation between the RSV of sun tanning and melanoma (51). Risk factors for melanoma, including exposure to sunshine, lighter clothing, and even sun tanning, might be responsible for this result (52, 53). The health prevention campaign in Australia also promisingly reduced the rates of indoor tanning among young adults and thus helped to decrease the incidence (54). For countries in the Northern Hemisphere, such as the United States and the United Kingdom, the peak RSV appeared in June (summer), and the educational campaign of public awareness month for skin cancers in May might be responsible for increasing the RSV (55).

The related topics illustrated the most concerning themes for the public. The top related topics were defined as the most frequently searched topics within the chosen category, time, or country. As a type of cancer, melanoma mostly originates from the skin; the terms "Skin," "Skin cancer," and "Metastasis" were reasonably ranked in the top 3 related topics. The differential diagnosis of melanoma from other diseases such as "Melanocytic nevus" and "nevus" also attracted attention. Even senior dermatologists had some difficulties in recognizing malignant features to distinguish melanoma from nevus in dermoscopic images (56), and the involvement of artificial intelligence in dermatology liberated dermatologists and made some contributions to solving the problem (57). The terms "Basal cell carcinoma" and "Squamous cell carcinoma" refer to common malignant tumors in the United States and hence have become hot topics (58). "Malignancy," "Prognosis," "Relapse," and "Survival rate" might be the most concerning topics for the patients and appeared in the list.

The rising related topics are of newly emerged public interest. The results marked "Breakout" represent tremendous increases of over 5,000% compared with the previous search, probably representing the rapid development of these topics. Immunotherapies are in the spotlight in this era. The systemic treatment of melanoma has completely changed since the first introduction of ipilimumab in 2011 (59). In less than 10 years, over 10 drugs have been proven or are being proven effective for treating unresectable melanoma and dramatically increase the predicted survival time of patients (60). A review recently summarized the historically published articles and guided clinicians regarding the use of systemic therapy for melanoma (40). The overall success explained the emergence of the public interest in immunotherapies in recent years. "Cancer staging," "Metastasis," "Malignancy," and "Survival rate" also attracted attention. The complete revolution of melanoma management has invigorated the public interest in the prognoses of patients. The popularization of the concept of personalized medicine caused the public to become more concerned with the outcomes of patients instead of short-term effects. Hence, it was necessary to formulate an individualized systemic medication plan according to the cancer stage and metastasis of the patients to achieve the maximum survival rate.

The annual top related topics were analyzed to reveal the trends in the topics of greatest interest during 2004 to 2019. Most of these topics were consistent with the above discussion, but some interesting terms also emerged. "Basal-cell carcinoma," "Birthmark," "Dysplastic nevus," "Eye neoplasm," "Freckle," "Kaposi's sarcoma," "Liver spot," "Lentigo," "Melancholia," "Melanosis," "Melasma," "Sarcoma," "Subungual hematoma," and "Vulvar cancer" were the diseases associated with or manifestations of melanoma (61–63). Ocular melanoma is the second most common type of melanoma and is often observed as an eye neoplasm. Lentigo maligna might eventually develop into invasive melanoma (64). "Melancholia," "Melanosis," and "Melasma" might have similar spellings as melanoma and hence confuse the searchers.

Treatment methods ranked second among the results. Terms associated with surgical methods including "Exeresis" and "Mohs surgery" refer to effective treatment modalities for early-stage noninvasive melanoma and therefore attract public interest (65, 66). Consistent with the bibliometric analysis, immunotherapies and risk genes attracted attention. In addition to those we discussed above, CTLA-4 was recently the focus of the public and appeared on the list. CTLA-4 is an immune checkpoint molecule that downregulates pathways of T cell activation (67), and "Ipilimumab" can inhibit CTLA-4 to improve survival in patients with metastatic melanoma (68).

Risk factors that had been discussed above, including sun tanning and melanin, illustrated the importance of public educational campaigns (69, 70). The evolution and broad adaption of dermatoscopy in clinical examinations also improved the diagnosis of benign and malignant cutaneous neoplasms compared with diagnosis with unaided eyes. Dermatoscopy also improved the ability of expert readers to make appropriate management decisions (71). Cell cultures can contribute to the diagnosis and development of melanoma management plans and function as an experimental tool to facilitate the development of new drugs (72). Interestingly, American Joint Committee on Cancer and a celebrity, Bob Marley, who died of the disease, also appeared on the list. The former association formulates the guidelines for the cancer staging of melanoma, and the latter reflects the celebrity effect, which can stimulate the recognition of the disease among the public.

Our study revealed the consistency between the research interest and the public interest. Both interests focused on the risk genes of melanoma and their inhibitors or blockers. These included PD-1, BRAF, CTLA-4, ipilimumab, nivolumab, dabrafenib, and trametinib. The use of social media has substantially increased among researchers and the public and could explain this corresponding relationship (73). In Australia, the SunSmart skin cancer prevention program has been demonstrated to contribute to the reduction of melanoma among younger cohorts (74). In addition to Australia, the Euromelanoma campaign also organized a yearly media campaign, which targets the public and focuses on different aspects of melanoma prevention. Euromelanoma Day has been held each year in May, both in university-based and hospital-based outpatient clinics and private dermatology surgeries (75). Patients and even the normal population can enhance their knowledge through these campaigns and become familiar with the latest research interest (76). In addition, the research interest might be influenced by social media, as reported by Pemmaraju (74), and the types of tweets about skin cancer have changed rapidly over time. The number of pharmaceutical companies that is discussed has been increasing, and the topic tags transitioned from "melanoma" to "immunotherapies" from 2011 to 2016 (74).

However, some differences still exist. The public did not show interest in the omics and microbiomes of melanoma that the research community studied. This was comprehensive because the public might not be familiar with these academic terms. More importantly, patients were mostly concerned with the symptoms, differential diagnosis, metastasis, and treatment of melanoma, especially newly emerged targeted drugs, which might improve prognosis and predict survival time. These aspects might become future directions for research and the popularization of science. Mechanisms, pathogenesis, pathophysiology, and epidemiological features were probably less important for patients because the complete elucidation of such factors could not alleviate symptoms, cure the disease, and decrease the high treatment expenses. Although these research fields might not provide patients and their families with hope in this era, they remain valuable for researchers. The development of new techniques and the discovery of key molecules in melanoma are crucial to guide future management. The prognosis of melanoma patients with regional metastases is influenced by the genomic classification, offering insights to further personalize therapeutic decision making (20). In addition, the commensal microbiome might have a mechanistic impact on antitumor immunity in melanoma patients (23). Such research findings might be included in educational campaigns in the future.

There are several limitations to the study. First, the public interest is restricted to Internet users who are conducting Google searches in English. There may be selection bias because the disease might not attract enough attention in underdeveloped areas. Although English remains the most popular official language worldwide, different languages and cultures could have different interests. In addition, other search engines could also be more popular than Google Trends in certain countries. For example, the Baidu engine is the main search engine in China. To compensate for the loss of data, we tried to use "topics" instead of "terms" as keywords, which may include some synonyms of melanoma in other languages. Second, only the Web of Science database was used to search for eligible articles, and some articles may be missed. Notably, fewer citations do not mean that an article is unimportant because it may lack the ability to be accessed by scholars.

CONCLUSION

This study used bibliometric and Google Trends analyses to update the topics and to compare the differences and similarities of research interest and public interest in melanoma. Regarding research interest, the top 15 most frequently cited articles each year focused on immunotherapy (n=8), omics (n=5), and the microbiome (n=2). Regarding public interest, diseases associated with or manifestations of melanoma, treatment options, risk factors, diagnostic tools, and prognosis were of the greatest interest to the public. The results revealed the trends in research interest and public interest in melanoma, which may pave the way for further research.

AUTHOR CONTRIBUTIONS

HZ and QS conceived and designed the study. HZ and YZW prepared the manuscript, and had equal contribution to the study. QZ and KT prepared the tables and figures. QZ, KT, RF, YCW, and QS reviewed and revised the manuscript. All authors contributed to the article and approved the submitted version.

ACKNOWLEDGMENTS

We thank AJE (https://www.aje.com/) for its linguistic assistance in editing the English text of the revised manuscript. The fee was funded by the authors.

REFERENCES

1. Schadendorf D, van Akkooi ACJ, Berking C, Griewank KG, Gutzmer R, Hauschild A, et al. Melanoma. *Lancet (London England)* (2018) 392 (10151):971–84. doi: 10.1016/s0140-6736(18)31559-9

2. The L. GLOBOCAN 2018: counting the toll of cancer. *Lancet (London England)* (2018) 392(10152):985. doi: 10.1016/s0140-6736(18)32252-9

3. Yang K, Fung TT, Nan H. An Epidemiological Review of Diet and Cutaneous Malignant Melanoma. *Cancer Epidemiol Biomarkers Prev* (2018) 27 (10):1115–22. doi: 10.1158/1055-9965.Epi-18-0243

4. Egghe L. A Heuristic Study of the First-Citation Distribution. *Scientometrics* (2000) 48(3):345–59. doi: 10.1023/a:1005688404778

5. Iftikhar PM, Ali F, Faisaluddin M, Khayyat A, De Gouvia De Sa M, Rao T. A Bibliometric Analysis of the Top 30 Most-cited Articles in Gestational Diabetes Mellitus Literature (1946-2019). *Cureus* (2019) 11(2):e4131. doi: 10.7759/cureus.4131

6. Zhang H, Tang K, Wang Y, Fang R, Sun Q. General interest in rosacea in the United States and China: a search engine-based pilot study. *Int J Dermatol Venereol* (2020) 03(04):248–9. doi: 10.1097/jd9.0000000000000118

7. Guo X, Gao L, Wang Z, Feng C, Xing B. Top 100 Most-Cited Articles on Pituitary Adenoma: A Bibliometric Analysis. *World Neurosurg* (2018) 116: e1153–e67. doi: 10.1016/j.wneu.2018.05.189

8. Wang Y, Zhang H, Fang R, Tang K, Sun Q. The top 100 most cited articles in rosacea: a bibliometric analysis. *J Eur Acad Dermatol Venereol* (2020) 34 (10):2177–82. doi: 10.1111/jdv.16305

9. Iglesia EGA, Stone CA Jr., Flaherty MG, Commins SP. Regional and temporal awareness of alpha-gal allergy: An infodemiological analysis using Google Trends. *J Allergy Clin Immunol In Pract* (2019) 8(5):1725–7. doi: 10.1016/ j.jaip.2019.12.003

10. Kwan Z, Yong SS, Robinson S. Analysis of Internet searches using Google Trends to measure interest in sun protection and skin cancer in selected South-East Asian populations. *Photodermatol Photoimmunol Photomed* (2020) 36(2):83–9. doi: 10.1111/phpp.12510

11. Hopkins ZH, Secrest AM. An international comparison of Google searches for sunscreen, sunburn, skin cancer, and melanoma: Current trends and public health implications. *Photodermatol Photoimmunol Photomed* (2019) 35 (2):87–92. doi: 10.1111/phpp.12425

12. Hopkins ZH, Secrest AM. Public Health Implications of Google Searches for Sunscreen, Sunburn, Skin Cancer, and Melanoma in the United States. *Am J Health Promot* (2019) 33(4):611–5. doi: 10.1177/0890117118811754

13. McDonald L, Simpson A, Graham S, Schultze A, Nordstrom B, Durani P, et al. Google searches do not correlate with melanoma incidence in majority English speaking countries. *NPJ Digit Med* (2018) 1:44. doi: 10.1038/ s41746-018-0050-4

14. Bloom R, Amber KT, Hu S, Kirsner R. Google Search Trends and Skin Cancer: Evaluating the US Population's Interest in Skin Cancer and Its Association With Melanoma Outcomes. *JAMA Dermatol* (2015) 151(8):903–5. doi: 10.1001/jamadermatol.2015.1216

15. Phillips CA, Barz Leahy A, Li Y, Schapira MM, Bailey LC, Merchant RM. Relationship Between State-Level Google Online Search Volume and Cancer Incidence in the United States: Retrospective Study. *J Med Internet Res* (2018) 20(1):e6. doi: 10.2196/jmir.8870

16. Wang Y, Zhang H, Zheng Q, Tang K, Sun Q. Public interest in Raynaud's phenomenon: A Google Trends analysis. *Dermatol Ther* (2020) 33(6):e14017. doi: 10.1111/dth.14017

17. Hu D, Lou X, Xu Z, Meng N, Xie Q, Zhang M, et al. More effective strategies are required to strengthen public awareness of COVID-19: Evidence from Google Trends. *J Global Health* (2020) 10(1):11003. doi: 10.7189/jogh.10.011003

18. Mavragani A, Ochoa G. Google Trends in Infodemiology and Infoveillance: Methodology Framework. *JMIR Public Health Surveill* (2019) 5(2):e13439. doi: 10.2196/13439

19. Barnett A, Dobson A. *Analysing Seasonal Health Data.* Vol. 10. Berlin, Germany: Springer (2010). doi: https://doi.org/10.1007/978-3-642-10748-1

20. Akbani R, Akdemir KC, Aksoy BA, Albert M, Ally A, Amin SB, et al. Genomic Classification of Cutaneous Melanoma. *Cell* (2015) 161(7):1681–96. doi: 10.1016/j.cell.2015.05.044

21. Gopalakrishnan V, Spencer CN, Nezi L, Reuben A, Andrews MC, Karpinets TV, et al. Gut microbiome modulates response to anti-PD-1 immunotherapy in melanoma patients. *Science* (2018) 359(6371):97–103. doi: 10.1126/ science.aan4236

22. Hugo W, Zaretsky JM, Sun L, Song C, Moreno BH, Hu-Lieskovan S, et al. Genomic and Transcriptomic Features of Response to Anti-PD-1 Therapy in Metastatic Melanoma. *Cell* (2016) 165(1):35–44. doi: 10.1016/j.cell.2016. 02.065

23. Matson V, Fessler J, Bao R, Chongsuwat T, Zha Y, Alegre M-L, et al. The commensal microbiome is associated with anti-PD-1 efficacy in metastatic melanoma patients. *Science* (2018) 359(6371):104–+. doi: 10.1126/ science.aao3290

24. Ott PA, Hu Z, Keskin DB, Shukla SA, Sun J, Bozym DJ, et al. An immunogenic personal neoantigen vaccine for patients with melanoma. *Nature* (2017) 547 (7662):217–+. doi: 10.1038/nature22991

25. Postow MA, Chesney J, Pavlick AC, Robert C, Grossmann K, McDermott D, et al. Nivolumab and Ipilimumab versus Ipilimumab in Untreated Melanoma. *N Engl J Med* (2015) 372(21):2006–17. doi: 10.1056/NEJMoa1414428

26. Robert C, Karaszewska B, Schachter J, Rutkowski P, Mackiewicz A, Stroiakovski D, et al. Improved Overall Survival in Melanoma with Combined Dabrafenib and Trametinib. N Engl J Med (2015) 372(1):30–9. doi: 10.1056/NEJMoa1412690

27. Robert C, Long GV, Brady B, Dutriaux C, Maio M, Mortier L, et al. Nivolumab in Previously Untreated Melanoma without BRAF Mutation. N Engl J Med (2015) 372(4):320–30. doi: 10.1056/NEJMoa1412082

28. Robert C, Schachter J, Long GV, Arance A, Grob JJ, Mortier L, et al. Pembrolizumab versus Ipilimumab in Advanced Melanoma. N Engl J Med (2015) 372(26):2521–32. doi: 10.1056/NEJMoa1503093

29. Van Allen EM, Miao D, Schilling B, Shukla SA, Blank C, Zimmer L, et al. Genomic correlates of response to CTLA-4 blockade in metastatic melanoma. Science (2015) 350(6257):207–11. doi: 10.1126/science.aad0095

30. Weber J, Mandala M, Del Vecchio M, Gogas HJ, Arance AM, Cowey CL, et al. Adjuvant Nivolumab versus Ipilimumab in Resected Stage III or IV Melanoma. N Engl J Med (2017) 377(19):1824–35. doi: 10.1056/NEJMoa1709030

31. Weber JS, D'Angelo SP, Minor D, Hodi FS, Gutzmer R, Neyns B, et al. Nivolumab versus chemotherapy in patients with advanced melanoma who progressed after anti-CTLA-4 treatment (CheckMate 037): a randomised, controlled, open-label, phase 3 trial. Lancet Oncol (2015) 16(4):375–84. doi: 10.1016/s1470-2045(15)70076-8

32. Wolchok JD, Chiarion-Sileni V, Gonzalez R, Rutkowski P, Grob JJ, Cowey CL, et al. Overall Survival with Combined Nivolumab and Ipilimumab in Advanced Melanoma. N Engl J Med (2017) 377(14):1345–56. doi: 10.1056/NEJMoa1709684

33. Zaretsky JM, Garcia-Diaz A, Shin DS, Escuin-Ordinas H, Hugo W, Hu-Lieskovan S, et al. Mutations Associated with Acquired Resistance to PD-1 Blockade in Melanoma. N Engl J Med (2016) 375(9):819–29. doi: 10.1056/NEJMoa1604958

34. Tirosh I, Izar B, Prakadan SM, Wadsworth MH,2, Treacy D, Trombetta JJ, et al. Dissecting the multicellular ecosystem of metastatic melanoma by single-cell RNA-seq. Science (2016) 352(6282):189–96. doi: 10.1126/science.aad0501

35. Huang Y, Liu Y, Liu H, Hong X, Guo X, Fang L. Top 100 most-cited articles on echocardiography: A bibliometric analysis. Echocardiography (Mount Kisco NY) (2019) 36(8):1540–8. doi: 10.1111/echo.14440

36. Adam D. The counting house. Nature (2002) 415(6873):726–9. doi: 10.1038/415726a

37. Salinas S, Munch SB. Where should I send it? Optimizing the submission decision process. PloS One (2015) 10(1):e0115451. doi: 10.1371/journal.pone.0115451

38. Liu W, Ma L, Song C, Li C, Shen Z, Shi L. Research trends and characteristics of oral lichen planus: A bibliometric study of the top-100 cited articles. Medicine (2020) 99(2):e18578. doi: 10.1097/md.0000000000018578

39. Sweileh WM. Bibliometric analysis of literature on toxic epidermal necrolysis and Stevens-Johnson syndrome: 1940 - 2015. Orphanet J Rare Dis (2017) 12(1):14. doi: 10.1186/s13023-017-0566-8

40. Terheyden P, Krackhardt A, Eigentler T. The Systemic Treatment of Melanoma. Dtsch Arztebl Int (2019) 116(29-30):497–504. doi: 10.3238/arztebl.2019.0497

41. Luke JJ, Flaherty KT, Ribas A, Long GV. Targeted agents and immunotherapies: optimizing outcomes in melanoma. Nat Rev Clin Oncol (2017) 14(8):463–82. doi: 10.1038/nrclinonc.2017.43

42. Zheng Q, Li J, Zhang H, Wang Y, Zhang S. Immune Checkpoint Inhibitors in Advanced Acral Melanoma: A Systematic Review. Front Oncol (2020) 10:602705(2661). doi: 10.3389/fonc.2020.602705

43. Tumeh PC, Harview CL, Yearley JH, Shintaku IP, Taylor EJ, Robert L, et al. PD-1 blockade induces responses by inhibiting adaptive immune resistance. Nature (2014) 515(7528):568–71. doi: 10.1038/nature13954

44. Moreira RS, Bicker J, Musicco F, Persichetti A, Pereira A. Anti-PD-1 immunotherapy in advanced metastatic melanoma: State of the art and future challenges. Life Sci (2020) 240:117093. doi: 10.1016/j.lfs.2019.117093

45. Liu-Smith F, Jia J, Zheng Y. UV-Induced Molecular Signaling Differences in Melanoma and Non-melanoma Skin Cancer. Adv Exp Med Biol (2017) 996:27–40. doi: 10.1007/978-3-319-56017-5_3

46. Rubin KM. MAPK Pathway-Targeted Therapies: Care and Management of Unique Toxicities in Patients With Advanced Melanoma. Clin J Oncol Nurs (2017) 21(6):699–709. doi: 10.1188/17.Cjon.699-709

47. Gibney GT, Atkins MB. Immunotherapy or molecularly targeted therapy: what is the best initial treatment for stage IV BRAF-mutant melanoma? Clin Adv Hematol Oncol (2015) 13(7):451–8.

48. McArthur GA, Ribas A. Targeting oncogenic drivers and the immune system in melanoma. J Clin Oncol (2013) 31(4):499–506. doi: 10.1200/jco.2012.45.5568

49. Geller AC, Sober AJ, Zhang Z, Brooks DR, Miller DR, Halpern A, et al. Strategies for improving melanoma education and screening for men age >or= 50 years: findings from the American Academy of Dermatological National Skin Cancer Sreening Program. Cancer (2002) 95(7):1554–61. doi: 10.1002/cncr.10855

50. Siegel RL, Miller KD, Jemal A. Cancer statistics, 2019. CA Cancer J Clin (2019) 69(1):7–34. doi: 10.3322/caac.21551

51. Kirchberger MC, Heppt MV, Eigentler TK, Kirchberger MA, Schuler G, Heinzerling L. The tanning habits and interest in sunscreen of Google users: what happened in 12 years? Photodermatol Photoimmunol Photomed (2017) 33(2):68–74. doi: 10.1111/phpp.12289

52. Suppa M, Gandini S. Sunbeds and melanoma risk: time to close the debate. Curr Opin Oncol (2019) 31(2):65–71. doi: 10.1097/cco.0000000000000507

53. Rastrelli M, Tropea S, Rossi CR, Alaibac M. Melanoma: epidemiology, risk factors, pathogenesis, diagnosis and classification. In Vivo (Athens Greece) (2014) 28(6):1005–11.

54. Falzone AE, Brindis CD, Chren MM, Junn A, Pagoto S, Wehner M, et al. Teens, Tweets, and Tanning Beds: Rethinking the Use of Social Media for Skin Cancer Prevention. Am J Prev Med (2017) 53(3s1):S86–s94. doi: 10.1016/j.amepre.2017.04.027

55. Kluger N, Bouchard LJ. A Comparative Study of Google Search Trends for Melanoma, Breast Cancer and Prostate Cancer in Finland. Dermatology (Basel Switzerland) (2019) 235(4):346–7. doi: 10.1159/000498987

56. Sboner A, Aliferis CF. Modeling clinical judgment and implicit guideline compliance in the diagnosis of melanomas using machine learning. AMIA Annu Symp Proc (2005) 2005:664–8.

57. Erkol B, Moss RH, Stanley RJ, Stoecker WV, Hvatum E. Automatic lesion boundary detection in dermoscopy images using gradient vector flow snakes. Skin Res Technol (2005) 11(1):17–26. doi: 10.1111/j.1600-0846.2005.00092.x

58. Hogue L, Harvey VM. Basal Cell Carcinoma, Squamous Cell Carcinoma, and Cutaneous Melanoma in Skin of Color Patients. Dermatol Clinics (2019) 37(4):519–26. doi: 10.1016/j.det.2019.05.009

59. Silva IP, Long GV. Systemic therapy in advanced melanoma: integrating targeted therapy and immunotherapy into clinical practice. Curr Opin Oncol (2017) 29(6):484–92. doi: 10.1097/cco.0000000000000405

60. Pulte D, Weberpals J, Jansen L, Brenner H. Changes in population-level survival for advanced solid malignancies with new treatment options in the second decade of the 21st century. Cancer (2019) 125(15):2656–65. doi: 10.1002/cncr.32160

61. Huh JW, Yoo J, Kim MS, Choi KH, Jue MS, Park HJ. Late-onset bulky naevocytoma of the perineum masquerading as a malignant melanoma. Clin Exp Dermatol (2017) 42(2):178–81. doi: 10.1111/ced.12971

62. Kim CC, Berry EG, Marchetti MA, Swetter SM, Lim G, Grossman D, et al. Risk of Subsequent Cutaneous Melanoma in Moderately Dysplastic Nevi Excisionally Biopsied but With Positive Histologic Margins. JAMA Dermatol (2018) 154(12):1401–8. doi: 10.1001/jamadermatol.2018.3359

63. Gupta V, Patra S, Arava S, Sethuraman G. Hidden acral lentiginous melanoma with cutaneous metastases masquerading as Kaposi's sarcoma in an HIV-positive Indian man. BMJ Case Rep (2016) 2016:bcr2015213529. doi: 10.1136/bcr-2015-213529

64. Volpini BMF, Maia M, Agi J, Vital JF, Lellis RF. Synchronous conjunctival melanoma and lentigo maligna melanoma. An Bras Dermatol (2017) 92(4):565–7. doi: 10.1590/abd1806-4841.20176015

65. Falk Delgado A, Zommorodi S, Falk Delgado A. Sentinel Lymph Node Biopsy and Complete Lymph Node Dissection for Melanoma. Curr Oncol Rep (2019) 21(6):54. doi: 10.1007/s11912-019-0798-y

66. Ellison PM, Zitelli JA, Brodland DG. Mohs micrographic surgery for melanoma: A prospective multicenter study. J Am Acad Dermatol (2019) 81(3):767–74. doi: 10.1016/j.jaad.2019.05.057

67. Melero I, Hervas-Stubbs S, Glennie M, Pardoll DM, Chen L. Immunostimulatory monoclonal antibodies for cancer therapy. Nat Rev Cancer (2007) 7(2):95–106. doi: 10.1038/nrc2051

68. Hodi FS, O'Day SJ, McDermott DF, Weber RW, Sosman JA, Haanen JB, et al. Improved survival with ipilimumab in patients with metastatic melanoma. N Engl J Med (2010) 363(8):711–23. doi: 10.1056/NEJMoa1003466

69. Brash DE. UV-induced Melanin Chemiexcitation: A New Mode of Melanoma Pathogenesis. *Toxicol Pathol* (2016) 44(4):552–4. doi: 10.1177/0192623316632072

70. Carr S, Smith C, Wernberg J. Epidemiology and Risk Factors of Melanoma. *Surg Clinics North Am* (2020) 100(1):1–12. doi: 10.1016/j.suc.2019.09.005

71. Weber P, Tschandl P, Sinz C, Kittler H. Dermatoscopy of Neoplastic Skin Lesions: Recent Advances, Updates, and Revisions. *Curr Treat Options Oncol* (2018) 19(11):56. doi: 10.1007/s11864-018-0573-6

72. Sztiller-Sikorska M, Hartman ML, Talar B, Jakubowska J, Zalesna I, Czyz M. Phenotypic diversity of patient-derived melanoma populations in stem cell medium. *Lab Invest J Tech Methods Pathol* (2015) 95(6):672–83. doi: 10.1038/labinvest.2015.48

73. Gage-Bouchard EA, LaValley S, Mollica M, Beaupin LK. Cancer Communication on Social Media: Examining How Cancer Caregivers Use Facebook for Cancer-Related Communication. *Cancer Nurs* (2017) 40 (4):332–8. doi: 10.1097/ncc.0000000000000418

74. Pemmaraju N, Thompson MA, Mesa RA, Desai T. Analysis of the Use and Impact of Twitter During American Society of Clinical Oncology Annual Meetings From 2011 to 2016: Focus on Advanced Metrics and User Trends. *J Oncol Pract* (2017) 13(7):e623–e31. doi: 10.1200/jop.2017.021634

75. Suppa M, Gandini S, Njimi H, Bulliard JL, Correia O, Duarte AF, et al. Prevalence and determinants of sunbed use in thirty European countries: data from the Euromelanoma skin cancer prevention campaign. *J Eur Acad Dermatol Venereol* (2019) 33 Suppl 2:13–27. doi: 10.1111/jdv.15311

76. Papachristou I, Bosanquet N. Improving the prevention and diagnosis of melanoma on a national scale: A comparative study of performance in the United Kingdom and Australia. *J Public Health Policy* (2020) 41(1):28–38. doi: 10.1057/s41271-019-00187-0

10

The Challenge of Melanocytic Lesions in Pediatric Patients: Clinical-Pathological Findings and the Diagnostic Value of PRAME

Giuseppina Rosaria Umano [1†], Maria Elena Errico [2†], Vittoria D'Onofrio [2], Giulia Delehaye [1], Letizia Trotta [1], Claudio Spinelli [3], Silvia Strambi [3], Renato Franco [4], Giuseppe D'Abbronzo [4], Andrea Ronchi [4*] and Alfonso Papparella [1]

[1] Department of Woman, Child and General and Specialized Surgery, University of Campania "Luigi Vanvitelli", Naples, Italy,
[2] Department of Pathology, Azienda Ospedaliera di Rilievo Nazionale (AORN) Santobono Pausilipon, Pediatric Hospital, Naples, Italy, [3] Pediatric, Adolescent and Young Adults Surgery Division, Department of Surgical, Medical, Pathological, Molecular and Critical Area, University of Pisa, Pisa, Italy, [4] Pathology Unit, Department of Mental and Physical Health and Preventive Medicine, University of Campania "Luigi Vanvitelli", Naples, Italy

*Correspondence:
Andrea Ronchi
Andrea.ronchi@unicampania.it

†These authors share first authorship

Pediatric melanoma is a rare disease especially in children aged younger than 10 years old. Recent estimates report a rise of disease incidence in both adults and children. Diagnostic work-up is challenging in pediatric melanoma, as it displays a wide range of clinical presentations. Immunohistochemical biomarkers have been reported as predictors of malignancy in melanoma, however data specific to pediatric melanoma are poor. Our study aims to contribute to provide evidence of pediatric melanoma clinical features and differential diagnosis in this patient population. We describe our experience with a retrospective case series of pigmented skin lesions including malignant melanoma, atypical spitzoid tumor, and benign nevi in children and adolescents aged less than 16 years. We described the clinical and demographic characteristics of the cohort and evaluated the immunohistochemical expression of the PReferentially expressed Antigen in MElanoma (PRAME) for differential diagnosis of melanoma in children. The series displayed a similar distribution of melanoma between males and females, and the most common site of melanoma onset were the upper and lower limbs. In our cohort, PRAME was negative in most cases. Focal and slight positivity (from 1 to 5% of the neoplastic cells) was observed in four cases (two Spitz nevi and two atypical Spitz tumors). A moderate positivity in 25% of the neoplastic cells was observed in one case of atypical Spitz tumor. Immunohistochemical expression of PRAME might be useful in the differential diagnosis of malignant melanoma.

Keywords: melanoma, children, atypical spitzoid tumor, PRAME, immunohistochemistry

INTRODUCTION

Malignant melanoma (MM) affects mainly the adult population, and about 14% of patients aged >18 years-old develop MM during their life according to recent studies (1). Although MM is rare in pediatric age, it is the most common form of skin cancer in children. The incidence increases with age: it is a rare neoplasm in children aged less than 10 years (annual incidence of 0.7–0.8 per million). However, this cancer cannot be considered a rare disease in teenagers, as its incidence is above two cases per million (2). Teenagers aged 15–19 years represent about 73% of pediatric MM cases; patients aged 10–14 years of age represent about 17%, while those aged 5–9 years and 1–4 old represent 6 and 4%, respectively (3). Overall, MM incidence in pediatric patients ranges from 1.1 per million in children younger than 5 years to 10.4 per million in those aged 15–19 years in the United States (4). However, data about trends in subjects aged less than 20 years are poor and contrasting (5, 6). In 2011, a literature review reported an incidence increase of 1–4% per year in the pediatric population (5). Conversely, Campbell et al. observed a decreased incidence in teenagers from 2004 to 2010 in the United States (6).

These data highlights how our understanding of pediatric MM is limited because clinical studies rarely involve children and adolescents. In addition, MM diagnosis in children is challenging, as it exhibits a wide range of clinical presentations (7). Clinical surveys have reported that MM in younger children might be amelanotic, uniformly pigmented, bleeding, thicker, and more frequently associated with lymph node metastasis compared to MM in adult patients, and thus displays a different biological behavior (8, 9).

A correct diagnosis is mandatory, as the patient's management and the correct therapy are directly dependent on diagnosis. Indeed, the therapeutic options for MM include not only surgery, but also targeted therapy using BRAF and MET inhibitors and immunotherapy. Moreover, a better understanding of the MM molecular landscape has led to the identification of new prognostic biomarkers (ALK, NTRK, MYC, C-KIT, and others) and will allow new targets for therapy in the near future (10). The diagnosis of melanocytic lesions is one of the most difficult aspects of dermatology and pathology. The development of dermoscopy in the last decades has improved the recognition of atypical lesions that need to be excised. However, the diagnosis still relies on histological examination, and the differential diagnosis in pediatric patients mainly includes Spitz nevus, atypical Spitz tumors, and Spitz melanoma. Histological diagnosis of melanocytic proliferations is certainly a challenge, as it mainly relies on morphological findings, which are almost partially subjective and requires trained pathologists with specific expertise (11). Recently, immunohistochemical and molecular biomarkers have been applied to the differential diagnosis, and have improved the diagnostic specificity.

Immunohistochemistry (IHC) is one of the most used techniques in pathology laboratories, as it is inexpensive, automatized, and can precisely evaluate the cellular population expressing a specific protein. Several immunohistochemical markers are tested on melanocytic neoplasms in everyday practice, mainly including HMB45, p16, and Ki67. Nevertheless, IHC plays an ancillary role in the diagnosis of melanocytic neoplasms in pediatric patients, and no immunohistochemical marker is entirely specific in differentiating benign from malignant neoplasms.

PRAME (PReferentially expressed Antigen in MElanoma) is a tumor-associated antigen recently identified in some neoplasms, including myxoid liposarcoma, synovial sarcoma, and MM (12). Current data suggest that PRAME is expressed by MM cells, but not by benign melanocytic neoplasms, and consequently it may be applied in the differential diagnosis of challenging melanocytic lesions. However, data about the expression of PRAME by melanocytic lesions in pediatric patients are limited. To fill the gap in this field, our study aims were twofold: first, to provide a description of cases presenting with suspected pigmented skin lesions and clinical findings of atypical melanocytic neoplasms including MM based on the experience of three hospital centers, and second, to evaluate the expression of PRAME in the subset of atypical spitzoid neoplasms in children.

MATERIALS AND METHODS

Patient Cohort

We retrospectively included clinical and histopathological data of children and adolescents referred to participating institutions for pigmented skin lesions suspected of melanoma. Three centers participated in the study: Santobono Hospital (Naples, Italy), the Pediatric Surgery Unit of University of Campania Luigi Vanvitelli (Naples, Italy), and the Pediatric, Adolescents and Young Adults Surgery Division of University of Pisa (Pisa, Italy). From databases containing data of patients subjected to excisional biopsy at these three centers, we selected patients satisfying the following criteria for inclusion in the study: 1) subjects referred to the participating centers from 2006 to 2020; 2) age ≤16 years; and 3) availability of demographic, clinical, surgical, and histopathological results. Data regarding benign pigmented skin lesions were obtained as a control group.

The present study was retrospectively conducted using archival biological samples. The diagnoses had already been rendered in all included cases. Approval by the participating institutions ethical review boards was collected.

At diagnosis, each patient received a baseline evaluation, which included medical history assessment and physical examination. Demographic and clinic characteristics included: sex, age, anatomical site of onset, signs of bleeding, itching, growth speed, and shape/color changes. Surgical characteristics recorded were removal of sentinel lymph node and sentinel lymph node state.

Through a telephone history we also obtained data about the presence of possible risk factors, such as clear skin phenotype, UV exposure levels, familiarity for skin melanoma in first degree relatives, number and presence of congenital nevi, dysplastic nevus syndrome, immunodeficiency status, and residence in polluted areas in patients that were diagnosed with either *in situ* or invasive MM.

This study was reviewed and approved by the ethics committee of University of Campania Luigi Vanvitelli (Naples, Italy).

Morphological Evaluation

Histological slides of all cases were reviewed by two experienced pathologists trained in melanocytic pathology. Histological studies were performed when necessary for diagnostic purposes. The histological review included immunohistochemical slides, when available. In some cases, further immunohistochemical markers were tested for diagnostic purposes, including HMB45 and p16. We applied diagnostic criteria defined in the most recent WHO classification of skin tumors (13).

PRAME Immunohistochemistry

Inclusion criteria for PRAME IHC included: 1) spitzoid morphology; and 2) availability of archived residual biomaterial in paraffin blocks. Immunocytochemistry was performed on 5-micron thick sections cut from formalin-fixed and paraffin-embedded (FFPE) tissue blocks. A commercially available anti-PRAME monoclonal antibody (dilution 1:200; EPR20330, Abcam, Cambridge, United Kingdom) was used on the Ventana Bench Mark Ultra System, (Ventana, Oro Valley, USA) autostainer platform, according to the manufacturer's instructions. The staining of PRAME IHC was recorded as the percentage of immunoreactive tumor cells with nuclear labeling per total number of tumor cells. A positive control was added to each slide, consisting in a PRAME-positive MM. The non-melanocytic tissue in the slide was considered the negative control.

The immunohistochemical slides were interpreted by two experienced dermatopathologists, evaluating both the intensity of the staining and the percentage of stained neoplastic cells on the total number of neoplastic cells. In cases where a consensus was not obtained, it was achieved through review by a third experienced pathologist. Intensity of the staining was graded as follows: score 1+: slight positivity; score 2+: moderate positivity; score 3+: intense positivity. The percentage of the positive cells was recorded, as well as the location of positive cells in the setting of the lesion (junctional *versus* intradermal).

RESULTS

Clinical and Pathological Findings

We evaluated a total of 63 lesions in 63 subjects. Eight of 63 lesions were diagnosed as MM, 17 as atypical Spitz tumor (AST), and 38 as benign nevi (**Figure 1**). Overall, 52% of subjects were males, and the mean age was 6.1 ± 3.3 years. MM lesions were more frequently located in the lower and upper limbs, whereas benign lesions were equally distributed between lower limbs and trunk (see **Table 1**). With regards to clinical characteristics, none of the benign lesions were associated with signs of bleeding and/or itching. One patient exhibited recent shape, dimensions, and color changes of the pre-existing lesion with asymmetry.

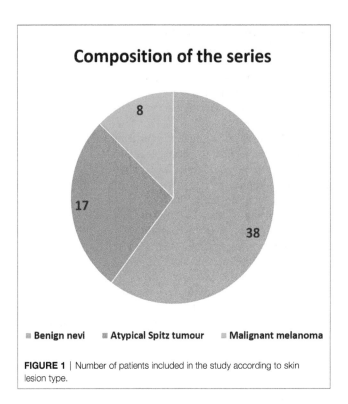

FIGURE 1 | Number of patients included in the study according to skin lesion type.

TABLE 1 | Clinical and demographic characteristics of the pediatric cohort according to lesion type.

Feature	Melanoma (n = 8)	Atypical Spitz Tumor (n = 17)	Benign Pigmented Skin Lesions (n = 38)
Sex			
Male	4	9	20
Signs/Symptoms			
Fast growth	5	17	28
Color changes	3	0	10
Asymmetry	1	0	1
Bleeding	0	0	0
Itching	0	0	0
Site of onset			
Trunk	2	2	12
Upper limb	4	4	7
Lower limb	3	11	12
Head/Neck	0	0	7

Moreover, two children presented an increased in size of the lesion. All lesions were diagnosed with cellular dysplasia on histopathologic examination. The remaining benign pigmented lesions underwent surgical excision because of recent fast growth and/or color changes on dermatologic consultation.

With regards to MM lesions, the majority did not arise from a pre-existing nevus and in four cases a rapid growth was reported. No cases of familial melanoma syndrome were observed. One melanoma developed from a congenital nevus and it presented with a rapid change in shape and color. No signs of itching and bleeding were reported.

In this group, a 5-year follow-up was carried out with a survival rate of 100% and neither relapses nor the appearance of metastases occurred. Only one patient underwent an additional surgical excision of a benign skin lesion.

PRAME Immunohistochemistry

PRAME immunohistochemistry was performed on 38 melanocytic neoplasms with spitzoid features, including 19 Spitz nevi, 17 ASTs, and 2 MMs. Six cases diagnosed as MM were not included in the immunohistochemical evaluation, as no residual bioptic material was available in paraffin blocks after the histological and molecular evaluations performed for diagnostic purposes.

Overall, the mean age of the tested population was 7 years, ranging from 1 to 16 years. For 20 of the 38 (52.6%) cases, lesions were located on the lower limbs, while in 7 (18.4%) cases lesions were located on the trunk, in 6 (15.8%) cases on the upper limbs, and 5 (13.2%) cases on the head and neck region.

Concerning the 19 cases diagnosed as Spitz nevi, the patients ranged in age from 1 to 10 years (mean age: 5.1 years). The lesions were located on the lower limbs in 7 patients (36.8%), on head and neck in 5 (26.3%), on the trunk in 4 (22.2%), and on the upper limbs in 3 (15.8%) patients. One of these patients was diagnosed with a desmoplastic Spitz nevus, with the lesion located on the dorsal trunk of the 8-year-old child (**Table 2**).

Regarding the 17 patients diagnosed as ASTs, ages ranged from 2 to 13 years (mean age: 7.2 years). Twelve of 17 (70.6%) patients presented lesions on the lower limbs, while in 3 (17.6%) and 2 (11.8%) lesions were located on the upper limbs and the trunk, respectively. The two cases diagnosed as MM presented lesions on the right foot of a 4-year-old child and on the dorsal trunk of a 10-year-old child (**Table 2**).

Overall, PRAME immunohistochemistry was negative in 33 of 38 (86.8%) cases. Two cases diagnosed with MM tested negative. Five of 38 (13.2%) cases showed some PRAME positivity. PRAME immunohistochemistry testing was positive in 25% of the neoplastic cells in a case of AST arising at the lower limb of an 8-year-old child. The intensity of the staining resulted in a score 2+, and the positive cells included both junctional and intradermal cells. The remaining four positive cases included two ASTs and two SN. In these cases, the percentage of positive cells ranged from 1 to 5%, and the intensity of the staining yielded a score of 1+. The positive cells were junctional in three cases and intradermal in one case (an AST located at the lower limb of a 2-year-old child) (**Figure 2**). The clinical and pathological features of the positive cases are listed in **Table 3**.

TABLE 2 | Clinical features of Spitz nevus and atypical Spitz tumor lesions subjected to PRAME immunohistochemistry testing.

Lesion	SN	AST
Cases	19	17
Age (mean age, range)	5.1; 1–10	7.; 2–13
Location (N, %)		
Head and neck	5 (26.3%)	0 (0%)
Trunk	4 (22.2%)	2 (11.8%)
Upper limbs	3 (15.8%)	3 (17.6%)
Lower limbs	7 (36.8%)	12 (70.6%)

SN, spitz nevi; AST, atypical Spitz tumors.

DISCUSSION

Although MM is relatively rare, it is the most common skin cancer in pediatric age. The estimated incidence in children under 10 years of age is 1.8 cases for 1 million in the United States (14). MM incidence increases during puberty, with a rate of 14 and 23 cases per million in adolescent males and females, respectively (15). Consequently, MM may be considered a rare tumor in pediatric patients, but the same cannot be said for adolescents. Although MM is a significant problem even in this population, clinical data are insufficient. Moreover, the differential diagnosis of melanocytic neoplasms remains a challenge, mainly in the setting of spitzoid lesions.

Herein, we analyzed a series of melanocytic lesions, and tested the expression of PRAME in a subset of cases. The first part of our study assessed the demographic and clinical presentation of suspected pigmented skin lesions. The ratio of pigmented lesions was equivalent between sexes and the most frequent site of onset was the limbs. The sex distribution of lesions was similar to that reported in previous case series including subjects of similar ages as our study (16). Conversely, in adolescents and youths, females were more frequently diagnosed with MM (17).

In our cohort, we more frequently observed malignant lesions in the lower and upper limbs. This finding is consistent with the data described by Dean et al. who reported the same body distribution for melanoma (16). This trend could be explained, as indicated by Strouse et al. (18), by the greater exposure of the upper and lower limbs to environmental disruptors and/or sunbathing. The latter is considered a risk factor also in adults, as well as phenotypic traits including red hair, blue eyes, and poor tanning ability (19). In addition, if we consider body surface distribution in children compared to adults, in pediatric subjects there is a relative higher prevalence on the upper and lower extremities over trunk surfaces. The common risk factors reported for pediatric melanoma, as well as giant melanocytic nevi, xeroderma pigmentosum, and neurocutaneous melanosis (19) were not detected in our cohort. Moreover, it has been reported in scientific literature that germline variants, such as MC1R, CDKN2A, and p16 gene variants are also associated with increased risk of melanoma (19).

Excisional biopsy is mandatory in cases of melanocytic lesions with atypical features in pediatric patients, and the diagnosis relies on histological examination. In this setting, the histological diagnosis of spitzoid neoplasms is one of the most difficult issues in dermatopathology. Despite a better understanding of the molecular biology underlying these neoplasms, the differential diagnosis between benign lesions and malignant lesions is still difficult, and largely based on qualitative and albeit, partially subjective findings (11). PRAME has recently emerged as a novel immunohistochemical marker able to distinguish benign from malignant melanocytic proliferations (20). However, the value of PRAME in the setting of differential diagnosis of spitzoid melanocytic neoplasms in pediatric patients is not well defined. We performed PRAME immunohistochemistry on a series of 38 spitzoid melanocytic neoplasms, including 19 Spitz nevi, 17 ASTs, and 2 MMs. Overall, PRAME was negative in 33 of 38 (86.8%) cases, including three ASTs and two SN. Notably, the

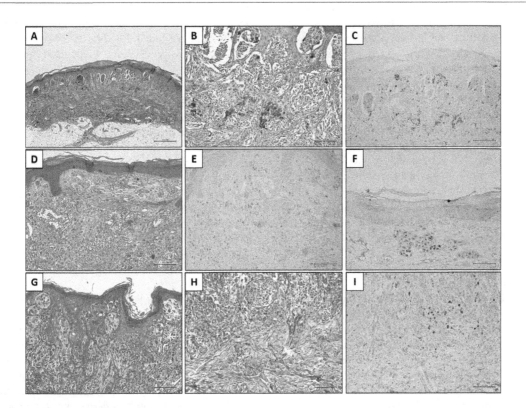

FIGURE 2 | PRAME immunostaining in three explicative lesions. Case 1 (Spitz nevus): a melanocytic lesion located on the right foot of an 8-year-old child. Histologically, the neoplasm was characterized by large junctional nests with peripheral clefting [**(A)** H&E, original magnification 40×]. Some junctional nests are confluent; smaller nests are present in the dermis, in addition to melanophages [**(B)** H&E, original magnification 200×]. PRAME immunostaining was negative [**(C)** immunostaining, original magnification 100×]. Case 2 (Atypical Spitz tumor): a melanocytic lesion located on the leg of an 8-year-old child. In this field, the melanocytic population is arranged in single epithelioid cells and small nests, located in the dermis [**(D)** H&E, original magnification 100×]. Overall, PRAME immunostaining was positive in about 25% of the melanocytic population [**(E)** immunostaining, original magnification 100×] with a moderate (score 2+) intensity [**(F)** immunostaining, original magnification 200×]. Case 3 (Spitz nevus): a melanocytic lesion located on the face of a 3-year-old child. Histologically, the junctional component was organized in confluent nests and constituted by epithelioid and spindle cells, in the context of a hyperplastic epidermis [**(G)** H&E, original magnification 200×]. The dermal component was organized in smaller nests, and peri-adnexal spread was present [**(H)** H&E, original magnification 200×]. PRAME immunostaining showed slight positivity (score 1+) in a few cells, corresponding to the 2% of the melanocytic population [**(I)** immunostaining, original magnification 200×].

TABLE 3 | Clinical and pathological features of PRAME-positive cases.

N.	Diagnosis	Location	Age (y)	% Positivity	Score	Location
1	AST	Lower limb	8	25	2+	Junctional and dermal
2	SN	H/N	3	2	1+	Junctional
3	AST	Upper limb	7	5	1+	Junctional
4	SN	Lower limb	2	1	1+	Junctional
5	AST	Lower limb	2	1	1+	Dermal

two cases diagnosed as MM tested negative as well. In five cases, including three ASTs and two SN, some PRAME positivity was observed. In particular, 25% of both junctional and intradermal neoplastic cells showed a score 2+ staining in an AST located at the lower limb of an 8-year-old child. In the remaining four cases, only a few cells resulted slightly positive (score 1+), ranging between 1 and 5% of the melanocytic population. To more decisively evaluate these results, it is mandatory to define a cut-off value to be applied for positive cases. PRAME stains mainly in the nucleus and consequently the results are of high

quality and are easily interpretable in all cases, despite the amount of melanin pigment. In our experience, PRAME staining is diffusely positive, in most neoplastic cells, and in both junctional and intradermal cells, in cases morphologically diagnosed as MM. Nonetheless, we are accustomed to defining negative cases with only few positive cells. Our experience matches observations reported by other studies. Lezcano et al. recently examined the immunohistochemical expression of PRAME in a heterogenous series of 400 melanocytic lesions. The Authors considered PRAME positivity significant when observed in ≥76% of neoplastic cells (20). Similarly, Raghavan et al. defined positive cases showing PRAME staining in at least 60% of the cells (21). Based on these data, in our series the positivity observed in the five cases does not appear to be significant, and we considered all cases tested as negative. Nevertheless, we might speculate that the data reported in literature relied on a higher cut-off value of cellular staining to define PRAME positivity.

Differential diagnosis in the setting of spitzoid melanocytic lesions is challenging, and ancillary tests may be useful. In this setting, PRAME immunohistochemistry is emerging as a novel immunohistochemical test that has been recently introduced in the routine diagnostic work-up of dermatopathologists. When faced with the diagnosis of a melanocytic lesion, a basic immunohistochemistry panel may include HMB45, p16, Ki67, and PRAME expression. However, data regarding the diagnostic value of PRAME in the setting of the spitzoid melanocytic lesions in pediatric patients are missing. In the single paper available in the literature, Raghavan et al. evaluated the expression of PRAME in a series of atypical melanocytic lesions, including 35 spitzoid neoplasms (20 SN, 13 ASTs, and 2 MMs). The authors found that PRAME was expressed in 7.7% of ASTs and in 4% of SNs (21). The study evaluated only two cases of MM, and PRAME expression was in one case (21). However, the series did not consider pediatric patients. In this study, we evaluated PRAME expression specifically focusing on spitzoid lesions in pediatric patients. In our series, PRAME tested negative in all cases. Although some cells showed PRAME expression in five lesions, its expression was focal (25% of the cells in one case and ≤5% in the remaining four cases) and did not reach the cut-off value for positivity. We can conclude that PRAME is not expressed in SN and ASTs in pediatric patients, and therefore it is not useful for the differential diagnosis of SN and AST in this clinical setting. Conversely, we tested only two MMs, and therefore no significant information could be obtained from our series relative to the expression of PRAME in MM lesions in pediatric patients.

In conclusion, in our case series we observed that pediatric MM equally affects young boys and girls, and that the limbs are the most common site of onset. These findings highlight the different clinical behavior of MM in children compared to adults. In addition, we tested PRAME expression in a series of 38 spitzoid melanocytic lesions in pediatric patients. Although PRAME is an emerging IHC marker for the characterization of melanocytic lesions in adults, data regarding its utility in the diagnosis of spitzoid lesions in pediatric patients are lacking. Herein, we demonstrated that PRAME is not expressed in either SN or ASTs in this clinical setting; thus PRAME positivity may be considered an element useful for the differential diagnosis of MM. However, there are insufficient data in pediatric populations about PRAME expression in MM with spitzoid morphology, as only two cases have been reported by a previous study, of which only one case resulted positive. Considering the paucity of clinical and histopathological data in pediatric cohorts, additional studies should be conducted in this field with the aim of identifying predictors of malignant forms.

AUTHOR CONTRIBUTIONS

AR, RF, and GD'A revised the histological and immunohistochemical slides and contributed to design the study. ME and GU contributed to design the study, contributed to write the manuscript and data analysis. VD'O, GD, LT, CS, and SS provided the clinical data and biological material, contributed to the analysis of the data. AP contributed to design the study and reviewed the manuscript. All authors contributed to the article and approved the submitted version.

REFERENCES

1. Cancer Today. Available at: https://gco.iarc.fr/today/online-analysis-table (Accessed March 26, 2021).

2. Ferrari A, Brecht IB, Gatta G, Schneider DT, Orbach D, Cecchetto G, et al. Defining and Listing Very Rare Cancers of Paediatric Age: Consensus of the Joint Action on Rare Cancers in Cooperation With the European Cooperative Study Group for Pediatric Rare Tumors. Eur J Cancer (2019) 110:120–26. doi: 10.1016/j.ejca.2018.12.031

3. Lange JR, Palis BE, Chang DC, Soong SJ, Balch CM. Melanoma in Children and Teenagers: An Analysis of Patients From the National Cancer Data Base. J Clin Oncol (2007) 25:1363–8. doi: 10.1200/JCO.2006.08.8310

4. United States Cancer Statistics, Cancer, CDC. Available at: https://www.cdc.gov/cancer/uscs/index.htm (Accessed March 26, 2021).

5. Paradela S, Fonseca E, Prieto VG. Melanoma in Children. Arch Pathol Lab Med (2011) 135:307–16. doi: 10.5858/2009-0503-ra.1

6. Campbell LB, Kreicher KL, Gittleman HR, Strodtbeck K, Barnholtz-Sloan J, Bordeaux JS. Melanoma Incidence in Children and Adolescents: Decreasing Trends in the United States. J Pediatr (2015) 166:1505–13. doi: 10.1016/j.jpeds.2015.02.050

7. Cordoro KM, Gupta D, Frieden IJ, McCalmont T, Kashani-Sabet M. Pediatric Melanoma: Results of a Large Cohort Study and Proposal for Modified ABCD Detection Criteria for Children. J Am Acad Dermatol (2013) 68:913–25. doi: 10.1016/j.jaad.2012.12.953

8. Kaste SC. Imaging of Pediatric Cutaneous Melanoma. Pediatr Radiol (2019) 49:1476–87. doi: 10.1007/s00247-019-04374-9

9. Livestro DP, Kaine EM, Michaelson JS, Mihm MC, Haluska FG, Muzikansky A, et al. Melanoma in the Young: Differences and Similarities With Adult Melanoma: A Case-Matched Controlled Analysis. Cancer (2007) 110:614–24. doi: 10.1002/cncr.22818

10. Ronchi A, Montella M, Cozzolino I, Argenziano G, Moscarella E, Piccolo V, et al. The Potential Diagnostic and Predictive Role of Anaplastic Lymphoma Kinase (ALK) Gene Alterations in Melanocytic Tumors. Eur Rev Med Pharmacol Sci (2020) 24:3829–38. doi: 10.26355/eurrev_202004_20849

11. Ronchi A, Pagliuca F, Zito Marino F, Argenziano G, Brancaccio G, Alfano R, et al. Second Diagnostic Opinion by Experienced Dermatopathologists in the Setting of a Referral Regional Melanoma Unit Significantly Improves the Clinical Management of Patients With Cutaneous Melanoma. Front Med (2021) 7:568946. doi: 10.3389/fmed.2020.568946

12. Hemminger JA, Toland AE, Scharschmidt TJ, Mayerson JL, Guttridge DC, Iwenofu OH. Expression of Cancer-Testis Antigens MAGEA1, Magea3, ACRBP, Prame, SSX2, and CTAG2 in Myxoid and Round Cell Liposarcoma. Mod Pathol (2014) 27:1238–45. doi: 10.1038/modpathol.2013.244

13. Xavier-Junior JCC, Ocanha-Xavier JP. Who (2018) Classification of Skin Tumors. Am J Dermatopathol (2019) 41:699–700. doi: 10.1097/DAD.0000000000001446

14. Cancer Statistics Review, 1975-2014 - SEER Statistics. Available at: https://seer.cancer.gov/archive/csr/1975_2014/ (Accessed March 26, 2021).

15. Pisani P, Buzzoni C, Crocetti E, Dal Maso L, Rondelli R, Alessi D, et al. Italian Cancer Figures - Report 2012: Cancer in Children and Adolescents. Epidemiol Prev (2013) 37:1–296.

16. Dean PH, Bucevska M, Strahlendorf C, Verchere C. Pediatric Melanoma: A 35-Year Population-Based Review. *Plast Reconstr Surg-Glob Open* (2017) 5:1–8. doi: 10.1097/GOX.0000000000001252

17. Kalani N, Guidry JA, Farahi JM, Stewart SB, Dellavalle RP, Dunnick CA. Pediatric Melanoma: Characterizing 256 Cases From the Colorado Central Cancer Registry. *Pediatr Dermatol* (2019) 36:219–22. doi: 10.1111/pde.13747

18. Strouse JJ, Fears TR, Tucker MA, Wayne AS. Pediatric Melanoma: Risk Factor and Survival Analysis of the Surveillance, Epidemiology and End Results Database. *J Clin Oncol* (2005) 23:4735–41. doi: 10.1200/JCO.2005.02.899

19. *Childhood Melanoma Treatment (Pdq®): Health Professional Version.* (Accessed March 26, 2021).

20. Lezcano C, Jungbluth AA, Nehal KS, Hollmann TJ, Busam KJ. Prame Expression in Melanocytic Tumors. *Am J Surg Pathol* (2018) 42:1456–65. doi: 10.1097/PAS.000000000000113

21. Raghavan SS, Wang JY, Kwok S, Rieger KE, Novoa RA, Brown RA. Prame Expression in Melanocytic Proliferations With Intermediate Histopathologic or Spitzoid Features. *J Cutan Pathol* (2020) 47:1123–31. doi: 10.1111/cup.13818

11

Melanoma of Unknown Primary: Evaluation of the Characteristics, Treatment Strategies, Prognostic Factors in a Monocentric Retrospective Study

Paolo Del Fiore [1*†], Marco Rastrelli [1,2†], Luigi Dall'Olmo [3†], Francesco Cavallin [4†], Rocco Cappellesso [5], Antonella Vecchiato [1], Alessandra Buja [6], Romina Spina [1], Alessandro Parisi [7], Renzo Mazzarotto [8], Beatrice Ferrazzi [9], Andrea Grego [2], Alessio Rotondi [10], Clara Benna [2], Saveria Tropea [1], Francesco Russano [1], Angela Filoni [1], Franco Bassetto [11], Angelo Paolo Dei Tos [5], Mauro Alaibac [12], Carlo Riccardo Rossi [1,2], Jacopo Pigozzo [13], Vanna Chiarion Sileni [13] and Simone Mocellin [1,2]

[1] Surgical Oncology Unit, Veneto Institute of Oncology IOV - IRCCS, Padua, Italy, [2] Department of Surgery, Oncology and Gastroenterology (DISCOG), University of Padua, Padua, Italy, [3] Emergency Department- Azienda Ospedaliera Padova, Padova, Italy, [4] Independent Statistician, Solagna, Italy, [5] Surgical Pathology and Cytopathology Unit, Department of Medicine (DIMED), University of Padua, Padua, Italy, [6] Department of Cardiological, Thoracic, Vascular Sciences and Public Health, University of Padua, Padua, Italy, [7] Radiotherapy Unit, Veneto Institute of Oncology, IOV-IRCCS, Padua, Italy, [8] Department of Radiotherapy, Ospedale Civile Maggiore, Azienda Ospedaliera Universitaria Integrata, Verona, Italy, [9] Postgraduate School of Occupational Medicine, University of Verona, Verona, Italy, [10] Department of Medicine (DIMED), University of Padua, Padua, Italy, [11] Clinic of Plastic Surgery, Department of Neuroscience, Padua University Hospital, University of Padua, Padua, Italy, [12] Unit of Dermatology, University of Padua, Padua, Italy, [13] Melanoma Oncology Unit, Veneto Institute of Oncology IOV-IRCCS, Padua, Italy

*Correspondence:
Paolo Del Fiore
paolo.delfiore@iov.veneto.it

†These authors have contributed equally to this work

Background: Melanoma of unknown primary (MUP), accounts for up to 3% of all melanomas and consists of a histologically confirmed melanoma metastasis to either lymph nodes, (sub)cutaneous tissue, or visceral sites without any evidence of a primary cutaneous, ocular, or mucosal melanoma. This study aimed to investigate the characteristics, treatment strategies, and prognostic factors of MUP patients, in order to shed some light on the clinical behavior of this malignancy.

Methods: All the consecutive patients with a diagnosis of MUP referring to our institutions between 1985 and 2018 were considered in this retrospective cohort study. The records of 173 patients with a suspected diagnosis of MUP were retrospectively evaluated for inclusion in the study. Patient selection was performed according to the Das Gupta criteria, and a total of 127 MUP patients were finally included in the study, representing 2.7% of the patients diagnosed with melanoma skin cancer at our institutions during the same study period. A second cohort of all consecutive 417 MKP patients with AJCC stages IIIB–IV, referring tions in the period considered (1985–2018), was included in the study to compare survival between MUP and MKP patients. All the diagnoses were based on histopathologic, cytologic and immunohistochemical examination of the metastases.

All tumors were re-staged according to the 2018 American Joint Committee on Cancer (AJCC) 8th Edition.

Results: Median follow-up was 32 months (IQR: 15–84). 3-year progression-free survival (PFS) was 54%, while 3-year overall survival (OS) was 62%. Worse OS and PFS were associated with older age (P = 0.0001 for OS; P = 0.008 for PFS), stage IV (P < 0.0001 for OS; P = 0.0001 for PFS) and higher Charlson Comorbidity Index (P < 0.0001 for OS and P = 0.01 for PFS). Patients with lymph node disease showed longer PFS (P = 0.001) and OS (P = 0.0008) than those with (sub)cutis disease. Complete lymph node dissection (CLND) was the most common surgical treatment; a worse OS in these patients was associated with the number of positive lymph nodes (P = 0.01), without significant association with the number of retrieved lymph nodes (P = 0.79). Survival rates were lower in patients undergoing chemotherapy (CT) and target therapy (TT), and higher in those receiving immunotherapy (IT). 417 patients with AJCC stages IIIB–IV of Melanoma Known Primary (MKP) were included for the survival comparison with MUP. 3-year PFS rates were 54 and 58% in MUP and MKP, respectively (P = 0.30); 3-year OS rates were 62 and 70% in MUP and MKP, respectively (P = 0.40).

Conclusions: The most common clinical scenario of our series was a male patient around 59 years with lymph node disease. We report that CLND associated with IT was the best treatment in terms of survival outcome. In the current era of IT and TT for melanoma, new studies have to clarify the impact of novel drugs on MUP.

Keywords: melanoma of unknown primary, occult primary melanoma, skin cancer, melanoma, MUP, melanoma treatment, immunotherapy, target therapy

INTRODUCTION

Melanoma of unknown primary (MUP) also known as occult primary melanoma accounts for up to 3% of all melanomas (1) and consists of a histologically confirmed melanoma metastasis to either lymph nodes, (sub)cutaneous tissue, or visceral sites. The diagnosis of MUP is definitive when a primary cutaneous, ocular, or mucosal melanoma is missing after a thorough physical examination and histological revision of previously excised melanocytic lesions. In 1963, Das Gupta and collaborators defined the diagnostic criteria for MUP (2). Such criteria exclude patients who do not receive complete physical examination (including anus/genitalia and ophthalmological visit); those with evidence of previous orbital enucleation, those without histological documentation of prior surgical or non-surgical procedures (e.g., for a mole, birthmark, freckle, chronic paronychia, or skin blemish), and those with nodal involvement and presence of a scar in the skin area drained by the lymphatic basin (2). Of note, according to Kamposioras, only 16% of publications on MUP applied the stringent Das Gupta's exclusion criteria, thus the remaining might have included as MUP some melanoma of known primary (MKP) (3). The peak incidence of MUP occurs between the fourth and fifth decade of age, which is comparable to that of MKP of the skin but earlier than those arising from the mucosa. MUP is also more common in men than women. The management of patients with MUP has been the same to the management of patients with metastatic melanoma and with MKP. Although the survival of patients with stage III–IV MUP as compared to patients with stage III–IV MKP has been richly explained (4–6) including the hypotheses attributable to immune-mediated control of the primary tumor in patients with MUP, a distinct signature of MUP that differentiate the treatment strategies for MUP and MKP has not been defined. To do this, more retrospective cohort studies such as ours are needed to compare outcomes between patients with MUP and stage-matched MKP during novel therapy.

This study aimed to investigate the characteristics, treatment strategies and prognostic factors of MUP patients, in order to shed some light on the clinical behavior of this rare type of melanoma. In addition, survival in MUP patients was compared with survival in MKP patients with the same stage and metastatic sites. The clinical impact of our study is to build a retrospective cohort study for the clinical features and behavior of MUP in the evolving era of immunotherapy, targeted therapies, and their combinations.

MATERIALS AND METHODS

Study Design

All the consecutive patients with a diagnosis of MUP referring to the Melanoma and Sarcoma Clinic of the Veneto Institute of Oncology (IOV) and the Department of Surgery Oncology and Gastroenterology (DISCOG) of the University of Padua (Italy)

between 1985 and 2018 were considered in this retrospective cohort study. IOV and DISCOG are level III referral institutions in Northeastern Italy. Most patients are referred for diagnosis and/or first-line treatment, while some patients are referred for disease progression after being treated in level I–II centers. The study was conducted according to the Helsinki Declaration principles and was approved by the local Ethics Committee (17/04/2020, approval No. 7254). All patients gave their consent for data collection and analysis for scientific purposes.

Patients

The records of 173 patients with a suspected diagnosis of MUP referring to IOV or DISCOG between 1985 and 2018 were retrospectively evaluated for inclusion in the study.

Patient selection was performed according to the Das Gupta criteria (2) (**Table 1**). Forty-six patients were excluded because of unclear information on primary melanoma (14 patients), misdiagnosis of MUP (medical history of previous cutaneous melanoma, 11 patients) or "evidence of previous skin excision or other surgical manipulation of a mole, freckle, birthmark, paronychia or skin blemish", or "evidence of metastatic melanoma in a draining lymph node with a scar in the area of skin supplying the lymph node basin" (21 patients) (1). A total of 127 MUP patients were finally included in the study, representing 2.7% of the patients diagnosed with melanoma skin cancer (127 out of 4,703 patients) at our institutions during the same study period.

A second cohort of all consecutive 417 MKP patients with AJCC stages IIIB–IV, referring to our institutions in the period considered (1985–2018), was included in the study to compare survival between MUP and MKP patients.

Diagnosis and Treatment

All the diagnoses were based on histopathologic, cytologic, and immunohistochemical examination of the metastases. All tumors were re-staged according to the 2018 American Joint Committee on Cancer (AJCC) 8th Edition—TNM staging system (7) was used for tumor staging.

Patients with melanoma metastases in the (sub)cutis, soft tissue, and/or lymph nodes, without a detectable primary tumor were diagnosed s stage III disease, while those with distant metastases including visceral metastases are diagnosed as stage IV.

The surgical treatment included wide resection (WR) in patients with (sub)cutis/soft tissue lesion, complete lymph node dissection (CLND) in those with lymph node metastasis

---

TABLE 1 | Das Gupta's exclusion criteria.

Das Gupta's exclusion criteria

Evidence of previous orbital exenteration or enucleation
Evidence of previous skin excision,electrodessication, cauterization or other surgical manipulation of a mole, freckle,birthmark, paronychia, or skin blemish.
Evidence of metastatic melanoma in a draining lymph node with a scar in the area of skin supplying that lymph node basin.
Lack of a nonthorough physical examination, including the absence of an ophthalmologic, anal, and genital exam.

---

and metastasectomy in those with complete, resectable distant/visceral location.

Radiation therapy (RT) was performed according to location, stage, surgical radicality, and residual disease load. Medical oncology treatments included target therapy (TT), immunotherapy (IT), and classic chemotherapy (CT). In some patients, electrochemotherapy (ECT) and hyperthermic limb perfusion (ILP) were also employed.

IT with high-dose interferon (IFN HD) was used as adjuvant treatment after radical surgery in stage III patients. Since 2012, stage IV patients were treated with targeted therapy (TT) if the melanoma carried the V600E BRAF mutation: in particular, the combination of BRAF and MEK inhibitors (Dabrafenib and Trametinib or Vemurafenib and Cobimetinib, respectively); in case of *BRAF* wild type disease, immune checkpoint blockade with anti-PD1 monoclonal antibodies (Pembrolizumab or Nivolumab) alone or in combination with anti-CTLA4 monoclonal antibodies (Ipilimumab) (8, 9).

Systemic CT (*i.e.* dacarbazine and bio-chemotherapy regimens) was administered before 2012.

Follow-up was performed every three months for the first two years, then every six months up to the 5th year, and once a year thereafter. Disease progression was defined as local disease recurrence, lymph node metastasis and/or distant metastasis.

Data Collection

All data were extracted from a prospectively maintained database. Demographics included age at diagnosis, gender and family history of cancer, while melanoma-related information included clinical presentation, metastasis size, and AJCC TNM stage (7). Tumor stage according to Balch's proposal (which includes stage IV non-visceral tumors in stage III) was also assessed (10). Comorbidity status was summarized using the age-adjusted Charlson Comorbidity Index (11). Neoplastic comorbidity and autoimmune comorbidity were evaluated separately. Information on treatment strategy included surgical therapy (WR, CLND, metastasectomy) and medical therapy (radiotherapy, target therapy, immunotherapy and chemotherapy). Follow-up information was extracted from the reports of scheduled visits. Overall survival was calculated from diagnosis to death (by any cause) or to the last visit, while recurrence/progression-free survival was calculated from diagnosis to recurrence/progression or to the last visit.

Statistical Analysis

Categorical data were summarized as frequency and percentage, while continuous data as median and interquartile range (IQR).

Survival curves were calculated using Kaplan–Meier method. Survival estimates were compared between MUP and MKP patients using the log-rank test.

The association between clinically relevant variables and survival was assessed using Cox regression models. Effects sizes were reported as hazard ratio (HR) with 95 per cent confidence interval (95% CI). Of note, the association between surgical treatments and survival was not evaluated because surgical treatments mirrored the clinical presentation of MUP.

Multivariable analysis of survival was performed with Cox regression models including a set of clinically relevant factors at diagnosis (*i.e.* age, Charlson Comorbidity Index, and tumor presentation). Metastasis size was not included in the analysis because this information was available only for lymph node metastases (but not skin metastases). In addition, some potential factors could not be included in the multivariable models due to collinearity with presentation (AJCC stage), rarity of the events (neoplastic and autoimmune comorbidity) or incomplete information (BRAF mutational status).

The association between medical treatments and tumor stage was evaluated using Fisher's exact test.

All tests were two-sided and a p-value less than 0.05 was considered statistically significant. Statistical analysis was performed using R 4.0 (R Foundation for Statistical Computing, Vienna, Austria) (12).

RESULTS

Patients
Of the 173 patients with MUP considered in this study, 46 were excluded, according to the Gupta's criteria. One hundred and twenty-seven patients (78 males and 49 females; median age 59 years) with a diagnosis of MUP between 1985 and 2018 were included in the analysis. Patient and tumor characteristics are shown in **Table 2**. There were 68 AJCC stage III tumors (Balch stage III) and 59 AJCC stage IV tumors, of whom 25 were non-visceral tumors (Balch stage III) and 34 were visceral tumors (Balch stage IV). *BRAF* was mutated in 38 out of 68 evaluable patients (56%).

Treatment
Treatment strategies are shown in **Figure 1**. Ninety-four patients (74%) underwent surgical treatment: 65 CLND, 14 WR, seven metastasectomy, and eight CLND+WR, while 30 patients underwent only medical treatment and three refused the treatment. CLND was performed in axilla (27 patients), groin

(eight patients) or neck (12 patients), with a median of 23 retrieved nodes (IQR 18–32) and a median of two positive nodes (IQR 1–5). Such information was not available for six patients.

Medical treatment was administered to 103 patients (81%), with 38 patients receiving more than one treatment, and 65 patients receiving only one treatment. Overall, 34 patients received chemotherapy, which was more frequent among stage IV patients (37 *vs.* 18% in stage III patients, p = 0.02). Seventy-four patients received immunotherapy, which was more frequent among stage III patients (72 *vs.* 42% in IV patients, p = 0.001). Target therapy was administered to 23 patients, with no statistically significant difference between stage III *vs.* IV patients (13 *vs.* 23%, p = 0.19). Twenty-five patients (20%) received radiotherapy, with no statistically significant difference between stage III *vs.* IV patients (23 *vs.* 15%, p = 0.34). Nine patients received chemo-radiotherapy.

Survival
Median follow-up was 32 months (IQR 15–84). At the analysis, seven patients had local recurrence, 39 had recurrence with clinical upstaging, and 19 had disease progression.

3-year recurrence/progression-free survival was 54%, while 3-year overall survival was 62% (**Figure 2**).

Univariate analyses of recurrence/progression-free survival and overall survival are reported in **Table 3**. Impaired recurrence/progression-free survival was associated with older age (HR 1.03, 95% CI 1.01 to 1.04; p = 0.008), stage IV (HR 2.77, 95% CI 1.66 to 4.63; p = 0.0001) and higher Charlson Comorbidity Index (HR 1.16, 95% CI 1.03 to 1.30; p = 0.01). Patients with lymph node metastasis showed longer recurrence/progression-free survival than those with (sub)cutis metastases (HR 0.37, 9%% CI 0.20 to 0.68; p = 0.002). Among patients who underwent RLND, overall survival was associated with the number of positive lymph nodes (HR 1.06, 95% CI 1.01 to 1.11; p = 0.01) but not with the number of retrieved nodes (HR 1.00, 95% CI 0.96 to 1.03; p = 0.79). Impaired overall survival was associated with older age (HR 1.04, 95% CI 1.02 to 1.06; p = 0.0001), stage IV (HR 3.43, 95% CI 2.00 to

TABLE 2 | Patient and tumor characteristics.

Variable			AJCC stage III	AJCC stage IV	
			Patient with lymph node metastases	Patient with (Sub)cutis metastases	Patient with visceral metastases
Demographics	N patients:	127	68	25	34
	Age at diagnosis, year[a]	59 (48–70)	57 (47–67)	60 (48–69)	62 (49–73)
	Sex:				
	Female	49 (39)	24 (35)	12 (48)	13 (38)
	Male	78 (61)	44 (65)	13 (52)	21 (62)
	Family history of cancer[b]	11 (12)	4 (8)	3 (19)	4 (15)
Tumor characteristics	Size of lymph node metastasis, cm[a,c]	4.0 (2.5–5.0)	4.0 (2.5–5.0)	–	4.0 (3.4–6.0)
	AJCC stage:				
	III	68 (54)	68 (100)	0	0
	IV	59 (46)	0	25 (100)	34 (100)
Comorbidity status	Charlson Comorbidity Index[a]	2 (1–3)	2 (0–3)	2 (1–3)	2 (1–4)
	Neoplastic comorbidity	19 (15)	10 (15)	2 (8)	7 (21)
	Autoimmune comorbidity	22 (17)	9 (13)	3 (12)	10 (29)

Data expressed as n (%) or [a]median (IQR). Data not available in [b]one and [c]29 patients.

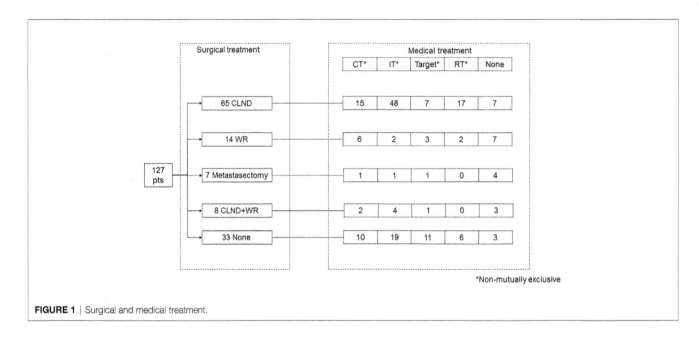

FIGURE 1 | Surgical and medical treatment.

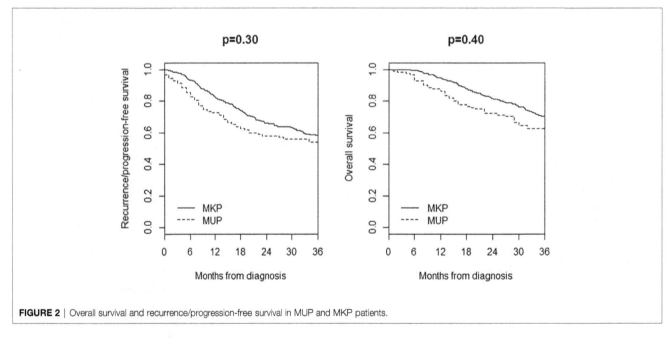

FIGURE 2 | Overall survival and recurrence/progression-free survival in MUP and MKP patients.

5.89; p < 0.0001) and higher Charlson Comorbidity Index (HR 1.25, 95% CI 1.12 to 1.40; p < 0.0001). Patients with lymph node metastasis showed longer overall survival than those with (sub) cutis metastases (HR 0.34, 9%% CI 0.18 to 0.65; p = 0.001). Among patients who underwent CLND, overall survival was associated with the number of positive lymph nodes (HR 1.06, 95% CI 1.01 to 1.11; p = 0.01) but not with the number of retrieved nodes (HR 1.00, 95% CI 0.96 to 1.03; p = 0.79).

Of note, survival was impaired in patients undergoing CT and target therapy and improved in those receiving immune therapy (**Table 3**).

Multivariable analysis identified only stage as independent predictor of survival among clinically relevant factors at

diagnosis (**Table 4**). Patients with lymph node metastases had longer recurrence/progression-free survival (HR 0.36, 95% CI 0.19 to 0.67; p = 0.001) and overall survival (HR 0.33, 9%% CI 0.17 to 0.63; p = 0.0008) than those with (sub)cutis metastases.

Comparison of Survival in MUP and MKP Patients

Four hundred and seventeen MKP patients (213 males and 204 females; median age 59 years, IQR 45–70) with AJCC stage IIIB–IV were included in the comparison of survival, 3-year recurrence/progression-free survival was 54% in MUP and 58% in MKP (p = 0.30), and 3-year overall survival was 62% in MUP and 70% in MKP (p = 0.40) (**Figure 3**).

TABLE 3 | Univariate analysis of survival.

Variable	Recurrence/progression-free survival		Overall survival	
	HR (95% CI)	p-value	HR (95% CI)	p-value
Age at diagnosis, years:	1.03 (1.01 to 1.04)	0.008	1.04 (1.02 to 1.06)	0.0001
Sex:				
Female	Reference	–	Reference	–
Male	1.05 (0.63 to 1.75)	0.86	1.37 (0.79 to 2.36)	0.26
Family history of cancer:				
No	Reference	–	Reference	–
Yes	2.10 (0.97 to 4.51)	0.06	1.52 (0.64 to 3.62)	0.34
Size of lymph node metastasis, cm[a]	1.09 (0.97 to 1.22)	0.15	1.09 (0.94 to 1.26)	0.27
AJCC stage:				
III	Reference	–	Reference	–
IV	2.77 (1.66 to 4.63)	0.0001	3.43 (2.00 to 5.89)	<0.0001
Charlson Comorbidity Index	1.16 (1.03 to 1.30)	0.01	1.25 (1.12 to 1.40)	<0.0001
Presentation:				
(Sub)cutis metastases	Reference	–	Reference	–
Lymph node metastases	0.37 (0.20 to 0.68)	0.002	0.34 (0.18 to 0.65)	0.001
Visceral metastases	1.03 (0.54 to 1.96)	0.94	1.36 (0.71 to 2.62)	0.36
Neoplastic comorbidity:				
No	Reference	–	Reference	–
Yes	1.40 (0.71 to 2.74)	0.34	1.73 (0.90 to 3.35)	0.10
Autoimmune comorbidity				
No	Reference	–	Reference	–
Yes	1.23 (0.64 to 2.37)	0.53	1.13 (0.57 to 2.23)	0.73
BRAF:				
Wild Type	Reference	–	Reference	–
Mutation	1.22 (0.65 to 2.29)	0.54	0.71 (0.35 to 1.43)	0.34
CT:				
No	Reference	–	Reference	–
Yes	2.76 (1.66 to 4.57)	<0.0001	2.23 (1.33 to 3.75)	0.002
Immune therapy:				
No	Reference	–	Reference	–
Yes	0.58 (0.35 to 0.95)	0.03	0.53 (0.32 to 0.89)	0.02
Target therapy:				
No	Reference	–	Reference	–
Yes	3.37 (1.94 to 5.87)	<0.0001	1.85 (1.01 to 3.40)	0.04
RT:				
No	Reference	–	Reference	–
Yes	1.35 (0.6 to 2.42)	0.31	1.13 (0.61 to 2.09)	0.71

[a]Among patients with lymph node metastases or visceral metastases.

TABLE 4 | Multivariable analysis of overall survival.

Variable	Recurrence/progression-free survival		Overall survival	
	HR (95% CI)	p-value	HR (95% CI)	p-value
Age at diagnosis, years:	1.01 (0.98 to 1.04)	0.42	1.03 (0.99 to 1.06)	0.11
Charlson Comorbidity Index	1.09 (0.89 to 1.32)	0.41	1.10 (0.91 to 1.33)	0.31
Presentation:				
(Sub)cutis metastases:	Reference	–	Reference	–
Lymph node metastases:	0.36 (0.19 to 0.67)	0.001	0.33 (0.17 to 0.63)	0.0008
Visceral metastases:	0.94 (0.49 to 1.80)	0.85	1.12 (0.89 to 2.17)	0.73

DISCUSSION

This study describes patient characteristics, therapeutic approaches, and prognosis of a series of 127 consecutive cases of melanoma of unknown primary (MUP).

The most common clinical scenario in this cohort was a male patient with a median age of 59 years, presenting with a melanoma localized at lymph nodes with neither a detectable primary tumor nor a history of previous melanoma removal, and satisfying all the Das Gupta's exclusion criteria for the definition of MUP.

The median size of lymph node involvement was 4 cm, irrespective of AJCC III or IV stage (*i.e.* with no difference in size between patients with nodal metastases alone, and those with concurrent nodal and visceral metastases). CLND was the most common surgical treatment, and the survival was

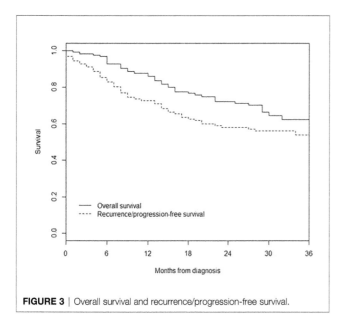

FIGURE 3 | Overall survival and recurrence/progression-free survival.

associated with the number of positive lymph nodes, without significant association with the number of retrieved lymph nodes, in agreement with other studies (13–16). As expected, our results show a worse survival for advanced stage of disease. Considering the staging, our data support AJCC staging system and suggest that the Balch proposal to consider subcutaneous disease as stage III could be not appropriate. In fact, in our series, patients with subcutaneous disease (AJCC stage IV, Balch stage III) had a worse survival than those with lymph nodes metastases (AJCC stage III, Balch stage III), supporting the inclusion of patients with subcutaneous metastases alone in AJCC stage IV.

In addition, the Charlson comorbidity status resulted to be associated with a worse survival in our series.

Considering stage and treatment of MUP, two milestones have been reported. In 2006, the routine use of combined PET/CT at diagnosis in MUP patients increased the shift from stage III to stage IV, and starting from 2011 the introduction of immune and targeted therapy changed the clinical outcome and long-term survival in advanced melanoma. However, in our center, as well in Italy, both therapies were available only in CRTs till 2014; therefore their impact in this series is limited at the last five years. In this historical context, a possible limitation of our study is the long period considered and the imaging and therapeutic changes introduced. Nevertheless, even pooling and considering as "immune-therapy" (IT) the classical interferon option and the novel immune-modulating opportunities (*i.e.* CTLA4 inhibitors and PDL1 inhibitors), IT was the medical treatment associated with the best survival outcome. The lower survival obtained in patients treated with traditional chemotherapy (CT) was in line with the significant superiority of IT compared to CT in all clinical studies. The lower effect of targeted therapy (TT) was due to selection or to more aggressive features in BRAF mutated patients, or could be related to the immune mechanism involved in the initial elimination of melanoma. Indeed a MUP could be considered a recurrence of an immune eliminated melanoma,

and IT could restore an effective immune response, and a greater effect of IT in patients with a "fable immunity" was often observed and reported in the literature in old patients and in immune deficient patients. The comparison of IT to TT in this type of melanoma should be tested in large cohorts and prospectively.

Additionally, the origin of MUP is still an open question, and future studies elucidate whether MUP has to be considered and treated as a melanoma with a known primary (MKP) or represents a different entity. As for survival, we could not demonstrate a difference among MUP and MKP as already reported by other groups. However many authors showed a significant improved survival of MUP compared with MKP (3–5, 17–22).

This was originally explained by Smith and Stehlin in 1965 with a phenomenon of immunological *spontaneous regression* of the primitive tumor (T of TNM). Of note, in contrast to this interpretation, a partial regression of the primary tumor at dermatoscopy has traditionally been recognized as a negative prognostic sign. Therefore linking *regression* to better survival seems at least in part a contradiction, as for melanoma. However the explanation by Smith and Stehlin has been re-proposed by many authors afterwards and is cited also by Anbari and coworkers in 1997 alongside with other criteria of exclusion of MUP (*i.e. a concurrent, unrecognized melanoma or a previously excised, misdiagnosed melanoma*). Indeed, the original contribution of the latter report at the end of last century was the proposal of a new explanation for the origin of MUP: it could represent a primary tumor (T of TNM) within a node rather than a metastatic process to the regional basin (N of TNM). This could explain the better prognosis of MUP patients when compared to MKP, but this does not explain subcutaneous metastases without nodes or visceral metastasis only.

Whatever the origin, it should be considered that the absence of cutaneous/mucosal malignancy in MUP patients could explain by itself their better prognosis for the lesser tumor load (*i.e.* lower amount of cancer stem cells able to metastasize and/or give rise to recurrent disease).

Recently, new reports tried to assess the existence of any correlation between mutations in the main genes (BRAF/NRAS) involved in melanoma initiation and progression (23); they have proposed a distinct molecular classification for MUP to explain the differences in patient outcomes. MUP patients presents consistently BRAF and TERT promoter mutations, suggesting a cutaneous origin. BRAF mutations rate in MUPs appears similar to MKPs; however, for MUPs the rate for V600K seems higher than the rate for MKPs (24). Melanomas with the V600K mutation are characterized by a lower dependence on the activation of the ERK pathway and greater use of alternative pathways; against these melanomas they have a higher mutational load and respond better to immunotherapy; this would concretely explain the better response to immunotherapy and the worse response to BRAFi/MEKi of the MUPs (25–27). The strengths of our study include the diagnosis of MUP based on Das Gupta's criteria (2), the sample size (one of the largest in MUP literature), the evaluation of Balch's staging proposal, and the evaluation of systemic treatments.

The present study has also some limitations. First, it is a single-center study, thus the generalizability of the findings is limited. Second, the retrospective nature of the study limited the availability of data (*e.g.* mutational status). Third, the included patients were treated with heterogeneous modalities because of the long period of inclusion. Fourth, the new medical options now available both in in the adjuvant as in the metastatic setting for all patients could make the distinction between MUP and MKP clinically needless.

AUTHOR CONTRIBUTIONS

Study concepts: PF, MR, SM. MA, VC, JP. Study design: PF, FC, SM, MA, CR. Data acquisition: PF, RS, FC, GA, AP, BF, AS. Quality control of data and algorithms: PF, FC. Data analysis and

interpretation: PF, FC, SM, DL, GA. Statistical analysis: FC. Manuscript preparation: PF, FC, SM, AB, RC, GA. Manuscript editing: PF, FC, SM, DL, MR. Manuscript review: SM, AB, AF, FB, MA, RM, CR. All authors contributed to the article and approved the submitted version.

ACKNOWLEDGMENTS

The authors thank "Piccoli Punti ONLUS", Giuseppe Valentini and "Fondazione Lucia Valentini Terrani" for the long-lasting support.

REFERENCES

1. Scott JF, Gerstenblith MR. "Melanoma of Unknown Primary". In: JF Scott, MR Gerstenblith, editors. *Non cutaneous Melanoma*. Brisbane (AU: Codon Publications (2018). Available at: http://www.ncbi.nlm.nih.gov/books/NBK506989/.
2. Dasgupta T, Bowden L, Berg JW. Malignant melanoma of unknown primary origin. *Surg Gynecol Obstet* (1963) 117:341–5.
3. Kamposioras K, Pentheroudakis G, Pectasides D, Pavlidis N. Malignant melanoma of unknown primary site. To make the long story short. A systematic review of the literature. *Crit Rev Oncol Hematol* (2011) 78:112–26. doi: 10.1016/j.critrevonc.2010.04.007
4. Bae JM, Choi YY, Kim DS, Lee JH, Jang HS, Lee JH, et al. Metastatic melanomas of unknown primary show better prognosis than those of known primary: a systematic review and meta-analysis of observational studies. *J Am Acad Dermatol* (2015) 72:59–70. doi: 10.1016/j.jaad.2014.09.029
5. Lee CC, Faries MB, Wanek LA, Morton DL. Improved survival for stage IV melanoma from an unknown primary site. *J Clin Oncol* (2009) 27:3489–95. doi: 10.1200/JCO.2008.18.9845
6. De Waal AC, Aben KK, van Rossum MM, Kiemeney LA. Melanoma of unknown primary origin: A population-based study in the Netherlands. *Eur J Cancer* (2013) 49:676–83. doi: 10.1016/j.ejca.2012.09.005
7. Gershenwald JE, Scolyer RA. Melanoma Staging: American Joint Committee on Cancer (AJCC) 8th Edition and Beyond [published correction appears in Ann Surg Oncol. 2018 Dec; 25(Suppl 3):993-994]. *Ann Surg Oncol* (2018) 25(8):2105–10. doi: 10.1245/s10434-018-6513-7
8. Ribero S, Pampena R, Bataille V, Moscarella E, Thomas L, Quaglino P, et al. Unknown Primary Melanoma: Worldwide Survey on Clinical Management. *Dermatology* (2016) 232(6):704–7. doi: 10.1159/000453592
9. Verver D, van der Veldt A, van Akkooi A, Verhoef C, Grünhagen DJ, Louwman WJ. Treatment of melanoma of unknown primary in the era of immunotherapy and targeted therapy: A Dutch population-based study. *Int J Cancer* (2020) 146(1):26–34. doi: 10.1002/ijc.32229
10. Balch CM, Soong SJ, Murad TM, Smith JW, Maddox WA, Durant JR. A multifactorial analysis of melanoma. IV. Prognostic factors in 200 melanoma patients with distant metastases (stage III). *J Clinoncol* (1983) 1(2):126–34. doi: 10.1200/JCO.1983.1.2.126
11. Charlson ME, Pompei P, Ales KL, MacKenzie CR. A new method of classifying prognostic comorbidity in longitudinal studies: development and validation. *J Chronic Dis* 40:373–83. doi: 10.1016/0021-9681(87)90171-8
12. R Core Team. *R: A language and environment for statistical computing.* Vienna, Austria: R Foundation for Statistical Computing (2020).
13. Jonk A, Kroon BB, Rümke P, Mooi WJ, Hart AA, van Dongen JA. Lymph node metastasis from melanoma with an unknown primary site. *Br J Surg* (1990) 77(6):665–8. doi: 10.1002/bjs.1800770625
14. Cormier JN, Xing Y, Feng L, Huang X, Davidson L, Gershenwald JE, et al. Metastatic melanoma to lymphnodes in patients with unknown primary sites. *Cancer* (2006) 106(9):2012–20. doi: 10.1002/cncr.21835

15. Lee CC, Faries MB, Wanek LA, Morton DL. Improved survival for stage IV melanoma from an unknown primary site. *J Clin Oncol* (2009) 26(4):3489–95. doi: 10.1200/JCO.2008.18.9845
16. Rutkowski P, Nowecki ZI, Dziewirski W, Zdzienicki M, Pieńkowski A, Salamacha M, et al. Melanoma without a detectable primary site with metastases to lymphnodes. *Dermatol Surg* (2010) 36(6):868–76. doi: 10.1111/j.1524-4725.2010.01562.x
17. Anbari KK, Schuchter LM, Bucky LP, Mick R, Synnestvedt M, Guerry D 4th, et al. Melanoma of unknown primary site: presentation, treatment, and prognosis–a single institution study. University of Pennsylvania Pigmented Lesion Study Group. *Cancer* (1997) 79(9):1816–21. doi: 10.1002/(sici)1097-0142(19970501)79:9<1816::aid-cncr26>3.0.co;2-.
18. Kuk D, Shoushtari AN, Barker CA, Panageas KS, Munhoz RR, Momtaz P, et al. Prognosis of Mucosal, Uveal, Acral, Non acral Cutaneous, and Unknown Primary Melanoma From the Time of First Metastasis. *Oncologist* (2016) 21(7):848–54. doi: 10.1634/theoncologist.2015-0522
19. Lopez R, Holyoke ED, Moore RH, Karakousis CP. Malignant melanoma with unknown primary site. *J Surg Oncol* (1982) 19(3):151–4. doi: 10.1002/jso.2930190308
20. Chang P, Knapper WH. Metastatic melanoma of unknown primary. *Cancer* (1982) 49(6):1106–11. doi: 10.1002/1097-0142(19820315)49:6<1106::aid-cncr2820490607>3.0.co;2-0
21. Panagopoulos E, Murray D. Metastatic malignant melanoma of unknown primary origin: a study of 30 cases. *J Surg Oncol* (1983) 23(1):8–10. doi: 10.1002/jso.2930230104
22. Nasri S, Namazie A, Dulguerov P, Mickel R. Malignant melanoma of cervical and parotid lymph nodes with an unknown primary site. *Laryngoscope* (1994) 104(10):1194–8.
23. Sini MC, Doneddu V, Paliogiannis P, Casula M, Colombino M, Manca A, et al. Genetic alterations in main candidate genes during melanoma progression. *Oncotarget* (2018) 9(9):8531–41. doi: 10.18632/oncotarget.23989
24. De Andrade JP, Wong P, O'Leary MP, Parekh V, Amini A, Schoellhammer HF, et al. Care for Melanoma of Unknown Primary: Experience in the Era of Molecular Profiling. *Ann Surg Oncol* (2020) 27(13):5240–7. doi: 10.1245/s10434-020-09112-2
25. Pires da Silva I, Wang KYX, Wilmott JS, Holst J, Carlino MS, Park JJ, et al. Distinct Molecular Profiles and Immunotherapy Treatment Outcomes of V600E and V600K *BRAF*-Mutant Melanoma. *Clin Cancer Res* (2019) 25(4):1272–9. doi: 10.1158/1078-0432.CCR-18-1680
26. Gambichler T, Chatzipantazi M, Schröter U, Stockfleth E, Gedik C. Patients with melanoma of unknown primary show better outcome under immune checkpoint inhibitor therapy than patients with known primary: preliminary results. *Oncoimmunology* (2019) 8(12):e1677139. doi: 10.1080/2162402X.2019.1677139
27. Beasley GM. Melanomas of Unknown Primary May Have a Distinct Molecular Classification to Explain Differences in Patient Outcomes. *Ann Surg Oncol* (2020) 27(13):4870–1. doi: 10.1245/s10434-020-09114-0

Immune Checkpoint Inhibitors in Advanced Acral Melanoma

Qingyue Zheng [1,2†], Jiarui Li [3†], Hanlin Zhang [1,2†], Yuanzhuo Wang [1,2] and Shu Zhang [1*]

[1] Department of Dermatology, Peking Union Medical College Hospital, Chinese Academy of Medical Sciences and Peking Union Medical College, Beijing, China, [2] Eight-year MD Program, Peking Union Medical College, Beijing, China, [3] Department of Medical Oncology, Peking Union Medical College Hospital, Chinese Academy of Medical Sciences and Peking Union Medical College, Beijing, China

*Correspondence:
Shu Zhang
zhangshu10666@pumch.cn

†These authors have contributed equally to this work and share first authorship

Introduction: Acral melanoma (AM) has different biological characteristics from cutaneous melanoma. Although systemic therapeutic strategies for advanced AM resemble those for advanced cutaneous melanoma, the evidence of the clinical use of immune checkpoint inhibitors (ICIs) for AM is still inadequate. We aimed to systematically analyze the therapeutic effects and safety profile of ICI treatments in advanced AM.

Methods: This systematic review was conducted in line with a previously registered protocol. Three electronic databases, conference abstracts, clinical trial registers, and reference lists of included articles were searched for eligible studies. The primary outcomes were therapeutic effects, and the secondary outcomes were the safety profiles.

Results: This systematic review included six studies investigating anti-CTLA-4 immunotherapy, 12 studies investigating anti-PD-1 immunotherapy, one study investigating the combination therapy of anti-CTLA-4 and anti-PD-1, and one study investigating anti-PD-1 immunotherapy in combination with radiotherapy. In most studies investigating ipilimumab, the anti-CTLA-4 antibody, the objective response rate ranged from 11.4 to 25%, the median progression-free survival ranged from 2.1 to 6.7 months, and the median overall survival was more than 7.16 months. For studies discussing anti-PD-1 immunotherapy with nivolumab, pembrolizumab, or JS001, the objective response rate ranged from 14 to 42.9%, the median progression-free survival ranged from 3.2 to 9.2 months, and the median overall survival was more than 14 months. The combination therapy of anti-CTLA-4 and anti-PD-1 immunotherapy showed better efficacy with an objective response rate of 42.9% than single-agent therapy. The retrospective study investigating the combination therapy of anti-PD-1 immunotherapy and radiation showed no overall response. Few outcomes regarding safety were reported in the included studies.

Conclusions: ICIs, especially anti-CTLA-4 monoclonal antibodies combined with anti-PD-1 antibodies, are effective systematic treatments in advanced AM. However, there remains a lack of high-level evidence to verify their efficacy and safety and support their clinical application.

Keywords: melanoma, immunotherapy, systematic review, ipilimumab, programmed cell death 1 receptor, radiotherapy, combination drug therapy

INTRODUCTION

Acral melanoma (AM), a relatively uncommon subtype of melanoma, affects palmar, plantar, and subungual surfaces. Although only comprising 2–3% of all melanoma cases, AM tends to be the most common melanoma subtype in Asian, African, and Hispanic patients, who are at lower risk for sun-related melanoma subtypes (1). Compared with other melanoma subtypes, AM is usually diagnosed at a more advanced stage, which has been proved by the study utilizing the Surveillance, Epidemiology and End Reports (SEER) database (2). Nearly two-thirds of AM was diagnosed at stage II or above, while only approximately one-third of cutaneous melanoma was diagnosed at stage II or above. Therefore, most patients have developed distant metastasis when diagnosed with AM, and systemic treatment for advanced AM is of great significance (3).

Unlike cutaneous melanoma, AM is generally not associated with UV-exposure, which partly accounts for its far lower mutational burdens than cutaneous melanoma. An Australian study demonstrated that three of the 35 (9%) acral melanomas were found to be UVR dominant. The three acral melanomas had biological characteristics similar to the cutaneous melanoma, including elevated total mutational burdens and lower levels of structural variations when compared with acral melanomas with a non-UVR signature (4). AM has different oncogenic drivers from the cutaneous melanoma, including fewer BRAF mutations (10–23%), inconstant *KIT* mutation rates (3–29%), *CCND1* and *CDK4* amplification, and deletion or mutations in different genes, such as *CDK2NA*, *PTEN*, *NF1*, and hTERT (2, 5). However, systemic treatment for advanced AM resembles those for advanced cutaneous melanoma, possibly on account of the limited number of clinical trials evaluating optimal interventions in AM. The responses of AM patients to BRAF-inhibitors are modest as AM has lower frequencies of BRAF mutations (6). AM had different kinds of mutations of KIT, such as copy number gains and activating mutations (7), but targeted therapies with inhibitors such as imatinib usually exert poor or non-durable responses (8). There still remains an urgent need for effective systemic treatment for advanced AM.

Recently, immune checkpoint inhibitors (ICIs) have been recommended as first-line treatment for advanced cutaneous melanoma (9). However, given the low incidence of AM worldwide, few clinical trials reported the therapeutic effects and safety profile of ICIs on the AM. To identify whether ICIs are beneficial for the patients of AM, we conducted this systematic review to analyze the therapeutic effects and safety profile of ICIs in advanced AM.

MATERIALS AND METHODS

This systematic review was conducted in line with the protocol registered online in the PROSPERO on May 1, 2020 (ID: CRD42020183476) and was designed in line with the PRISMA guidelines (10).

Literature Search

Considering the rarity of AM worldwide, we identified all randomized controlled trials (RCTs), prospective observational studies, retrospective studies, and expanded access programs of advanced AM treated with ICIs. Single case reports and narrative reviews were not included. Only the articles published in English or Chinese were included.

Three electronic databases: PubMed, Cochrane Central Register of Controlled Trials (CENTRAL), and EMBASE were searched to identify possibly related studies (from January 1, 1990 to July 20, 2020). Besides, clinical trial registers, conference abstracts, and reference lists of the included studies were also checked for additional possibly relevant studies. The search strategies were shown in the **Supplementary Material**.

Data Collection and Analysis

In the screening progress, two authors (ZQ and LJ) independently screened the titles and abstracts of the articles identified from the three electronic databases. The articles considered to be potentially relevant would come to the next step, assessing the eligibility. Two authors (ZQ and LJ) assessed the articles according to their full texts. An additional author (ZS) was consulted and resolved possible disagreements. One author (ZH) searched the clinical trial registers, conference abstracts and references of the included studies, and then assessed the eligibility of the records. The included studies must report the response of the patients with unresectable, metastatic, advanced or stage III or IV AM. Two authors (ZQ and LJ) extracted data independently, and a third author (ZS) reviewed the extracted data and made the decision through discussion whenever discrepancies arose. One author (ZQ) used quality assessment tool for before-after (pre-post) studies with no control group, described by the National Heart, Lung, and Blood Institute (NHLBI) (https://www.nhlbi.nih.gov/health-topics/study-quality-assessment-tools), to evaluate the methodological quality of the included studies and the risk of bias.

The primary and secondary outcome data were extracted. The objective response rate (ORR) counted from the sum of complete response (CR) and partial response (PR), median progression-free survival (PFS), median overall survival (OS), the incidence of one-year progression-free survival and the incidence of one-year overall survival were extracted as the primary outcomes to demonstrate the efficacy of the ICIs. As for the safety of ICIs, immune-related adverse event (irAE) rate of all grades and irAE rate of grade 3 or more were extracted as the secondary outcomes. The irAEs were graded in line with the Common Terminology Criteria for Adverse Events (CTCAE).

RESULTS

We initially identified 247 records in the literature search process. After removing duplicates, 200 of them remained. After screening, 37 potentially relevant studies were selected, and the full texts were obtained for eligibility assessment. Finally, the primary and secondary outcomes of the 18 records meeting the eligibility criteria were extracted and systemically analyzed (**Figure 1**). The extracted data from the included studies were listed in **Table 1**.

Anti-CTLA-4 Immunotherapy

In the field of anti-CTLA-4 monotherapy, six studies with 177 AM patients treated with ipilimumab were identified (**Table 1**) (11–16). The ORRs for ipilimumab monotherapy ranged from 11.4 to 25%, the median PFS ranged from 2.1 to 6.7 months, and the median OS was more than 7.16 months, demonstrating the therapeutic effects of anti-CTLA-4 immunotherapy in AM. The only study investigating the safety profile of anti-CTLA-4 immunotherapy in AM showed that the frequency of irAEs was 57%, and the frequency of grade 3 or above irAEs was 17%. There remains an unmet need for randomized controlled trials evaluating the anti-CTLA-4 antibodies in AM.

In a prospective, non-interventional, non-controlled, multi-center (146 institutions), observational study, 107 Japanese patients with radically unresectable acral lentiginous melanoma (ALM) receiving ipilimumab had a median OS of 7.16 months (95% CI, 4.99–10.32 months) (11), which was significantly lower than that in other included studies. One possible reason is that the other studies reporting OS all investigated anti-CTLA-4 antibodies as first-line therapy, but this prospective study involved different lines of treatment, in which the patients'

overall health condition was worse. In the results of a published expanded access program, five patients with unresectable stage III/IV AM received 3 mg/kg ipilimumab for up to four cycles. None of them was untreated, and two (40%) patients had a PR (12). A retrospective review of 35 AM patients receiving ipilimumab either 3 mg/kg or 10 mg/kg was conducted in America. One patient achieved CR (2.9%), three achieved PR (8.6%), and four achieved stable disease (SD) (11.4%). The ORR was 11.4%, and the clinical benefit rate (CR + PR + SD) was 22.9%. Of note is that all patients with positive responses were in the 3 mg/kg ipilimumab group. The median PFS was 2.5 months (95% CI, 2.3–2.7months). The median OS was 16.7 months (95% CI, 10.9–22.5 months). In this study, 20 patients (57%) had irAEs of any grade, and 17% patients had grade 3 or 4 events, including colitis (n = 2), hypophysitis (n = 2), hepatotoxicity (n = 1), and skin toxicity (n = 1). No patients died of irAEs (13). In a retrospective analysis of 17 patients with metastatic AM treated with ipilimumab as first-line therapy, the ORR was 17.8%. The median PFS was 6.7 months (95% CI, 2.8–17.2 months), and the median OS was 38.7 months (95% CI, 7.8–61.6 months) (14). A single-center retrospective cohort study conducted in Switzerland involved 8 advanced ALM patients with ipilimumab as the first-line treatment. The ORR was 25%. The median PFS and median OS were 2.1 months and 21 months, respectively (15). A retrospective study conducted in Germany evaluated the therapeutic effects of anti-CTLA-4 and

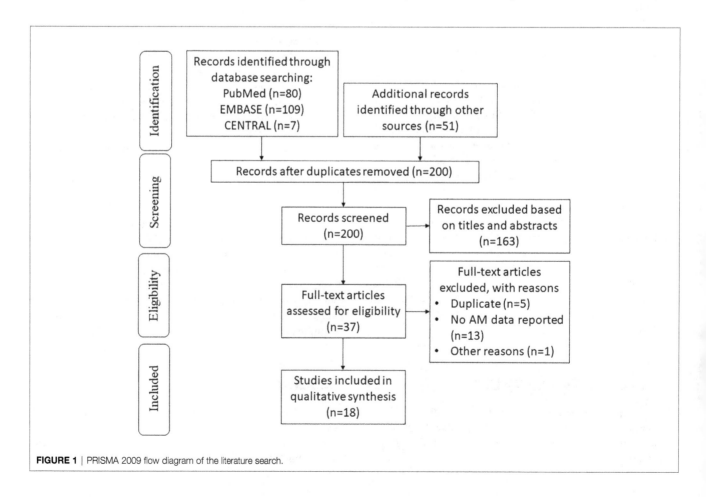

FIGURE 1 | PRISMA 2009 flow diagram of the literature search.

TABLE 1 | Characteristics of the 18 studies included in the qualitative review.

First author and year	Registration ID	Study design	Population	Location	Intervention (mg/kg)	Line of immunotherapy	Record type	ORR	PR	CR	PFS (median)	OS (median)	1-year PFS	1-year OS	All grades irAEs	Grade 3+ irAEs	Methodological quality
															Secondary outcomes		
Yamazaki 2020 (11)	NCT02717364	prospective, non-interventional, multi-center, observational study	n = 547 (total), n = 107 (<co-ALM-</x>)	Japan	ipilimumab(3)	1+	journal article	NR	NR	NR	NR	7.16 months (95% CI, 4.99–10.32 months)	NR	NR	NR	NR	good
Shaw 2012 (12)	NA	EAP	n = 27 (total), n = 5 (AM)	UK	ipilimumab(3)	2+	conference abstract	NR	2 (40%)	NR	NR	NR	NR	NR	NR	NR	poor
Johnson 2015 (13)	NA	retrospective uncontrolled	n = 35 (AM only)	America	ipilimumab(3 or 10)	NR	journal article	11.40%	3 (8.6%)	1 (2.9%)	2.5 months (95% CI, 2.3–2.7 months)	16.7 months (95% CI, 10.9–22.5 months)	NR	NR	20 (57%)	6 (17%)	good
Saberian 2020 (14)	NA	retrospective uncontrolled	n = 44 (AM only)	America	ipilimumab or pembrolizumab or nivolumab	1	conference abstract	17.8% (anti-CTLA-4, n = 17, 40% (anti-PD-1, n = 15)	NR	NR	6.7 months (95% CI, 2.8–17.2 months, anti-CTLA-4), 9.2 months (95% CI, 2.7–19.7 months, anti-PD-1)	38.7 months (95% CI, 7.8–61.6 months, anti-CTLA-4), 60.1 months (95% CI, 12.4–67.4 months, anti-PD-1)	NR	NR	NR	NR	fair
Hafliger 2018 (15)	NA	retrospective uncontrolled	n = 8 (ALM only)	Switzerland	ipilimumab	1	journal article	25%	NR	NR	2.1 months	21 months	NR	NR	NR	NR	fair
Zaremba 2019 (16)	NA	retrospective uncontrolled	n = 21 (AM)	German	anti-PD-1 and anti-CTLA-4 checkpoint inhibitor, respectively	1	journal article	NR	NR	NR	NR	98 months (anti-PD-1, n=16), 95 months (anti-CTLA-4, n=5)	NR	NR	NR	NR	fair
Nathan 2019 (17)	NCT02156804	open-label, single-arm, multi-center phase II study	n = 1,008 (total), n = 55 (AM)	Europe	nivolumab(3)	2+	journal article	NR	NR	NR	NR	25.8 months (95% CI, 15.1–30.6 months)	NR	35 (63.64%)	42 (76.4%)	14 (25.5%)	fair
Yamazaki 2019 (18)	JapicCTI-142533	open-label, single-arm, multicenter phase II study	n = 23 (total), n = 7 (ALM)	Japan	nivolumab(3)	1	journal article	28.6% (90% CI, 10.0–59.1%)	NR	NR	NR	NR	NR	5 (71.4%)	NR	NR	fair
Maeda 2019 (19)	NA	retrospective uncontrolled	n = 68 (total), n = 16 (ALM)	Japan	nivolumab	NR	research letter	19%	3	0	197 days	421 days	NR	NR	NR	NR	fair
Si 2019 (20)	NCT02821000	open-label, non-randomized, multicenter, phase Ib study	n = 102 (total), n = 38 (AM)	China	Pembrolizumab (2)	2	journal article	15.8% (95% CI, 6.0–31.3%)	6 (15.8%)	0	NR	NR	NR	NR	NR	NR	fair
Tang 2019 (21)	NCT02836795	single-center, phase 1, open-label, 2-part (part A dose-escalation and part B dose-expansion) study	n = 36 (total), n = 13 (AM)	China	JS001(1 or 3 or10)	2+	journal article	23%	2	1	NR	NR	NR	NR	NR	0	good
Tang 2020 (22)	NCT03013101	single-center, single arm, open-label phase II registration study	n = 128 (total), n = 50 (AM)	China	JS001(3)	2+	journal article	14.00%	NR	NR	3.2 months (95% CI, 1.8–3.6 months)	16.9 months (95% CI, 10.9–not estimable months)	5 (10%)	28 (56%)	NR	NR	good
Nakamura 2020 (23)	NA	retrospective, single arm	n = 193 (AM only)	Japan	anti-PD-1 antibody	1+	conference abstract	16.60%	13.50%	3.10%	NR	18.1 months	NR	NR	NR	27 (14.0%)	fair
Betof 2020 (24)	NA	retrospective uncontrolled	n = 396 (total), n = 50 (AM)	America	pembrolizumab or nivolumab	NR	journal article	NR	NR	6 (12%)	NR	NR	NR	NR	NR	NR	good
Shoushtari 2016 (25)	NA	multi-institutional, retrospective cohort analysis	n = 60 (total), n = 25 (AM)	America	nivolumab(0.3 to 10) or pembrolizumab (2 or 10)	1+	journal article	32% (95% CI, 15–54%)	6 (24%)	2 (8%)	4.1 months	31.7 months	5 (20%)	5 (20%)	NR	NR	good
Zhao 2019 (26)	NA	retrospective uncontrolled	n = 51 (total), n = 16 (AM)	China	nivolumab(3) or pembrolizumab (2)	1+	journal article	18.75%	3	0	5.3 months (95% CI, 2.4–8.2 months)	NR	NR	NR	NR	NR	fair
Namikawa 2018 (27)	JapicCTI-152869	open-label, single-arm, multi-center phase II study	n = 30 (total), n = 7 (AM)	Japan	nivolumab(1) and ipilimumab (3)	1	journal article	42.9% (95% CI, 9.9–81.6)	NR	NR	NR	NR	3 (43%)	6 (86%)	NR	NR	good
Kato 2019 (28)	NA	retrospective uncontrolled	n = 10 (total), n = 3 (AM)	Japan	radiotherapy and nivolumab (3 or 2) or pembrolizumab (2)	NR	journal article	0	0	0	NR	NR	NR	NR	NR	0	fair

NA, Not Applicable; NR, Not Reported.

anti-PD-1/PDL1 checkpoint inhibitors, respectively. The five AM patients receiving anti-CTLA-4 monoclonal antibodies as first-line therapy had an OS of 95 months, which was significantly higher in comparison with BRAF inhibitors, MEK inhibitors, and chemotherapy in this study (16).

Anti-PD-1 Immunotherapy

In the field of anti-PD-1 monotherapy, 12 studies with 494 AM patients treated with anti-PD-1 monoclonal antibodies were identified (**Table 1**). The extracted statistics demonstrated that immunotherapy targeting the interaction between PD-L1 and PD-1 had nearly the same effect as the antibodies targeting CTLA-4 in AM. The ORR ranged from 14 to 40.0%, the median PFS ranged from 3.2 to 9.2 months, and the median OS was more than 421 days in these studies. The only two studies assessing the safety profile of the anti-PD-1 monotherapy in AM patients showed that the rate of grade 3 or above irAEs was between 14.0 and 25.5%. One patient died of grade 5 myasthenia gravis, which should not be neglected. IrAEs should be taken into serious consideration in clinical practice. As the two studies exploring the safety of the anti-PD-1 monotherapy in AM patients involved 193 and 55 AM patients, respectively, the results were relatively convincing (17, 29). These outcomes demonstrated that anti-PD-1 monotherapy could extend the lifespan with tolerable toxicities in part of the patients with advanced AM. However, some patients might encounter serious adverse events, such as grade 3 or above irAEs leading to discontinuation of the therapy and even death.

Three studies assessed nivolumab monotherapy (17–19). In an open-label, single-arm, multi-centered phase II study in Europe (CheckMate 172), 55 patients with unresectable AM and disease progression or recurrence after prior treatment including anti-cytotoxic T-lymphocyte antigen 4 (CTLA-4) monoclonal antibodies received nivolumab intravenously 3 mg/kg every 2 weeks for up to 2 years until progressive disease or intolerable adverse events was observed. The median OS was 25.8 months (95% CI, 15.1–30.6), which was similar to that of patients with non-acral cutaneous melanoma [25.3 months (95% CI, 20.9–28.9)]. The 1-year OS rate was 63.64%. The rate of treatment-related AEs was 76.4%, and the rate of grade 3 or 4 treatment-related AEs was 25.5% (17). Another open-label, single-arm, multi-centered phase II study conducted in Japan explored the nivolumab as first-line treatment in unresectable stage III/IV or recurrent AM. The patients received nivolumab via intravenous infusion 3 mg/kg every 2 weeks in a 6-week cycle until disease progression or unacceptable toxicity happened. The ORR was 28.6% (90% CI, 10.0–59.1%) for the seven ALM patients participating in this study. The 1-year OS rate was 71.4% (18). In a retrospective uncontrolled study to explore the efficacy of nivolumab monoclonal antibodies in ALM in Japan, the 16 ALM patients receiving nivolumab monotherapy had an ORR of 19%. Three of the ALM patients achieved a partial response, and none of them achieved a complete response. The estimated median OS and PFS were 421 and 197 days, respectively. Of note is that among the 13 ALM patients with visceral metastasis, only one achieved a partial response. In

comparison, two of the three ALM patients without visceral metastasis achieved a partial response. This phenomenon indicated that the efficacy of nivolumab monotherapy for AM patients might differ in different subgroups (19).

Pembrolizumab was independently assessed in one study (20). In an open-label, non-randomized, multi-centered phase Ib study in China, 38 AM patients received pembrolizumab 2 mg/kg via intravenous infusion on day 1 of each 3-week cycle for up to 35 cycles as second-line therapy until disease progression, the onset of intolerable toxicity, investigator decision to discontinue treatment, or voluntary withdrawal of informed consent. As none of the AM patients achieved CR, and six of them achieved PR, the ORR was only 15.8% (95% CI, 6.0–31.3%).

JS001, also known as toripalimab, was independently assessed in two studies, both of which were conducted in China (21, 22). One was a single-center, phase 1, open-label, 2-part (part A dose-escalation and part B dose-expansion) study. Among 13 AM patients refractory to standard systemic treatment, one confirmed CR, two confirmed PR, and three confirmed SD were achieved, with an ORR of 23.1% and a disease control rate of 46.2%. No grade 3 or above irAEs were observed in the involved AM patients, which indicated that JS001 was well-tolerated in this study (21). The other study is a multi-centered, single-arm, open-label phase II registration study. Fifty previously treated advanced AM patients received JS001 3 mg/kg once every two weeks intravenously until disease progression, intolerable toxicity, or voluntary withdrawal of informed consent. The median OS was 16.9 months (95% CI, 10.9–not estimable months), and the median PFS was 3.2 months (95% CI, 1.8–3.6 months). The 1-year OS rate was 56%, and the 1-year PFS rate was 10% (22).

Six retrospective studies evaluated nivolumab and pembrolizumab together (14, 16, 23–26). A study involving 21 Japanese institutions evaluated the efficacy of anti-PD-1 antibodies in 193 advanced AM patients. The CR was 3.1%, and the PR was 13.5%. As a consequence, the ORR was 16.6%. The median OS was reported to be 18.1 months, and irAEs of grades 3 to 5 occurred in 27 patients (14.0%). One patient (0.5%) died of grade 5 myasthenia gravis (23). A study conducted in America involved 50 patients with unresectable stage III or stage IV AM. Six patients (12%) achieved CR (24). A multi-institutional, retrospective cohort analysis conducted in America involved 25 AM patients. Eight of them received nivolumab 0.3 mg/kg to 10 mg/kg intravenously every 2 to 3 weeks. Seventeen AM patients received pembrolizumab either 2 mg/kg every 3 weeks or 10 mg/kg every 2 to 3 weeks. As two AM patients had a CR, and six had a PR, the ORR was 32% (95% CI, 15–54%). The median PFS was 4.1 months, and the median OS was 31.7 months. The 1-year PFS rate was 20%, and the 1-year OS rate was also 20% (25). A study involving 16 metastatic AM patients was conducted in China. The patients received nivolumab 3 mg/kg every 2 weeks, or received pembrolizumab 2 mg/kg every 3 weeks by intravenous infusion. None of the patients achieved CR, and three patients achieved PR. The median PFS was 5.3 months (95% CI, 2.4–8.2 months) (26). Another study conducted in Germany evaluated the efficacy of anti-PD-1/PDL1 and anti-CTLA-4 monoclonal antibodies, respectively. The 16 AM patients receiving anti-PD-1 antibodies as first-line therapy had an OS of 98 months, which was significantly higher in comparison with BRAF inhibitors, MEK inhibitors, and chemotherapy in this study (16). In an analysis of 15 patients with metastatic AM who received pembrolizumab or nivolumab as the first-line treatment, the ORR was 40%. The median PFS of the 15 patients was 9.2 months (95% CI, 2.7–19.7 months), and the median OS was 60.1 months (95% CI, 12.4–67.4 months) (14).

Combination Therapy of Anti-CTLA-4 and Anti-PD-1 Monoclonal Antibodies

One study involving seven AM patients assessed combination therapy of ipilimumab and nivolumab (**Table 1**) (27). An open-label, single-arm, multi-centered phase II study conducted in Japan treated patients with confirmed unresectable stage III/IV or recurrent AM with two doses of nivolumab (1 mg/kg) intravenously plus ipilimumab (3 mg/kg) per cycle for two 3-week cycles, then 6-week cycles with biweekly nivolumab (3 mg/kg) as first-line therapy. The ORR was 42.9% (95% CI, 9.9–81.6), and the number of patients with 1-year PFS and 1-year OS was 3 (43%) and 6 (86%), respectively.

Combination Therapy of Anti-PD-1 Immunotherapy and Radiotherapy

The efficacy and safety of anti-PD-1 immunotherapy and radiotherapy were investigated in one retrospective study conducted in Japan. Three AM patients received one of the following regimens: 3 mg/kg nivolumab every 2 weeks; 2 mg/kg nivolumab every 3 weeks; or 2 mg/kg pembrolizumab every 3 weeks. They were all treated with radiotherapy after the progression of anti-PD-1. None of the patients achieved PR or SD, and two patients achieved SD. There was no grade 3 or above irAEs (28).

DISCUSSION

This systematic review included 16 studies with 542 advanced AM patients and provided a general overview of the efficacy and safety profile of immune checkpoint inhibitors in advanced AM. We conclude that ICIs generally demonstrated remarkable clinical efficacy and acceptable irAEs for most patients.

Anti-CTLA-4 Monotherapy and Anti-PD-1 Monotherapy

High-level evidence of the therapeutic effects and safety profile of anti-CTLA-4 and anti-PD-1 monotherapy in AM is still limited, and its therapeutic effects need to be confirmed *via* high-quality randomized controlled trials. There are three uncompleted clinical trials evaluating anti-PD-1 antibodies for AM patients, which involve different kinds of antibodies from different companies, such as IBI308, IBI310, and pembrolizumab. Two of them were randomized controlled trials. The NCT04277663 will study IBI310 combined with IBI308 in comparison to high-dose interferon in AM removed by surgery. The NCT03698019 will study pembrolizumab in stage III or IV high-risk melanoma before and after surgery. With more clinical trials, the therapeutic effects and safety profile of anti-PD-1 monotherapy will be illustrated more clearly.

Combination Therapy of Anti-CTLA-4 and Anti-PD-1 Immunotherapy

Previous research in cutaneous melanoma showed that the combination of anti-CTLA-4 monoclonal antibodies and anti-PD-1 monoclonal antibodies was more effective but more toxic than single-agent therapy (30, 31). The only study evaluating the therapeutic effects of anti-CTLA-4 (ipilimumab) in combination with anti-PD-1 (nivolumab) in advanced AM showed an ORR of 42.9%, a 1-year PFS rate of 43%, and a 1-year OS rate of 86%, which were all much higher than those of anti-CTLA-4 or anti-PD-1 immunotherapy alone, demonstrating that administering nivolumab plus ipilimumab may provide a more hopeful treatment choice for patients with AM than either agent alone.

However, as the number of patients involved in the study was not enough to exert a convincing conclusion, more clinical trials evaluating the therapeutic effects and safety profile of the combined therapy of anti-CTLA-4 and anti-PD-1 are needed. The NCT02978443 is an uncompleted biomarker study of advanced mucosal melanoma or ALM treated with the combination of ipilimumab and nivolumab.

Combination Therapy of Anti-PD-1 Immunotherapy and Radiotherapy

Radiotherapy is now seldom used due to the remarkable success of targeted therapy and immunotherapy, as well as melanoma's low susceptibility to radiotherapy. Nevertheless, several studies discovered that radiation combined with immune checkpoint inhibitors had a synergistic effect in advanced cutaneous melanoma (32, 33). This systematic review included one retrospective study that assessed the anti-PD-1 immunotherapy combined with radiation (28). The ORR was 0, and the rate of grade 3 or above irAEs was also 0. As only three AM patients were involved in this study, the credibility and convincement of this evidence are poor, calling for more relevant studies to solve this problem. In theory, radiotherapy can enhance the transport of T cells to tumor tissues and enhance the strength of specific anti-tumor immune responses (34), so the combination of ICIs and radiotherapy may be more effective than monotherapy.

Combination Therapy of Tyrosine Kinase Inhibitor and ICIs

As melanomas often overexpress VEGF, which may play a significant role in disease progression, anti-angiogenesis targeting VEGF is a meaningful strategy in treating melanoma (35). Although there is no completed clinical trial investigating the combination of tyrosine kinase inhibitor and ICIs in AM, some clinical trials are recruiting patients, which will fill the gaps in this field. The NCT03955354 investigates the combination of anti-PD-1 monoclonal antibody SHR-1210 and Apatinib as first-line therapy in advanced AM. The NCT03991975 studies the TQB2450, a kind of PD-L1 antibodies, combined with Anlotinib in patients with advanced AM.

Different Effects of ICIs in AM and Non-Acral Cutaneous Melanoma

Some studies identified in this systematic review compared the therapeutic effects of immune checkpoint inhibitors in AM and other subtypes of melanoma. A retrospective study found that in anti-PD-1 monotherapy, patients with AM (12%) were less likely to have a CR compared to cutaneous melanoma (30.9%) (24). In an open-label, nonrandomized, multi-centered, phase Ib study evaluating the efficacy of pembrolizumab as second-line therapy, the ORR was 15.8% (95% CI, 6.0–31.3%) in AM, 19.5% (95% CI, 8.8–34.9%) in non-acral melanoma (20). An open-label, single-arm, multi-centered phase II study showed that in combination therapy of anti-CTLA-4 and anti-PD-1 immunotherapy, the ORR of patients with AM (42.9%) was much lower than that of patients with non-acral cutaneous melanoma (75.0%) (27). However, a retrospective study found that therapy containing pembrolizumab had the same effect in AM (ORR 26.7%) as in the non-acral cutaneous subtype (ORR 26.7%) (36). Although the quality and size of each one of the studies was not enough to provide strong evidence, the evidence that supports AM has worse efficacy outcomes when treated with ICIs compared with cutaneous melanoma overweighs the few evidence for the same efficacy outcomes. Although the exact reason for the worse efficacy outcomes in AM compared to cutaneous melanoma in most studies was unclear, several studies have revealed unique biological characteristics of AM, which may contribute to uncovering the underlying reason. Unlike cutaneous melanoma, AM is generally not linked to UV-exposure, which results in its far lower mutational burdens than cutaneous melanoma. A study using whole-genome sequencing showed that single-nucleotide variant were 1.02–3.68 per Mb in AM, which is much lower than that in cutaneous melanoma (37). The frequencies of somatic structural variants were more in acral than in cutaneous melanomas, and greater proportions of the acral and mucosal melanoma genomes had copy number variation (38, 39). AM also has different oncogenic drivers from cutaneous melanoma, including inconstant *KIT* mutation rates (3–29%), *CCND1* and *CDK4* amplification, and deletion or mutations in different genes, such as *CDK2NA*, *PTEN*, *NF1*, and hTERT (2). A few studies suggested that the response to immunotherapy is associated with tumor mutational burden, and increased tumor neoantigen load may predict the objective response (40–43). This may partly explain why the efficacy of ICIs for AM is lower than that for the non-acral cutaneous subtype.

A possible reason is that PD-L1 expression is lower in AM than that in the non-acral cutaneous subtype. One study reported the expression of the PD-L1 in different subtypes of melanoma. 33% of AM had PD-L1 expression, compared with 62% of the sun-damaged melanomas (44). As anti-PD-1 antibodies target the interaction between PD-1 and PD-L1, the PD-L1 expression might be a biomarker predictive of the response to ICIs (45, 46).

The tumor microenvironment may also play a role. In a study, grade III TILs were more frequent in cutaneous non-ALM than in ALM (33.3 vs. 22.6%, p = 0.033), and lower TIL levels (p = 0.031) were significantly associated with shorter OS (47). However, in a study from Korea, there was no significant association between nodular melanoma, superficial spreading melanoma, and ALM with respect to the presence of lymphocytes or LS and DFS and OS (48). So whether there is a difference in TIL in the tumor microenvironment between AM and cutaneous melanomas remains to be determined. As the skin in acral sites is strikingly different from the skin in other anatomical sites, including differences of melanocyte differentiation and the absence of hair follicles and sebaceous glands, the differences between the microenvironment of AM and cutaneous melanoma may suggest a different response rate for ICIs.

Limitations and Prospects

We recognized several limitations in this systematic review. First, the methodological quality of 11 out of 18 studies included in this systematic review was evaluated as poor or fair, and 10 out of 18 studies were retrospective, together with the lack of randomized controlled trials, may result in biases. The number of studies involved in this review was also small due to the limited exploration in this field. Second, the ICIs were applied in mixed lines of therapy in most studies. Nevertheless, ICIs may have variable efficacy and safety outcomes as first-line and further-line treatment of AM. For instance, a prospective study showed that the OS result in treatment-naive AM patients was longer than in those who had received prior treatment when treated with anti-CILA-4 antibodies (11). The conclusion would be more convincing if the studies separated the patients into different subgroups according to the lines of treatment when they received ICIs. Third, most of the studies did not report the primary location of AM, or did not analyze the outcomes of different subgroups of primary sites, but the response to treatment might differ in different primary site of AM. According to a multi-center retrospective study in China, there exist differences in survival in different primary locations in AM. Compared with AM arising from sole, AM arising from palm and nail bed subgroup has a better prognosis (49). AM in different anatomical positions may have variable mutation profiles, which is exemplified by the study result that BRAF mutations were more often found in AM located on the feet. Comparing AM arising from dorsal acral sites with AM on palms and soles, lower frequencies of NRAS (25 *versus* 39.1%) and NF1 (0 *versus* 17.3%) and higher frequencies of BRAF (75 *versus* 21.7%) and TERT promoter (50 *versus* 8.6%) mutations were observed (16). As the variable genetic changes in varying anatomical positions likely influence biological behavior and therapeutic response, it is worthwhile to evaluate the therapeutic effects and safety profile of ICIs in AM arising from specific primary sites. Last, most included studies did not report the outcomes concerning the irAEs of ICIs in AM separately, so the safety of ICIs in AM remains an unsettled question that needs to be further explored.

There remain several directions of exploration in the application of ICIs in the AM. First, the most suitable clinical setting for the ICIs must be defined to achieve satisfactory outcomes. High-quality clinical trials focusing on ICIs in combination with radiotherapy, chemotherapy, or other immunotherapies in the treatment for AM are in urgent need, especially the randomized controlled trials involving statistically sufficient patients. In addition, the appropriate neoadjuvant and adjuvant therapy also needs to be explored, which could not be accomplished without the efforts and contributions of countries including China where AM is one of the most prevalent melanoma subtypes. Second, there lack laboratory models of AM, which hinders the development of new treatments such as ICIs. Third, prognostic biomarkers that can predict the response of AM to ICIs should be further explored. Tumor neoantigen load and PD-L1 expression level are regarded as promising biomarkers, but the reliability of them in AM needs to be verified, as they might not be applied in the actual situation (50). In a retrospective study, the PD-L1 expression level was not associated with anti-PD-1 ORR ($p = 0.982$) in AM (14). Besides the two markers, lower infiltration of cancer-associated fibroblasts and expression of cancer-associated fibroblast markers are linked to the positive response to anti-PD-1 monoclonal antibodies in AM (51), which is worth further exploring. Finally, possibly effective treatments for AM after the ICI treatment fails also need to be considered. Targeted therapy, or other immunotherapies, even other kinds of ICIs might be effective. In a clinical trial, nivolumab had desirable efficacy and safety results after tumor progression on prior ipilimumab (17), which brought hope to these patients.

CONCLUSIONS

In conclusion, ICIs generally demonstrated remarkable clinical efficacy and acceptable irAEs in patients with advanced AM. ICIs, especially anti-CTLA-4 immunotherapy combined with anti-PD-1 immunotherapy, are promising therapeutic strategy for advanced AM. Nevertheless, there remains a lack of high-level proof to verify their safety and support their clinical application. The effect of ICIs in AM from different primary sites should also be further elucidated in future studies. We hope that this systematic review could benefit physicians and patients, and pave the way for further research on the treatment of advanced AM.

AUTHOR CONTRIBUTIONS

QZ and JL conceived and designed this review. QZ, JL, and HZ conducted the literature search and collected the data. QZ drafted the manuscript and figures. SZ, HZ, JL, and YW reviewed and revised the manuscript. All authors contributed to the article and approved the submitted version.

REFERENCES

1. Redi U, Marruzzo G, Lovero S, Khokhar HT, Lo Torto F, Ribuffo D. Acral lentiginous melanoma: A retrospective study. J Cosmet Dermatol (2020). doi: 10.1111/jocd.13737

2. Chen YA, Teer JK, Eroglu Z, Wu JY, Koomen JM, Karreth FA, et al. Translational pathology, genomics and the development of systemic therapies for acral melanoma. Semin Cancer Biol (2020) 61:149–57. doi: 10.1016/j.semcancer.2019.10.017

3. Namikawa K, Yamazaki N. Targeted Therapy and Immunotherapy for Melanoma in Japan. Curr Treat Options Oncol (2019) 20(1):7. doi: 10.1007/s11864-019-0607-8

4. Rawson RV, Johansson PA, Hayward NK, Waddell N, Patch AM, Lo S, et al. and non-UVR mutation burden in some acral and cutaneous melanomas. Lab Invest (2017) 97(2):130–45. doi: 10.1038/labinvest.2016.143

5. Ravaioli GM, Dika E, Lambertini M, Chessa MA, Fanti PA, Patrizi A. Acral melanoma: correlating the clinical presentation to the mutational status. G Ital Dermatol Venereol (2019) 154(5):567–72. doi: 10.23736/s0392-0488.18.05791-7

6. Bai X, Mao LL, Chi ZH, Sheng XN, Cui CL, Kong Y, et al. BRAF inhibitors: efficacious and tolerable in BRAF-mutant acral and mucosal melanoma. Neoplasma (2017) 64(4):626–32. doi: 10.4149/neo_2017_419

7. Curtin JA, Busam K, Pinkel D, Bastian BC. Somatic activation of KIT in distinct subtypes of melanoma. J Clin Oncol (2006) 24(26):4340–6. doi: 10.1200/jco.2006.06.2984

8. Guo J, Si L, Kong Y, Flaherty KT, Xu X, Zhu Y, et al. open-label, single-arm trial of imatinib mesylate in patients with metastatic melanoma harboring c-Kit mutation or amplification. J Clin Oncol (2011) 29(21):2904–9. doi: 10.1200/jco.2010.33.9275

9. Li J, Kan H, Zhao L, Sun Z, Bai C. Immune checkpoint inhibitors in advanced or metastatic mucosal melanoma: a systematic review. Ther Adv Med Oncol (2020) 12:1758835920922028. doi: 10.1177/1758835920922028

10. Moher D, Liberati A, Tetzlaff J, Altman DG, Grp P. Preferred Reporting Items for Systematic Reviews and Meta-Analyses: The PRISMA Statement. PloS Med (2009) 6(7):264–9, w64. doi: 10.1371/journal.pmed.1000097

11. Yamazaki N, Kiyohara Y, Uhara H, Tsuchida T, Maruyama K, Shakunaga N, et al. Real-world safety and efficacy data of ipilimumab in Japanese radically unresectable malignant melanoma patients: A postmarketing surveillance. J Dermatol (2020) 47:834–48. doi: 10.1111/1346-8138.15388

12. Shaw H, Larkin J, Corrie P, Ellis S, Nobes J, Marshall E, et al. Ipilimumab for advanced melanoma in an expanded access programme (EAP): ocular, mucosal and acral subtype UK experience. Ann Oncol (2012) 23:ix374–. doi: 10.1093/annonc/mds404

13. Johnson DB, Peng C, Abramson RG, Ye F, Zhao S, Wolchok JD, et al. Clinical Activity of Ipilimumab in Acral Melanoma: A Retrospective Review. Oncologist (2015) 20(6):648–52. doi: 10.1634/theoncologist.2014-0468

14. Saberian C, Ludford K, Roszik J, Gruschkus S, Johnson DH, Bernatchez C, et al. Analysis of tumor mutation burden (TMB), PD-L1 status and clinical outcomes with checkpoint inhibitors (CPI) in acral melanoma (AM). Pigment Cell Melanoma Res (2020) 33(1):226–7. doi: 10.1111/pcmr.12834

15. Hafliger EM, Ramelyte E, Mangana J, Kunz M, Kazakov DV, Dummer R, et al. Metastatic acral lentiginous melanoma in a tertiary referral center in Switzerland: a systematic analysis. Melanoma Res (2018) 28(5):442–50. doi: 10.1097/cmr.0000000000000465

16. Zaremba A, Murali R, Jansen P, Moller I, Sucker A, Paschen A, et al. Clinical and genetic analysis of melanomas arising in acral sites. Eur J Cancer (2019) 119:66–76. doi: 10.1016/j.ejca.2019.07.008

17. Nathan P, Ascierto PA, Haanen J, Espinosa E, Demidov L, Garbe C, et al. Safety and efficacy of nivolumab in patients with rare melanoma subtypes who progressed on or after ipilimumab treatment: a single-arm, open-label, phase II study (CheckMate 172). *Eur J Cancer* (2019) 119:168–78. doi: 10.1016/j.ejca.2019.07.010

18. Yamazaki N, Kiyohara Y, Uhara H, Uehara J, Fujisawa Y, Takenouchi T, et al. Long-term follow up of nivolumab in previously untreated Japanese patients with advanced or recurrent malignant melanoma. *Cancer Sci* (2019) 110 (6):1995–2003. doi: 10.1111/cas.14015

19. Maeda T, Yoshino K, Nagai K, Oaku S, Kato M, Hiura A, et al. Efficacy of nivolumab monotherapy against acral lentiginous melanoma and mucosal melanoma in Asian patients. *Br J Dermatol* (2019) 180(5):1230–1. doi: 10.1111/bjd.17434

20. Si L, Zhang X, Shu Y, Pan H, Wu D, Liu J, et al. A Phase Ib Study of Pembrolizumab as Second-Line Therapy for Chinese Patients With Advanced or Metastatic Melanoma (KEYNOTE-151). *Transl Oncol* (2019) 12(6):828–35. doi: 10.1016/j.tranon.2019.02.007

21. Tang B, Yan X, Sheng X, Si L, Cui C, Kong Y, et al. Safety and clinical activity with an anti-PD-1 antibody JS001 in advanced melanoma or urologic cancer patients. *J Hematol Oncol* (2019) 12(1):7. doi: 10.1186/s13045-018-0693-2

22. Tang B, Chi Z, Chen YB, Liu X, Wu D, Chen J, et al. Safety, Efficacy and Biomarker Analysis of Toripalimab in previously treated advanced melanoma: results of the POLARIS-01 multicenter phase II trial. *Clin Cancer Res* (2020) 26:5048. doi: 10.1158/1078-0432.Ccr-19-3922

23. Nakamura Y, Namikawa K, Yoshino K, Yoshikawa S, Uchi H, Goto K, et al. Anti-PD1 checkpoint inhibitor therapy in acral melanoma: A multicentre study of 193 Japanese patients. *Ann Oncol Off J Eur Soc Med Oncol* (2020) 31:1198–206. doi: 10.1016/j.annonc.2020.05.031

24. Betof Warner A, Palmer JS, Shoushtari AN, Goldman DA, Panageas KS, Hayes SA, et al. Long-Term Outcomes and Responses to Retreatment in Patients With Melanoma Treated With PD-1 Blockade. *J Clin Oncol* (2020) 38:Jco1901464. doi: 10.1200/jco.19.01464

25. Shoushtari AN, Munhoz RR, Kuk D, Ott PA, Johnson DB, Tsai KK, et al. The efficacy of anti-PD-1 agents in acral and mucosal melanoma. *Cancer* (2016) 122(21):3354–62. doi: 10.1002/cncr.30259

26. Zhao L, Yang Y, Ma B, Li W, Li T, Han L, et al. Factors Influencing the Efficacy of Anti-PD-1 Therapy in Chinese Patients with Advanced Melanoma. *J Oncol* (2019) 2019:6454989. doi: 10.1155/2019/6454989

27. Namikawa K, Kiyohara Y, Takenouchi T, Uhara H, Uchi H, Yoshikawa S, et al. Efficacy and safety of nivolumab in combination with ipilimumab in Japanese patients with advanced melanoma: An open-label, single-arm, multicentre phase II study. *Eur J Cancer* (2018) 105:114–26. doi: 10.1016/j.ejca.2018.09.025

28. Kato J, Hida T, Someya M, Sato S, Sawada M, Horimoto K, et al. Efficacy of combined radiotherapy and anti-programmed death 1 therapy in acral and mucosal melanoma. *J Dermatol* (2019) 46(4):328–33. doi: 10.1111/1346-8138.14805

29. Nakamura Y, Namikawa K, Yoshino K, Yoshikawa S, Uchi H, Goto K, et al. Real-world efficacy of anti-PD-1 antibodies in advanced acral melanoma patients: A retrospective, multicenter study (JAMP study). *J Clin Oncol* (2019) 37:9529. doi: 10.1200/JCO.2019.37.15_suppl.9529

30. Pasquali S, Hadjinicolaou AV, Chiarion Sileni V, Rossi CR, Mocellin S. Systemic treatments for metastatic cutaneous melanoma. *Cochrane Database Syst Rev* (2018) 2:Cd011123. doi: 10.1002/14651858.CD011123.pub2

31. Wolchok JD, Chiarion-Sileni V, Gonzalez R, Rutkowski P, Grob JJ, Cowey CL, et al. Overall Survival with Combined Nivolumab and Ipilimumab in Advanced Melanoma. *N Engl J Med* (2017) 377(14):1345–56. doi: 10.1056/NEJMoa1709684

32. Liniker E, Menzies AM, Kong BY, Cooper A, Ramanujam S, Lo S, et al. Activity and safety of radiotherapy with anti-PD-1 drug therapy in patients with metastatic melanoma. *Oncoimmunology* (2016) 5(9):e1214788. doi: 10.1080/2162402x.2016.1214788

33. Filippi AR, Fava P, Badellino S, Astrua C, Ricardi U, Quaglino P. Radiotherapy and immune checkpoints inhibitors for advanced melanoma. *Radiother Oncol* (2016) 120(1):1–12. doi: 10.1016/j.radonc.2016.06.003

34. Lugade AA, Moran JP, Gerber SA, Rose RC, Frelinger JG, Lord EM. Local Radiation Therapy of B16 Melanoma Tumors Increases the Generation of Tumor Antigen-Specific Effector Cells That Traffic to the Tumor. *J Immunol* (2005) 174(12):7516–23. doi: 10.4049/jimmunol.174.12.7516

35. Gorski DH, Leal AD, Goydos JS. Differential expression of vascular endothelial growth factor-A isoforms at different stages of melanoma progression. *J Am Coll Surg* (2003) 197(3):408–18. doi: 10.1016/s1072-7515(03)00388-0

36. Wen X, Ding Y, Li J, Zhao J, Peng R, Li D, et al. The experience of immune checkpoint inhibitors in Chinese patients with metastatic melanoma: a retrospective case series. *Cancer Immunol Immunother* (2017) 66(9):1153–62. doi: 10.1007/s00262-017-1989-8

37. Furney SJ, Turajlic S, Stamp G, Thomas JM, Hayes A, Strauss D, et al. The mutational burden of acral melanoma revealed by whole-genome sequencing and comparative analysis. *Pigment Cell Melanoma Res* (2014) 27(5):835–8. doi: 10.1111/pcmr.12279

38. Hayward NK, Wilmott JS, Waddell N, Johansson PA, Field MA, Nones K, et al. Whole-genome landscapes of major melanoma subtypes. *Nature* (2017) 545(7653):175–80. doi: 10.1038/nature22071

39. Krauthammer M, Kong Y, Ha BH, Evans P, Bacchiocchi A, McCusker JP, et al. Exome sequencing identifies recurrent somatic RAC1 mutations in melanoma. *Nat Genet* (2012) 44(9):1006–14. doi: 10.1038/ng.2359

40. Snyder A, Makarov V, Merghoub T, Yuan J, Zaretsky JM, Desrichard A, et al. Genetic basis for clinical response to CTLA-4 blockade in melanoma. *N Engl J Med* (2014) 371(23):2189–99. doi: 10.1056/NEJMoa1406498

41. Yarchoan M, Hopkins A, Jaffee EM. Tumor Mutational Burden and Response Rate to PD-1 Inhibition. *N Engl J Med* (2017) 377(25):2500–1. doi: 10.1056/NEJMc1713444

42. Cristescu R, Mogg R, Ayers M, Albright A, Murphy E, Yearley J, et al. Pan-tumor genomic biomarkers for PD-1 checkpoint blockade-based immunotherapy. *Science* (2018) 362(6411):eaar3593. doi: 10.1126/science.aar3593

43. Xu-Monette ZY, Zhang M, Li J, Young KH. PD-1/PD-L1 Blockade: Have We Found the Key to Unleash the Antitumor Immune Response? *Front Immunol* (2017) 8:1597:1597. doi: 10.3389/fimmu.2017.01597

44. Kaunitz GJ, Cottrell TR, Lilo M, Muthappan V, Esandrio J, Berry S, et al. Melanoma subtypes demonstrate distinct PD-L1 expression profiles. *Lab Invest* (2017) 97(9):1063–71. doi: 10.1038/labinvest.2017.64

45. Havel JJ, Chowell D, Chan TA. The evolving landscape of biomarkers for checkpoint inhibitor immunotherapy. *Nat Rev Cancer* (2019) 19(3):133–50. doi: 10.1038/s41568-019-0116-x

46. Daud AII, Wolchok JD, Robert C, Hwu WJ, Weber JS, Ribas A, et al. Programmed Death-Ligand 1 Expression and Response to the Anti-Programmed Death 1 Antibody Pembrolizumab in Melanoma. *J Clin Oncol* (2016) 34(34):4102–9. doi: 10.1200/jco.2016.67.2477

47. Castaneda CA, Torres-Cabala C, Castillo M, Villegas V, Casavilca S, Cano L, et al. Tumor infiltrating lymphocytes in acral lentiginous melanoma: a study of a large cohort of cases from Latin America. *Clin Transl Oncol* (2017) 19 (12):1478–88. doi: 10.1007/s12094-017-1685-3

48. Park CK, Kim SK. Clinicopathological significance of intratumoral and peritumoral lymphocytes and lymphocyte score based on the histologic subtypes of cutaneous melanoma. *Oncotarget* (2017) 8(9):14759–69. doi: 10.18632/oncotarget.14736

49. Wei X, Wu D, Li H, Zhang R, Chen Y, Yao H, et al. The Clinicopathological and Survival Profiles Comparison Across Primary Sites in Acral Melanoma. *Ann Surg Oncol* (2020) 27:3478–85. doi: 10.1245/s10434-020-08418-5

50. Tang B, Chi Z, Guo J. Toripalimab for the treatment of melanoma. *Expert Opin Biol Ther* (2020) 20:863–9. doi: 10.1080/14712598.2020.1762561

51. Yu J, Xie Y, Wu X, Cheng Z, Yin T, Guo J, et al. Targeting cancer-associated fibroblasts synergizes with anti-PD-1 immunotherapy in advanced acral melanoma. *Pigment Cell Melanoma Res* (2020) 33(1):196–7. doi: 10.1111/pcmr.12834

The WHO 2018 Classification of Cutaneous Melanocytic Neoplasms: Suggestions from Routine Practice

Gerardo Ferrara[1]* and Giuseppe Argenziano[2]

[1] Anatomic Pathology Unit, Macerata General Hospital, Macerata, Italy, [2] Department of Dermatology, 'Luigi Vanvitelli' University School of Medicine, Naples, Italy

*Correspondence:
Gerardo Ferrara
gerardo.ferrara@libero.it

The "multidimensional" World Health Organization (WHO) classification 2018 of melanocytic tumors encompasses nine melanoma pathways (seven of which for cutaneous melanoma) according to a progression model in which morphologically intermediate melanocytic tumors are cosidered as simulators and/or precursors to melanoma. These "intermediates" can be subclassified into: i) a "classical" subgroup (superficial/thin compound: dysplastic nevus), which is placed within the morphologic and molecular progression spectrum of classical (Clark's and McGovern's) melanoma subtypes (superficial spreading and, possibly, nodular); and ii) a "non-classical" subgroup (thick compound/dermal: "melanocytomas") whose genetic pathways diverge from classical melanoma subtypes. Such a progression model is aimed at giving a conceptual framework for a histopathological classification; however, routine clinicopathological practice strongly suggests that most melanomas arise *de novo* and that the vast majority of nevi are clinically stable or even involuting over time. Clinicopathological correlation can help identify some severely atypical but benign tumors (*e.g.*: sclerosing nevus with pseudomelanomatous features) as well as some deceptively bland melanomas (*e.g.*: lentiginous melanoma; nested melanoma), thereby addressing some ambiguous cases to a correct clinical management. The recently available adjuvant therapy regimens for melanoma raise the problem of a careful distinction between severely atypical (high grade) melanocytoma and "classical" melanoma: conventional morphology can guide an algorithmic approach based on an antibody panel (anti-mutated BRAF, BAP1, PRAME, ALK, TRKA, MET, HRAS-WT, ROS; beta catenin; R1alpha; p16; HMB45; Ki67), a first-line molecular study (identification of hot spot mutations of *BRAF* and *NRAS*) and an advanced molecular study (sequencing of *NF1, KIT, BRAF, MAP2K1, GNAQ, GNA11, PLCB4, CYSLTR2, HRAS*; fusions studies of *BRAF, RET, MAP3K8, PRKCA*); as a final step, next-generation sequencing can identify melanocytic tumors with rare genetic signatures and melanocytic tumors with a high tumor mutation burden which should be definitely ascribed to the category of classical melanoma with the respective therapeutic options.

Keywords: melanoma, melanocytoma, dysplastic nevus, clinicopathological correlation, histopathology, immunohistochemistry, molecular biology

INTRODUCTION

The histopathological diagnosis and classification of melanocytic skin tumors is probably the greatest conceptual and practical challenge in modern dermatopathology and is expected to rapidly evolve in the next future, with the WHO 2018 classification being the basis for the forthcoming studies (1). One major problem, however, is that the histopathological diagnosis itself is not based upon the search of a single (or a few), objective, and easily reproducible morphological diagnostic feature(s) but rather, it is born by a constellation of diagnostic criteria whose implementation, meaning, and relative weight considerably vary case by case and is responsible for a worrisome list of diagnostic pitfalls (**Table 1**). Thus, the histopathological diagnosis of melanocytic skin neoplasms, being based upon the simultaneous evaluation of several criteria, is no more than an *assessment of probability* and, as such, is often a matter of a sizable disagreement and inter-observer variability (2). In addition, and even more importantly, the time-honored "unifying concept of melanoma" (melanoma as a single entity evolving with a well-defined and repetitive "sequence of events") (3) has been questioned, because both clinicopathological (4) and molecular studies (5) point toward the existence of melanocytic neoplasms of low malignant potential (putative low-grade melanocytic malignancies different from "classical" melanoma).

In order to face with these problems in routine histopathological practice, the WHO Working Group supports the use of descriptive and provisional terminology, *i.e:* i) "intraepidermal atypical melanocytic proliferation of uncertain significance (IAMPUS)": a melanocytic neoplasms raising the differential diagnosis with melanoma *in situ*; ii) "superficial atypical melanocytic proliferation of uncertain significance (SAMPUS)": a thin compound melanocytic neoplasm whose differential diagnosis is with early invasive, radial growth phase (thin non-mitogenic and non-tumorigenic) melanoma; iii) "melanocytic tumor of uncertain malignant potential (MELTUMP)": a compound or dermal-based neoplasm whose differential diagnosis includes melanoma in vertical growth phase (typified by dermal mitotic figures and/or

---

TABLE 1 | Main settings of diagnostic difficulties in melanocytic skin neoplasms.

1. Unrecognized melanoma on partial (shave/punch) biopsies
2. Nevoid melanoma *vs.* "common" or "congenital" compound/dermal nevus
3. Desmoplastic melanoma *vs.* desmoplastic nevus *vs.* scar
4. Recurrent/persistent nevus *vs.* (recurrent) melanoma
5. Spindle cell melanoma *vs.* spindle cell nevus
6. Spitz/spitzoid melanoma *vs.* atypical Sptz nevus/tumor *vs.* Spitz nevus
7. Superficial spreading melanoma *vs.* dysplastic nevus
8. Superficial spreading melanoma *vs.* haloed nevus
9. Melanoma (in special site) *vs.* nevus with site-related atypia
10. Melanoma with regression *vs.* compound nevus with regression-like fibrosis
11. Melanoma with regression *vs.* melanosis
12. Melanoma *in situ* in chronic sun-damaged skin *vs.* melanocytic hyperplasia/photoactivation
13. Dermal melanoma over congenital nevus *vs.* proliferative nodule in congenital nevus
14. Cellular blue nevus *vs.* animal-type melanoma *vs.* blue nevus-like metastatic melanoma
15. Deep penetrating nevus *vs.* deep penetrating nevus-like melanoma
16. Pigmented epithelioid melanocytoma *vs.* animal-type melanoma

by dermal nests/sheets which are larger than the larger junctional nest) (6). Based on the these definitions, such a descriptive terminology applies to simulators (morphologically atypical nevi and deceptively bland melanomas) (2) as well as to biological "intermediates" (melanocytic neoplasms of low malignant potential) (4); and a strong suggestion is made that several neoplasms belonging to both categories may be in fact precursors to melanoma. The present review is aimed at giving some suggestions in the multidisciplinary approach based on the WHO 2018 classification.

THE PATHWAYS TO MELANOMA

The WHO 2018 classification of melanocytic tumors sets forth nine pathways to melanoma (6), seven of which being primary cutaneous (**Table 2**), by largely transposing a previously proposed "multidimensional" pathogenetic scheme based on: i) the role of ultraviolet (UV) radiation; ii) the cell (or tissue) of origin; iii) driving and/or recurrent genomic changes (7).

The most common melanomas in Whites arise from epithelium-associated melanocytes in cutaneous sites with some degree of cumulative sun damage (CSD); these neoplasms are characterized by a high number of point mutations, mostly consisting in the so-called "UV signature" (cytosine to thymidine transitions at dipyrimidine sites); as a rule, the higher the degree of CSD the higher the tumor mutation burden (TMB) (on average: 30 mutations/megabase in high-CSD melanoma; 15 mutations/megabase in low-CSD melanoma) (10). Desmoplastic melanoma is a subtype of high-CSD characterized by a particularly high TMB (on average: 62 mutations/megabase) (11). The degree of CSD is related with the histopathological evidence of dermal solar elastosis, graded according to a three-tiered scale (grade 1: single elastic fibers; grade 2: bunches of fibers; grade 3 basophilic masses) (6).

The other subtypes of melanoma are UV-unrelated. The most common melanomas in non-White population arise from epithelium-asssociated melanocytes on acral skin (palms, soles, nail apparatus) or mucous membranes and are characterized by an early onset of major chromoscomal rearrangements, such as chromotripsis, with gene copy number changes, including multiple high-level amplifications (8). Spitz melanoma and melanomas arising from non-epithelium associated melanocytes (uveal melanoma, melanoma arising in blue nevus and in congenital nevus) also have a very low TMB, but lack the highly rearranged genomes of acral and mucosal melanomas (7, 20). The separation among melanomas with different TMBs is clinically relevant because the TMB may be predictive of response to immune checkpoint inhibitors (21, 22); parenthetically, the assessment of the TMB may be even proposed as a tool for the management of some cases of severely atypical MELTUMP (see below).

Next generation sequencing (NGS) studies have identified many recurrently mutated genes in melanoma, incuding well known genes (*PTEN, MAP2K1-2, RB1*) and recently identified genes (*ARID2, PPP6C, RAC1, DDX3X, IDH1*) (23, 24); however,

TABLE 2 | The WHO 2018 classification of melanoma according to pathways.

Relationship with sun exposure/sun damage	Pathway n.	Subtype	Genetic hallmarks
Melanomas arising in sun-exposed skin	1	*Low-CSD melanoma/superficial spreading melanoma*	High frequency of *BRAF* p.V600 mutations (7–9)
	2	*High-CSD melanoma (including lentigo maligna melanoma and high-CSD nodular melanoma)*	Predominating mutually exclusive *NF1*, *NRAS*, other *BRAF* (non-p.V600E), and perhaps *KIT* mutations (7–9)
	3	*Desmoplastic melanoma*	Recurrent inactivating *NF1* mutations, *NFKBIE* promoter mutations, and several different activating mutations in the MAPK pathway (e.g.: *MAP2K1*) (9–11)
Melanomas arising at sun-shielded sites or without known etiological associations with UV radiation exposure	4	*Malignant Spitz tumor (Spitz melanoma)*	Mutations in *HRAS* and kinase fusions in *ROS1*, *NTRK1*, *NTRK3*, *ALK*, *BRAF*, *MET*, and *RET*; *CDKN2A* homozygous deletion, *TERT* promoter mutations and *MAP3K8* fusions/truncating mutations only in aggressive or lethal variants (7, 12–15)
	5	*Acral melanoma (including nodular melanoma in acral skin)*	Multiple amplifications of *CCND1*, *KIT*, and *TERT*; mutations of *BRAF*, *NRAS*, and *KIT*; kinase fusions of *ALK* or *RET* in a few cases (7, 8)
	6	*Mucosal melanoma*	Numerous copy number and structural variations; uncommonly, *KIT* and *NRAS* mutations (16)
	7	*Melanoma arising in congenital nevus*	In large to giant congenital nevi: *NRAS* mutation; in small to medium-sized congenital nevi, *BRAF* mutations (17, 18)
	8	*Melanoma arising in blue nevus*	Initiating mutations in the Gαq signalling pathway (*GNAQ*, *GNA11*, *CYSLTR2*, *PLCB4*); monosomy 3 (associated with loss of *BAP1*) and chromosome 8q gains in aggressive cases; additional secondary copy number aberrations in *SF3B1* and *EIF1AX* (7, 19)
	9	*Uveal melanoma*	Mutually exclusive mutations in the Gαq pathway (*GNAQ*, *GNA11*, *PLCB4*, *CYSLTR2*); *BAP1*, *SF3B1*, and *EIF1AX* mutations during progression (16)

most of these genes are involved in melanoma progression, rather than in melanoma initiation. Based on the presence of specific driver mutations, The Cancer Genome Atlas (TCGA) classified melanomas into four molecular subtypes: *BRAF*-mutated, *RAS*-mutated, *NF1*-mutated, and triple wild-type (lack of mutations in all three genes); among the latter were cases characterized by *KIT* mutations and by early onset of somatic copy number variations in terms of both gene amplifications in *KIT*, *CCND1*, *CDK4*, *MITF*, and *TERT* and gene deletion/loss-of-function of *TP53* and *CDKN2A* (9).

TCGA molecular subtypes correspond to most cases of the classical (Clark's and McGovern's) (25, 26) types of melanoma and roughly identify melanoma pathways 1–3 of the WHO 2018 classification; melanoma arising in congenital nevus may be also genetically related to classical melanoma because they harbor multiple DNA copy number changes (17) superimposed to *NRAS* mutation. By contrast, the genetic profiles of Spitz melanoma (mutations in *HRAS* and kinase fusions in *ROS1*, *NTRK1*, *NTRK3*, *ALK*, *BRAF*, *MET*, and *RET*) (12, 13) as well as of melanoma arising in blue nevus (mutations in the Gαq signalling pathway) (19, 27) are not encompassed within the TCGA classification. Such cases will unlikely harbor numerous DNA copy number changes or a high TMB; thus they may be genetically considered as "non-classical" subtypes of melanoma.

NEVI AS POTENTIAL PRECURSORS TO MELANOMA

As a rule, all nevi may be virtually simulators of melanoma (and *vice versa*). In addition, the recent identification of the presence

of shared genomic abnormalities between some melanomas and associated nevi has provided support for a potential role of some nevi (28) as both simulators and precursors. However, only some of the WHO 2018 pathways to melanoma may have their putative startpoint in nevi harboring the same mutation:

- Pathway 1: the vast majority of acquired nevi possess single driver mutations of either *BRAF* V600E or *NRAS* Q61R/L (29);
- Pathway 4: some Spitz nevi harbor *HRAS* mutation or translocations with kinase gene fusions involving *ALK*, *ROS*, *RET*, *MET*, and *NTRK* (12, 13).
- Pathway 7: *NRAS* mutation is most frequently observed in congenital melanocytic nevi (18);
- Pathway 8: some blue nevi harbor the *GNAQ* or *GNA11* mutation (19, 27).

In contrast to melanomas, which acquire additional driver mutations, nevi usually enter a suppressive state of replicative senescence which is regulated by the tumor suppressor gene *CDKN2A via* its proteins, p14 and p16, and various transcriptional controls of the cell cycle (30, 31). Therefore, the above-listed mutations, as a single event, appear to be insufficient for melanomagenesis, but bear partially transformed melanocytes which may have an increased susceptibility to additional pathogenic mutation(s) (16). Such a progression model also encompasses neoplasms that have an intermediate number of pathogenetic mutations between nevi and melanomas: within this category, the WHO Working Group lists atypical junctional/thin compound neoplasms (dysplastic nevus and melanoma *in situ*) as well as papulonodular tumorigenic dermal proliferations ("melanocytomas"), and both categories are subclassified into low-grade and high-grade (16). Like Pathway 1 to melanoma, dysplastic nevi are associated with activating mutations of *BRAF* or *NRAS* (18, 29); additional mutation of the *TERT* promoter and, sometimes, hemizygous loss of *CDKN2A* are involved in the morphological progression to a "classical" (superficial spreading) melanoma *in situ* (32).

Many melanocytomas are instead dermal-based, thick, "combined" melanocytic tumors in which an activating mutation of *BRAF* (or, much less commonly, *NRAS*) is followed by a second genetic hit with expansion of a morphologically peculiar ("non-classical") clone of melanocytes. Morphology of this secondary clone strictly depends on the type of second genetic hit: inactivation of the *BAP1* (*BRCA1*-associated protein) gene is the hallmark of *BAP1*-inactivated nevus (BIN) (33, 34); gain-of-function mutations of *CTNNB1* or loss of *APC* is found in deep penetrating nevus (DPN) (35, 36); loss-of-function of *PRKAR1A* is typical of pigmented epithelioid melanocytoma (PEM) (37, 38). However, several melanocytomas arise *de novo* (without a pre-exsisting common nevus): for example, cases of "pure" (non-combined) PEM are also genetically peculiar because often they harbor kinase (most commonly *PRKA*, but also *NTRK1* and *NTRK3*) (38) fusions as the initiating event. Most of these dermal-based tumors are clinically stable; however, they can display various degrees of histopathological atypia (39–42). Increasing atypical histopathological features may correlate with increased risk of disease progression (43), but available data are too weak because of the relative rarity of these tumors and the need of long-term follow-up data. Since the initiating genetic change of such neoplasms is often an activating mutation of *BRAF* or *NRAS*, the three above-mentioned types of melanocytomas are placed within Pathway 1 of melanomagenesis, whose endpoint is superficial spreading melanoma; however, cases of superficial spreading melanoma dysplaying the genetic signature of the above-listed melanocytomas are exceedingly rare. Therefore, in real life such melanocytomas are probably unrelated to the vast majority of classical (Clark's and McGovern's) (25, 26) types of melanoma. **Figure 1** shows a case of early superficial spreading melanoma over a combined BIN, with the malignant component being BAP1-positive, and being thus unrelated with the dermal melanocytoma.

According to Table 2.06 of the WHO classification (16), even the other pathways to melanoma starting from the respective nevi have their own "melanocytomas", namely: atypical Spitz tumor (Pathway 4), (atypical proliferative) nodule in congenital nevus (Pathway 7), and (atypical) cellular blue nevus (Pathway 8). It has been suggested that these entities share with BIN, DPN, and PEM the existence of a "spectrum within the spectrum" (43), namely: a set of atypical histopathological features which can be variously combined with each other, thereby bearing a "spectrum" of lesions with increasing risk of disease progression up to overtly malignant neoplasms. However, the WHO Working Group underlines that regarding Pathway 7, there is no convincing evidence that *bona fide* proliferative nodules in congenital nevi evolve into melanoma (44); and that regarding Pathway 8, a histopathological diagnosis of malignancy is straightforward for melanoma arising in blue

nevus (45). Instead, regarding atypical Spitz tumor, it is acknowledged that there is the need of a "risk stratification" (46), evidently because neoplasms belonging to the Spitz lineage distribute along a spectrum of increasing histopathological atypia, with their malignant end being Spitz melanoma (14, 15).

Interestingly, atypical Spitz tumor shares at least with PEM a peculiar biological behavior, featuring a high incidence of nodal metastases with a very low incidence of distant metastases (41, 47): such as unique biological property that strongly favors ultrasonograpy monitoring over sentinel node biopsy in the clinical management of such cases (47, 48). Based on these data, PEM and atypical Spitz tumor might represent melanocytic tumors of low-grade (mostly lymphotropic) malignancy different from "classical" melanoma: it seems thus reasonable to include atypical Spitz tumor into the "melanocytoma" rubric, as suggested since the beginning (49). Interestingly enough, the list of putative low-grade melanocytic malignancies with a peculiar genetic and morphologic profile has been growing for the last years and has thus been increasingly supporting the concept itself (50–53). An example of CRTC1-TRIM11 (50) fused melanocytoma is provided in **Figure 2**; like several other melanocytomas, such a putatively low-grade malignant melanocytic tumor does not likely progress from a common nevus.

For the above, intermediate melanocytic tumors may be subclassified into: i) a "classical" subgroup (dysplastic nevus and melanoma *in situ*), which is placed within the morphologic and molecular progression spectrum of "classical" melanoma subtypes (superficial spreading and, possibly, nodular; WHO 2018 Pathway 1); and ii) a "non-classical" subgroup ("melanocytomas") whose genetic pathways diverge from "classical" melanoma subtypes. Among the latter are probably low-grade melanocytic malignancies whose list has been increasing for the last years and whose risk stratification needs a careful and systematic approach (48).

Not surprisingly, neoplasms belonging to the WHO 2018 intermediate category are prone to a lower interobserver agreement and are classified as ambiguous by multiple pathologists. Thus, the intermediate rubric also encompasses the provisional categories IAMPUS, SAMPUS, and MELTUMP (6), whose definitions (see above) imply a "subjective" diagnostic uncertainty, rather than a morphologic subset of melanocytic neoplasms. Immunohistochemical and genetic investigations may help classify the WHO 2018 provisional entities into the proper subgroup of melanocytic tumors: this goal is of paramount importance because the "provisional" terminology should be adopted as less as possible (48).

THE WHO 2018 PROGRESSION MODEL: WHAT MATTERS IN ROUTINE PRACTICE

The WHO 2018 progression model is aimed at giving a framework for a histopathological classification; it is therefore a relatively simplifed linear scheme which must be accepted with the awareness that not only are there multiple pathways to

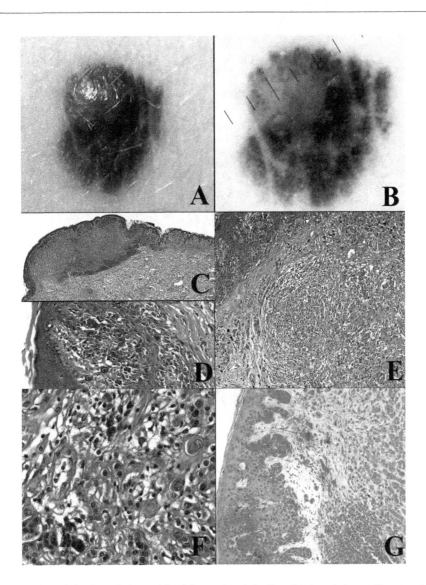

FIGURE 1 | Man, 54 years; a severely atypical melanocytic tumor of the abdomen characterized by a flat pigmented area with an eccentric nodule (A). On dermoscopy, the flat area is typified by a prominent and focally irregular pigment network, whereas the nodular area is characterized by an atypical vascular pattern (B). Histopathologically, the tumor is strikingly asymmetric (C; hematoxylin–eosin, ×25), with a broad highly cellular "shoulder" composed by junctional melanocytes arranged in irregular nests and in single unit (D; hematoxylin–eosin, ×400); the severely atypical junctional component spans above the dermal nodule, the latter being characterized by a lymphoid cell infiltrate (E; hematoxylin–eosin, ×250) and nests of nevocytes intermingled with moderately pleomorphic epithelioid melanocytes with "inclusion-like" cytoplasms (F; hematoxylin–eosin, ×400); all the melanocytic components of this tumor were BRAFv600e mutated protein positive (not shown) and only the dermal epithelioid cell component disclosed loss of the nuclear expression of BAP1 (G; ×250). The tumor was interpreted as an early melanoma developing as a neoplastic progression of a common nevus and not as a progression of a BIN.

melanomagenesis but also that some of the intermediate steps may be bypassed and that other non-linear pathways exist. The most frequent and most important non-linear pattern is by far melanoma *de novo* of the "classical" type. In a meta-analysis carried out by Pampena et al. on 38 observational cohort and case–control studies, only 29.1% of melanomas likely arose from a preexisting nevus and 70.9% arose *de novo* (54). Studies on nevus-associated melanoma based on histopathology alone may have several biases: a benign component may be absent in the tissue levels examined or, else, it may be completely destroyed by the malignant growth; on the contrary, peripheral or deep areas

of melanoma may have a deceptive "nevus-like" appearance ("pseudomaturation"). Dermoscopy and dermoscopic digital monitoring can help differentiate between melanoma characterized by a homogeneous remodeling of the tumor (likely melanoma *de novo*; **Figures 3A–D**) and melanoma characterized by focal changes ("dermoscopic island"; likely nevus-associated melanoma) (55) (**Figures 3E–H**). An early melanoma may be missed if grossing of the specimen is carried out blind to the clinicodermoscopic features of a given melanocytic lesion (56). Dermoscopic digital monitoring also shows that the overwhelming majority of nevi are stable and are

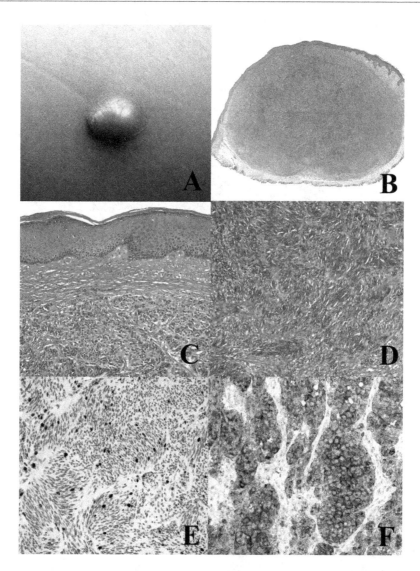

FIGURE 2 | Woman, 44 years; a reddish nodule of the thigh (**A**). Histopathology shows an expansile dermal nodule (**B** hematoxylin–eosin, ×25) composed by nests of epithelioid cells (**C** hematoxylin–eosin, ×250) and fascicles of spingle cells separated by thin fibrotic bands (**D** hematoxylin–eosin, ×250); the proliferation rate (Ki67-positive cells) is 5%, with no clusters of proliferating cells (**E**; ×250); the tumor cells are diffusely positive for TRKA (**F**; ×400). Molecular studies allowed to exclude the possibility of a dermal clear cell sarcoma and to establish a diagnosis of CRTC1-TRIM1 fused melanocytoma. Courtesy of Dr. Arnaud de la Fouchardière, Lyon, F.

more likely to involute according to one of the following: i) a fading pattern (progressive replacement of the nevus by normal skin); ii) a haloed pattern (progressive replacement of the nevus by centripetal extension of a peripheral white vitiligo-like ring); iii) a regression-like pattern (replacement of the nevus by dermoscopic regression structures (peppering, white scarlike ares) (57). The regression-like pattern is seldom documented with dermoscopic monitoring, but is peculiar enough to allow a clinicopathological differential diagnosis between melanoma with regression and its main benign simulator, the so-called "sclerosing nevus with pseudomelanomatous features" or "compound nevus with regression-like fibrosis" (58, 59). The latter is a kind of "chronically recurrent nevus" following chronic unnoticed trauma, and has been described mainly, albeit not

exclusively, in the convex area of the back of young to middle aged patients. Histopathologically, this neoplasm is usually large and asymmetric with a typical "trizonal" pattern featuring: i) an irregular junctional component with irregular epidermal hyperplasia and areas of prevailing single cell proliferation; ii) a significant area of dermal sclerosis with architecturally atypical melanocytic nests; iii) a residual, bland-appearing nevus tissue (very often with congenital nevus-like features) around and deep into the cicatricial tissue (**Figure 4**). The presence of a clear-cut benign dermal component is the main clue to the diagnosis, because regressing melanoma is usually not associated with a nevus. Such a severely atypical melanocytic tumor, in our experience often cautiously diagnosed as MELTUMP, can be indeed diagnosed with confidence when considering the proper

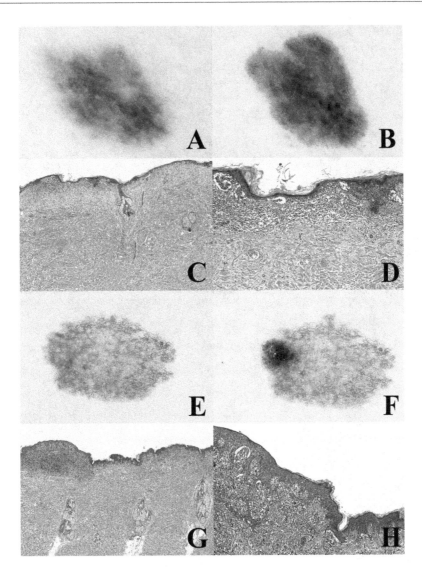

FIGURE 3 | **(A–D)** man, 53 years; a pigmented lesion of the back with a slightly irregular pigment network **(A)**; after six months, the tumor appears as uniformly enlarged, with increasingly irregular pigment network **(B)**. Histopathologically, the tumor is strikingly asymmetric (**C**; hematoxylin–eosin, ×25), with a lichenoid infiltrate at the base of its more severely atypical half (**D**; hematoxylin–eosin, ×100). Even if the histopathological picture might be interpreted as a melanoma *in situ* developing in the background of a dysplastic nevus, the homogeneous remodeling of the tumor documented with dermoscopic digital monitoring favored the diagnosis of melanoma *de novo*. E-H: Woman, 35 years; a pigmented lesion of the back with a thin and regular pigment network at the baseline **(E)**; after eight months, a raised bluish areas is evident at the periphery ("dermoscopic island") **(F)**. Histopathologically the tumor shares with the previous case the striking asymmetry **(G)** hematoxylin–eosin, ×25) and the presence of a lichenoid infiltrate at the base of its more severely atypical half **(H)** hematoxylin–eosin, ×100). However, dermoscopic digital follow up data clarify that this case likely represents an early melanoma *in situ* over a junctional dysplastic nevus.

clinicopathological setting; together with the many nevi in special sites (nevi with site-related atypia), it is an example of histopathological atypia probably unrelated with a signficantly higher risk of progression toward melanoma. This entity also underlines the role of clinically identifiable "environmental modifiers" (trauma, epilation, acute sun exposure) which may increase the histopathological features of atypia in nevi (2, 34) presumably without any impact in melanomagenesis.

As also underlined by the WHO Working Group in a paper published shortly after the 2018 Classification, the risk of an individual nevus progressing to melanoma has been estimated to be in the order of one in 33,000 or less per year (60). Therefore, from a practical point of view, we can conclude that:

1. the vast majority of nevi are, at worst, clinicopathological simulators and not precursors to melanoma;
2. besides esthetic reasons, indication to their excision is solely related to the impossibility to rule out melanoma on clinical grounds alone;
3. with the possible (but not universally accepted) exception of medium (1.5–20 cm) and large/giant (>20 cm) congenital nevi, which carry a definite size-related melanoma risk [up to

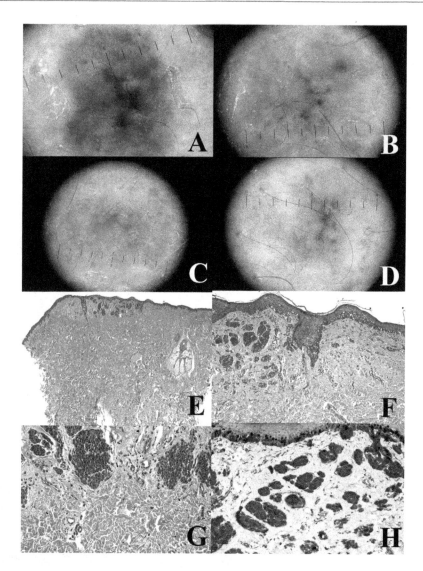

FIGURE 4 | Man, 38 years at the time of the surgical excision of a pigmented lesion of the scapular area; at the baseline, the tumor shows a a relatively regular peripheral pigment network associated with slightly eccentric globules and a central bluish area **(A)** the tumor shows a progressive and relatively symmetric fading after 1 year **(B)**, four years **(C)**, and 6 years **(D)**. The tumor discloses a "trizonal" histopathological pattern **(E**; hematoxylin–eosin, ×25), with an atypical junctional component, a scar-like dermal thickening **(F**; hematoxylin–eosin, ×100) and a very bland-appearing deep dermal component **(G**; hematoxylin–eosin, ×100); the proliferation rate (Ki67-positive dermal melanocytes, evaluated with a KI67/MART1 double stain) is very low **(H**; ×250). These histopathological features are consistent with the so-called "sclerosing nevus with pseudomelanomatus features". Such a histopathological diagnosis is in keeping with the slowly progressive and relatively symmetrical involution of the tumor, as documented with dermoscopic digital monitoring. Clinical images provided by Dr. Luigi Ligrone, Salerno, I.

15% (61)], by no means the excision of a nevus must be viewed as a tool of primary prevention ("prophylactic excision").

These statements also apply to dysplastic nevus and dysplastic nevus syndrome. The WHO Working Group defines dysplastic nevus as a clinically atypical, histopathologically benign junctional or compound melanocytic tumor, >4 mm in breadth on fixed sections (>5 mm clinically), with architectural disorder plus cytological atypia (62). The former is typified by irregular (horizontally oriented, bridging adjacent rete, and/or varying in shape and size) and/or dyscohesive nests of intraepidermal melanocytes plus increased density of non-nested junctional melanocytes (*e.g.* more melanocytes than keratinocytes in an area ≥1 mm^2); the latter is evaluated on the basis of the highest degree of cytological atypia present in more than a few melanocytes as low grade (nuclei ≤1.5× larger than basilar keratinocytes, with small or absent nucleoli and uniformly hyperchromatic or dispersed chromatin, and with "random" variation in size and shape) or high grade (nuclei ≥ larger than basilar keratinocytes, with prominent nucleoli and coarse or peripherally condensed chromatin, and with slightly confluent variation in size and shape) (62). It is stated that nevi with high-grade dysplasia and/or with additional genetic alterations such as TERT promoter mutation should be considered for complete excision (62); this implies that a nevus with high-grade displasia needs no re-excision if already excised with clear margins.

Some studies are reported in which the degree of dysplasia is related with an increased melanoma risk (63–66); however, with the sole exception of a retrosective review considering the personal history of melanoma (66), these studies were histopathologically based, i.e.: they did not take into account the clinical features of risk of the individual patients (familial history of melanoma, skin type, personal history of sunburns, number of nevi, number of clinically atypical nevi). Thus, from a practical point of view, a histopathological diagnosis of dysplastic nevus must be evaluated in the clinical context in order to assess the risk of the individual patient to develop a melanoma; and, since genetic findings are relatively inconsistent to date (62), the diagnosis of dysplastic nevus syndrome (aka: Familial Atypical Multiple Mole and Melanoma, FAMMM; OMIN #155600) is largely based on clinical criteria, i.e.: number of nevi, number of clinically atypical and/or large nevi, personal/famlial history of melanoma (64, 66).

Excluded from the rubric of dysplastic nevus is lentiginous nevus, because being very common, unassociated with a relevant risk of progression to melanoma, and prone to poor diagnostic riproducibility (67). Lentiginous nevus is defined as a benign, junctional, or compound melanocytic tumor, <4 mm in width (on fixed sections), usually symmetrical but with poorly defined borders, with increased density of regularly spaced, non-nested junctional melanocytes around the tips and sides of the rete ridges, with no to mild cytological atypia and minor/variable features also seen in dysplastic nevi (67). These definitional features must be kept in mind because not uncommon in clinical practice are broad and irregular lentiginous melanocytic proliferations of the trunk and the proximal limbs, mostly found in elderly patients, which are probably the clinicopathological counterpart of lentigo maligna on non-chronically sun-exposed skin and are called lentiginous melanoma (68, 69). Dermoscopic digital monitoring of some of these lesions has demonstrated a homogeneous remodelling over many years, thereby suggesting that these are very slow-growing melanomas de novo and not the evolution to melanoma from lentiginous nevi (**Figures 5A–E**). In our experience on lentiginous melanoma, histopathological criteria alone are often weak and may result in a provisional diagnosis of IAMPUS or SAMPUS; the clinical picture of these cases is, however, very often unequivocal for melanoma and must be therefore incorporated into the decision-making process regarding their management.

Nested melanoma (of the elderly) is another example of deceptively bland melanoma (70) whose recognition often depends on a thorough clinicopathological correlation. Like lentiginous melanoma, it is often removed from the trunk and limbs in elderly patients as being large, growing and dermoscopically atypical flat pigmented tumor (71); histopathology features a junctional nesting which is not invariably irregular enough to allow a confident histopathological diagnosis; thus, the result is often a provisionla diagnosis of high-grade dysplasia, IAMPUS, or SAMPUS which, however, is not consistent with the clinical picture. Dermoscopic features of nested melanoma (70) suggest that it conceivably a slow growing melanoma de novo, rather than a melanoma evolving from a nevus (**Figures 5F–I**).

A MANAGEMENT-BASED APPROACH: THE MPATH-DX SYSTEM AND BEYOND

A histopathological diagnosis is aimed at giving a Mutidisciplinary Team the main (albeit not the sole) information for the clinical management. However, such an approach centered on histopathology having some major limitations, more or less explicitly underlined by the WHO Working Group, namely:

1. the diagnostic terminology varies depending on the individual cultural background and on local giudelines (72);
2. the diagnostic interobserver reproducibility is poor even among experts (73);
3. all the available evidence-based clinical guidelines are set upon a dichotomic diagnostic approach (all melanocytic tumors are either nevi or melanomas) and upon a unifying concept of melanoma (all melanocytic malignancies have the same biological behavior which can be predicted on the basis of a universally applicable set of histopathological parameters) (3).

In 2014, the Melanocytic Pathology Assessment Tool and Hierarchy for Diagnosis (MPATH-Dx) schema was proposed in an effort to reduce uncertainty and offer guidelines, mostly for melanocytic tumors different from melanoma (the "classical" melanocytic malignancy with its own evidence-based guidelines) (74): notably, the original schema excluded some melanocytic tumors (pigmented spindle cell; Spitz; epithelioid blue; cellular blue; deep penetrating/plexiform spindle cell) from Class 1 (no apparent risk), thereby anticipating the WHO 2018 concept of intermediate melanocytic tumors. The MPAT-Dx system stratified melanocytomas into four classes (Classes 2 to 5) of melanocytic tumors, with the first two being discriminated on the basis of the degree of histopathological atypia, and the last two discriminated on the basis of Breslow's thickness. The latter criterion, however, should not be applied to melanocytomas, because they are morphologically, genetically, and biologically different from "classical" melanoma with its "classical" prognostic parameters.

In order to specifically address the clinical management of dermal-based tumorigenic "intermediate" melanocytic tumors, practical recommendations have been delivered by the ESP, the EORTC, and the EURACAN (48). Morphological evaluation of these tumors is based on the evaluation of a list of general criteria, both architectural (diameter >6 mm; asymmetry; epidermal effacement; ulceration; high dermal cellularity; tumor clones; loss of grenz zone; absence of vertical "maturation"; expansile nodule formation; destriucive growth pattern; deep subcutaneous extension; pagetoid spread) and cytological (cellular pleomorphism; macro-eosinophilic

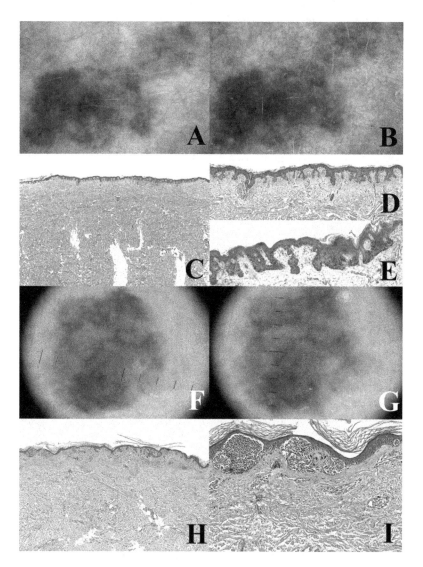

FIGURE 5 | (A–E) Man 52 years. Dermoscopy of a large pigmented lesion of the back with an irregular pigment network at the baseline **(A)** after one year, the lesion shows an increase in size with a homogeneous remodeling and a more prominent pigment network **(B)** such a slow clinical evolution is akin to a lentigo maligna of chronically sun-exposed skin and virtually excludes a diagnosis of nevus. Histopathologically, the tumor has a dysplastic nevus-like silhouette **(C**; hematoxylin–eosin, ×25**)** but is severely atypical because of the striking predominance of tightly packed single melanocytes at the junction **(D**; hematoxylin–eosin, ×100**)**. PRAME immunostain shows a strong and diffuse nuclear positivity in intraepidermal melanocytes **(E)** ×250, as expected in melanoma. Clinicopathological features of the lesion are diagnostic for lentiginous melanoma *in situ*. **(F–I)** Man, 59 years. A large pigmented lesion of the abdomen, dermoscopically characterized by tiny eccentically grouped globules and structureless peripheral areas **(F)** after seven months the peripheral strucureless areas show a clear-cut increase in size **(G)**. Histopathologically there are some areas with a dysplastic nevus-like silhouette, but the epidermis is largely atrophic **(H**; hematoxylin–eosin, ×25**)** and junctional nests are very large and irregular **(I**; hematoxylin–eosin, ×250**)**. These features suggest a diagnosis of melanoma *in situ* with a focally "nested" architecture.

nucleoli; variable density of nuclear chromatin; irregular nuclear membrane; >1 mitosis/mm^2; overlapping nuclei; tumor necrosis). Melanocytomas are then stratified into "low-grade" (few criteria present) and "high grade" (roughly up to half of them present), with excision margins estimated as adequate at 2 mm for the former and at 5–10 mm for the latter. Since a 2-mm excision margin is recommended for every melanocytic tumor, no further excision is required for low-grade melanocytomas. Pigmented epithelioid melanocytoma is by definition an intermediate-high-grade tumor; sentinel node staging is

recommended only for "unclassified atypical dermal tumors" and for cases in which a Spitz melanoma cannot be ruled out; cases labeled as MELTUMP should be managed as per melanoma of the same thickness.

The ESP-EORTC-EURACAN recommendations concerning Spitz melanoma should be applied also on the basis of the recent observation that a "spitzoid" morphology is not invariably associated with a "Spitz" genetic signature (14, 15); in other words, malignant Spitz tumor (Spitz melanoma) is different from "spitzoid" melanoma, which can be regarded as a melanocytic malignancy with "Spitz-like" morphology but genetically ascribed to a "classical" melanoma subtype because of the presence of a specific driver mutation, or numerous DNA copy number changes, or a high TMB. **Figure 6** illustrates the clinicopathological features of an ulcerated melanocytic malignancy histopathologically composed of large epithelioid cells with Spitz-like features, but immunohstichemically typified as a "classical" melanoma because of its immunohistochemical positivity to the anti-BRAF mutated protein VE1 antibody. Parenthetically, PEM-like (75, 76) and DPN-like melanomas (77, 78) might be differentiated from their "melanocytoma counterpart" based on immunohistochemical and/or genetic findings akin to "classical" melanoma.

Based on the above, a new problem is thus rising in dermatopathology, *i.e.*: the differential diagnosis between severely atypical melanocytoma and melanocytoma-like "classical" melanoma. This is not merely a speculative problem, because both a severely atypical melanocytoma and a melanocytoma-like "classical" melanoma will likely spread to the regional nodes, but only the latter will be candidates to sentinel node biopsy and, possibly, to an adjuvant therapy with *BRAF*-inhibitors or with immune checkpoint inhibitors (79, 80). This means that underdiagnosing a "classical" melanoma as a severely atypical melanocytoma may address the patient to an improper wait-and-watch strategy. Many melanocytomas (comprising Spitz tumors) currently lack an identifiable genetic

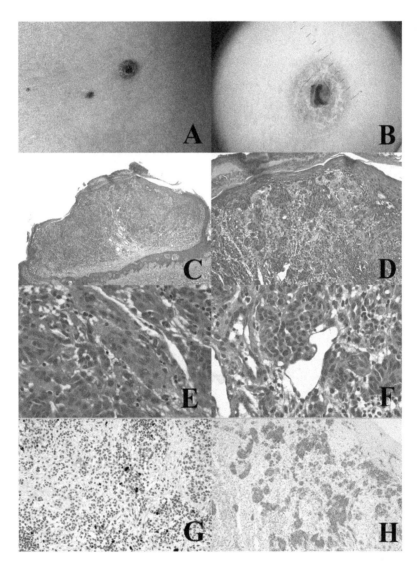

FIGURE 6 | Woman, 22 years. An ulcerated nodule of the right flank **(A)** dermoscopically characterized by keratoacanthoma-like features with vessels surrounded by a white halo **(B)**. Histopathologically, the tumor has an irregularly nodular, exophytic silhouette with an epidermal "collarette", a superficial crust, and a "brisk" inflammatory infiltrate in the dermis **(C**; hematoxylin–eosin, ×25); the superficial nests are very irregularly confluent with no sharp circumscription from the overlying epidermis **(D**; hematoxylin–eosin, ×250); dermal melanocytes show a "spitzoid" morphology, with spindle **(E**; hematoxylin–eosin, ×400) and epthelioid **(F**; hematoxylin–eosin, ×400) cells, both with reatively abundant and eosinophilic cytoplasms. In spite of the severe architectural atypia, the proliferation rate of the tumor (Ki67-positive dermal melanocytes) is low **(G)** ×250); however, the tumor is not an atypical Spitz tumor, but a classical nodular melanoma because it is positive to the antibody anti-BRAFv600e-mutated protein **(H)** ×250).

"signature"; by definition, however, they lack *BRAF*-mutation and a high TMB which are predictive parameters for neoadjuvant therapy (79, 80). Thus, the differential diagnosis between a severely atypical melanocytoma with no known genetic signature and a classical "melanocytoma-like" melanoma may be approached by looking for predictive (rather than diagnostic) paramenters; the same might apply for cases provisionally labeled as MELTUMP or as unclassified atypical dermal lesion (48).

A THERAPY-ORIENTED DIAGNOSTIC APPROACH

When dealing with an atypical melanocytic tumor of the skin, the first step can be the differential diagnosis between a "classical" type of melanocytic tumor and a "melanocytoma" (comprising

Spitz tumor). Immunohistochemistry can assist such a differential diagnosis as follows:

- The anti BRAF-mutated protein VE1 antibody identifies the subset of melanocytic tumors of the "classical" type harboring the *BRAF*^{v600e} mutation (or a "combined" melanocytoma) (48, 81);
- The immunostain for BAP1 can document loss of the consitutive nuclear immunoreactivity in BAP1-inactivated melanocytic tumors (33, 34);
- The anti PRAME immunostain can assist the differential diagnosis between benign and malignant "traditional" melanocytic tumors (82); in our experience, particularly for lentiginous neoplasms and for the differential diagnosis between congenital nevus and nevoid melanoma;
- The anti-ALK, anti-TRKA, anti-MET, anti-HRAS-WT, and anti-ROS1 antibodies identify the subset of melanocytic tumors of the Spitz lineage with the respective kinase gene changes (48, 83, 84);

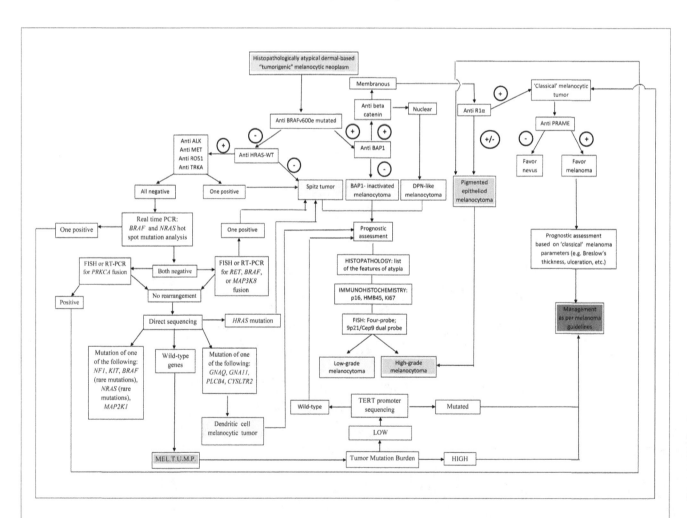

FIGURE 7 | A flow chart illustrating a therapy-oriented morphomolecular approach to atypical dermal-based tumorigenic melanocytic neoplasms. Of paramount importance are: i) the distinction between melanocytomas (recognized as such by specific genetic signatures) and melanocytic tumors of uncertain malignant potential (MEL.T.U.M.P.; provisionally defined as tumors with unknown driver mutations); ii) among melanocytomas, the distinction between low-grade and high-grade tumors; iii) among MELTUMP, the distinction between tumors with a low tumor mutation burden and tumors with a a high tumor mutation burden, the latter being best managed as per "classical" melanoma.

- The anti-beta catenin immunostain identifies the aberrant nuclear positivity definitional for DPN and related tumors (36);
- Tha anti-R1alpha can document loss of constitutive nuclear immunoreactivity in PEM with inactivating mutation or epigenetic inactivation of *PRKAR1A* (85).

An immunohistochemical panel aimed at a risk stratification can encompass:

- p16, which may disclose uneven immunoreactivity or "clonal" loss as an atypical feature (2, 48);
- HMB45, which may be unevenly distributed, with loss of the "gradient" pattern seen in benign tumors (2);
- Cell cycle-related protein Ki67, which may show a high rate of expression and/or "proliferative clusters" in atypical lesions (2).

The traditional four-probe (targeting *MYB*, *RREB*, *Cep6*, and *CCND11*) plus the anti-*CDKN2A/Cep9* dual probe FISH examination may help refine the risk stratification of melanocytic tumors as recently proposed (86).

If morphology and immunohistochemistry are not contributory in assigning the melanocytic tumor to a given lineage, molecular analysis guided by morphology may be implemented as follows:

- Identification of hotspot mutations of *BRAF* (codon 600) and *NRAS* [exon 2 (odons 12, 13), exon 3 (codons 59, 61), and of exon 4 (codons 117, 146)];
- Sequencing techniques for the following: *NF1*, *KIT* (exons 11, 13, 17, and 18), *BRAF* (rare mutations), *NRAS* (rare mutations), and *MAP2K1* (exons 2 and 3; in-frame deletion) for "classical" melanocytic tumors; *GNAQ* (exons 4 and 5), *GNA11* (exons 4 and 5), *PLCB4*, and *CYSLTR2* for dendritic melanocytic tumors (WHO 2018 Pathways 8 and 9); *HRAS* (exons 2 and 3) for a subset of Sptz tumors; TERT promoter for a subset of aggressive malignencies (some characterized by a 'Spitz-like' morphology);
- Fluorescence *in situ* hybridization (FISH) or reverse transcriptase polymerase chain reaction (RT-PCR) examination for fusions involving: *BRAF* and *RET* for Spitz tumors; *MAP3K8* for

morphologically malignant epithelioid cell Spitz neoplasms (87, 88); *PRKCA* for PEM.

As per ESP-EORTC-EURACAN guidelines, if the immunohistochemical screening implies additional procedures, immuno-positive cases (of Spitz neoplasms) should be confirmed for the respective genomic aberration by molecular examinations (48); this is, however, a theroretically uncommon scenario.

As a final step for an approach akin to tumor-agnostic therapy, NGS analysis can help identify melanocytic tumors with "rare" genetic signatures, and—even more important— melanocytic tumors with a high TMB which should be definitely ascribed to the category of classical melanoma with the relative therapeutic options. Specialized referral centers must be involved for sequencing, fusion studies, and NGS examination (48).

A visual summary of the above-proposed algorithmic diagnostic approach is given in **Figure 7**.

TAKE-HOME MESSAGE

The traditional "dichotomic" (benign *vs* malignant) view of melanocytic tumors and the concept of melanoma as a "unique" clinicopathological entity no longer fit with the routine diagnostic approach. Along with "classical" (Clark's and McGovern's) subtypes of melanoma, other melanocytic malignancies, each charcaterized by peculiar biological behavior probably exist, must be distinguished from "classical" melanoma subtypes and require specific clinical guidelines. Clinicopathological correlation can allow both reducing the histopathological diagnostic uncertainty and addressing patients to a proper management.

AUTHOR CONTRIBUTIONS

Both authors listed have made a substantial, direct, and intellectual contribution to the work and approved it for publication.

REFERENCES

1. Elder DE, Massi D, Scolyer RA, Willemze R. *Who Classification of Skin Tumours, 4th Edition*. Lyon: IARC (2018).
2. Ferrara G. "The Histopathological Gray Zone". In: G Argenziano, A Lallas, C Longo, E Moscarella, A Kyrgidis, G Ferrara, editors. *Cutaneous Melanoma: A Pocket Guide for Diagnosis and Management*. London, UK: Academic Press (2017). p. 155–89.
3. Ackerman AB. Malignant Melanoma: A Unifying Concept. *Hum Pathol* (1980) 11:591–5. doi: 10.1016/s0046-8177(80)80069-4
4. Cerroni L, Barnhill R, Elder D, Gottlieb G, Heenan P, Kutzner H, et al. Melanocytic Tumors of Uncertain Malignant Potential: Results of a Tutorial Held at the XXIX Symposium of the International Society of Dermatopathology in Graz, October 2008. *Am J Surg Pathol* (2010) 34:314–26. doi: 10.1097/PAS.0b013e3181cf7fa0

5. Harbst K, Staaf J, Lauss M, Karlsson A, Måsbäck A, Johansson I, et al. Molecular Profiling Reveals Low- and High-Grade Forms of Primary Melanoma. *Clin Cancer Res* (2012) 18:4026–36. doi: 10.1158/1078-0432.CCR-12-0343
6. Elder DE, Barnhil R, Bastian BC, Cook MG, de la Fouchardière A, Gerami P, et al. "Melanocytic Tumour Classification and the Pathway Concept". In: DE Elder, D Massi, RA Scolyer, R Willemze, editors. *Who Classification of Skin Tumours, 4th Edition*. Lyon, F: IARC (2018). p. 66–71.
7. Bastian BC. The Molecular Pathology of Melanoma: An Integrated Taxonomy of Melanocytic Neoplasia. *Annu Rev Pathol* (2014) 9:239–71. doi: 10.1146/annurev-pathol-012513-104658
8. Curtin JA, Fridyland J, Kageshita T, Patel HN, Busam K, Kutzner H, et al. Distinct Sets of Genetic Alterations in Melanoma. *N Engl J Med* (2005) 353:2135–47. doi: 10.1056/NEJMoa050092
9. Cancer Genome Atlas N. Genomic Classification of Cutaneous Melanoma. *Cell* (2015) 161:1681–96. doi: 10.1016/j.cell.2015.05.044

10. Krauthammer M, Kong Y, Bacchiocchi A, Evans P, Pomputtapong N, Wu C, et al. Exome Sequencing Identifies Recurrent Mutations in NF1 and RASopathy Genes in Sun-Exposed Melanomas. *Nat Genet* (2015) 47:996–1002. doi: 10.1038/ng.3361

11. Shain AH, Garrido M, Botton T, Talevich E, Yeh I, Sanborn IZ, et al. Exome Sequencing of Desmoplastic Melanoma Identifies Recurrent NFKBIE Promoter Mutations and Diverse Activating Mutations in the MAPK Pathway. *Nat Genet* (2015) 47:1194–9. doi: 10.1038/ng.3382

12. van Dijk MC, Bernsen MR, Ruiter DJ. Analysis of Mutations in B-RAF, N-RAS, and H-RAS Genes in the Differential Diagnosis of Spitz Nevus and Spitzoid Melanoma. *Am J Surg Pathol* (2005) 29:1145–51. doi: 10.1097/01.pas.0000157749.18591.9e

13. Wiesner T, He J, Yelensky R, Esteve-Puig R, Botton T, Yeh I, et al. Kinase Fusions are Frequent in Spitz Tumours and Spitzoid Melanomas. *Nat Commun* (2014) 5:3116. doi: 10.1038/ncomms4116

14. Lazova R, Pornputtapong N, Halaban R, Bosenberg M, Bai Y, Chai H, et al. Spitz Nevi and Spitzoid Melanomas: Exome Sequencing and Comparison With Conventional Melanocytic Nevi and Melanomas. *Mod Pathol* (2015) 30:640–9. doi: 10.1038/modpathol.2016.237

15. Raghavan SS, Peternel S, Mully TW, North JP, Pincus LB, LeBoit PE, et al. Spitz Melanoma is a Distinct Subset of Spitzoid Melanoma. *Mod Pathol* (2020) 33:1122–34. doi: 10.1038/s41379-019-0445-z

16. Bastian BC, de la Fouchardière A, Elder DE, Gerami P, Lazar AJ, Massi D, et al. "Genomic Landscape of Melanoma". In: DE Elder, D Massi, RA Scolyer, R Willemze, editors. *Who Classification of Skin Tumours, 4th Edition*. Lyon, F: IARC. (2018) p. 72–5.

17. Bastian BC, Xiong J, Frieden IJ, Williams ML, Chou P, Busam K, et al. Genetic Changes in Neoplasms Arising in Congenital Melanocytic Nevi: Differences Between Nodular Proliferations and Melanoma. *Am J Pathol* (2002) 161:1163–9. doi: 10.1016/S0002-9440(10)64393-3

18. Bauer J, Curtin JA, Pinkel D, Bastian BC. Congenital Melanocytic Nevi Frequently Harbor NRAS Mutations But No BRAF Mutations. *J Invest Dermatol* (2007) 127:179–82. doi: 10.1038/sj.jid.5700490

19. Pérez-Alea M, Vivancos A, Caratú G, Matito J, Ferrer B, Hernandez-Losa J, et al. Genetic Profile of GNAQ-mutated Blue Melanocytic Neoplasms Reveals Mutations in Genes Linked to Genomic Instability and the PI3K Pathway. *Oncotarget* (2016) 7:28086–95. doi: 10.18632/oncotarget.8578

20. Newell F, Wilmott JS, Johanson PA, Nones K, Addala V, Mukhopadhyay P, et al. Whole-Genome Sequencing of Acral Melanoma Reveals Genomic Complexity and Diversity. *Nat Commun* (2020) 11:5259. doi: 10.1038/s41467-020-18988-3

21. Boussemart L, Johnson A, Schrock AB, Pal SK, Frampton GM, Fabrizio D, et al. Tumor Mutational Burden and Response to PD-1 Inhibitors in a Case Series of Patients With Metastatic Desmoplastic Melanoma. *J Am Acad Dermatol* (2019) 80:1780–2. doi: 10.1016/j.jaad.2018.12.020

22. Chan TA, Yarchoan M, Jafee E, Swanton C, Quezada SA, Stenzinger A, et al. Development of Tumor Mutation Burden as an Immunotherapy Biomarker: Utility for the Oncology Clinic. *Ann Oncol* (2019) 30:44–56. doi: 10.1093/annonc/mdy495

23. Palmieri G, Ombra M, Colombino M, Casula M, Sini M, Manca A, et al. Multiple Molecular Pathways in Melanomagenesis: Characterization of Therapeutic Targets. *Front Oncol* (2015) 5:183. doi: 10.3389/fonc.2015.00183

24. Palmieri G, Colombino M, Casula M, Manca A, Mandalà M, Cossu A. Molecular Pathways in Melanomagenesis: What We Learned From Next-Generation Sequencing Approaches. *Curr Oncol Rep* (2018) 20:86. doi: 10.1007/s11912-018-0733-7

25. Clark WHJr., From L, Bernardino EA, Mihm MC. The Histogenesis and Biologic Behaviour of Primary Human Malignant Melanoma of the Skin. *Cancer Res* (1969) 29:705–27.

26. McGovern VJ. The Classification of Melanoma and Its Relationship With Prognosis. *Pathology* (1970) 2:85–98. doi: 10.3109/00313027009077330

27. Van Raamsdonk CD, Bezrookove V, Green G, Bauer J, Gaugler L, O'Brien JM, et al. Frequent Somatic Mutations of GNAQ in Uveal Melanoma and Blue Naevi. *Nature* (2009) 457:599–602. doi: 10.1038/nature07586

28. Shain AH, Yeh I, Kovalyshyn I, Sriharan A, Talevich E, Gagnon A, et al. The Genetic Evolution of Melanoma From Precursor Lesions. *N Engl J Med* (2015) 373:1926–36. doi: 10.1056/NEJMoa1502583

29. Colebatch AJ, Ferguson P, Newell F, Kazakoff S. Molecular Genomic Profiling of Melanocytic Nevi. *J Invest Dermatol* (2019) 139:1762–8. doi: 10.1016/j.jid.2018.12.033

30. LaPak KM, Burd CE. The Molecular Balancing Act of 16^{INK4a} in Cancer and Aging. *Mol Cancer Res* (2014) 12:167–83. doi: 10.1158/1541-7786.MCR-13-0350

31. Ross AL, Sanchez MI, Grichnik JM. Nevus Senescence. *ISRN Dermatol* (2011) 2011:642157. doi: 10.5402/2011/642157

32. Shain AH, Yeh I, Kovalyshin I, Sriharan A, Talevich E, Gagnon A, et al. The Genetic Evolution of Melanoma From Precursor Lesions. *N Engl J Med* (2015) 373:1926–36. doi: 10.1056/NEJMoa1502583

33. Zhang AJ, Rush PS, Tsao H. Duncan LM BRCA1-Associated Protein (BAP1)-Inactivated Melanocytic Tumors. *J Cutan Pathol* (2019) 46:965–72. doi: 10.1111/cup.13530

34. Ferrara G, Mariani MP, Auriemma M. BAP1-Inactivated Melanocytic Tumour With Borderline Histopathological Features (BAP1-Inactivated Melanocytoma): A Case Report and a Reappraisal. *Australas J Dermatol* (2021) 62:e88–91. doi: 10.1111/ajd.13408.

35. Yeh I, Lang UE, Durieux E, Tee MK, Jorapur A, Shain H, et al. Combined Activation of MAP Kinase Pathway and β-Catenin Signaling Cause Deep Penetrating Nevi. *Nat Commun* (2017) 8:644. doi: 10.1038/s41467-017-00758-3

36. de la Fouchardière A, Caillot C, Jacquemus J, Durieux E, Houlier A, Haddad V, et al. β-Catenin Nuclear Expression Discriminates Deep Penetrating Nevi From Other Cutaneous Melanocytic Tumors. *Virchows Arch* (2019) 474:539–50. doi: 10.1007/s00428-019-02533-9

37. Cohen JN, Joseph NM, North JP, Onodera C, Zembowicz A, LeBoit PE. Genomic Analysis of Pigmented Epithelioid Melanocytomas Reveals Recurrent Alterations in PRKAR1A, and PRKCA Genes. *Am J Surg Pathol* (2017) 41:1333–46. doi: 10.1097/PAS.0000000000000902

38. Isales MC, Mohan LS, Quan VL, Garfield EM, Zhang B, Shi K, et al. Distinct Genomic Patterns in Pigmented Epithelioid Melanocytoma: A Molecular and Histologic Analysis of 16 Cases. *Am J Surg Pathol* (2019) 43:480–8. doi: 10.1097/PAS.0000000000001195

39. Yélamos O, Navarrete-Dechent C, Marchetti MA, Rogers T, Apalla Z, Bahadoran P, et al. Clinical and Dermoscopic Features of Cutaneous BAP1 Inactivated Melanocytic Tumors: Results of a Multicenter Case-Control Study by the International Dermoscopy Society (Ids). *J Am Acad Dermatol* (2019) 80:1585–93. doi: 10.1016/j.jaad.2018.09.014

40. Cosgarea I, Griewank KG, Ungureanu L, Tamayo A, Siepman T. Deep Penetrating Nevus and Borderline Deep Penetrating Nevus: A Literature Review. *Front Oncol* (2020) 10:837. doi: 10.3389/fonc.2020.00837

41. Zembowicz A, Carney JA, Mihm MC. Pigmented Epithelioid Melanocytoma: A Low-Grade Melanocytic Tumor With Metastatic Potential Indistinguishable From Animal-Type Melanoma and Epithelioid Blue Nevus. *Am J Surg Pathol* (2004) 28:31–40. doi: 10.1097/00000478-200401000-00002

42. Cohen JN, Yeh I, Mully TW, LeBoit PE, McCalmont TH. Genomic and Clinicopathologic Characteristics of PRKAR1A-Inactivated Melanomas: Toward Genetic Distinctions of Animal-type Melanoma/Pigment Synthesizing Melanoma am. *J Surg Pathol* (2020) 44:805–16. doi: 10.1097/PAS.0000000000001458

43. Ferrara G, Bradamante M. Melanocytic Skin Tumors: Does the Molecular Progression Model Fit With the Routine Clinicopathological Practice? *Dermatol Pract Concept* (2019) 10:e2020001. doi: 10.5826/dpc.1001a01

44. Massi G, Bastian BC, PE L, VG P, Xu X. "Proliferative Nodules in Congenital Melanocytic Naevus". In: (WHO Classification of Skin Tumours, *4th Edition*, eds. D. E. Elder, D. Massi, R. A. Scolyer, R Willemze (F. Lyon F: IARC), (2018). p. 136.

45. de la Fouchardière A, Scolyer R, Calonje E, Fullen DR, Gerami P, Requena L, et al. "Melanoma Arsing in Blue Naevus". In: (WHO Classification of Skin Tumours, *4th Edition*, eds. D. E. Elder, D. Massi, R. A. Scolyer, R Willemze (F. Lyon F: IARC), (2018). p. 124–5.

46. Barnhill R, Bahrami A, Bastian BC, Busam KJ, Cerroni L, de la Fouchardière A, et al. "Malignant Spitz Tumor (Spitz Melanoma)". In: (WHO Classification of Skin Tumours, *4th Edition*, eds. D. E. Elder, D. Massi, R. A. Scolyer, R Willemze (F. Lyon F: IARC), (2018). p. 108–10.

47. Lallas A, Kyrgidis A, Ferrara G, Kittler H, Apalla Z, Castagnetti F, et al. Atypical Spitz Tumours and Sentinel Lymph Node Biopsy: A Systematic Review. *Lancet Oncol* (2014) 15:e176–83. doi: 10.1016/S1470-2045(13)70608-9

48. de la Fouchardiere A, Blokx W, van Kempen LC, Luzar B, Piperno-Neumann S, Puig S, et al. Esp, EORTC, and EURACAN Expert Opinion: Practical Recommendations for the Pathological Diagnosis and Clinical Management of Intermediate Melanocytic Tumors and Rare Melanoma Variants. *Virch Arch* (2021). doi: 10.1007/s00428-020-03005-1. Online ahead of print.

49. Zembowicz A, Scolyer RA. Nevus/Melanocytoma/Melanoma: An Emerging Paradigm for Classification of Melanocytic Neoplasms? *Arch Pathol Lab Med* (2011) 135:300–6. doi: 10.1043/2010-0146-RA.1

50. Cellier L, Perron E, Pissaloux D, Karanian M, Haddad V, Alberti L, et al. Cutaneous Melanocytoma With CRTC1-TRIM11 Fusion: Report of 5 Cases Resembling Clear Cell Sarcoma. *Am J Surg Pathol* (2018) 42:382–91. doi: 10.1097/PAS.0000000000000996

51. Macagno N, Pissaloux D, Etchevers H, Haddad V, Vergier B, Sierra-Fortuny S, et al. Cutaneous Melanocytic Tumors With Concomitant NRAS^{Q61R} and IDH1^{R132C} Mutations. A Report of Six Cases. *Am J Surg Pathol* (2020) 44:1398–405. doi: 10.1097/PAS.0000000000001500

52. de la Fouchardiere A, Pissaloux D, Tirode F, Karanian M, Fletcher CDM, Hanna J. Clear Cell Tumor With Melanocytic Differentiation and ACTIN-MITF Translocation: Report of 7 Cases of a Novel Entity. *Am J Surg Pathol* (2020) 45:962–8. doi: 10.1097/PAS.0000000000001630

53. de la Fouchardiere A, Pissaloux D, Tirode F, Hanna J. Clear Cell Tumor With Melanocytic Differentiation and MITF-CREM Translocation: A Novel Entity Similar to Clear Cell Sarcoma. *Virchows Arch* (2021). doi: 10.1007/s00428-021-03027-3. Online ahead of print.

54. Pampena R, Kyrgidis A, Lallas A, Moscarella E, Argenziano G, Longo C. A Meta-Analysis of Nevus-Associated Melanoma: Prevalence and Practical Implications. *J Am Acad Dermatol* (2017) 77:938–45. doi: 10.1016/j.jaad.2017.06.149

55. Borsari S, Longo C, Ferrari C, Benati E, Bassoli S, Schianchi S, et al. Dermoscopi Island: A New Descriptor for Thin Melanoma. *Arch Dermatol* (2010) 146:1257–62. doi: 10.1001/archdermatol.2010.311

56. Ferrara G, Argenziano G, Giorgio CM, Zalaudek I, Kittler H. Dermoscopic-Pathologic Correlation: Apropos of Six Equivocal Cases. *Semin Cutan Med Surg* (2009) 28:157–64. doi: 10.1016/j.sder.2009.06.003

57. Terushkin V, Scope A, Halpern AC, Marghoob AA. Pathways to Involution of Nevi: Insights From Dermoscopic Follow-Up. *Arch Dermatol* (2010) 146:459–60. doi: 10.1001/archdermatol.2010.20

58. Fabrizi G, Pennacchia I, Pagliarello C, Massi G. Sclerosing Nevus With Pseudomelanomatous Features. *J Cutan Pathol* (2008) 35:995–1002. doi: 10.1111/j.1600-0560.2008.01176.x

59. Ferrara G, Amantea A, Argenziano G, Broganelli P, Cesinaro AM, Donati P, et al. Sclerosing Nevus With Pseudomelanomatous Features and Regressing Melanoma With Nevoid Features. *J Cutan Pathol* (2009) 36:913–5. doi: 10.1111/j.1600-0560.2008.01176.x

60. Elder DE, Bastian BC, Cree IA, Massi D, Scolyer RA. The 2018 World Health Organization Classification of Cutaneous, Mucosal, and Uveal Melanoma. Detailed Analysis of 9 Distinct Subtypes Defined by Their Evolutionary Patter. *Arch Pathol Lab Med* (2020) 144:500–22. doi: 10.5858/arpa.2019-0561-RA

61. Marghoob AA. Congenital Melanocytic Nevi. Evaluation and Management. *Dermatol Clin* (2002) 20:697–16. doi: 10.1016/s0733-8635(02)00030-x. viii.

62. Elder DE, Barnhill R, Bastian BC, Duncan LM, Massi D, Mihm MC Jr, et al. "Dysplastic Naevus". In: (WHO Classification of Skin Tumours, *4th Edition*, eds. D. E. Elder, D. Massi, R. A. Scolyer, R Willemze (F. Lyon F: IARC), (2018). p. 82–6.

63. Shors AR, Kim S, White A, Arenyi Z, Barnhill RL, Duray P, et al. Dysplastic Naevi With Moderate to Severe Histological Dysplasia: A Risk Factor for Melanoma. *Br J Dermatol* (2006) 155:988–93. doi: 10.1111/j.1365-2133.2006.07466.x

64. Xiong MY, Rabkin MS, Piepkorn MW, Barnhill RL, Argenyi Z, Erickson L, et al. Diameter of Dysplastic Nevi is a More Robust Biomarker of Increased Melanoma Risk Than Degree of Histologic Dysplasia: A Case-Control Study. *J Am Acad Dermatol* (2014) 71:1257–68.e4. doi: 10.1016/j.jaad.2014.07.030

65. Arumi-Uria M, McNutt NS, Finnerty B. Grading of Atypia in Nevi: Correlation With Melanoma Risk. *Mod Pathol* (2003) 16:764–71. doi: 10.1097/01.MP.0000082394.91761.E5

66. Slade J, Marghoob AA, Salopek TG, Rigel DS, Kopf AW, Bart RS. Atypical Mole Syndrome: Risk Factor for Cutaneous Malignant Melanoma and Implications for Management. *J Am Acad Dermatol* (1995) 32:479–94. doi: 10.1016/0190-9622(95)90073-x

67. Wick MR, Elenitsas R, Kim J, Kossard R. Simple Lentigo and Lentiginous Melanocytic Naevus. In: (WHO Classification of Skin Tumours, *4th Edition*, eds. D. E. Elder, D. Massi, R. A. Scolyer, R Willemze (F. Lyon F: IARC), (2018). p. 78–9.

68. King R, Page RN, Googe PB, Mihm MCJr. Lentiginous Melanoma: A Histologic Pattern of Melanoma To Be Distinguished From Lentiginous Nevus. *Mod Pathol* (2005) 18:1397–401. doi: 10.1038/modpathol.3800454

69. Ferrara G, Zalaudek I, Argenziano G. Lentiginous Melanoma: A Distinctive Clinicopathological Entity. *Histopathology* (2008) 52:523–5. doi: 10.1111/j.1365-2559.2008.02943.x

70. Kutzner H, Metzler G, Argenyi Z, Requena L, Palmedo G, Mentzel T, et al. Histological and Genetic Evidence for a Variant of Superficial Spreading Melanoma Composed Predominantly of Large Nests. *Mod Pathol* (2012) 25:838–45. doi: 10.1038/modpathol.2012.35

71. Dri A, Conforti C, Zelin E, Toffoli L, Signoretto D, Zacchi A, et al. Nested Melanoma: When Dermoscopy Turns Histopathology Into Question. *Int J Dermatol* (2020) 60:e70–2. doi: 10.1111/ijd.15218

72. Piepkorn MW, Longton GM, Reisch LM, Elder DE, Pepe MS, Kerr KF, et al. Assessment of Second-Opinion Strategies for Diagnoses of Cutaneous Melanocytic Lesions. *JAMA Netw Open* (2019) 10:e1912597. doi: 10.1001/jamanetworkopen.2019.12597

73. Ferrara G, Argenyi Z, Argenziano G, Cerio R, Cerroni L, Di Blasi A, et al. The Influence of Clinical Information in the Histopathologic Diagnosis of Melanocytic Skin Neoplasms. *PlosONE* (2009) 4:e5375. doi: 10.1371/journal.pone.0005375

74. Piepkorn MW, Barnhill RL, Elder DE, Knezevich SR, Carney PA, Reish LM, et al. The MPATH-Dx Reporting Schema for Melanocytic Proliferations and Melanoma. *J Am Acad Dermatol* (2014) 70:131–41. doi: 10.1016/j.jaad.2013.07.027

75. Cohen J, Spies J, Ross FNP-C, Bolke A, McCalmont T. Heavily Pigmented Epithelioid Melanoma With Loss of Protein Kinase A Regulatory Subunit-α Expression. *Am J Dermatopathol* (2020) 40:912–6. doi: 10.1097/DAD.0000000000001185

76. Cohen JN, Yeh I, Mully TW, LeBoit PE, McCalmont TH. Genomic and Clinicopathologic Characteristics of PRKAR1A-inactivated Melanomas: Toward Genetic Distinctions of Animal-Type Melanoma/Pigment Synthesizing Melanoma. *Am J Surg Pathol* (2020) 44:805–16. doi: 10.1097/PAS.0000000000001458

77. Magro CM, Abraham RM, Guo R, Li S, Wang X, Proper S, et al. Deep Penetrating Nevus-Like Borderline Tumors: A Unique Subset of Ambiguous Melanocytic Tumors With Malignant Potential and Normal Cytogenetics. *Eur J Dermatol* (2014) 24:594–602. doi: 10.1684/ejd.2014.2393

78. Isales MC, Khan AU, Zhang B, Compres EV, Kim D, Tan TL, et al. Molecular Analysis of Atypical Deep Penetrating Nevus Progressing to Melanoma. *J Cutan Pathol* (2020) 47:1150–4. doi: 10.1111/cup.13775

79. Baetz TD, Fletcher GG, Knight G, McWhirter E, Rajagopal S, Song X, et al. Systemic Adjuvant Therapy for Adult Patients At High Risk for Recurrent Melanoma: A Systematic Review. *Cancer Treat Rev* (2020) 87:102032. doi: 10.1016/j.ctrv.2020.102032

80. Pham TV, Boichard A, Goodman A, Riviere P, Yeerna H, Tamayo P, et al. Role of Ultraviolet Mutational Signature Versus Tumor Mutation Burden in Predicting Response to Immunotherapy. *Mol Oncol* (2020) 14:1680–94. doi: 10.1002/1878-0261.12748

81. Long GV, Wilmott JS, Capper D, Preusser M, Zhang YE, Thompson JF, et al. Immunohistochemistry is Highly Sensitive and Specific for the Detection of V600E BRAF Mutation in Melanoma. *Am J Surg Pathol* (2013) 37:61–5. doi: 10.1097/PAS.0b013e31826485c0

82. Lezcano C, Jungbluth AA, Nehal KS, Hollman TJ. PRAME Expression in Melanocytic Tumors. *Busam KJ Am J Surg Pathol* (2018) 42:1456–65. doi: 10.1097/PAS.0000000000001134

83. Kiuru M, Jungbluth A, Kutzner H, Wiesner T, Busam KJ. Spitz Tumors: Comparison of Histological Features in Relationship to Immunohistochemical Staining for ALK and NTRK1. *Int J Surg Pathol* (2016) 24:200–6. doi: 10.1177/1066896916630375

84. Quan VL, Panah E, Zhang B, Shi K, Mohan LS, Gerami P. The Role of Gene Fusions in Melanocytic Neplasms. *J Cutan Pathol* (2019) 46:878–87. doi: 10.1111/cup.13521

85. Zembowicz A, Knoepp SM, Bei T, Stergiopoulos S, Eng C, Mihm MC, et al. Loss of Expression of Protein Kinase a Regulatory Subunit 1alpha in Pigmented Epithelioid Melanocytoma But Not in Melanoma or Other Melanocytic Lesions. *Am J Surg Pathol* (2007) 31:1764–75. doi: 10.1097/PAS.0b013e318057faa7

86. Ferrara G, De Vanna AC. Fluorescence in Situ Hybridization for Melanoma Diagnosis: A Review and a Reappraisal. *Am J Dermatopathol* (2016) 38:253–69. doi: 10.1097/DAD.0000000000000380

87. Houlier A, Pissaloux D, Masse I, Tirose F, Karanian M, Pincus LB, et al. Melanocytic Tumors With MAP3K8 Fusions: Report of 33 Cases With Morphological-Genetic Correlations. *Mod Pathol* (2019) 33:846–57. doi: 10.1038/s41379-019-0384-8

88. Newman S, Pappo A, Raimondi S, Zhang J, Barnhill E, Bahrami A. Pathologic Characteristics of Spitz Melanoma With MPA3K8 Fusion or Truncated in a Pediatric Cohort. *A J Surg Pathol* (2019) 43:1631–7. doi: 10.1097/PAS.0000000000001362

Malignant Melanoma in Children and Adolescents Treated in Pediatric Oncology Centers: An Australian and New Zealand Children's Oncology Group (ANZCHOG) Study

Anne L. Ryan[1*], Charlotte Burns[2], Aditya K. Gupta[3], Ruvishani Samarasekera[4], David S. Ziegler[4], Maria L. Kirby[5], Frank Alvaro[6], Peter Downie[2,7], Stephen J. Laughton[8], Siobhan Cross[9], Timothy Hassall[10], Geoff B. McCowage[3], Jordan R. Hansford[2,11], Rishi S. Kotecha[1,12,13] and Nicholas G. Gottardo[1,12*]

[1] Department of Haematology, Oncology and Bone Marrow Transplant, Perth Children's Hospital, Perth, WA, Australia, [2] Children's Cancer Centre, The Royal Children's Hospital, Melbourne, VIC, Australia, [3] Cancer Centre for Children, The Children's Hospital at Westmead, Westmead, NSW, Australia, [4] Kids Cancer Centre, Sydney Children's Hospital, Randwick, NSW, Australia, [5] Department of Haematology/Oncology, Women's and Children's Hospital, Adelaide, SA, Australia, [6] Department of Haematology/Oncology, John Hunter Children's Hospital, Newcastle, NSW, Australia, [7] Department of Haematology/Oncology, Monash Children's Hospital, Melbourne, VIC, Australia, [8] Starship Blood and Cancer Centre, Starship Children's Hospital, Auckland, New Zealand, [9] Children's Haematology/Oncology Centre, Christchurch Hospital, Christchurch, New Zealand, [10] Department of Haematology/Oncology, Queensland Children's Hospital, Brisbane, QLD, Australia, [11] Murdoch Children's Research Institute; Department of Pediatrics, University of Melbourne, Melbourne, VIC, Australia, [12] Telethon Kids Cancer Centre, Telethon Kids Institute, Perth, WA, Australia, [13] Curtin Medical School, Curtin University, Perth, WA, Australia

*Correspondence:
Anne L. Ryan
anne.ryan@health.wa.gov.au
Nicholas G. Gottardo
nick.gottardo@health.wa.gov.au

Objectives: Unlike adults, malignant melanoma in children and adolescents is rare. In adult melanoma, significant progress in understanding tumor biology and new treatments, including targeted therapies and immunotherapy have markedly improved overall survival. In sharp contrast, there is a paucity of data on the biology and clinical behavior of pediatric melanoma. We report a national case series of all pediatric and adolescent malignant melanoma presenting to ANZCHOG Childhood Cancer Centers in Australia and New Zealand.

Methods: A retrospective, descriptive, multi-center study was undertaken to identify patients less than 18 years of age treated for cutaneous malignant melanoma over a twenty-year period (1994 to 2014). Data on clinical characteristics, histopathology, and extent of disease, treatment and follow-up are described.

Results: A total of 37 cases of malignant melanoma were identified from all of the Australasian tertiary Childhood Cancer Centers. The median age was 10 years (range 1 month – 17 years). Clinically, the most common type of lesion was pigmented, occurring in sixteen (57%) patients, whilst amelanotic was seen in 7 patients (25%). In 11 (27.9%) the Breslow thickness was greater than 4mm. A total of 11 (29.7%) patients relapsed and 90% of these died of disease. Five-year event free survival (EFS) and overall survival were 63.2 (95% CI: 40.6 – 79.1) and 67.7% (95% CI: 45.1 – 82.6) respectively.

Conclusion: Our data confirms that melanoma is a rare presentation of cancer to tertiary Australasian Childhood Cancer Centers with only 37 cases identified over two decades. Notably, melanoma managed in Childhood Cancer Centers is frequently at an advanced stage, with a high percentage of patients relapsing and the majority of these patients who relapsed died of disease. This study confirms previous clinical and prognostic information to support the early multidisciplinary management in Childhood Cancer Centers, in conjunction with expert adult melanoma centers, of this rare and challenging patient group.

Keywords: cutaneous melanoma, childhood, dermatology, outcome, rare tumors

INTRODUCTION

Cutaneous melanoma in children and adolescents is rare, with an incidence ranging between 0.3 and 1 per 100 000 children a year, and only a small percentage occurring before puberty (1–4). Pediatric melanoma has not been studied as extensively as adult melanoma and our current understanding of the outcomes for melanoma presenting in children and adolescents is limited to mainly single-institution review series and a recent prospective European rare pediatric cancer consortium registry study (3–7). In Australia <2% of all cases of cutaneous melanoma occur before the age of 25 years (1, 7–9). Given that certain geographical areas of Australia and New Zealand have been reported to have the highest rates of adult melanoma in the world, it is important to review pediatric data and evaluate specific factors that influence prognosis and overall survival (7–9).

The rarity of pediatric melanoma combined with differences in the clinical presentation compared to adults (10), especially in young children can make diagnosis challenging. Moreover, histopathological diagnosis is complicated due to the similar histological appearance of malignant melanoma with more benign lesions in childhood, such as spitz nevi, atypical spitz nevi and the concept of melanocytic tumors of uncertain prognosis (MELTUMP). Molecular diagnostic tools, such as fluorescent *in situ* hybridization and genomic testing, are now assisting pathologists to distinguish between these different entities (11, 12).

Over the past decade, significant advances have been made in elucidating the molecular pathogenesis of adult melanoma. Approximately 60% of adult melanoma patients have identifiable oncogenic mutations in the *BRAF* gene, whilst another 20% have oncogenic *NRAS* mutations (13). These genetic discoveries have been translated into the clinic, with mitogen-activated protein kinase (MAPK) pathway inhibitors such as BRAF and mitogen-activated protein kinase/extracellular signal-regulated kinase (MEK) inhibitors inducing dramatic responses and significantly improving survival (14, 15). In addition, the highly immunogenic nature of melanoma has successfully been exploited using immunotherapy, with major improvements in patient outcomes (16).

Despite these advances, melanoma that has spread to distant sites remains incurable in the majority of patients. Clinical trials are ongoing to develop novel and more effective targeted therapies and immunotherapies to treat metastatic melanoma (16–19). The management of pediatric melanoma patients has been extrapolated from the treatment of adults with melanoma. However, the limited understanding surrounding the diagnosis and prognosis of childhood melanoma initially led to the almost uniform exclusion of these patients from clinical trials offered to adult patients; a strategy that has hampered research efforts and access to treatment in this population (20). The increased use of precision medicine to molecularly characterize tumors in children has further guided specific treatments including molecular target therapies and immunotherapy. In Australia this is being undertaken through the Precision Medicine in Children with Cancer (PRISM) clinical trial (https:// clinicaltrials.gov/ct2/show/NCT03336931).

For these reasons, we evaluated the clinical characteristics and outcomes of all pediatric and adolescent malignant melanoma patients managed at pediatric oncology centers in Australia and New Zealand over the past two decades.

METHODS

We undertook a retrospective, descriptive, multicenter study of children and adolescents with malignant melanoma. All ten pediatric oncology centers in the Australia and New Zealand Children's Oncology Group (ANZCHOG) participated in the study. Patients aged less than 18 years and treated for malignant melanoma between 1994 and 2014 were included. A detailed review of each patient chart was undertaken and data collected for each case included age, gender, ethnicity, site of disease, staging, extent of disease (including Breslow thickness), ulceration and *BRAF* status. Treatment outcomes, mode of follow-up, relapse and cause of death were also recorded. All data were all collected in accordance with the approval of institutional research ethics boards.

The number of cases of pediatric and adolescent melanoma patients was compared to the number of cases published in the national cancer registry, for both Australia and New Zealand, over the same timeframe.

Data has been presented as medians and ranges and as percentages. The overall survival (OS) has been calculated according to the Kaplan-Meier method: from the date of diagnosis to the date of death or latest follow-up for patients still alive. The event free survival (EFS) has been calculated from the date of diagnosis to the date of disease recurrence, death or latest follow-up for patients still alive and in complete remission.

RESULTS

Thirty-seven patients with malignant melanoma were identified over the twenty-year period timeframe. The ratio of males to females was 1:1 and the median age at diagnosis was 10 years age (range 1 month to 17 years). A total of 16 (43%) patients were less than 10 years old. The majority of patients were of Caucasian ethnicity (83.7%) with only five New Zealand Maori (n=3), African (n=1) and Australian Aboriginal (n=1) patients. Tumors were located on the head and neck (n = 14, 37.8%), trunk (n = 10, 27%), upper limb (n = 5, 13.5%) and lower limb (n = 5 cases, 13.5%). The primary location was unknown in two patients (**Table 1**).

The Australia and New Zealand cancer registries reported 1,778 children and adolescents with melanoma over the same twenty-year time period (**Table 2**).

Melanoma arose from congenital nevi in six patients (16.3%) and two patients had a history of malignancy with one patient being treated for acute leukemia, including total body radiation conditioning for an allogeneic bone marrow transplant and another patient with previous anaplastic astrocytoma and leukemia and known Li Fraumeni Syndrome.

A description of lesions at clinical presentation was available in 28 patients. The majority (16 cases, 55%) had a pigmented lesion reported, whilst seven (25%) had amelanotic lesions which were described as scaly, warty or friable in appearance. Two (7%) patients presented with subungal nodular lesions on the toe and index finger and three (11%) patients had nodal enlargement as the presenting clinical feature.

Histologically the most common melanoma subtypes were nodular and Spitzoid, with eight cases (21.6%) reported for each group respectively. Breslow thickness was reported in 25 cases and nearly 30% (11 cases) had thick lesions with a measurement greater than 4mm at presentation.

Based on the American Joint Committee on Cancer (AJCC) classification, our study found that eight patients (21.6%) were stage I, nine patients (24.3%) were stage II, four patients were stage III (10.8%) and the remaining were stage IV (11 cases, 29.7%) at diagnosis. For five patients, no exact staging classification was possible. *BRAFV600E* testing was conducted in seven (18%) patients and was positive for one patient. There was also one patient who was tested for and found positive for an *NRAS* exon 3 mutations.

Initial Treatment

All but three patients underwent initial surgical resection of their tumor. Of the three patients who did not receive surgical resection, one had an unknown primary lesion; one initially had a shave biopsy before proceeding to further surgery and one had a fine needle aspirate of an enlarged lymph node before

TABLE 1 | Patient characteristics and Clinical Features of the 37 patients with malignant melanoma in Australia and New Zealand 1st January 1995 – 31st December 2014.

	N (%)
Gender: Male/Female	18/19 (48.6/51.4)
Age:	
0 – 4 years	5 (13.6)
5 – 9 years	11 (29.7)
10 – 14 years	13 (35.1)
15 – 18 years	8 (21.6)
Ethnicity:	
Caucasian	31 (83.7)
African	1 (2.7)
Aboriginal	1 (2.7)
Maori	3 (8.1)
Unknown	1 (2.7)
Site of Disease:	
Trunk	10 (27)
Head and Neck	14 (37.8)
Extremity - Upper	5 (13.5)
Extremity - Lower	5 (13.5)
Other	1 (2.7)
Unknown	2 (5.6)
Histology:	
Superficial Spreading	4 (10.8)
Nodular	8 (21.6)
On congenital naevus	6 (16.3)
Spitzoid	8 (21.6)
Not classified	11 (29.7)
Breslow Thickness:	
≤ 1.00mm	4 (10.8)
1.01 – 2.00mm	4 (10.8)
2.01 – 4.00mm	6 (16.3)
> 4.00mm	11 (29.7)
Unknown	12 (32.4)
AJCC Stage at diagnosis:	
Stage I	8 (21.6)
Stage II	9 (24.3)
Stage III	4 (10.8)
Stage IV	11 (29.7)
Unknown	5 (13.6)

subsequent nodal excision. Primary re-excision, in order to obtain adequate margins, was performed in seven (19%) of patients. Lymph node biopsy was undertaken in 13 (35%) patients and lymphoscintigraphy was performed in 1 patient. Lymph nodes were positive following biopsy in five (38%) patients. Among the cases with positive lymph node biopsies, three had nodular histology and two were associated with congenital nevi. All but one of these patients relapsed and subsequently died of the disease.

Chemotherapy was used in five patients, following initial surgical resection, and included interferon in four patients (3 patients stage III and 1 stage IV) and a combination of cisplatin, dacarbazine and fotemustine in another patient (stage IV).

Relapses and Treatment

Eleven patients (29.7%) relapsed, with a median time from diagnosis to first relapse of 22 months (range 2 months – 9 years). All but one of the 11 patients who relapsed died from malignant melanoma. Among the patients who relapsed, 3 (27%) had melanoma arising from a congenital nevus, four (37%) had

TABLE 2 | Incidence Count from 1st Jan 1994 – 31st Dec 2013, based on Australia and New Zealand national cancer registry data.

0 – 4 years	19
5 – 9 years	43
10 – 14 years	198
15 – 19 years	1289
Number of Deaths: Australia 1st Jan 1994 – 31st Dec 2013	
0 – 4 years	1
5 – 9 years	2
10 – 14 years	3
15 – 19 years	26
Incident Count: New Zealand 1st Jan 1994 – 31st December 2013	
0 – 4 years	3
5 – 9 years	3
10 – 14 years	30
15 – 19 years	193
Number of Deaths: New Zealand 1st Jan 2007 – 31st December 2012	
0 – 4 years	1
5 – 9 years	0
10 – 14 years	1
15 – 19 years	8

Mean population of children 0 - 19 years in Australia and New Zealand over the duration of the study = 3, 069, 745 per annum (http://www.stats.govt.nz/topics/population, https://abs.gov.au/statistics/people/population.

nodular histology, one (9%) had superficial spreading histology and in three (27%) patients the histology was unknown. The site of relapse was in regional lymph nodes for five patients, local cutaneous for two patients and metastatic in four patients. A summary of relapsed treatment can be found in **Table 3**. Relapsed treatments were varied and included surgery, when feasible (five cases), but more predominately chemotherapy (seven cases) and palliative radiotherapy (five cases). Targeted therapy was used in two patients and included immunotherapy with ipilimumab and pembrolizomab in one patient and the combination of targeted therapy with the *BRAF* inhibitor dabrafinab followed by ipilimumab in the other patient.

Survival Outcomes

At the end of the follow-up period 10 patients (27%) had died of disease (**Table 3**). A total of 26 patients were still in first Complete Response (CR) and one in second CR. **Figures 1** and **2** show Kaplan-Meier curves for EFS and OS. After a median follow-up of 5.8 years (2 months – 16.5 years) the 5 year EFS and OS were 63.2 (95% CI: 40.6 – 79.1) and 67.7% (95% CI: 45.1 – 82.6) respectively.

DISCUSSION

We report here a retrospective case series of all malignant melanomas occurring in children and adolescents in Australia and New Zealand from the ANZCHOG, who were managed at tertiary pediatric oncology centers over two decades. Patients were referred from various other health professionals, including dermatologists, primary health care physicians general and plastic surgeons, often after initial surgery.

Our finding that only 37 pediatric patients were treated at tertiary pediatric oncology centers over a twenty-year period is in stark contrast with national registry data, where the total incidence of malignant melanoma among children and adolescents in Australia and New Zealand over the same time period was 1,778 across both registries. These data reveal that malignant melanoma in children and adolescents is rarely treated at pediatric oncology centers in Australia and New Zealand. In keeping with our data, a recent Italian study estimated that only one in three children and one in ten adolescents with melanoma are treated in tertiary pediatric referral centers (3). However, there is a paucity of similar data for other countries.

Another important aspect of our findings concerns the stage of the melanoma in referred patients. Our data shows that a large percentage (29.7%) of patients referred to tertiary oncology centers had stage IV disease at presentation. Our findings strongly suggest that patients are usually referred to tertiary oncology centers only when harboring advanced stages of the disease, which likely also explain the relatively high death rate of 27% that was observed. Consistent with our hypothesis, Réguerre et al., analyzed 52 cases of malignant melanoma in children and adolescents and suggested that the relatively poor prognosis noted in their cohort could be explained by having selected patients referred to expert oncology hospitals (21). Compared to other published series, patients reported by Réguerre et al. had more advanced stages or the worst initial presentations, such as metastatic relapse after the excision of a supposedly benign lesion.

For a cancer like melanoma, early diagnosis is a crucial factor determining the outcome of a patient. For both adults and children, the successful management of melanoma is stage dependent and surgical treatment alone, with adequate margins, is curative for both adult and pediatric patients who present with early-stage localized disease (22, 23). In addition, early diagnosis has also been shown to significantly improve the quality of life for patients with melanoma. For example, a study of 395 melanoma patients evaluated with the EQ-5D-5L questionnaire showed that postoperative stage I–II melanoma patients experienced better health outcomes >2 years after treatment, compared to patients with stage III melanoma (24, 25).

The morphological appearance of lesions is also of paramount significance. The presence of thick lesions (>4mm) is associated with a higher risk of disease spread, and these patients may benefit from additional chemotherapy (26). In a large pediatric series of melanoma, Brecht et al., reported that the presence of histological ulceration, nodular histology, Breslow thickness of more than 2mm and AJCC classification of III or IV, were indicative of a poor prognosis (27). Our data, although contained a relatively small number of cases, is consistent with these findings, with tumor thickness, nodular histology and advanced stage having worst survival outcomes (All six patients with known nodular histology and Breslow thickness of >2mm died of disease). However, these histological factors need to be evaluated further in larger cohorts of children and adolescents with melanoma before their true prognostic value can be evaluated. The presence of

TABLE 3 | Relapse characteristics.

Site of Primary Disease	Site of Relapse	Age at Diagnosis	Time to relapse	Histology	Breslow Thickness	AJCC Stage at Diagnosis	Therapy for Relapse	Outcome
Subungal	Metastatic (Scalp, lymph nodes)	7 years, 3 months	21 months	Nodular	3.5mm	II	Chemotherapy Radiotherapy	DOD
Trunk	Trunk	20 months	2 months	On congenital naevus	8mm	IV	Chemotherapy Radiotherapy	DOD
Ear	Metastatic (lymph nodes, Lung)	11 years, 7 months	18 months	Nodular	10mm	IV	Surgery Chemotherapy Immunotherapy	DOD
Trunk	Trunk	5 years, 7 months	10 months	On congenital naevus	7.4mm	IV	Surgery Radiotherapy	DOD
Scalp	Metastatic (lymph nodes, bone, liver)	15 years, 4 months	8 months	Superficial Spreading	3.2mm	IV	Surgery, Chemotherapy, Immunotherapy Radiotherapy	DOD
Lymph node	Lymph nodes	17 years, 3 months	2 years, 4 months	Unknown	Unknown	IV	Chemotherapy	DOD
Scalp	Lymph nodes	13 years, 6 months	1 year, 2 months	Nodular	7.5mm	II	Chemotherapy	DOD
Trunk	Lymph nodes	16 years, 2 months	9 months	Nodular	6.4mm	II	Chemotherapy Immunotherapy	DOD
Meninges	Lymph nodes	3 years, 9 months	1 year, 5 months	Unknown	Unknown	Unknown	Surgery	DOD
Trunk	Metastatic (lymph nodes, liver, bone)	1 year, 6 months	9 months	On congenital naevus	11.4mm	II	Radiotherapy	DOD

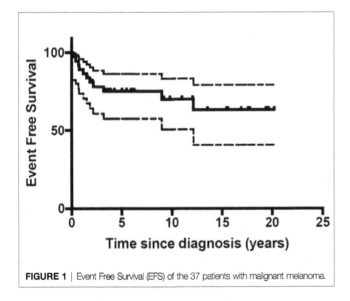

FIGURE 1 | Event Free Survival (EFS) of the 37 patients with malignant melanoma.

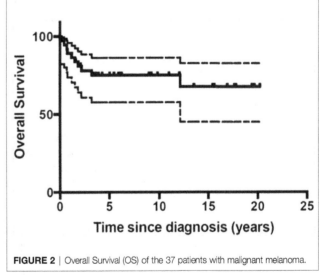

FIGURE 2 | Overall Survival (OS) of the 37 patients with malignant melanoma.

ulceration was rarely documented and its prognostic significance should be stressed in the histopathological work-up of such cases in the future. Lymph node evaluation with the use of sentinel node biopsy was not routinely documented in this cohort but would offer additional important prognostic information for childhood melanoma patients. In addition, other missing information relating to comorbidities, family history and further details of treatment such as surgical techniques and margins would have been valuable to evaluate in relation to survival outcomes. Another important aspect concerns treatment location. It is difficult to ascertain whether the location of diagnosis and treatment for children and adolescents with malignant melanoma ultimately influences

outcome. It is well recognized that children and adolescents diagnosed with cancer benefit from access to a specialized multidisciplinary team with ongoing systematic clinical reviews and surveillance imaging (21, 28, 29). A recent Italian study that analyzed nationwide hospital discharge of adolescents with melanoma found that patients were dispersed across a large number of hospitals, not always in a pediatric oncology center. The study identified 418 adolescents diagnosed with cutaneous melanoma between 2007 and 2014. These patients were referred to 137 different hospitals, where they were treated in various units, such as pediatric and adult oncology, adult general surgery and dermatology. These findings highlight the need to develop better ways to manage melanoma patients, to ensure that they are referred to an appropriate specialized clinic (28).

Given the association between childhood and adolescent malignant melanoma and the presence of an underlying cancer predisposition syndrome, any such case should be considered for referral to clinical genetics and for genetic counseling (30–32).

As in adults, changes in the appearance of a pigmented lesion should alert to the possibility of melanoma. However, the ABCDE clinical rule (asymmetry, border, irregularity, color variability and diameter >6mm and evolving), often used to identify concerning skin lesions in adults, may be difficult to apply to children (33). Common benign lesions such as Spitz nevi and benign nevi that grow as the child grows often have these clinical features. A study by Cordoro et al. showed that 60% of children aged 0 to10 years and 40% of children aged 11 to 19 years with melanoma did not present with the conventional ABCDE criteria, but rather with amelanosis, bleeding, uniform color and *de novo* development were the most common clinical presentations (33). In our cohort, while the majority of patients had pigmented lesions, a large number were described as amelanotic and associated with non-specific skin changes or bleeding. The low index of clinical suspicion for malignant melanoma in such lesions has been reported as the cause of delays or misdiagnosis in 50 to 60% of patients (21, 26).

Despite the advances in targeted therapies of adult melanoma, the genomic landscape of pediatric melanoma has only recently been explored. Only 18% of our cohort underwent analysis of *BRAF* V600E mutation, which was present in only one case. In addition, a patient in which melanoma arose from a congenital nevus was positive for an *NRAS* mutation. The limited molecular information in this study reflects the era over which many of the patients were treated; molecular analyses, especially for tumors such as melanoma, were still in their infancy and not widely available. Such molecular information is now essential and should be collected in future prospective clinical studies to fully characterize this rare childhood malignancy and to potentially guide treatment with targeted therapies a. Indeed, a study by Lu et al. provides the most comprehensive genomic analysis of pediatric melanoma to date (34) and shows that there are three distinct groups of childhood melanoma, each with a unique clinical behavior and molecular profile. The first group is the conventional melanoma that shares the histopathological and clinical features of adult melanoma, where 50 – 60% of patients harbor the *BRAF* V600E mutation and the condition rarely develops before puberty. The second group arises in association with congenital nevi, where approximately 5 – 10% of all patients with large or giant congenital nevi develop melanoma. The condition arises most often in the first decade of life and harbors *NRAS* mutations. Finally, the third group is Spitzoid melanoma, where *NRAS* and *BRAF* mutations are absent and the lesions often have a less aggressive clinical course (34).

Collectively, the data from these initial genomic studies suggest that the therapeutic targets for genotype specific melanoma in adults might be applicable to some cases of melanoma in children. What remains to be determined is the safety and efficacy of targeted therapies currently used in adults in children and adolescents with malignant melanoma. Consequently, it is critical that the molecular pathogenesis of future cohorts of pediatric melanoma lesions be evaluated to continue to resolve these important clinical issues.

Due to the rarity of malignant melanoma in young people, it has been difficult to conduct prospective clinical trials tailored to children. In addition, most adult treatment protocols are generally not accessible to children. Recent approval and early phase trials with immune checkpoint inhibitors, such as ipilimumab and nivolumab, *BRAF* inhibitors (e.g. Dabrafanib) and MEK inhibitors (e.g. Binimetinib) has begun for adolescents with advanced malignant melanoma at selected pediatric centers (35). In this study, only 2 out of the 11 children with relapsed disease were treated with immunotherapy. This was due to them being treated in an era prior to immunotherapy being an established treatment for metastatic melanoma and not due to contraindications to the use of immunotherapy.

CONCLUSION

Whilst the limited number of cases identified in this study precludes any definitive conclusions on the clinical behavior of melanoma in children and adolescents, some important observations can be made. Consistent with previous reports, the diagnosis of malignant melanoma is challenging, especially in young children as their clinical and histopathological features are poorly characterized. The cases we identified have been compared to published national cancer registry data and build on previous international studies revealing that only a small proportion of children and adolescents with malignant melanoma are managed in tertiary oncology centers (3, 21, 28). Malignant melanoma patients treated in these centers often have more advanced disease and subsequent poor prognosis.

As with many rare pediatric cancers, the diagnosis and subsequent treatment of malignant melanoma is challenging. This study confirms previous clinical and prognostic information in pediatric melanoma to support the early multidisciplinary management in Childhood Cancer Centers, in conjunction with expert adult melanoma centers, of this rare and challenging patient group (21, 25, 28). Scientific advancement together with growing collaborative efforts provide opportunities to advance understanding and treatment (34–36). Further progress involves taking advantage of sophisticated molecular analysis and application of this knowledge in the clinical setting, such that a therapeutic multi-center prospective trial, which includes the collection of tumor samples, be considered in the near future.

AUTHOR CONTRIBUTIONS

AR: conception design, data acquisition, analysis and interpretation, and manuscript drafting. CB: data acquisition. AG: data acquisition. DZ: conception designs and data acquisition. MK: data acquisition and manuscript drafting. FA: data acquisition. PD: data acquisition. SL: data acquisition. SC: data acquisition, and analysis and interpretation. TH: data acquisition, and analysis and interpretation. GM: data acquisition, and analysis and interpretation. JH: conception design, data acquisition, analysis and interpretation, and manuscript drafting. RSK: conception design and manuscript

drafting. NG: conception design, data acquisition, analysis and interpretation, and manuscript drafting. All authors contributed to the article and approved the submitted version.

ACKNOWLEDGMENTS

RK is supported by a Fellowship from NHMRC Australia (APP1142627) and the Children's Leukaemia and Cancer Research Foundation (CLCRF, Australia).
NG is supported by the Stan Perron Chair of Paediatric Haematology and Oncology.

REFERENCES

1. Wallingford SC, Iannacone MR, Youlden DR, Baade PD, Ives A, Verne J, et al. Comparison of melanoma incidence and trends among youth under 25 years in Australia and England, 1990-2010. *Int J Cancer* (2015) 137:2227-33. doi: 10.1002/ijc.29598

2. Campbell LB, Kreicher KL, Gittleman HR, Strodtbeck K, Barnholtz-Sloan J, Bordeaux J. Melanoma Incidence in Children and Adolescents: Decreasing Trends in the United States. *J Pediatr* (2015) 166:1505-13. doi: 10.1016/j.jpeds.2015.02.050

3. Ferrari A, Bisogno G, Cecchetto G, Santinami M, Maurichi A, Bono A, et al. Cutaneous melanoma in children and adolescents: the Italian rare tumors in pediatric age project experience. *J Pediatr* (2014) 164:376-82.e1-2. doi: 10.1016/j.jpeds.2013.10.012

4. Strouse JJ, Fears TR, Tucker MA, Wayne AS. Pediatric melanoma: risk factor and survival analysis of the surveillance, epidemiology and end results database. *J Clin Oncol* (2005) 23:4735-41. doi: 10.1200/JCO.2005.02.899

5. Kalani N, Guidry JA, Farahi JM, Stewart SB, Dellavalle RP, Dunnick AC. Pediatric melanoma: Characterizing 256 cases from the Colorado Central Cancer Registry. *Pediatr Dermatol* (2019) 36:219-22. doi: 10.1111/pde.13747

6. Brecht IB, De Paoli A, Bisogno G, Orbach D, Schneider DT, Leiter U, et al. Pediatric patients with cutaneous melanoma: A European study. *Pediatr Blood Cancer* (2018) 65:e26974. doi: 10.1002/pbc.26974

7. Iannacone MR, Youlden DR, Baade PD, Aitken JF, Green AC. Melanoma incidence trends and survival in adolescents and young adults in Queensland, Australia. *Int J Cancer* (2015) 136(3):603-9. doi: 10.1002/ijc.28956

8. Xu JX, Koek S, Lee S, Hanikeri M, Lee M, Beer T, et al. Juvenile melanomas: Western Australian Melanoma Advisory Service experience. *Australas J Dermatol* (2017) 58:299-303. doi: 10.1111/ajd.12661

9. MacLennan R, Green AC, McLeod GR, Martin NG. Increasing incidence of cutaneous melanoma in Queensland, Australia. *J Natl Cancer Inst* (1992) 84:1427-32. doi: 10.1093/jnci/84.18.1427

10. Ferrari A, Bono A, Baldi M, Collini P, Casanova M, Pennacchioli E, et al. Does melanoma behave differently in younger children than in adults? A retrospective study of 33 cases of childhood melanoma from a single institution. *Pediatrics* (2005) 115:649-54. doi: 10.1542/peds.2004-0471

11. Gammon B, Gerami P. Fluorescence in situ hybridization for ambiguous melanocytic tumors. *Histol Histopathol* (2012) 27:1539-42. doi: 10.14670/hh-27.1539

12. Gerami P, Busam K, Cochran A, Cook MG, Duncan LM, Elder DE, et al. Histomorphologic assessment and interobserver diagnostic reproducibility of atypical spitzoid melanocytic neoplasms with long-term follow-up. *Am J Surg Pathol* (2014) 38:934-40. doi: 10.1097/pas.0000198

13. Lee JH, Choi JW, Kim YS. Frequencies of BRAF and NRAS mutations are different in histological types and sites of origin of cutaneous melanoma: a

meta-analysis. *Br J Dermatol* (2011) 164:776-84. doi: 10.1111/j.1365-2133.2010.10185.x

14. Chapman PB, Hauschild A, Robert C, Haanen JB, Ascierto P, Larkin J, et al. Improved survival with vemurafenib in melanoma with BRAF V600E mutation. *New Engl J Med* (2011) 364:2507-16. doi: 10.1056/NEJMoa1103782

15. Smalley KS, Sondak VK. Targeted therapy for melanoma: is double hitting a home run? *Nat Rev Clin Oncol* (2013) 10:5-6. doi: 10.1038/nrclinonc.2012.215

16. Weber J, Mandala M, Del Vecchio M, Gogas HJ, Arance AM, Cowey CL, et al. Adjuvant nivolumab versus ipilimumab in resected stage III or IV melanoma. *New Engl J Med* (2017) 377:1824-35. doi: 10.1056/NEJMoa1709030

17. Hodi FS, O'Day SJ, McDermott DF, Weber RW, Sosman JA, Haanen JB, et al. Improved survival with ipilimumab in patients with metastatic melanoma. *N Engl J Med* (2010) 363:711-23. doi: 10.1056/NEJMoa1003466

18. Ralli M, Botticelli A, Visconti IC, Angeletti D, Fiore M, Marchetti P, et al. Immunotherapy in the Treatment of Metastatic Melanoma: Current Knowledge and Future Directions. *J Immunol Res* (2020) 2020:9235638. doi: 10.1155/2020/9235638

19. Furue M, Ito T, Wada N, Wada M, Kadono T, Uchi H. Melanoma and Immune Checkpoint Inhibitors. *Curr Oncol Rep* (2018) 20:29. doi: 10.1007/s11912-018-0676-z

20. Indini A, Brecht I, Del Vecchio M, Sultan I, Signoroni S, Ferrari A. Cutaneous melanoma in adolescents and young adults. *Pediatr Blood Cancer* (2018) 65:e27292. doi: 10.1002/pbc.27292

21. Reguerre Y, Vittaz M, Orbach D, Robert C, Bodemer C, Mateus C, et al. Cutaneous malignant melanoma in children and adolescents treated in pediatric oncology units. *Pediatr Blood Cancer* (2016) 63:1922-7. doi: 10.1002/pbc.26113

22. Saenz NC, Saenz-Badillos J, Busam K, LaQuaglia MP, Corbally M, Brady MS. Childhood melanoma survival. *Cancer* (1999) 85:750-4. doi: 10.1002/(SICI)1097-0142(19990201)85:3<750::AID-CNCR26>3.0.CO;2-5

23. Paradela S, Fonseca E, Pita-Fernandez S, Kantrow SM, Diwan AH, Herzog C, et al. Prognostic factors for melanoma in children and adolescents: a clinicopathologic, single-center study of 137 Patients. *Cancer* (2010) 116:4334-44. doi: 10.1002/cncr.25222

24. Tromme I, Devleesschauwer B, Beutels P, Richez P, Leroy A, Baurain JF, et al. Health-related quality of life in patients with melanoma expressed as utilities and disability weights. *Br J Dermatol* (2014) 171:1443-50. doi: 10.1111/bjd.13262

25. Schlesinger-Raab A, Schubert-Fritschle G, Hein R, Stolz W, Volkenandt M, Hölzel D, et al. Quality of life in localised malignant melanoma. *Ann Oncol* (2010) 21:2428-35. doi: 10.1093/annonc/mdq255

26. Pappo AS. Melanoma in children and adolescents. *Eur J Cancer* (2003) 39:2651-61. doi: 10.1016/j.ejca.2003.06.001

27. Brecht IB, Garbe C, Gefeller O, Pfahlbery A, Bauer J, Eigentler TK, et al. 443 paediatric cases of malignant melanoma registered with the German Central

Malignant Melanoma Registry between 1983 and 2011. *Eur J Cancer* (2015) 51:861–8. doi: 10.1016/j.ejca.2015.02.014

28. Ferrari A, Bernasconi A, Sironi G, Botta L, Chiaravalli S, Casanova M, et al. Where are adolescents with cutaneous melanoma treated? An Italian nationwide study on referrals based on hospital discharge records. *Pediatr Blood Cancer* (2020) 68:e28566. doi: 10.22541/au.159050481.13629196

29. Halalsheh H, Kaste SC, Navid F, Bahrami A, Shulkin B, Roa B, et al. The role of routine imaging in pediatric cutaneous melanoma. *Pediatr Blood Cancer* (2018) 65:e27412. doi: 10.1002/pbc.27412

30. Soura E, Eliades PJ, Shannon K, Stratigos AJ, Tsao H. Hereditary melanoma: Update on syndromes and management: Emerging melanoma cancer complexes and genetic counseling. *J Am Acad Dermatol* (2016) 74:411–20. doi: 10.1016/j.jaad.2015.08.037

31. De Simone P, Valiante M, Silipo V. Familial melanoma and multiple primary melanoma. *G Ital Dermatol Venereol* (2017) 152:262–65. doi: 10.23736/S0392-0488.17.05554-7

32. Sreeraman KR, Messina JL, Reed D, Navid F, Sondak VK. Pediatric Melanoma and Atypical Melanocytic Neoplasms. *Cancer Treat Res* (2016) 167:331–69. doi: 10.1007/978-3-319-22539-5_15

33. Cordoro KM, Gupta D, Frieden IJ, McCalmont T, Kashani-Sabet M. Pediatric melanoma: results of a large cohort study and proposal for modified ABCD detection criteria for children. *J Am Acad Dermatol* (2013) 68:913–25. doi: 10.1016/j.jaad.2012.12.953

34. Lu C, Zhang J, Nagahawatte P, Easton J, Lee S, Lui Z, et al. The genomic landscape of childhood and adolescent melanoma. *J Invest Dermatol* (2015) 135:816–23. doi: 10.1038/jid.2014.425

35. McCormack CR, Scolyer R, Bhabha F, Smith S. Cancer Council Australia Melanoma Guidelines Working Party. In: . *How Should melanoma in children be managed*. Sydney: Cancer Council Australia (2019). Available at: https://wiki.cancer.org.au/australia/Guidelines:Melanoma.

36. Pappo AS, Furman WL, Schultz KA, Ferrari A, Helman L, Krailo M. Rare Tumors in Children: Progress Through Collaboration. *J Clin Oncol* (2015) 33:3047–54. doi: 10.1200/JCO.2014.59.3632

15

Favorable Response to the Tyrosine Kinase Inhibitor Apatinib in Recurrent Merkel Cell Carcinoma

Yiyi Feng, Xin Song* and Renbing Jia*

Department of Ophthalmology, Ninth People's Hospital, Shanghai Jiao Tong University School of Medicine, Shanghai Key Laboratory of Orbital Diseases and Ocular Oncology, Shanghai, China

*Correspondence:
Renbing Jia
renbingjia@sjtu.edu.cn
Xin Song
drsongxin@163.com

Background: As angiogenesis is an essential step in tumor growth and metastasis, the tyrosine kinase inhibitor (TKI) apatinib has become a revolutionary anticancer therapy across various malignancies. However, its efficiency and safety in Merkel cell carcinoma (MCC) are uncertain.

Case presentation: The current study described the case of a 91-year-old man who presented with a 3.2 × 3.0 × 2.2 cm rapidly growing, solitary tumor of the right lower eyelid. It was diagnosed as MCC pathologically. Twenty-seven days after the surgery, the patient returned to the hospital with recurrent MCC. Apatinib was then administered to this patient. The patient had a complete response (CR) to apatinib after 4.4 months of targeted therapy. Twenty-seven months of progression-free survival (PFS) was achieved with controllable treatment-related adverse events (AEs).

Conclusion: Treatment with apatinib demonstrated clinical benefit in our patient with recurrent MCC, highlighting its potential utility in other MCC patients. Further clinical trials are needed to determine the efficacy and safety of apatinib in MCC patients.

Keywords: Merkel cell carcinoma, tyrosine kinase inhibitor, apatinib, eyelid, targeted therapy

INTRODUCTION

Merkel cell carcinoma (MCC) is a rare but highly aggressive cutaneous malignancy with neuroendocrine features that has 33–46% mortality (1, 2). Heath M et al. (3) summarized the clinical features of MCC in an acronym: AEIOU—Asymptomatic/lack of tenderness, Expanding rapidly, Immune suppression, Older than age 50, and ultraviolet (UV)-exposed site on a person with fair skin. The incidence rate of MCC varies across the world, with approximately 2,488 cases per year diagnosed in the United States (4). Merkel cell polyomavirus (MCPyV) and UV exposure play a major role in the pathogenesis of MCC (2). The most common primary sites of MCC are head and neck (45%), and eyelid tumors represent only 2.5% of cases (5).

Wide excision of the tumor in combination with adjuvant radiation therapy to the primary site is the first-line strategy (6). Chemotherapy and immunotherapy can be used to treat metastatic or unresectable MCC (6). In immunotherapy, immune checkpoint inhibitors targeting programmed cell death protein 1 (PD-1) or its ligand (PD-L1) are the favored agents. In addition, as tumor angiogenesis is one of the features of cancer, the inhibition of vascular endothelial growth factor (VEGF) signaling pathway has become a revolutionary anticancer approach across various malignancies (7). However, its efficacy and safety in MCC patients are unknown. Here, we report an elderly male who developed MCC of the eyelid and was treated with apatinib, a small molecule inhibitor of vascular endothelial growth factor receptor-2 (VEGFR-2).

CASE PRESENTATION

The study was carried out according to the principles of the Declaration of Helsinki; informed consent has been obtained from the patient.

A 91-year-old Chinese man presented in the Ninth People's Hospital, Shanghai Jiao Tong University School of Medicine, on May 7, 2018, with a rapidly growing, solitary tumor of the right lower eyelid, which was initially noted in March 2018 without tenderness. Clinically, the tumor was a violet-colored nodule of 3.2 × 3.0 × 2.0 cm with pigmentation and an irregular ulcer in the center (**Figure 1A**). Fine needle aspiration biopsy was performed at Hua Shan Hospital, Fu Dan University, on April 17, 2018, which confirmed the diagnosis of MCC. The patient suffered from prostate cancer, hypertension, coronary heart disease (CHD), chronic cardiac insufficiency (NYHA, II–III) and chronic renal insufficiency and had received treatments of Enantone (3.75 mg, H,

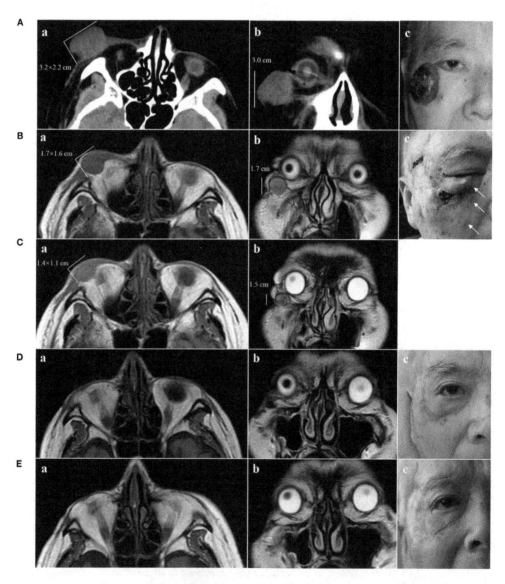

FIGURE 1 | Clinical presentation of MCC and changes on imaging. **(A)** May 2018. **A**(a) and **A**(b) CT scans showing a tumor of 3.2 × 2.2 × 3.0 cm without destruction of bone. **A**(c) Solitary violet-colored nodule of the right lower eyelid with pigmentation and an irregular ulcer in the center. **(B)** June 2018. **B**(a) and **B**(b) MRI showing a tumor of 1.7 × 1.6 × 1.7 cm. **B**(c) Recurrence of the MCC. The white arrows show three hard, subcutaneous nodules. **(C)** July 2018, 2 weeks after treatment with apatinib. **C**(a) and **C**(b) MRI showing regression of the MCC (1.4 × 1.1 × 1.5 cm). **(D)** November 2018, 4 months after treatment with apatinib. **D**(a) and **D**(b) MRI showing MCC disappearance with a favorable response to apatinib. **D**(c) Only a scar with pigmentation was observed. **(E)** November 2019, 17 months after treatment with apatinib. **E**(a) and **E**(b) MRI showing no sign of recurrence. **E**(c) The pigmentation gradually subsided, leaving a pink scar.

q4w), Adalat (30 mg, po, qd), Diovan (80 mg, po, qd), Furosemide (30 mg, po, qd) and spironolactone (20 mg, po, qd). He also had a history of pulmonary tuberculosis when he was young. Ultrasound and computed tomography (CT) were performed to clinically assess the tumor and cervical lymph nodes, and no signs of cervical lymph node metastasis were found. Clinical detection of lymph nodes or metastatic disease was performed *via* inspection and palpation, as the patient could not tolerate the long time required to complete the imaging examination. The physical examination was negative. After a multidisciplinary meeting, we decided to treat this patient with surgery, and sentinel lymph node biopsy (SLNB) was not considered due to the negative results of the imaging examination. Mohs micrographic surgery with a 1 cm excision margin was performed on May 10, 2018. The tumor had infiltrated the periosteum, and all the infiltrated soft tissue was removed together with the tumor. After confirmation of negative margins, reconstruction was performed. A rotation flap was designed to repair skin defects. Histologically small, monomorphic, round-to-oval, low-differentiated cells with a vesicular nucleus and scant cytoplasm were observed, which invaded the muscle, nerve and blood vessels (**Figure 2**). Necrosis was prominent (**Figure 2**). The immunohistochemistry results indicated the following patterns: CK (+), CK20 (+), SYN (+), CAM5.2 (+), CD34 (+), Ki67 (80%+), Vim (−), LCA (−), S100 (−), CD99 (−), DES (−), and CHGA (−) (**Figures 2, 3**). According to the American Joint Committee on Cancer (AJCC) staging system, the final clinical diagnosis was MCC of the lower right eyelid, IIB. Postoperative radiotherapy was strongly recommended. However, the patient refused.

On June 6, 2018, several subcutaneous, hard nodules were observed at the primary site of surgery (**Figure 1B**). Chest CT, ultrasonography of the liver and kidneys, inspection and palpation of skin and lymph nodes ruled out distant metastasis. Considering the patient's physical condition, surgery was abandoned after a multidisciplinary discussion. Ultimately, apatinib was used to treat MCC in this patient from June 26, 2018 (0.25 g, po, bid). As the treatment was well tolerated by the patient, two days later, we changed the dose of apatinib (0.5 g, po, qd). Blood pressure, routine blood tests, renal function, and liver function were carefully monitored (**Figure 4**). The MCC showed a strong response to apatinib, and the efficacy was significant (**Figure 1C**). However, on July 20, 2018, exacerbated proteinuria and thrombocytopenia led us to reduce the dose of apatinib (0.25 g, po, qd). The patient was treated with leucogen (20 mg, po, tid), and his thrombocytopenia resolved. On September 14, 2018, we stopped the use of apatinib due to a high serum creatinine level (182 μmol/L). Hand–foot syndrome also occurred. However, these treatment-related adverse events (AEs) were well controlled with symptomatic treatment. On October 1, 2018, after another multidisciplinary meeting, we restarted treatment (0.125 g, po, five times a week). After two cycles, we changed the dose of apatinib (0.125 g, po, four times a week) to a low maintenance dose. On November 9, 2018, 4.4 months after the first administration of apatinib, the patient had a complete response (CR) (**Figure 1D**). We continued administering low-dose apatinib for the treatment of MCC. In

the following follow-up, the patient's condition was stable (**Figure 1E**). Unfortunately, the patient died on October 4, 2020 due to heart failure and respiratory failure with no sign of recurrence or distant metastasis.

DISCUSSION

To the best of our knowledge, we report the first case of MCC of the eyelid treated with apatinib. As previously described, this case of MCC had a strong response to apatinib with few AEs. In addition, the effect was durable. Finally, the progression-free survival (PFS) of this patient was 27 months.

MCC is an aggressive skin cancer that is associated with exposure to UV radiation and MCPyV, with a median interval to recurrence of 8–9 months (8, 9). Wide excision is the first choice for the treatment of MCC. The National Comprehensive Cancer Network (NCCN) Merkel Cell Carcinoma Panel recommends adjuvant radiotherapy to the primary site for all patients with large primary tumors (≥1 cm) and risk factors such as lymphovascular invasion (LVI) or immunosuppression (6). Whether to apply radiotherapy to the draining nodal basin depends on the result of SLNB (negative or positive). Patients who do not undergo SLNB or LN dissection are also recommended to receive radiotherapy. The dosage of radiotherapy depends on the pathology of the resection margins and the result of SLNB. In this case, SLNB was not performed, and as infiltration of muscle, nerve and blood vessels was observed histologically, radiotherapy was recommended according to the NCCN MCC guidelines. However, the patient refused.

For unresectable MCC and metastatic MCC, systemic therapy is the choice, including chemotherapy and immunotherapy. The effect of chemotherapy varies from study to study. The objective response rate (ORR) for first-line chemotherapy ranged from 29.4 to 55%, and the durability of response (DOR) was 2.8–6.7 months (10–12). In patients who received one or more prior lines of chemotherapy, the ORR was 10.3–28.6%, and the DOR was 1.9–3.4 months (10–12). The PFS was 3.1–4.6 months for those patients receiving first-line chemotherapy and as low as 2–3 months in patients who received one or more prior lines of chemotherapy. In addition to the low response rates and limited durability, chemotherapy may cause toxicity, and it is not a suitable choice for elderly people with many underlying diseases, who have a higher risk of developing AEs. In this case report, the patient was 91 years old and had multiple underlying diseases, and chemotherapy was not chosen to treat the recurrent MCC. Regarding immunotherapy, PD-1 and PD-L1 are immune checkpoint molecules that control tumor growth. Immune checkpoint inhibitors (ICIs), such as avelumab (anti-PD-L1 antibody), nivolumab (anti-PD-1 antibody), and pembrolizumab (anti-PD-1 antibody), are used for the treatment of MCC. Some clinical trials of therapeutic antibodies against PD-1 or PD-L1 have showed high and durable response rates (2, 13, 14). The results of a multicenter, phase II trial of first-line use of pembrolizumab in patients with unresectable advanced MCC

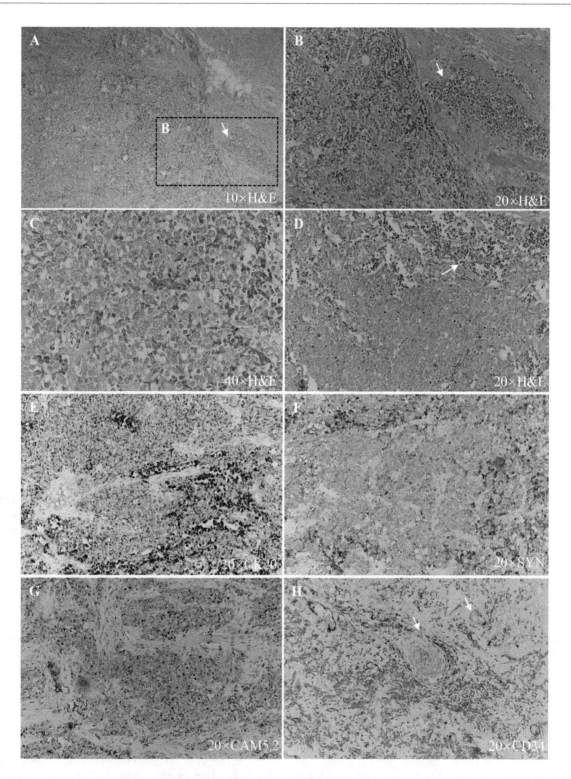

FIGURE 2 | Histopathologic features. **(A)**, **(B)**, and **(C)** Hematoxylin–eosin staining, showing small, monomorphic, round-to-oval, low-differentiated cells with a vesicular nucleus and scant cytoplasm with muscle infiltration (arrow). **(D)** Hematoxylin–eosin staining, showing necrosis (arrow). **(E)** CK20 (+). **(F)** SYN (+). **(G)** CAM5.2 (+). **(H)** CD34 (+), blood vessels and tumor cells within them are indicated with arrows.

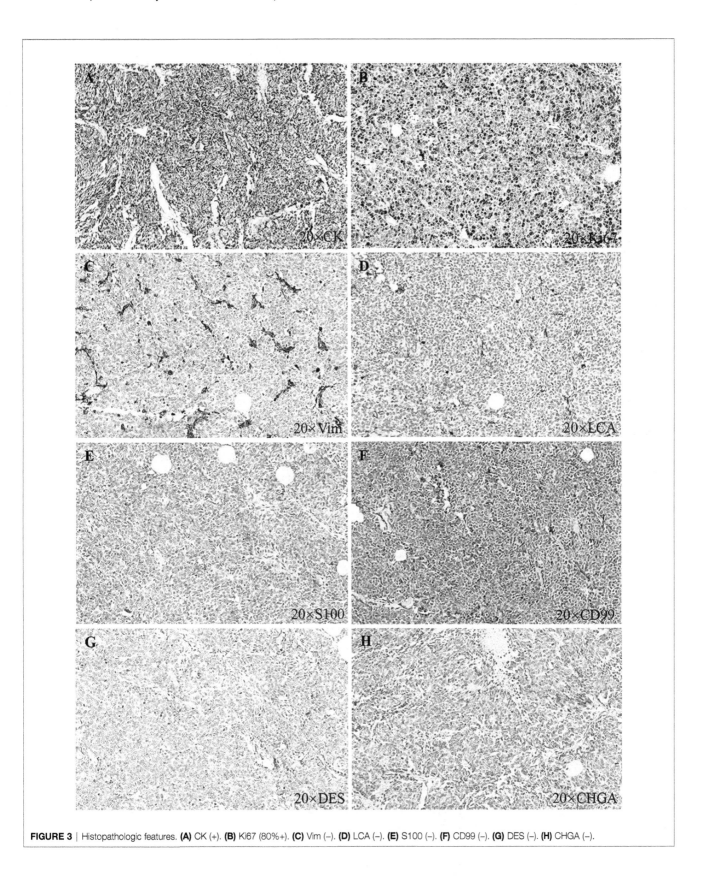

FIGURE 3 | Histopathologic features. **(A)** CK (+). **(B)** Ki67 (80%+). **(C)** Vim (–). **(D)** LCA (–). **(E)** S100 (–). **(F)** CD99 (–). **(G)** DES (–). **(H)** CHGA (–).

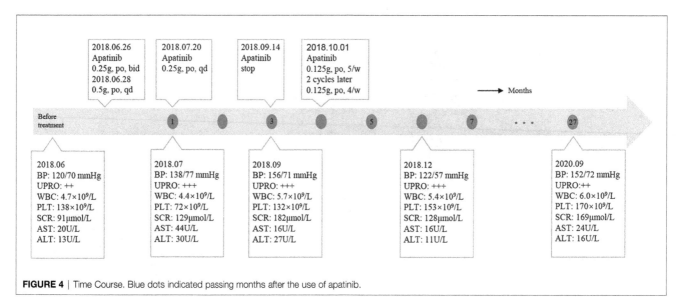

FIGURE 4 | Time Course. Blue dots indicated passing months after the use of apatinib.

demonstrated an ORR of 56% and a DOR of 2.2–9.7 months (NCT02267603) (13). An international, multicenter clinical trial of first-line use of avelumab in metastatic MCC indicated an ORR of 62.1% and a DOR of at least 3 months (93%) (14).

Angiogenesis is a necessary step in tumor growth and metastasis. Among angiogenic factors, VEGF is the most potent. There are three molecular subtypes of the VEGF receptor (VEGFR), including VEGFR-1, VEGFR-2, and VEGFR-3. These receptors are type II transmembrane proteins characterized by tyrosine kinase (TK) activity (7). Among them, VEGFR-2 is the principal subtype of VEGF-induced angiogenic signaling (7). Several studies showed that VEGF and VEGFR-2 were overexpressed in MCC (15–17), and the upregulation of VEGF was associated with aggressive tumor behavior (15). Hence, VEGF and VEGFR can be potential targets for targeted therapy and have attracted increasing attention for the treatment of MCC. One study showed the efficacy of an anti-VEGF antibody (bevacizumab) in MCC in a mouse model (18), however, it has not yet been studied in clinical trials. Tyrosine kinase inhibitors (TKIs) are another potential choice, and their efficacy in other malignancies is impressive. However, little is known about their clinical benefit in MCC. To date, only one clinical trial of TKIs (NCT02036476) has been registered (19); however, due to toxicity and a lack of response, it was closed prematurely. In addition,

some case reports have demonstrated the efficiency of TKIs, such as pazopanib and cabozantinib (20, 21). In this case report, we report impressive tumor regression in a patient with recurrent unresectable MCC during treatment with apatinib. Apatinib is a new inhibitor of VEGFR-2 TK activity targeting the intracellular ATP binding site of the receptor (22). The most frequent adverse events of apatinib included hypertension, proteinuria, and hand–foot syndrome, which were also observed in our patient. However, they could be controlled clinically. Our patient had an impressive response to apatinib, and he tolerated the treatment well with controllable AEs.

In conclusion, apatinib had a favorable effect with great durability in this patient, highlighting its potential utility in other MCC patients, especially those who cannot tolerate chemotherapy and those who do not respond to immunotherapy. Further clinical trials are needed to determine the efficacy and safety of apatinib in MCC patients.

AUTHOR CONTRIBUTIONS

XS and RJ provided direction and guidance throughout the preparation of this manuscript. XS and YF extracted all data. YF drafted the paper. All authors contributed to the article and approved the submitted version.

REFERENCES

1. Schadendorf D, Lebbé C, Zur Hausen A, Avril MF, Hariharan S, Bharmal M, et al. Merkel cell carcinoma: Epidemiology, prognosis, therapy and unmet medical needs. *Eur J Cancer* (2017) 71:53–69. doi: 10.1016/j.ejca.2016.10.022
2. Becker JC, Stang A, DeCaprio JA, Cerroni L, Lebbé C, Veness M, et al. Merkel cell carcinoma. *Nat Rev Dis Primers* (2017) 3:17077. doi: 10.1038/nrdp.2017.77
3. Heath M, Jaimes N, Lemos B, Mostaghimi A, Wang LC, Peñas PF, et al. Clinical characteristics of Merkel cell carcinoma at diagnosis in 195 patients: the AEIOU features. *J Am Acad Dermatol* (2008) 58(3):375–81. doi: 10.1016/j.jaad.2007.11.020

4. Paulson KG, Park SY, Vandeven NA, Lachance K, Thomas H, Chapuis AG, et al. Merkel cell carcinoma: Current US incidence and projected increases based on changing demographics. *J Am Acad Dermatol* (2018) 78(3):457–63.e2. doi: 10.1016/j.jaad.2017.10.028
5. Lemos BD, Storer BE, Iyer JG, Phillips JL, Bichakjian CK, Fang LC, et al. Pathologic nodal evaluation improves prognostic accuracy in Merkel cell carcinoma: analysis of 5823 cases as the basis of the first consensus staging system. *J Am Acad Dermatol* (2010) 63(5):751–61. doi: 10.1016/j.jaad.2010.02.056
6. Bichakjian CK, Olencki T, Aasi SZ, Alam M, Andersen JS, Blitzblau R, et al. Merkel Cell Carcinoma, Version 1.2018, NCCN Clinical Practice Guidelines in Oncology. *J Natl Compr Canc Netw* (2018) 16(6):742–74. doi: 10.6004/jnccn.2018.0055
7. Zhang H. Apatinib for molecular targeted therapy in tumor. *Drug Des Devel Ther* (2015) 9:6075–81. doi: 10.2147/DDDT.S97235

8. Santamaria-Barria JA, Boland GM, Yeap BY, Nardi V, Dias-Santagata D, Cusack JC. Merkel cell carcinoma: 30-year experience from a single institution. *Ann Surg Oncol* (2013) 20(4):1365–73. doi: 10.1245/s10434-012-2779-3

9. Hui AC, Stillie AL, Seel M, Ainslie J. Merkel cell carcinoma: 27-year experience at the Peter MacCallum Cancer Centre. *Int J Radiat Oncol Biol Phys* (2011) 80(5):1430–5. doi: 10.1016/j.ijrobp.2010.04.061

10. Iyer JG, Blom A, Doumani R, Lewis C, Tarabadkar ES, Anderson A, et al. Response rates and durability of chemotherapy among 62 patients with metastatic Merkel cell carcinoma. *Cancer Med* (2016) 5(9):2294–301. doi: 10.1002/cam4.815

11. Becker JC, Lorenz E, Ugurel S, Eigentler TK, Kiecker F, Pfohler C, et al. Evaluation of real-world treatment outcomes in patients with distant metastatic Merkel cell carcinoma following second-line chemotherapy in Europe. *Oncotarget* (2017) 8(45):79731–41. doi: 10.18632/oncotarget.19218

12. Cowey CL, Mahnke L, Espirito J, Helwig C, Oksen D, Bharmal M. Real-world treatment outcomes in patients with metastatic Merkel cell carcinoma treated with chemotherapy in the USA. *Future Oncol (London England)* (2017) 13 (19):1699–710. doi: 10.2217/fon-2017-0187

13. Nghiem PT, Bhatia S, Lipson EJ, Kudchadkar RR, Miller NJ, Annamalai L, et al. PD-1 Blockade with Pembrolizumab in Advanced Merkel-Cell Carcinoma. *N Engl J Med* (2016) 374(26):2542–52. doi: 10.1056/NEJMoa1603702

14. D'Angelo SP, Russell J, Lebbe C, Chmielowski B, Gambichler T, Grob JJ, et al. Efficacy and safety of first-line avelumab treatment in patients with stage IV metastatic Merkel cell carcinoma: a preplanned interim analysis of a clinical trial. *JAMA Oncol* (2018) 4(9):e180077. doi: 10.1001/jamaoncol.2018.0077

15. Fernández-Figueras MT, Puig L, Musulén E, Gilaberte M, Lerma E, Serrano S, et al. Expression profiles associated with aggressive behavior in Merkel cell

16. carcinoma. *Mod Pathol* (2007) 20(1):90–101. doi: 10.1038/modpathol.3800717

16. Brunner M, Thurnher D, Pammer J, Geleff S, Heiduschka G, Reinisch CM, et al. Expression of VEGF-A/C, VEGF-R2, PDGF-alpha/beta, c-kit, EGFR, Her-2/Neu, Mcl-1 and Bmi-1 in Merkel cell carcinoma. *Mod Pathol* (2008) 21 (7):876–84. doi: 10.1038/modpathol.2008.63

17. Kukko H, Koljonen V, Lassus P, Tukiainen E, Haglund C, Böhling T. Expression of vascular endothelial growth factor receptor-2 in Merkel cell carcinoma. *Anticancer Res* (2007) 27(4C):2587–9.

18. Kervarrec T, Gaboriaud P, Tallet A, Leblond V, Arnold F, Berthon P, et al. VEGF-A Inhibition as a Potential Therapeutic Approach in Merkel Cell Carcinoma. *J Invest Dermatol* (2019) 139(3):736–9. doi: 10.1016/j.jid.2018.08.029

19. Rabinowits G, Lezcano C, Catalano PJ, McHugh P, Becker H, Reilly MM, et al. Cabozantinib in Patients with Advanced Merkel Cell Carcinoma. *Oncologist* (2018) 23(7):814–21. doi: 10.1634/theoncologist.2017-0552

20. Davids MS, Davids M, Charlton A, Ng SS, Chong ML, Laubscher K, et al. Response to a novel multitargeted tyrosine kinase inhibitor pazopanib in metastatic Merkel cell carcinoma. *J Clin Oncol* (2009) 27(26):e97–100. doi: 10.1200/JCO.2009.21.8149

21. Tarabadkar ES, Thomas H, Blom A, Parvathaneni U, Olencki T, Nghiem P, et al. Clinical Benefit from Tyrosine Kinase Inhibitors in Metastatic Merkel Cell Carcinoma: A Case Series of 5 Patients. *Am J Case Rep* (2018) 19:505–11. doi: 10.12659/AJCR.908649

22. Roviello G, Ravelli A, Polom K, Petrioli R, Marano L, Marrelli D, et al. Apatinib: A novel receptor tyrosine kinase inhibitor for the treatment of gastric cancer. *Cancer Lett* (2016) 372(2):187–91. doi: 10.1016/j.canlet.2016.01.014

16

Clinical and Dermoscopic Factors for the Identification of Aggressive Histologic Subtypes of Basal Cell Carcinoma

Riccardo Pampena[1], Gabriele Parisi[2], Mattia Benati[2], Stefania Borsari[1], Michela Lai[1,2], Giovanni Paolino[3,4], Anna Maria Cesinaro[5], Silvana Ciardo[2], Francesca Farnetani[2], Sara Bassoli[2], Giuseppe Argenziano[6], Giovanni Pellacani[2] and Caterina Longo[1,2*]

[1] Centro Oncologico ad Alta Tecnologia Diagnostica, Azienda Unità Sanitaria Locale - IRCCS di Reggio Emilia, Reggio Emilia, Italy, [2] Department of Dermatology, University of Modena and Reggio Emilia, Modena, Italy, [3] Unit of Dermatology, IRCCS Ospedale San Raffaele, Milano, Italy, [4] Clinica Dermatologica, La Sapienza University of Rome, Rome, Italy, [5] Department of Pathological Anatomy, Modena University Hospital, Modena, Italy, [6] Dermatology Unit, University of Campania Luigi Vanvitelli, Naples, Italy

*Correspondence:
Caterina Longo
longo.caterina@gmail.com
orcid.org/0000-0002-8218-3896

Background: Infiltrative basal cell carcinoma (BCC) has a higher risk for post-surgical recurrence as compared to the most common low-aggressive superficial and nodular BCC. Independent diagnostic criteria for infiltrative BCC diagnosis have not been still defined. Improving the pre-surgical recognition of infiltrative BCC might significantly reduce the risk of incomplete excision and recurrence.

Objective: The aim of this study is to define clinical and dermoscopic criteria that can differentiate infiltrative BCC from the most common low-aggressive superficial and nodular BCC.

Methods: Clinical and dermoscopic images of infiltrative, superficial, and nodular BCC were retrospectively retrieved from our database and jointly evaluated by two experienced dermoscopists, blinded for the histologic subtype. Pairwise comparisons between the three histologic subtypes were performed and multivariable logistic regression models were constructed in order to define clinical and dermoscopic factors independently associated with each subtype. To validate our findings, two experienced dermoscopists not previously involved in the study were asked to evaluate clinical and dermoscopic images from an external dataset, guessing the proper BCC subtype between infiltrative, nodular and superficial, before and after being provided with the study results.

Result: A total of 481 histopathologically proven BCCs (51.4% nodular, 33.9% superficial, and 14.8% infiltrative) were included. We found that infiltrative BCC mostly appeared on the head and neck as an amelanotic hypopigmented plaque or papule, displaying ulceration on dermoscopic examination, along with arborizing and fine superficial telangiectasia. Shiny white structures were also frequently observed. Multivariate regression analysis allowed us to define a clinical-dermoscopic profile of infiltrative BCC.

Conclusions: We defined the clinical-dermoscopic profile of infiltrative BCC, allowing to differentiate this variant from superficial and nodular BCC. This will improve pre-surgical recognition of infiltrative forms, reducing the risk for post-surgical recurrence.

Keywords: basal cell carcinoma, subtype, infiltrative, superficial, nodular, dermoscopy

INTRODUCTION

Basal cell carcinoma (BCC) is a keratinocyte carcinoma with low aggressive behavior and represents the most common tumor of human being (1). The diagnosis of BCC is generally straightforward integrating clinical and dermoscopic examination, although in a minority of cases BCC may simulate other benign and malignant tumors (2–6). Several histologic classification have been described for BCC being the superficial (sBCC), nodular (nBCC), and infiltrative (iBCC) forms the most commonly referred to. A minority of BCCs belong to a mixed pattern with more than one histotype simultaneously (7, 8). Basically, BCC histotypes can be classified as non-aggressive and aggressive depending on their behavior to deep infiltration, perineural invasion and recurrence after surgical excision (9). Among the three most common BCC histotypes, infiltrative forms are the most aggressive and it has been reported as an independent risk factor for post-surgical recurrence (10). Superficial and nodular BCCs are instead non-aggressive forms, with a very low surgical recurrence (1). Several studies described clinical and dermoscopic criteria associated to different BCC subtypes (11–15), although specific criteria allowing to differentiate the infiltrative subtype from nodular and superficial forms have not been fully elucidated (4, 6, 7, 11–13). The aim of the current study is to define clinical and dermoscopic criteria that can help to differentiate iBCC from the most common low-aggressive sBCC and nBCC.

MATERIALS AND METHODS

Study Population

We retrospectively selected high-quality clinical and dermoscopic images of histopathologically proven BCCs from the digital databases of the Department of Dermatology of the University of Modena and Reggio Emilia (Research Project NET-2011-02347213). BCCs undergoing only partial biopsy or with more than one subtype at histopathological examination were excluded. We focused our analysis on the following histologic subtypes: infiltrative, superficial, nodular. Other subtypes only represented a minority of our case and were therefore excluded. Clinical images were taken *via* conventional clinical photography. Dermoscopic images were taken *via* polarized light contact dermoscopy (DermLite Photo 3Gen, San Juan Capistrano, CA, USA, mounted on a Canon G16 camera). Demographics and clinical data were also retrieved (i.e., skin phototype, maximum diameter and body site). This work was supported in part by Research Project NET-2011-02347213, Italian Ministry of Health. Funding source was not involved in

design and conduct of the study, collection, management, analysis and interpretation of data, preparation, review, or approval of the manuscript, or decision to submit the manuscript for publication.

Study Workflow

All clinical and dermoscopic images were jointly evaluated by two of us with different degree of expertise in dermoscopy [GaPa (novice) and RP (expert with 5 years of practice)]. Evaluators were aware of demographics and clinical data, but were blinded for the histological subtype. The following clinical parameter were evaluated: color (white, pink, red, brown, blue, black-gray) and palpability (flat, elevated, nodular) together with 12 BCC-specific dermoscopic criteria: arborizing telangiectasia, superficial fine telangiectasias, blue-gray ovoid nests, blue-gray ovoid globules, ulceration, maple leaf-like, spoke-wheel areas, concentric structures, multiple small erosion, in-focus dots, shiny red-white/structureless areas, short white streaks (chrysalis) (4). Evaluators were finally asked to classify each enrolled lesion, on clinical and dermoscopic basis, as amelanotic, light, normally or heavy pigmented according to the area covered by brown-black colors (0%, <25%, 25–75%, and >75%, respectively). To assess practical implications of our results in improving BCC histotype recognition, we selected 90 BCCs (30 iBCC, 300 nBCC, and 30 sBCC) from the database of the "Centro Oncologico ad Alta Tecnologia Diagnostica" of Reggio Emilia. Clinical and dermoscopic images of this external dataset were evaluated by two experienced Clinicians with more than 10 years training in dermoscopy (GA and GiPa) not previously involved in the study, together with demographics data. They were first blinded for study results and were asked to guess the proper histologic subtype between sBCC, nBCC, and iBCC. After a washout period of 2 weeks, they were provided with study results and repeated the same evaluation.

Statistical Analysis

Quantitative variables were assessed for normal distribution and then compared using the Student's T or the Mann-Whitney U test. For qualitative variables the chi-square or Fisher's exact tests were instead used. Data were descriptively displayed and compared according to the BCC's histologic subtype. Pairwise comparisons between the three histologic subtypes were conducted for demographics, clinical, and dermoscopic variables. Three multivariable logistic regression models were subsequently constructed, one for each pairwise comparison among histologic subtypes, to define which demographics and clinical variables and which dermoscopic features were independently associated with each of the three subtypes. Alpha level was set at 0.05, while an alpha level of 0.10 was used as cut-off for variable inclusion in multivariable models.

TABLE 1 | Demographics, clinical and dermoscopic variables according to the basal cell carcinoma histologic subtype with pairwise comparisons.

Variables		Histologic subtype			Total	p value superf vs. infiltrative	p value nodular vs. infiltrative	p value superf vs. nodular
		Infiltrative	Nodular	Superficial				
Age	Median (IQR)	71 (58–79)	67 (52–76)	61 (50–71)	65 (51–75)	<0.001	0.034	0.023
Diameter	Median (IQR)	7 (5–10)	6 (4–8)	6 (5–10)	6 (5–10)	0.267	<0.001	<0.001
Sex	M	33	128	80	241	0.714	0.427	0.587
		46.50%	51.80%	49.10%	50.1%			
	F	38	119	83	240			
		53.50%	48.20%	50.90%	49.9%			
Phototype	2	51	167	111	329	0.707	0.629	0.972
		71.80%	67.60%	68.10%	68.4%			
	3	20	78	51	149			
		28.20%	31.60%	31.30%	31.0%			
	4	0	2	1	3			
		0.00%	0.80%	0.60%	0.6%			
Location	HN	56	138	31	225	<0.001	<0.001	<0.001
		78.90%	55.90%	19.00%	46.8%			
	Trunk	4	79	92	175			
		5.60%	32.00%	56.40%	36.4%			
	Upper limbs	2	23	16	41			
		2.80%	9.30%	9.80%	8.5%			
	Lower limbs	9	7	24	40			
		12.70%	2.80%	14.70%	8.3%			
Palpability	Macule	5	7	52	64	<0.001	<0.001	
		7.00%	2.80%	31.90%	13.31%			
	Plaque	55	136	108	299			
		77.50%	55.10%	66.30%	62.16%			
	Papule	11	104	3	118			
		15.50%	42.10%	1.80%	24.53%			
Colors clinical	White	36	75	46	157	0.001	0.002	0.641
		50.70%	30.40%	28.20%	32.6%			
	Pink	66	200	146	412	0.414	0.016	0.019
		93.00%	81.00%	89.60%	85.7%			
	Red	37	98	28	163	<0.001	0.062	<0.001
		52.10%	39.70%	17.20%	33.9%			
	Brown	15	44	47	106	0.219	0.527	0.009
		21.10%	17.80%	28.80%	22.0%			
	Blue	12	62	34	108	0.484	0.15	0.321
		16.90%	25.10%	20.90%	22.5%			
	Black-gray	18	81	23	122	0.038	0.446	<0.001
		25.40%	32.80%	14.10%	25.4%			
Degree of clinical pigmentation	Non-pigmented	36	93	69	198	0.134	0.056	0.016
		50.70%	37.70%	42.30%	41.2%			
	Light pigmented	17	64	58	139			
		23.90%	25.90%	35.60%	28.9%			
	Pigmented	12	37	16	65			
		16.90%	15.00%	9.80%	13.5%			
	Heavy pigmented	6	53	20	79			
		8.50%	21.50%	12.30%	16.4%			
Degree of dermatoscopic pigmentation	Non-pigmented	31	55	44	130	0.084	0.002	0.069
		43.70%	22.30%	27.00%	27.0%			
	Light pigmented	20	80	53	153			
		28.20%	32.40%	32.50%	31.8%			
	Pigmented	11	42	37	90			
		15.50%	17.00%	22.70%	18.7%			
	Heavy pigmented	9	70	29	108			
		12.70%	28.30%	17.80%	22.5%			
Dermocopy	Arborizing (treelike)	51	202	11	264	<0.001	0.067	<0.001
		71.80%	81.80%	6.70%	54.9%			
	Short fine superficial telangiectasias	14	8	122	144	<0.001	<0.001	<0.001
		19.70%	3.20%	74.80%	29.9%			

(Continued)

TABLE 1 | Continued

Variables		Histologic subtype			Total	p value superf vs. infiltrative	p value nodular vs. infiltrative	p value superf vs. nodular
		Infiltrative	Nodular	Superficial				
	Blue-gray ovoid nests	16	95	10	**121**	<0.001	0.013	<0.001
		22.50%	38.50%	6.10%	**25.2%**			
	Multiple blue-gray globules	28	141	104	**273**	0.001	0.009	0.175
		39.40%	57.10%	63.80%	**56.8%**			
	Ulceration	35	60	9	**104**	<0.001	<0.001	<0.001
		49.30%	24.30%	5.50%	**21.6%**			
	Maple leaf-like	6	46	60	**112**	<0.001	0.041	<0.001
		8.50%	18.60%	36.80%	**23.3%**			
	Spoke-wheel areas	1	2	18	**21**	0.013	.533*	<0.001
		1.40%	0.80%	11.00%	**4.4%**			
	Concentric structures	0	5	16	**21**	.004*	.591*	<0.001
		0.00%	2.00%	9.80%	**4.4%**			
	Multiple small erosion	1	2	30	**33**	<0.001	.533*	<0.001
		1.40%	0.80%	18.40%	**6.9%**			
	In-focus dots	4	14	13	**31**	0.526	>0.99*	0.357
		5.60%	5.70%	8.00%	**6.4%**			
	Shiny red-white, structureless areas	49	149	141	**339**	0.002	0.183	<0.001
		69.00%	60.30%	86.50%	**70.5%**			
	Short white streaks (chrysalis)	55	153	65	**273**	<0.001	0.015	<0.001
		77.50%	61.90%	39.90%	**56.8%**			
Total		**71**	**247**	**163**	**481**			

IQR, interquartile range.

Sensitivity, specificity, positive and negative predictive values (PPV and NPV) were calculated to define the diagnostic accuracy of the two evaluators asked to guess the proper BCC histologic subtype before and after being provided with the study results. Statistical analyses were performed using the IBM SPSS 26.0 package (Statistical Package for Social Sciences, IBM SPSS Inc., Chicago, Ill.).

RESULTS

A total of 526 BCCs were initially retrieved. After exclusion of 45 (8.6%) cases with mixed histotypes, 481 BCCs were enrolled belonging to 443 patients [mean age 65 years, interquartile range (IQR): 51–75 years; 218, 49.2% males and 225, 50.8% females]. Three hundred twenty-nine lesions (68.4%) belonged to patients with phototype II, 149 (31.30%) to phototype III, and 3 (0.6%) to phototype IV. Concerning histologic subtype, the majority of the enrolled BCCs were nodular (247/481; 51.4%), followed by superficial (163/481; 33.9%) and infiltrative (71/481; 14.8%) forms. Individual lesions were mainly located on the head/neck (225/481; 46.8%) and trunk (175/481; 36.4%), while only a minority arose on the limbs (upper = 41/481; 8.5%, lower = 40/481; 8.3%). Specific head and neck locations were specified in **Supplementary Table 1**. The iBCC was more frequently located on the temple and the cheek as compared to the other two histotypes. Both iBCC and the nBCC were more frequently seen on the nose than sBCC, with iBCC mainly appearing on the tip and nBCC on the nose wings. The median diameter of the enrolled lesions was 6 mm (IQR: 5–10 mm). Concerning the

degree of clinical pigmentation, we found a predominance of amelanotic (198/481) and light pigmented lesions (139/481), with pink as the most widely observed color (412/481; 85.7%), followed by red (163/481; 33.9%), white (157/481; 32.6%), black-gray (122/481; 25.4%), blue (108/481; 22.5%), and brown (106/481; 22%). Dermoscopically, we found a lower number of completely amelanotic lesions (130/481; 27%), while the number of pigmented lesions proportionally increased, as compared to clinical evaluation, with a predominance of light pigmented BCCs (139/481; 28.9%). On dermoscopic examination, the most frequently observed criterion in all cases was shiny red-white structureless areas, in 339/481 (70.5%) BCCs. Multiple blue-gray globules and short white streaks were both detected in 273/481 (56.8%) lesions, arborizing telangiectasia in 264/481 (54.9%) and superficial fine telangiectasias in 144/481 (29.9%) lesions. In all, 121 (25.2%) and 112 (23.3%) out of the 481 BCCs showed blue-gray ovoid nests and maple leaf-like areas, respectively; 104/481 (21.6%) showed ulceration and 33/481 (6.9%) multiple small erosion. Other pigmented criteria, such as in focus dots, spoke-wheel areas, and concentric structures were observed only in a minority of cases. Pairwise comparisons among the three histologic subtypes are reported in **Table 1** according to demographics, clinical, and dermoscopic variables. To evaluate predictors of each BCC histologic subtype, three multivariable logistic regression models were constructed, one for each pairwise comparison. In the models of **Table 2A** demographics and clinical variables were included, together with the degree of dermoscopic pigmentation. In the models of **Table 2B** single dermoscopic criteria were instead included. We found that, as

TABLE 2 | Multivariate logistic regression analysis. Factors associated with each basal cell carcinoma histologic subtypes (infiltrative, nodular, and superficial): pairwise comparisons. Model a) demographic, clinical, and degree of pigmentation; model b) dermoscopic criteria.

A	Histotype comparison	Variables		OR	95% C.I. for OR		p value
					Lower	Upper	
Superficial *vs.* Infiltrative*	Age		1.04	1.01	1.07	0.019
	Location	HN	ref.			<0.001
		Trunk	0.01	0.00	0.05	<0.001
		Upper limbs	0.03	0.00	0.20	<0.001
		Lower limbs	0.16	0.05	0.49	0.001
	Clinical color	White color	3.37	1.34	8.46	0.01
		Red color	7.61	2.66	21.80	<0.001
	Surface	Flat	ref.			0.007
		Elevated	3.77	1.12	12.77	0.033
		Nodular	30.05	3.48	259.36	0.002
Nodular *vs.* infiltrative**	Location	HN	ref.			<0.001
		Trunk	0.137	0.047	0.405	<0.001
		Upper limbs	0.187	0.041	0.853	0.03
		Lower limbs	2.197	0.715	6.748	0.169
	Surface	Flat	ref.			0.001
		Elevated	0.605	0.16	2.286	0.459
		Nodular	0.143	0.033	0.618	0.009
Superficial *vs.* nodular***	Age		1.021	1.002	1.041	0.029
	Diameter (mm)		0.935	0.889	0.983	0.009
	Location	HN	ref.			<0.001
		Trunk	0.193	0.103	0.361	<0.001
		Upper limbs	0.493	0.201	1.208	0.122
		Lower limbs	0.078	0.024	0.254	<0.001
	Clinical color	Red color	2.587	1.318	5.077	0.006
		Black-gray color	3.138	1.591	6.189	0.001
	Surface	Flat	ref.			<0.001
		Elevated	7.107	2.827	17.866	<0.001
		Nodular	165.1	37.67	723.86	<0.001

B	Histotype comparison	Dermatoscopic variables	OR	95% C.I. for OR		p value
				Lower	Upper	
Superficial *vs.* infiltrative*	Arborizing (treelike)	17.60	5.01	61.89	<0.001
	Superficial fine telangiectasias	0.22	0.06	0.78	0.019
	Multiple blue-gray globules	0.25	0.08	0.77	0.015
	Ulceration	10.83	3.33	35.25	<0.001
	Short white streaks (chrysalis)	2.49	0.92	6.78	0.074
	Concentric structures	0.00	0.00	nc	0.998
	Multiple small erosion	0.08	0.01	0.99	0.049
Nodular *vs.* infiltrative**	Superficial fine telangiectasias	5.96	2.22	15.97	<0.001
	Multiple blue-gray globules	0.53	0.30	0.96	0.035
	Ulceration	3.36	1.87	6.04	<0.001
	Blue-gray ovoid nests	0.49	0.25	0.95	0.036
Superficial *vs.* nodular***	Arborizing (treelike)	15.13	6.01	38.14	<0.001
	Superficial fine telangiectasias	0.07	0.03	0.18	<0.001
	Blue-gray ovoid nests	6.61	2.33	18.74	<0.001
	Ulceration	3.13	0.92	10.73	0.069
	Maple leaf-like	0.32	0.12	0.80	0.015
	Concentric structures	0.20	0.04	1.05	0.057
	Multiple small erosion	0.04	0.00	0.62	0.021

a) *Variables entered on step 1: age. Location, white color, red color, black-gray color. Degree of dermatoscopic pigmentation. Palpability. **Variables entered on step 1: age. Location, white color, red color, pink color. Degree of dermatoscopic pigmentation. Palpability. ***Variables entered on step 1: age. Diameter (mm). Location, pink color, red color, brown color, black-gray color. Degree of clinical pigmentation. Degree of dermatoscopic pigmentation. Palpability.
b) *Variable(s) entered on step 1: arborizing (treelike) telangiectasia. Superficial fine telangiectasias. Ulceration. Maple leaf-like. Short white streaks (chrysalis). Blue-gray ovoid nests. Spoke-wheel areas. Concentric structures. Multiple small erosion. Shiny red-white structureless areas. Multiple blue-gray globules. **Variable(s) entered on step 1: arborizing (treelike) telangiectasia. Superficial fine telangiectasias. Ulceration. Maple leaf-like. Short white streaks (chrysalis). Blue-gray ovoid nests. Multiple blue-gray globules. ***Variable(s) entered on step 1: arborizing (treelike) telangiectasia. Superficial fine telangiectasias. Ulceration. Maple leaf-like. Short white streaks (chrysalis). Blue-gray ovoid nests. Spoke-wheel areas. Concentric structures. Multiple small erosion. Shiny red-white structureless areas.

compared with sBCC, iBCC had increased odds to be elevated or nodular than flat. Clinically, iBCC also more probably occurred in older individuals, more on the head and neck region than in other body sites and more frequently displayed white and red color. Concerning dermoscopic criteria, iBCC more frequently displayed arborizing telangiectasia and ulceration than sBCCs, which was instead more characterized by superficial fine telangiectasia and multiple blue-gray globules. Comparing iBCC with nBCC, we found higher odds for nBCC to be located on the trunk and upper limbs, while iBCC more frequently appeared on the head and neck. Furthermore, nBCC more frequently appeared as a papule than iBCC. Regarding dermoscopy, superficial fine telangiectasia and ulceration were more associated with iBCC, while multiple blue-gray globules and blue-gray ovoid nests with the nBCC. Finally, we also compared superficial and nodular BCCs, showing higher odds for sBCC to be a macule and to have a larger diameter. The sBCC was also more frequently seen on the trunk and lower limbs and more frequently displayed superficial fine telangiectasia, maple-leaf areas, and multiple small erosion upon dermoscopy. The nBCC, instead, was more frequently characterized by red and black-gray color at clinical examination and by arborizing telangiectasia and blue-gray ovoid nets. The main clinical and dermoscopic differences highlighted among BCC histologic subtypes are illustrated in **Table 3 (Figure 1).** The diagnostic accuracy of the two external readers before and after being instructed for study results is reported in **Table 4**. We registered increased levels of sensitivity and specificity and increased PPV and NPV for each of the three BCC subtypes. Baseline sensitivity for iBCC diagnosis was low for both the evaluators, with only 33.3% of cases correctly identified. After being provided with the study results almost a half of iBCC were instead correctly diagnosed.

DISCUSSION

In this monocentric retrospective observational study, we describe the main clinical and dermoscopic features of the iBCC subtype, as compared to sBCCs and nBCCs. Clinically, we found that iBCC generally appeared as an amelanotic or hypopigmented plaque or papule, located on the head and neck, in particular on the temple, cheek, and tip of the nose. Dermoscopically, iBCC frequently displayed ulceration and a mix of arborizing and superficial fine telangiectasia. Shiny white structures were also frequently observed, such as short white streaks and red-white structureless areas. When compared with

TABLE 3 | Infiltrative. nodular and superficial basal cell carcinoma clinical and dermoscopic profiles. Symbols (+, −, and ≈) were attributed according to the multivariate analysis results.

Variables		Infiltrative BCC vs.		Nodular BCC vs.
		Superficial	Nodular	Superficial
Age		+	≈	+
Diameter		≈	≈	−
Location	HN	++++	++*	+++
	Trunk	----	--	--
	Upper limbs	----	−	≈
	Lower limbs	--	≈	----
Color (clinical)	White	+	≈	≈
	Pink	≈	≈	≈
	Red	++	≈	+
	Brown	≈	≈	≈
	Black-gray	≈	≈	+
Surface	Macule	----	++	----
	Plaque	+	≈	++
	Papule	++++	--	+++++
Dermoscopic criteria	Arborizing vessels	+++	≈	+++
	Superficial fine telangiectasia	-	++	----
	Ulceration	++	+	+
	Multiple blue-gray globules	−	−	≈
	Blue-gray ovoid nests	≈	−	++
	Maple leaf-like	≈	≈	−
	Short white streaks	≈	≈	≈
	Spoke-wheel areas	≈	≈	≈
	Concentric structures	≈	≈	≈
	Multiple small erosion	≈	≈	----
	Shiny red-white structureless areas	≈	≈	≈
	Multiple blue-gray globules	≈	≈	≈
Degree of pigmentation	Clinical	≈	≈	≈
	Dermoscopic	≈	≈	≈

*Infiltrative more on the temple. Cheek and tip of the nose; nodular more on the nose wings. Green color highlights the strongest associations, yellow is for intermediate and orange for the weakest.

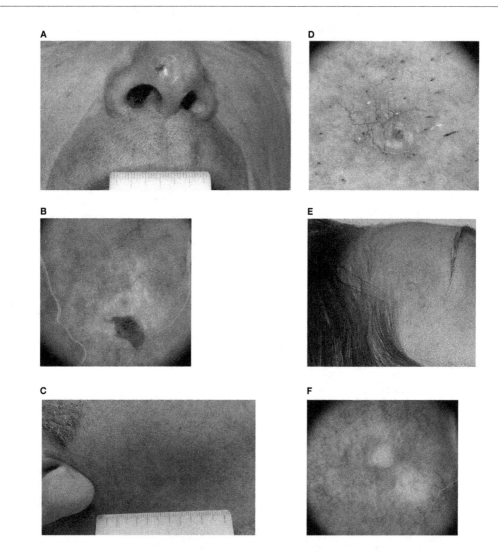

FIGURE 1 | Clinical and dermoscopic images of three cases of infiltrative basal cell carcinoma. **(A)** A man in his 60s with a 7 mm amelanotic plaque located on the tip of his nose. **(B)** Dermoscopically the lesion was ulcerated, with a pinkish-whitish background. Both short white streaks and red-white structureless areas could be seen, together with superficial fine telangiectasia. **(C)** A man in his 50s with a 5 mm pinkish papule located in his right cheek. **(D)** On dermoscopic examination both classic arborizing and more superficial fine telangiectasia are seen on a pinkish background, together with a small ulceration. **(E)** A woman in her 40s with a whitish 8 mm papule located on her right temple. **(F)** Dermoscopy highlights the presence of mixed red and white structureless areas with peripheral white streaks and superficial fine telangiectasia.

the other two histotypes, we found that patients with iBCC were slightly older than those with sBCC, but no age differences were observed with nBCC. Also, the iBCC was more often located on the head and neck and significantly less on the trunk and upper limbs, compared to the other non-aggressive histotypes. Concerning the degree of pigmentation seen on dermoscopy, iBCC was significantly more amelanotic and less heavy pigmented than nBCC in univariate analysis. However, when controlling for age, location, palpability, and clinical color in multivariate analysis no significant differences were observed. As expected, iBCC was more frequently palpable (plaque or papule) than the sBCC and less than nBCC.

Regarding dermoscopic examination, we found a prevalence of arborizing telangiectasia in iBCC, as compared to sBCC, in which superficial fine telangiectasia were instead more frequently seen. No significant differences in arborizing telangiectasia were instead observed between iBCC and nBCC, while in the former superficial fine telangiectasia were more frequently observed. Ulceration was more often reported in iBCC than both sBCC and nBCC, while multiple blue-gray globules and blue-gray ovoid nests were rarely seen among iBCCs. The definition of a specific Clinicians are dermoscopic profile for iBCC, sBCC, and nBCC, allowed external readers to increase their diagnostic accuracy in differentiating these histotypes after being provided with our study results. In particular, they were able to correctly identify a higher number of iBCCs (increased sensitivity). with a reduction of iBCCs misdiagnosed as sBCCs or nBCCs (false negative cases).

TABLE 4 | Diagnostic accuracy of two expert reviewers in diagnosing infiltrative, superficial and nodular basal cell carcinoma (BCC).

BCC histotype		I evaluator		II evaluator		Total	
		Before	After	Before	After	Before	After
Infiltrative	Sens	36.7%	50.0%	30.0%	46.7%	33.3%	48.3%
	Spec	80.0%	81.7%	76.7%	81.7%	78.3%	81.7%
	PPV	47.8%	57.7%	39.1%	56.0%	43.5%	56.8%
	NPV	71.6%	76.6%	68.7%	75.4%	70.1%	76.0%
Superficial	Sens	66.7%	70.0%	60.0%	63.3%	63.3%	66.7%
	Spec	80.0%	88.3%	80.0%	78.3%	80.0%	83.3%
	PPV	62.5%	75.0%	60.0%	59.4%	61.3%	67.2%
	NPV	82.8%	85.5%	80.0%	81.0%	81.4%	83.3%
Nodular	Sens	70.0%	76.7%	66.7%	73.3%	68.3%	75.0%
	Spec	76.7%	78.3%	71.7%	81.7%	74.2%	80.0%
	PPV	60.0%	63.9%	54.1%	66.7%	57.0%	65.3%
	NPV	83.6%	87.0%	81.1%	86.0%	82.4%	86.5%

Before and after being provided with the study results. Evaluation were performed on an external dataset of 90 BCCs (30 infiltrative, 30 nodular, and 30 superficial).
Sens, sensitivity; spec, specificity; PPV, positive predictive value; NPV, negative predictive value.

In clinical practice, this would improve pre-surgical recognition of iBCC, allowing the surgeon to keep wider margins and reducing the risk of recurrence. Previous studies mainly defined clinical, demographic and dermoscopic features associated with sBCC (11–13). However, little is known about factors allowing to differentiate sBCC from iBCC. The sBCC has been shown to occur in younger patients than the other BCC histotypes and to be mainly located in non-chronically sun-exposed areas, such as the trunk (16). Concerning dermoscopy, multiple small erosions, superficial fine telangiectasia and structures corresponding to dermo-epidermal pigmentation were shown to predict sBCC subtype. However, the presence of blue-gray ovoid nests seems to exclude the diagnosis of sBCC (12). Dermoscopic criteria more associated with iBCC have been previously reported. However, these findings are mainly based on descriptive analysis and expert opinions, while independent clinical and dermoscopic predictors have not been defined by multivariable analysis so far (4, 6, 11–13, 17). In 2014, Longo and colleagues reported on a study population of 22 iBCCs, 22 nBCC and 44 sBCC, that infiltrative forms were featured by arborizing telangiectasia, superficial fine telangiectasia and shiny white-red structureless areas (11). However, none of these criteria was significantly more observed in iBCC as compared to the other histotypes because of the small number of cases analyzed. Furthermore, multivariable logistic regression analysis was only performed to define confocal criteria predictive of each histotype.

Our study fills this gap by focusing on clinical and dermoscopic criteria independently associated with sBCC, nBCC and iBCC subtypes. In 2020, Conforti and colleagues defined the dermoscopic criteria independently associated with the sclerodermiform BCC subtype as compared to the other subtypes (sBCC + nBCC). They found in multivariate analysis, that ulceration was significantly more frequently seen in sclerodermiform BCC, followed by fine arborizing telangiectasia, pink-white areas and multiple blue-gray dots and globules (14). Recently, a systematic review pointed out that no very specific dermoscopic criteria allow to differentiate different BCC histotypes (7). The authors reported that nBCC was more

characterized by arborizing telangiectasia (75%), shiny white structures (43%), and ulceration (31%), while iBCC mainly presented arborizing telangiectasia (76%), ulceration (44%), and short-fine telangiectasia (40%). Only two dermoscopic structures appeared to be relatively unique for one subtype: leaf-like areas and shiny white-red structureless background in sBCC. In our study we failed to find these two criteria as more associated with sBCC, however, we confirmed that sBCC is easier to differentiate from both nBCC and iBCC. Wider differences were indeed observed in multivariable analysis in term of anatomic location, palpability and dermoscopic criteria, when comparing sBCC with nBCC and iBCC. Furthermore, we also reported significant differences between nBCC and iBCC. In particular iBCC was more frequently located on the head and neck as a macule, while nBCC was more frequently seen on the trunk as a papule. Upon dermoscopy, the most important difference regarded the highest occurrence of superficial fine telangiectasia in iBCC. This confirms previous observations, describing the telangiectasia of iBCC as having smaller caliber and less tendency to branch than those of nBCC (6). However, we didn't find significant differences in classic arborizing telangiectasia between iBCC and nBCC. Thus, we can conclude that in iBCC superficial fine and arborizing telangiectasia often coexist in the same lesion.

Some limitations of the current study include the retrospective design, the exclusion of minor BCC histotypes and lack of histopathological specimens' re-assessment. The latter limitation could have influenced the histotype recognition as well as the proportion of lesions showing more than one histotype. We partially controlled for this limitation by asking the pathologist (AMC) for re-assessment in case of doubtful lesions. Another limitation of the current study is the over-representation of patients with photo-type II or III, which is due to the phenotypic characteristics of the Italian population.

To conclude, we defined a clinical-dermoscopic profile of iBCC, allowing to differentiate this variant from sBCC and nBCC when Clinicians are trained on the results of the dermoscopic findings of our study.

AUTHOR CONTRIBUTIONS

CL, RP, GaPa equally contributed to the study concept and design, data analysis and interpretation, and writing of the report. RP did the statistical analysis. AC did the histopathological reassessment of doubtful cases. SBo, ML, GiPa, AC, SC, FF, SBa, GA, GiPe contributed to the data interpretation and provided expert insight into the writing of the report. All authors contributed to the article and approved the submitted version.

REFERENCES

1. Longo C, Borsari S, Pampena R, Benati E, Bombonato C, Raucci M, et al. Basal cell carcinoma: the utility of in vivo and ex vivo confocal microscopy. *J Eur Acad Dermatol Venereol* (2018) 32(12):2090–6. doi: 10.1111/jdv.14984

2. Lombardi M, Pampena R, Borsari S, Bombonato C, Benati E, Pellacani G, et al. Dermoscopic Features of Basal Cell Carcinoma on the Lower Limbs: A Chameleon! *Dermatology* (2017) 233(6):482–8. doi: 10.1159/000487300

3. Pampena R, Lai M, Piana S, Pellacani G, Longo C. Basal cell carcinoma or melanoma, that is the question! *J Eur Acad Dermatol Venereol* (2020) 34(8): e425–7. doi: 10.1111/jdv.16373

4. Lallas A, Apalla Z, Argenziano G, Longo C, Moscarella E, Specchio F, et al. The dermatoscopic universe of basal cell carcinoma. *Dermatol Pract Concept* (2014) 4(3):11–24. doi: 10.5826/dpc.0403a02

5. Peccerillo F, Mandel VD, Di Tullio F, Ciardo S, Chester J, Kaleci S, et al. Lesions Mimicking Melanoma at Dermoscopy Confirmed Basal Cell Carcinoma: Evaluation with Reflectance Confocal Microscopy. *Dermatology* (2019) 235(1):35–44. doi: 10.1159/000493727

6. Pampena R, Peccerillo F, Marghoob NG, Piana S, Longo C. Peritumoural clefting as a key feature in differentiating basal cell carcinoma from trichoblastoma through in vivo reflectance confocal microscopy. *J Eur Acad Dermatol Venereol* (2019) 33(5):e201–3. doi: 10.1111/jdv.15467

7. Reiter O, Mimouni I, Dusza S, Halpern AC, Leshem YA, Marghoob AA. Dermoscopic features of basal cell carcinoma and its subtypes: A systematic review. *J Am Acad Dermatol* (2019) S0190-9622(19)33008-7. doi: 10.1016/j.jaad.2019.11.008

8. Sexton M, Jones DB, Maloney ME. Histologic pattern analysis of basal cell carcinoma: study of a series of 1039 consecutive neoplasms. *J Am Acad Dermatol* (1990) 23(6):1118e26. doi: 10.1016/0190-9622(90)70344-H

9. Moon HR, Park TJ, Ro KW, Ryu HJ, Seo SH, Son SW, et al. Pigmentation of basal cell carcinoma is inversely associated with tumor aggressiveness in Asian patients. *J Am Acad Dermatol* (2019) 80(6):1755–7. doi: 10.1016/j.jaad.2018.06.059

10. Armstrong LTD, Magnusson MR, Guppy MPB. Risk factors for recurrence of facial basal cell carcinoma after surgical excision: A follow-up analysis. *J Plast Reconstr Aesthet Surg* (2017) 70(12):1738–45. doi: 10.1016/j.bjps.2017.04.006

11. Longo C, Lallas A, Kyrgidis A, Rabinovitz H, Moscarella E, Ciardo S, et al. Classifying distinct basal cell carcinoma subtype by means of dermatoscopy and reflectance confocal microscopy. *J Am Acad Dermatol* (2014) 71(4):716–24.e1. doi: 10.1016/j.jaad.2014.04.067

12. Lallas A, Tzellos T, Kyrgidis A, Apalla Z, Zalaudek I, Karatolias A, et al. Accuracy of dermoscopic criteria for discriminating superficial from other subtypes of basal cell carcinoma. *J Am Acad Dermatol* (2014) 70(2):303–11. doi: 10.1016/j.jaad.2013.10.003

13. Ahnlide I, Zalaudek I, Nilsson F, Bjellerup M, Nielsen K. Preoperative prediction of histopathological outcome in basal cell carcinoma: flat surface and multiple small erosions predict superficial basal cell carcinoma in lighter skin types. *Br J Dermatol* (2016) 175(4):751–61. doi: 10.1111/bjd.14499

14. Conforti C, Pizzichetta MA, Vichi S, Toffolutti F, Serraino D, Di Meo N., et al. Sclerodermiform basal cell carcinomas vs. other histotypes: analysis of specific demographic, clinical and dermatoscopic features. *J Eur Acad Dermatol Venereol* (2020). doi: 10.1111/jdv.16597

15. Zalaudek I, Kreusch J, Giacomel J, Ferrara G, Catricalà C, Argenziano G. How to diagnose nonpigmented skin tumors: a review of vascular structures seen with dermoscopy: part II. Nonmelanocytic skin tumors. *J Am Acad Dermatol* (2010) 63(3):377–86; quiz 387-8. doi: 10.1016/j.jaad.2009.11.697

16. Suppa M, Micantonio T, Di Stefani A, Soyer HP, Chimenti S, Fargnoli MC, et al. Dermoscopic variability of basal cell carcinoma according to clinical type and anatomic location. *J Eur Acad Dermatol Venereol* (2015) 29(9):1732–41. doi: 10.1111/jdv.12980

17. Altamura D, Menzies SW, Argenziano G, Zalaudek I, Soyer HP, Sera F, et al. Dermatoscopy of basal cell carcinoma: morphologic variability of global and local features and accuracy of diagnosis. *J Am Acad Dermatol* (2010) 62(1):67–75. doi: 10.1016/j.jaad.2009.05.035

17

Are Molecular Alterations Linked to Genetic Instability Worth to Be Included as Biomarkers for Directing or Excluding Melanoma Patients to Immunotherapy?

Giuseppe Palmieri[1†], Carla Maria Rozzo[1†], Maria Colombino[2], Milena Casula[2],
Maria Cristina Sini[2], Antonella Manca[1], Marina Pisano[1], Valentina Doneddu[3],
Panagiotis Paliogiannis[3] and Antonio Cossu[3*]

[1] Institute of Genetic and Biomedical Research (IRGB), National Research Council (CNR), Sassari, Italy, [2] Institute of
Biomolecular Chemistry (ICB), National Research Council (CNR), Sassari, Italy, [3] Department of Medical, Surgical, and
Experimental Sciences, University of Sassari, Sassari, Italy

*Correspondence:
Antonio Cossu
cossu@uniss.it

[†]These authors have contributed
equally to this work

The improvement of the immunotherapeutic potential in most human cancers, including melanoma, requires the identification of increasingly detailed molecular features underlying the tumor immune responsiveness and acting as disease-associated biomarkers. In recent past years, the complexity of the immune landscape in cancer tissues is being steadily unveiled with a progressive better understanding of the plethora of actors playing in such a scenario, resulting in histopathology diversification, distinct molecular subtypes, and biological heterogeneity. Actually, it is widely recognized that the intracellular patterns of alterations in driver genes and loci may also concur to interfere with the homeostasis of the tumor microenvironment components, deeply affecting the immune response against the tumor. Among others, the different events linked to genetic instability—aneuploidy/somatic copy number alteration (SCNA) or microsatellite instability (MSI)—may exhibit opposite behaviors in terms of immune exclusion or responsiveness. In this review, we focused on both prevalence and impact of such different types of genetic instability in melanoma in order to evaluate whether their use as biomarkers in an integrated analysis of the molecular profile of such a malignancy may allow defining any potential predictive value for response/resistance to immunotherapy.

Keywords: melanoma, microsatellite instability, aneuploidy, tumor mutation burden, immunotherapy response

INTRODUCTION

The increasing efficacy of immunotherapy with immune checkpoint inhibitors (ICIs) has deeply changed life expectancy for different types of fatal cancer: melanoma, lung cancer, renal carcinoma, advanced squamous cell carcinoma of the head and neck or skin districts, some colorectal cancers, and refractory lymphomas (1–5). At the same time, it is widely recognized that the therapeutic indication of ICI cannot be extended to all subtypes of tumor histology since it has been observed that majority of patients are not responsive (6). Therefore, the identification of biomarkers able to accurately predict either response or resistance to the treatment represents a crucial need in cancer immunotherapy.

Although the introduction into clinical practice of validated immuno-oncological biomarkers is currently limited by the heterogeneity of the types of specimens analyzed, because of the diversity of the used methodologies and the absence of a real sharing of the produced data, it is necessary to continue to support the efforts in conducting biomarker-driven trials (7). In recent years, multidisciplinary approaches have significantly increased the quest for an even more accurate molecular classification through the assessment of the mutational status in multiple oncogenes and tumor suppressor genes; in the immuno-oncological field, such efforts have already produced some approved tests (PD-L1 expression and microsatellite instability rates) and other advanced tests yet to be fully proven for efficacy (tumor mutation load, neoantigen pattern, intratumor T-cell infiltration rate) (5, 8–10).

Toward a holistic approach aimed at implementing precision oncology for treatment of "difficult" human cancers, should evaluation of genetic instability be included into the patients' molecular classification, probably even for the cancer types—like cutaneous melanoma—with a recognized low prevalence of such an alteration? In supporting a positive answer to this question, it has been recently demonstrated that a detailed tumor molecular profiling with identification of all low-frequency actionable alterations in pancreatic cancer—a definitely difficult-to-treat tumor—may produce a significant benefit from receiving a matched therapy (11). Before moving in this sense, we retain

to firstly go through the features bringing to the classification of an unstable genome.

GENETIC INSTABILITY

The accumulation and fixation of mutations into the genome, both in the transcribed or regulatory sequences and in those apparently inactive, is one of the most important ways through which evolution is carried out (12). Excluding mutations having deleterious effects with functional consequences, the great majority of sequence variants often display an undefined role (neither harmful nor beneficial) in disease pathogenesis (13). These apparently neutral genetic variants can spread and become fixed in a population, making a large contribution to the evolutionary change in genomes. Focusing on single individuals, the establishment of germinal mutations or the accumulation of somatic mutations can lead to serious cell dysfunctions. **Figure 1** represents the main mechanisms inducing the increase of the mutations' content in cancer cells.

An accurate and articulated system of control and repair of genomic DNA integrity has evolved into the cells (14, 15). The DNA damage can be caused by genetic instability that may exist at two distinct mechanistic levels. In most cases, genomic instability is observed at the chromosomal level as whole chromosome or segmental/focal aneuploidy; in a more limited fraction of tumors, instability is observed at the nucleotide level and is revealed by the presence of alterations in particular highly repeated DNA sequences with a uniform nucleotide composition, the satellite DNA loci (16, 17). Such satellite

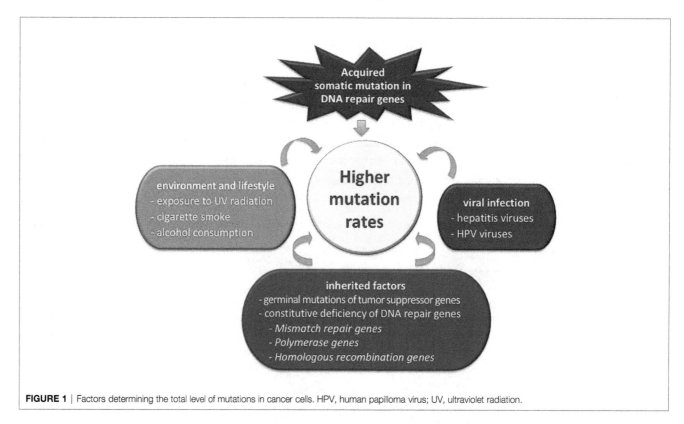

FIGURE 1 | Factors determining the total level of mutations in cancer cells. HPV, human papilloma virus; UV, ultraviolet radiation.

DNA regions are classified as minisatellite or microsatellite DNA, depending on the length of the repeated sequences (18–21). Minisatellites consist of repetitive motifs that range in length from 10 to over 100 base pairs. They are located mainly at the centromeres and at the sub-telomeric and telomeric chromosome regions (telomeres itself are constituted by tandem repeats). Minisatellites may play a role in modifying levels of transcription, alternative splicing, or imprinting changes; therefore, they can participate in cell functioning as regulators of gene expression (18, 19, 22). Microsatellites consist of tandem repeats of 1 to 6 base pairs, often organized in long strings, which are subject to mutational events such as insertions and deletions (18, 19, 21).

Aneuploidy—which is due to a genomic imbalance in terms of gain or loss of chromatid or chromosome regions—can be actually classified as a somatic copy number alteration (SCNA), being demonstrated to play a critical role during the process of tumorigenesis and prognosis (23). Occurrence of aneuploidy/ SCNA seems to contribute to immune evasion through the reduction of a cytotoxic immune infiltrate into the tumor microenvironment (TME); on this regard, TME can be immunosuppressive *per se*, facilitating tumor progression through mobilization of cytokines, chemokines, and inhibitory factors (24). Moreover, the TME can also recruit immunosuppressive immune cells including regulatory T cells (TREGs), myeloid-derived suppressor cells (MDSCs), and tumor-associated macrophages (TAMs) to evade immune clearance (25). The aneuploid status may potentiate the immunosuppressive TME activity by also negatively interfering with the presentation of the antigens of the major histocompatibility complex (MHC), which represents a fundamental moment into the recognition of the tumor by the immune system (26). The content of peptide neoantigens seems to vary based on the levels of tumor SCNAs, with a relative concentration that is significantly lower in aneuploid tumors than diploid ones acting in an opposite way from the increased overall mutation load and correspondent tumor neoantigen expression levels, which are both positively correlated with the induction of cytotoxic immune infiltrates (27).

Microsatellite instability (MSI) seems to be usually due to deficient DNA damage repair; it has been associated with promotion of a higher load of tumor mutations (28, 29). The MSI occurrence (MSI+) is subsequent to impairment of at least one main gene regulating the different DNA repair mechanisms: homologous recombination (involving *BLM, BRCA1/2, BRIP1, PALB2, RAD50/51,* Fanconi Anemia genes), mismatch repair (*MLH1, MSH2, MSH6, PMS2*), cell cycle checkpoints (*ATM, CHEK1/2*), base excision repair (*POLE*) (30, 31). A high tumor mutation burden (TMB-high) is generally defined as the >10–20 mutations per megabase of genomic area (threshold is deeply varying according to the cancer type) and can somehow act as a surrogate marker of the neoantigen load (32–34). Tumor specific peptide epitopes, which are usually absent in the normal human genome, can be recognized and targeted by the immune system (33–35). Both MSI+ and TMB-high have been both associated with favorable outcome to ICI therapy in some cancer types (33, 34, 36), but their role in predicting overall survival is still

controversial. Vast majority of MSI+ samples present with TMB-high (83%), but the converse is not true, since only 16% of samples with TMB-high are classified as MSI+ (37).

Overall, next-generation sequencing (NGS) analysis through a whole genome or exome screening is being used for detecting the high-level SCNAs, the MSI+ status, and the TMB-high in tumor tissues. The MSI+ and TMB-high conditions have been associated with the long-term response to ICI treatment in different human malignancies—including melanoma, lung and renal/bladder cancer, head and neck squamous cell carcinoma (38–45). Conversely, occurrence of aneuploidy/SCNA negatively correlates with the presence of a favorable immune signature, conferring resistance to ICI treatment (26). **Figure 2** summarizes the effects exerted by the different conditions on the activity of the immune system.

Although additional factors are involved in augmenting the adaptive immunity under ICI therapy—such as the histocompatibility leukocyte antigen (HLA) evolution pattern and tumor-infiltrating lymphocyte (TIL) reactivity (27), the simultaneous assessment of the SCNA burden and the rates of TMB and MSI in tumor tissue sections might be strongly useful for classifying patients who are more or less likely to respond to immunotherapies (46). Despite such recognized predictive values, the NGS-based test was not yet routinely included in

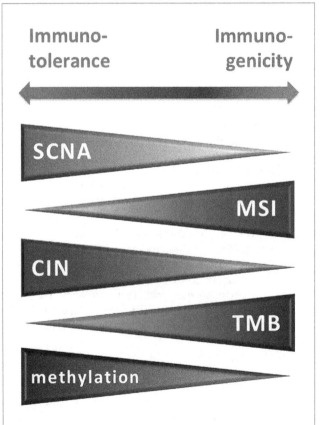

FIGURE 2 | Molecular alterations from genetic instability and immune reactivity. CIN, chromosomal instability; MSI, microsatellite instability; SCNA, somatic copy number alteration; TMB, tumor mutation burden.

clinics due to the required high level of technical expertise, the lack of standardization, the high cost, and the pretty-long time required to perform an extensive genomic screening (47, 48). Recently, the combination of reducing the costs of NGS technologies and developing large but manageable multi-gene panels has contributed to facilitate continuous implementations for the use of NGS-based assays in daily clinical practice (49). In other words, the aim of simplifying the sequencing of multiple genes per tumor sample, in order to detect targetable genomic alterations, is becoming a reality and NGS is presenting a really good analytical validity, with an increasingly favorable cost–benefit ratio. To achieve the most currently accurate molecular classification for guiding treatment decisions among cancer patients, recommendations on how multi-gene NGS assays should be used to profile human tumors for improving patients' management are being provided by scientific societies (50).

Aneuploidy: Mechanism and Effects

Aneuploidy can be mostly considered as the result of the impairment of the cell cycle checkpoints, which consist of mechanisms that verify DNA replication accuracy and control the cell cycle progression, detecting errors in DNA repair, DNA synthesis, and chromosome segregation (51). Occurrence of structural alterations significantly affecting the genome integrity constitutes a signal sent to the replication/segregation machinery in order to repair the damage (52).

Several cyclin-dependent kinases (CDKs) physiologically drive cell division and regulate the different phases of the cell cycle through phosphorylation of a complex network of substrates and activation of cascades of transduction signals (53). In case of genomic DNA damage, the cell cycle checkpoints arrest the G1/G2 and G2/M transitions by repressing the CDK activity. Hyperactive CDKs, caused by mutations in genes controlling the DNA damage response pathway, lead to the progression into the cell cycle and cell survival (52). On this regard, inactivating mutations in TP53 gene have a permissive role, strongly contributing to the propagation of genetic errors in descendant daughter cells (54). As consequence, deregulation of the TP53-driven pathway—also including impairment of the activity of its downstream effectors (i.e., RB1)—contributes to aneuploidy (55). A number of cancers with mutated TP53 are chromosomal stable and show MSI+, whereas TP53 loss-of-function is predominant in non-hypermutated tumors (54–56). Indeed, the TP53 inactivation is mostly dependent on whether or not mutations in this gene affect the function of p53 on repressing the activity of the Cyclin D1–CDK2 system controlling centrosome duplication and preventing aneuploidy (53).

Activating mutations in oncogenes (such as CCND1, EGFR, PIK3CA, KRAS, BRAF) and inactivating changes in tumor suppressor genes—like RB1, APC, and WNT signaling pathway components (CHK1 and CHK2-BRCA1)—can dramatically enhance cell proliferation and increase the replication stress levels, causing double-strand breaks in the DNA, with consequent genomic instability that affects tumor progression (57). This seems due to the fact that the unbalanced activity of the driver genes involved in promotion of cell proliferation and survival leads to a sort of oncogene-induced mitotic stress status (58). The enormous variation of segregation errors among different malignancies is indeed a strong indicator that mitotic events act as important players in aneuploidy occurrence (59). Deregulation of the centrosome duplication may indeed promote the formation of multiple centrosomes, which in turn leads to multipolar spindles and aneuploidy (58, 59). Molecular alterations favoring instability of centromeres can thus lead to chromosome segregation defects.

Actually, assessment of aneuploidy is mostly based on measuring SCNA rates in malignancies through bioinformatics approach, the allele-specific copy number analysis of tumors (ASCAT), using data generated by whole-genome/exome sequencing strategies (60). The rates of intratumor karyotype heterogeneity can accurately be determined by simultaneous estimation of the allele-specific total copy number after adjusting for both tumor ploidy—including gains, losses, copy number-neutral events, and loss of heterozygosity (61).

Individual chromosome arm-level alterations were found to be related to expression changes in immune and cell-cycle markers, independent of aneuploidy level; however, increased arm- and chromosome-level SCNA burdens were associated with proliferation signatures and immune evasion profiles (62). Moreover, tumor aneuploidy is likely to increase intratumor heterogeneity, which may inhibit tumor immunity (63). Many solid cancers presenting with a high somatic copy alteration burden exhibit features of immune exclusion, whereas tumors displaying low rates of aneuploidy present an immune active profile (26, 27, 64). High-level SCNAs are classified through bioinformatic approaches as events where focal copy number gain (or loss) are higher (or lower) than the maximum (or minimum) median arm-level copy number gain (or loss), hence avoiding artifacts or false positives after comparison with low-level SCNAs linked to the ploidy of tumor samples and thus obtaining more reliable thresholds (65, 66). High-level SCNA profile in activating beta-catenin signaling pathway elements including CTNNB1, APC, and AXIN1-2 genes has been reported in metastatic melanoma but not in primary melanoma (67). A significantly higher concordance between mutated SCNA profiles in beta-catenin signaling pathway activated samples with a low level of T-cell tumor inflammation has been demonstrated, thus suggesting that SCNA signature may act as a progression marker in advanced melanoma (67). For its prediction of the T-cell-inflamed gene expression signature, the SCNA score is worth to be included in molecular tests aimed at somehow anticipating probabilities of resistance to immunotherapies. Further supporting this, the SCNA level has been found lower in lung cancer patients with a responsive disease than those with stable or progressive disease under ICI treatment (68).

Finally, SCNAs can be intrinsically linked to complex structural variants (CSVs) in affecting the efficacy of ICI treatment in melanoma. In particular, CSVs—which are represented by deletions, duplications, translocations, or inversions and arise through the breakage and fusion of one or two genomic locations—are particularly reported in acral melanoma (69). In bioinformatic analysis of NGS-generated data, SCNAs and CSVs are detected as changes in sequencing read depth and in junction-spanning read pairs across the candidate genomic loci (70).

Microsatellite Instability

MSI is characterized by small insertions or deletions within short tandem repeats in tumor DNA when compared with the corresponding normal DNA. In other words, regions that contain sequences of repeated nucleotides are intrinsically unstable and the insertion of inappropriate nucleotide(s) or the slippage events during DNA replication give rise to the insertion or deletion of single bases or small tandem DNA sequences (56). These alterations, which are normally recognized and repaired, in the absence of an efficient MMR function, are maintained giving origin to alleles of different sizes during the successive replication cycles. The accumulation of unpaired alleles is at the basis of such a genome-wide genetic instability, which is recognized as MSI+ phenotype and observed at higher prevalence in gastrointestinal and endometrial cancers (37, 44, 56, 71). **Table 1** report frequencies of MSI+ in different tumor types, as inferred taking into the consideration the main published studies (72–76).

In colorectal carcinoma (CRC), the MSI+ phenotype has been long evaluated for its impacts on disease pathogenesis and behavior as well as for correlations with prognostic effects. While some distinct clinical and pathological features (proximal location, poor differentiation, mucinous histology) have been consistently associated with the occurrence of MSI, more controversial data have been produced on the prognostic role of this alteration (77). In early stage CRC, the MSI+ phenotype has been described in patients with a better

prognosis; conversely, detection of unstable microsatellites seems to confer a negative prognosis in patients with metastatic disease (77–79).

MSI reflects a defect in genes involved in DNA replication fidelity and mostly, is due to inactivation of the mismatch repair (MMR) genes (29, 31). The MMR genes may be impaired by inactivating or down-regulating genetic mutations as well as by gene-silencing epigenetic changes (80). The result of such alterations is the expression of normal levels of functionally deficient MMR proteins or lack of the MMR protein expression, both conditions progressively inducing genetic instability and somehow providing a selective advantage during neoplastic transformation and progression (80). The important components of the DNA mismatch repair system are represented by seven specific ATP-binding proteins that work coordinately in sequential steps to initiate repair of DNA mismatches in genomic DNA: MLH1, MSH2, MLH3, MSH3, MSH6, PMS2, and PMS1 (81). Inactivation of MLH1 and MSH2 was detected in more than 85% of the MSI+ tumors (80, 81). Nearly all MMR genes contain a mononucleotide repeat and thus represent the first target of inactivating mutations when the MSI+ phenotype coexists (71).

The real breakthrough in defining a more impacting role of the MSI in the clinic practice for the management of neoplastic patients has been registered in 2017, when the U.S. Food and Drug Administration (FDA) granted approval of an immune checkpoint inhibitor (the anti-PD-1 pembrolizumab) for treatment of patients with cancers carrying MSI or deficient-MMR (82). The approval by FDA of the anti-PD-1 treatment for all advanced MSI+ solid tumors still represents the first regulatory authorization based exclusively on the use of a specific biomarker, regardless of the anatomic location in the body where the tumor originated ("tumor agnostic") (83). The MSI and the mutation load underlie the response to PD-1 blockade immunotherapy in deficient-MMR human tumors; the extent of response seems to be particularly associated with the accumulation of insertion-deletion (indel) mutational load (84). In a recent meta-analysis of patients with MSI+ cancer, the ICI treatment was significantly confirmed to be associated with high activity independent of tumor type and drug used and MSI status assessment may have a predictive value for the selection of patients to be addressed to immunotherapy (85).

Epigenomic studies have shown that tumors with MSI exhibit hypermethylation of key genes implicated in tumor development (75, 86). The hypermethylated promoters were identified in some genes that regulate some main molecular signaling cascades (75, 76, 87): WNT (in the absence of WNT-signals, β-catenin—a key downstream effector of this pathway—is targeted for degradation through phosphorylation; the WNT signals thus stabilize the intracellular levels of β-catenin and subsequently increase transcription of downstream target genes in many human cancers), hedgehog (essential for embryonic and postnatal development, this pathway remains in the quiescent state in adult tissues but gets activated upon inflammation and injuries), and PTEN (its inactivation through mixed genetic/epigenetic mechanisms results in persistent activation of PI3K effectors, with an important impact on cell proliferation, apoptosis resistance, angiogenesis, metabolism regulation, genomic

TABLE 1 | MSI+ frequency in different tumor types.

Cancer	Number	MSI+	%
Endometrial carcinoma	1426	401	28.1
Gastric adenocarcinoma	573	117	20.4
Colorectal adenocarcinoma	1,456	196	13.5
Thyroid carcinoma	584	18	3.1
Hepatocellular carcinoma	375	11	2.9
Kidney renal clear cell carcinoma	278	6	2.2
Cutaneous melanoma	359	7	1.9
Ovarian carcinoma	63	1	1.6
Prostate adenocarcinoma	463	3	0.6
Lung nonsquamous cell adenocarcinoma	480	3	0.6
Head and neck squamous cell carcinoma	506	3	0.6
Lung squamous cell carcinoma	443	2	0.5
Urothelial carcinoma	253	1	0.4
Glioblastoma	262	1	0.4
Glioma	513	1	0.2
Kidney papillary cell carcinoma	207	0	0.0
Breast carcinoma	266	0	0.0
TOTAL	**8,507**	**771**	**9.1**

Total numbers and percentages were obtained summing data from literature (see text for references).

instability, cellular senescence, and cell migration). The hypermethylated status is also tightly correlated with the occurrence of somatic mutations in *BRAF* oncogene, overall causing a strong inhibition of the senescence mechanisms and a consequent promotion of an uncontrolled cell proliferation and survival (88, 89). Hypermethylation has also been related to the facilitation of tumor escape by repressing transcriptional expression of interferon (IFN) regulatory factors (90). Indeed, demethylating agents and histone deacetylases are being combined with ICI treatments in numerous clinical trials and types of malignancies (91, 92).

Several additional factors, other than those mainly underlying MSI, have been shown to be involved in determining a hypermutated status, such as inactivating mutations in the DNA polymerases as well as exposure to external (cigarette smoke, UV radiation, chemicals) and endogenous (reactive oxygen species) mutagens (93, 94). The hypermutated condition may be related to driver mutations in the DNA *polymerase ε* (*POLE*) and *δ1* (*POLD1*) genes among different tumor types, including colorectal, endometrial, and other cancers such as melanoma and lung cancer (95, 96). Deleterious mutations in *POLE/POLD1* genes compromise proofreading of genomic DNA during cell replication and the timing of their onset may vary, with constitutional defective MMR followed by acquired secondary *POLE/POLD1* defects or *vice versa* (97). It has been shown that the presence of mutations in *POLE* may promote a high level of non-synonymous single-nucleotide variations (ns-SNVs), not tightly associated with the presence of a MSI+ phenotype (the highest mutation rates were observed in MSS tumors) (71). The *POLD1* gene has been found silenced in several cancer types—mostly, in conjunction with a defective *POLE* gene—with increased genome instability and DNA damage effects (98–100). POLD1 is involved in different forms of DNA repair induced by exposure to mutagens, including nucleotide excision repair, double strand break repair, base excision repair, and mismatch repair (101). The coexistence of MSI+ and mutated *POLE* may be associated with higher densities of CD8+ TILs, PD-1-expressing CD8+ TILs, and tumor-infiltrating immune cells with a Th1 phenotype in the TME, strongly predicting response to checkpoint inhibitors (102).

As mentioned above, tumors with the hypermutated status present similar sensitivity to ICI. Indeed, a strong correlation was found between increased load of non-synonymous mutations and clinical benefits to PD-1 inhibition in non-small cell lung cancer (39) or to cytotoxic T-lymphocyte antigen T 4 (CTLA-4) blockade in melanoma (103). Considering such reported outcomes, one can speculate that increased production of neoepitopes predicting response to ICI might be even generated in cohorts of patients with low (<10% of case) or very low (<1%) prevalence of MSI (**Table 1**).

The hypermutated status can be actually defined with more extensively detailed approaches such as NGS or mass spectrometry assays (104). Among strategies not requiring to match normal DNA material, the single-molecule molecular inversion probe (smMIP) assay is able to detect the existence of an impaired intracellular capability of correcting smMIP-induced errors (105). All these screening strategies are useful in a

research context, but technically difficult to translate into clinical practice for routine diagnostic application, since either requiring an extensive bioinformatics analysis of the obtained results either remaining still expensive methods (48–50). Conversely, a simple method to directly detect MSI on formalin-fixed paraffin embedded tumor tissue sections is represented by the Idylla™ test, a fully automated PCR-based assay including a high-resolution melting curve analysis. The Idylla™ MSI test is able to detect mutations in seven tumor-specific MSI loci (ACVR2A, BTBD7, DIDO1, MRE11, RYR3, SEC31A, and SULF2), not requiring the analysis of paired normal tissue samples. For more extensive and detailed information about the methodologies aimed at investigating the MSI status, one can refer to the recent report from our group (106, 107).

The contextual assessment of the MSI+ phenotype and the hypermutated status may be strongly indicative for the existence of a higher tumor immunogenicity, though none of the alterations described as immediate biological effects of the MSI+ phenotype and the hypermutated status—the mutation load, the neoantigen prediction, and the intratumor immune cell infiltration rate—may be considered as a reliable predictor of response to anti-PD-1 treatment (108). Several additional molecular factors are suggested to be involved in immune response. Occurrence of mutations inactivating *JAK1*—within the JAK-STAT pathway that regulates different cellular processes—has been reported to confer resistance to the anti-PD-1 treatment by reducing both the PD-L1 expression and the ability to promote the IFN-γ driven response (109, 110). The relationship between such *JAK1* mutations and MSI status is however complex. In patients with tumors characterized by a low prevalence of MSI—including cutaneous melanoma, invasive breast cancer, and prostate adenocarcinoma—deleterious *JAK1* mutations are associated with unfavorable prognosis (109, 110). In MSI+ tumors, *JAK1* silencing seems to instead impair the tumor growth, playing a positive prognostic role (109, 110). This further confirms that often the same molecular alterations occurring in different tumor types have a distinct impact on biological behavior according to the different genetic backgrounds.

Classification of Melanoma Patients for Genetic Instability

According to their mutational status inferred by NGS analysis at somatic level, one could classify melanoma patients using:

- "qualitative" parameters, aimed at discriminating all classes of sequence changes or structural alterations (non-synonymous single-nucleotide variants/ns-SNVs, indels, copy number variations/CNVs, fusions, and splice variants) in tumor suppressor genes and/or oncogenes. These alterations occur at high frequency in melanoma samples. Research efforts should be aimed at defining the clinical role of the distinct mutational patterns of driver ns-SNVs as well as whether the increased load may rather represent the consequence of the sequential accumulation of "passenger" mutations in specific pathways during disease progression;

- "quantitative" parameters, aimed at defining the above described threshold-depending parameters representing the main immuno-oncology content (SCNA, MSI, and TMB). These alterations occur at low frequency in melanoma samples (**Figure 3**).

Most of such key features are actually achieved using large NGS-based panels, which usually include over 400 unique driver genes in correspondent genomic loci for the achievement of a comprehensive and simultaneous genomic profiling (**Table 2**).

MSI Detection on Liquid Biopsies

In cancer patients, the assessment of PD-L1 status in circulating tumor cells (CTC) and the determination of specific somatic mutations in circulating tumor DNA (ctDNA) represent non-invasive tools acting as predictive markers of the efficacy of the therapeutic response to ICI. The technology for CTC isolation is not widely available, whereas genomic analyzes on ctDNA are methodologically feasible. In NSCLC, undetectable ctDNA levels

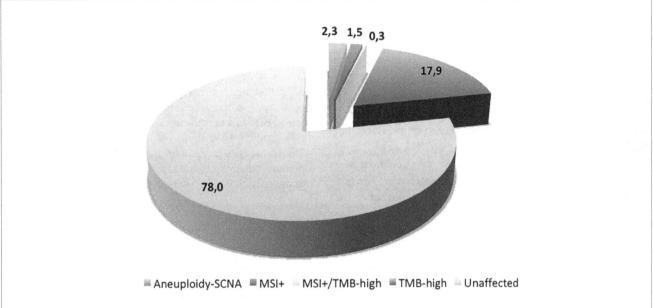

FIGURE 3 | Distribution of molecular alterations linked to genetic instability in melanoma samples. Numbers indicate the percentages of cases reported in literature (see text for references).

TABLE 2 | Molecular alterations underlying genetic instability useful in cancer patients' stratification for immunotherapy.

Type	Detection method	Identified alteration
SCNA	whole genome sequencing (WGS)	gene/locus gain or loss
	whole exome sequencing (WES)	copy number variation
	targeted multiple-gene NGS assays (panels)	complex structural variants
		loss of heterozygosity (LOH)
MSI	Bethesda panel assay (5 microsatellite loci)	genome-wide instability
	≥ 2 unstable markers (different microsatellite lengths between tumor and normal samples)	
	extended Bethesda panel (8 microsatellite loci and 2 homo-polymer markers: BAT25, BAT26, BAT40, D5S346, D17S250, D2S123, TGFB, D18S58, D17S787, D18S69 or BAT25, BAT26, BAT40, D2s123, D10s197, D13s153, D17s250, D18s58, D5s346, Mycl)	genome-wide instability
	≥30% unstable markers	mutations in seven MSI loci (ACVR2A, BTBD7, DIDO1, RYR3, MRE11, SEC31A, and SULF2)
	real-time PCR by Idylla™ MSI Test	
	≥ 1 mutated locus	
dMMR	protein expression by immunohistochemistry	lack of MMR protein(s)
	targeted multiple-gene NGS assays	mutations inactivating MMR genes (MLH1, MSH2, MLH3, MSH3, MSH6, PMS2, PMS1)
CIN	comparative genomic hybridization (CGH) fluorescence in-situ hybridization (FISH)	whole chromosome or segmental/focal aneuploidy
	gene fusion (mRNA) microarrays	
TMB	whole exome sequencing	mutations per megabase of genomic area
	targeted multiple-gene NGS assays	mutations inactivating DNA polymerases (POLE, POLD1)
Methylation	whole genome methylation	genome-wide DNA methylation with RRBS
	gene promoter methylation	methylation levels of candidate gene promoters

SCNA, somatic copy number alteration; MSI, microsatellite instability; dMMR, deficient mismatch repair; CIN, chromosomal instability; TMB, tumor mutation burden; NGS, next-generation sequencing; RRBS, reduced representation bisulfite sequencing.

after two months of ICI were demonstrated to be associated with a marked and lasting response to therapy, while an increase in ctDNA load after initiation of ICI was associated with poorer survival (111, 112). In melanoma, detectable ctDNA at baseline and post-surgical tumour removal may predict a shorter median disease-specific survival among stage III melanoma patients (113, 114) a s w e l l a s detection of persistent or increasing ctDNA levels during follow-up was shown to predict worse prognosis when compared to patients with undetectable or falling ctDNA levels (115, 116). Currently, plasma-based commercially available assays ("liquid biopsies") c a n be used to assess the MSI or the mismatch repair deficiency (dMMR) through genomic analysis by realt-time PCR or DNA sequencing assays in a large variety of cancer types (117–119). From the practical point of view, the real-time PCR is mainly based on the Idylla™ MSI assay (Biocartis, Bruxelles, Belgium; catalog n. A0101/ 6), which includes a set of seven MSI biomarkers consisting of short homo-polymers located in the above mentioned genes. The NGS tests on ctDNA are performed using complex multigene panels (i.e. the Oncomine Comprehensive Assay Plus panel, which provides highly multiplexed target selection of >400 genes implicated in cancer pathogenesis, carried out on the Ion GeneStudio S5 System)(120). These NGS-based tests are now feasible in clinical practice and they have very high concordance, sensitivity and specificity and a detection limit of 0.1% tumor content for MSI-H status. Moreover, such panels allow identification of further genomic alterations (i.e. the tumor mutation burden or TMB) with potential implications for predicting response to immunotherapy.

CONCLUSIVE REMARKS

Considering the steadily increasing advances in the knowledge of the molecular mechanisms underlying the genetic instability at the chromosomal and nucleotide levels as well as the recognized ascertainment of their clinical impact on cancer management, selection of the subgroups of patients according to the type of instability (SCNA+ vs. SCNA−, MSI+ vs. MSI−) or mutational composition (TMB-high vs. TMB-low; neoantigen-high vs. neoantigen-low) present is becoming mandatory. Further advancements will be however achieved by increasing correlations between such molecular features—through a continuous dissemination of the methodologies to be used for their assessment into the clinical practice—and all disease-related and therapy-dependent parameters. These efforts should facilitate the development of innovative diagnostic, predictive, and/or prognostic tools for a better molecular classification of cancer patients, even in a malignancy like melanoma with lower rates of such alterations. Nevertheless, more extensive applications of the NGS technologies could improve the assessment of all driver alterations putatively acting as disease markers to be transferred into the daily clinical practice.

AUTHOR CONTRIBUTIONS

All authors contributed to the conception, design, and writing of the manuscript. All authors contributed to the article and approved the submitted version.

REFERENCES

1. Fusi A, Dalgleish A. The Importance for Immunoregulation for Long-Term Cancer Control. Future Oncol (2017) 13(18):1619–32. doi: 10.2217/fon-2017-0085

2. Gelsomino F, Lamberti G, Parisi C, Casolari L, Melotti B, Sperandi F, et al. The Evolving Landscape of Immunotherapy in Small-Cell Lung Cancer: A Focus on Predictive Biomarkers. Cancer Treat Rev (2019) 79:101887. doi: 10.1016/j.ctrv.2019.08.003

3. Kok PS, Cho D, Yoon WH, Ritchie G, Marschner I, Lord S, et al. Validation of Progression-Free Survival Rate At 6 Months and Objective Response for Estimating Overall Survival in Immune Checkpoint Inhibitor Trials: A Systematic Review and Meta-Analysis. JAMA Netw Open (2020) 3(9): e2011809. doi: 10.1001/jamanetworkopen.2020.11809

4. Hu X, Yu H, Zheng Y, Zhang Q, Lin M, Wang J, et al. Immune Checkpoint Inhibitors and Survival Outcomes in Brain Metastasis: A Time Series-Based Meta-Analysis. Front Oncol (2020) 10:564382. doi: 10.3389/fonc.2020.564382

5. Wu X, Gu Z, Chen Y, Chen B, Chen W, Weng L, et al. Application of PD-1 Blockade in Cancer Immunotherapy. Comput Struct Biotechnol J (2019) 17:661–74. doi: 10.1016/j.csbj.2019.03.006

6. Datta M, Coussens LM, Nishikawa H, Hodi FS, Jain RK. Reprogramming the Tumor Microenvironment to Improve Immunotherapy: Emerging Strategies and Combination Therapies. Am Soc Clin Oncol Educ Book (2019) 39:165–74. doi: 10.1200/EDBK_237987

7. Ascierto PA, Bifulco C, Palmieri G, Peters S, Sidiropoulos N. Preanalytic Variables and Tissue Stewardship for Reliable Next-Generation Sequencing (NGS) Clinical Analysis. J Mol Diagn (2019) 21(5):756–67. doi: 10.1016/j.jmoldx.2019.05.004

8. Grasso CS, Giannakis M, Wells DK, Hamada T, Mu X, Quist M, et al. Genetic Mechanisms of Immune Evasion in Colorectal Cancer. Cancer Discovery (2018) 8:730–49. doi: 10.1158/2159-8290.CD-17-1327

9. Nava Rodrigues D, Rescigno P, Liu D, Yuan W, Carreira S, Lambros MB, et al. Immunogenomic Analyses Associate Immunological Alterations With Mismatch Repair Defects in Prostate Cancer. J Clin Invest (2018) 128:4441–53. doi: 10.1172/JCI121924

10. Travert C, Barlesi F, Greillier L, Tomasini P. Immune Oncology Biomarkers in Lung Cancer: An Overview. Curr Oncol Rep (2020) 22(11):107. doi: 10.1007/s11912-020-00970-3

11. Pishvaian MJ, Blais EM, Brody JR, Lyons E, DeArbeloa P, Hendifar A, et al. Overall Survival in Patients With Pancreatic Cancer Receiving Matched Therapies Following Molecular Profiling: A Retrospective Analysis of the Know Your Tumor Registry Trial. Lancet Oncol (2020) 21(4):508–18. doi: 10.1016/S1470-2045(20)30074-7

12. Xue C, Chen H, Yu F. Base-Biased Evolution of Disease-Associated Mutations in the Human Genome. Hum Mutat (2016) 37(11):1209–14. doi: 10.1002/humu.23065

13. Albert FW, Kruglyak L. The Role of Regulatory Variation in Complex Traits and Disease. Nat Rev Genet (2015) 16(4):197–212. doi: 10.1038/nrg3891

14. Scott SP, Pandita TK. The Cellular Control of DNA Double-Strand Breaks. *J Cell Biochem* (2006) 99(6):1463–75. doi: 10.1002/jcb.21067

15. Hustedt N, Durocher D. The Control of DNA Repair by the Cell Cycle. *Nat Cell Biol* (2016) 19(1):1–9. doi: 10.1038/ncb3452

16. Giam M, Rancati G. Aneuploidy and Chromosomal Instability in Cancer: A Jackpot to Chaos. *Cell Div* (2015) 10(3):1–12. doi: 10.1186/s13008-015-0009-7

17. Vodicka P, Musak L, Vodickova L, Vodenkova S, Catalano C, Kroupa M, et al. Genetic Variation of Acquired Structural Chromosomal Aberrations. *Mutat Res* (2018) 836(Pt A):13–21. doi: 10.1016/j.mrgentox.2018.05.014

18. Lengauer C, Kinzler KW, Volgestein B. Genetic Instabilities in Human Cancers. *Nature* (1998) 396:643–49. doi: 10.1038/25292

19. Catasti P, Chen X, Mariappan SV, Bradbury EM, Gupta G. DNA Repeats in the Human Genome. *Genetics* (1999) 106(1-2):15–36. doi: 10.1023/A:1003716509180

20. Schlotterer C. Evolutionary Dynamics of Microsatellite DNA. *Chromosome* (2000) 109:365–71. doi: 10.1007/s004120000089

21. Toth G, Gaspari Z, Jurka J. Microsatellites in Different Eukaryotic Genomes: Survey and Analysis. *Genome Res* (2000) 10:967–81. doi: 10.1101/gr.10.7.967

22. Bois P, Jeffreys AJ. Minisatellite Instability and Germline Mutation. *Cell Mol Life Sci* (1999) 55(12):1636–48. doi: 10.1007/s000180050402

23. Orr B, Godek KM, Compton D. Aneuploidy. *Curr Biol* (2015) 25:R538–42. doi: 10.1016/j.cub.2015.05.010

24. O'Donnell JS, Teng MWL, Smyth MJ. Cancer Immunoediting and Resistance to T Cell-Based Immunotherapy. *Nat Rev Clin Oncol* (2019) 16:151–67. doi: 10.1038/s41571-018-0142-8

25. Xiao Q, Nobre A, Piñeiro P, Berciano-Guerrero MÁ, Alba E, Cobo M, et al. Genetic and Epigenetic Biomarkers of Immune Checkpoint Blockade Response. *J Clin Med* (2020) 9(1):286. doi: 10.3390/jcm9010286

26. Davoli T, Uno H, Wooten EC, Elledge SJ. Tumor Aneuploidy Correlates With Markers of Immune Evasion and With Reduced Response to Immunotherapy. *Science* (2017) 355:eaaf8399. doi: 10.1126/science.aaf8399

27. Litchfield K, Reading JL, Puttick C, Thakkar K, Abbosh C, Bentham R, et al. Meta-Analysis of Tumor- and T Cell-Intrinsic Mechanisms of Sensitization to Checkpoint Inhibition. *Cell* (2021) 184(3):596–614. doi: 10,21203/rs.3.rs-76464/v1

28. Salem ME, Puccini A, Grothey A, Raghavan D, Goldberg RM, Xiu J, et al. Landscape of Tumor Mutation Load, Mismatch Repair Deficiency, and PD-L1 Expression in a Large Patient Cohort of Gastrointestinal Cancers. *Mol Cancer Res* (2018) 16(5):805–12. doi: 10.1158/1541-7786.MCR-17-0735

29. Ballhausen A, Przybilla MJ, Jendrusch M, Haupt S, Pfaffendorf E, Seidler F, et al. The Shared Frameshift Mutation Landscape of Microsatellite-Unstable Cancers Suggests Immunoediting During Tumor Evolution. *Nat Commun* (2020) 11(1):4740. doi: 10.1038/s41467-020-18514-5

30. Budczies J, Seidel A, Christopoulos P, Endris V, Kloor M, Győrffy B, et al. Integrated Analysis of the Immunological and Genetic Status in and Across Cancer Types: Impact of Mutational Signatures Beyond Tumor Mutational Burden. *Oncoimmunology* (2018) 7(12):e1526613. doi: 10.1080/2162402X.2018.1526613

31. Marmorino F, Boccaccino A, Germani MM, Falcone A, Cremolini C. Immune Checkpoint Inhibitors in pMMR Metastatic Colorectal Cancer: A Tough Challenge. *Cancers (Basel)* (2020) 12(8):2317. doi: 10.3390/cancers12082317

32. Chalmers ZR, Connelly CF, Fabrizio D, Gay L, Ali SM, Ennis R, et al. Analysis of 100,000 Human Cancer Genomes Reveals the Landscape of Tumor Mutational Burden. *Genome Med* (2017) 9(1):34. doi: 10.1186/s13073-017-0424-2

33. Samstein RM, Lee CH, Shoushtari AN, Hellmann MD, Shen R, Janjigian YY, et al. Tumor Mutational Load Predicts Survival After Immunotherapy Across Multiple Cancer Types. *Nat Genet* (2019) 51(2):202–6. doi: 10.1038/s41588-018-0312-8

34. Sha D, Jin Z, Budczies J, Kluck K, Stenzinger A, Sinicrope FA. Tumor Mutational Burden as a Predictive Biomarker in Solid Tumors. *Cancer Discovery* (2020) 10(12):1808–25. doi: 10.1158/2159-8290.CD-20-0522

35. Schumacher TN, Schreiber RD. Neoantigens in Cancer Immunotherapy. *Science* (2015) 348(6230):69–74. doi: 10.1126/science.aaa4971

36. Mei P, Freitag CE, Wei L, Zhang Y, Parwani AV, Li Z. High Tumor Mutation Burden is Associated With DNA Damage Repair Gene Mutation

in Breast Carcinomas. *Diagn Pathol* (2020) 15(1):50. doi: 10.1186/s13000-020-00971-7

37. Schrock AB, Ouyang C, Sandhu J, Sokol E, Jin D, Ross JS, et al. Tumor Mutational Burden is Predictive of Response to Immune Checkpoint Inhibitors in MSI-high Metastatic Colorectal Cancer. *Ann Oncol* (2019) 30 (7):1096–103. doi: 10.1093/annonc/mdz134

38. Le DT, Uram JN, Wang H, Bartlett BR, Kemberling H, Eyring AD, et al. PD-1 Blockade in Tumors With Mismatch-Repair Deficiency. *N Engl J Med* (2015) 372:2509–20. doi: 10.1056/NEJMoa1500596

39. Rizvi NA, Hellmann M, Snyder A, Kvistborg P, Makarov V, Havel J. Cancer Immunology. Mutational Landscape Determines Sensitivity to PD-1 Blockade in non-Small Cell Lung Cancer. *Science* (2015) 348:124–8. doi: 10.1126/science.aaa1348

40. Goodman AM, Kato S, Bazhenova L, Patel SP, Frampton GM, Miller V, et al. Tumor Mutational Burden as an Independent Predictor of Response to Immunotherapy in Diverse Cancers. *Mol Cancer Ther* (2017) 16(11):2598–608. doi: 10.1158/1535-7163.MCT-17-0386

41. Hellmann MD, Nathanson T, Rizvi H, Creelan BC, Sanchez-Vega F, Ahuja A, et al. Genomic Features of Response to Combination Immunotherapy in Patients With Advanced non-Small-Cell Lung Cancer. *Cancer Cell* (2018) 33:843–52.e4. doi: 10.1016/j.ccell.2018.03.018

42. Rizvi H, Sanchez-Vega F, La K, Chatila W, Jonsson P, Halpenny D, et al. Molecular Determinants of Response to Anti-Programmed Cell Death (PD)-1 and Anti-Programmed Death-Ligand 1 (PD-L1) Blockade in Patients With non-Small-Cell Lung Cancer Profiled With Targeted Next-Generation Sequencing. *J Clin Oncol* (2018) 36(7):633–41. doi: 10.1200/JCO.2017.75.3384

43. Macherla S, Laks S, Naqash AR, Bulumulle A, Zervos E, Muzaffar M. Emerging Role of Immune Checkpoint Blockade in Pancreatic Cancer. *Int J Mol Sci* (2018) 19:3505. doi: 10.3390/ijms19113505

44. Abida W, Cheng ML, Armenia J, Middha S, Autio KA, Vargas HA, et al. Analysis of the Prevalence of Microsatellite Instability in Prostate Cancer and Response to Immune Checkpoint Blockade. *JAMA Oncol* (2019) 5:471–8. doi: 10.1001/jamaoncol.2018.5801

45. Priestley P, Baber J, Lolkema MP, Steeghs N, de Bruijn E, Shale C, et al. Pan-cancer Whole-Genome Analyses of Metastatic Solid Tumours. *Nature* (2019) 575(7781):210–6. doi: 10.1038/s41586-019-1689-y

46. Xiang L, Fu X, Wang X, Li W, Zheng X, Nan K, et al. A Potential Biomarker of Combination of Tumor Mutation Burden and Copy Number Alteration for Efficacy of Immunotherapy in KRAS-mutant Advanced Lung Adenocarcinoma. *Front Oncol* (2020) 10:559896. doi: 10.3389/fonc.2020.559896

47. van Nimwegen KJ, van Soest RA, Veltman JA, Nelen MR, van der Wilt GJ, Vissers LE, et al. Is the $1000 Genome as Near as We Think? A Cost Analysis of Next-Generation Sequencing. *Clin Chem* (2016) 62(11):1458–64. doi: 10.1373/clinchem.2016.258632

48. Weymann D, Laskin J, Roscoe R, Schrader KA, Chia S, Yip S, et al. The Cost and Cost Trajectory of Whole-Genome Analysis Guiding Treatment of Patients With Advanced Cancers. *Mol Genet Genom Med* (2017) 5(3):251–60. doi: 10.1002/mgg3.281

49. Marino P, Touzani R, Perrier L, Rouleau E, Kossi DS, Zhaomin Z, et al. Cost of Cancer Diagnosis Using Next-Generation Sequencing Targeted Gene Panels in Routine Practice: A Nationwide French Study. *Eur J Hum Genet* (2018) 26(3):314–23. doi: 10.1038/s41431-017-0081-3

50. Mosele F, Remon J, Mateo J, Westphalen CB, Barlesi F, Lolkema MP, et al. Recommendations for the Use of Next-Generation Sequencing (NGS) for Patients With Metastatic Cancers: A Report From the ESMO Precision Medicine Working Group. *Ann Oncol* (2020) 31(11):1491–505. doi: 10.1016/j.annonc.2020.07.014

51. Kaushal S, Freudenreich CH. The Role of Fork Stalling and DNA Structures in Causing Chromosome Fragility. *Genes Chromosomes Cancer* (2019) 58 (5):270–83. doi: 10.1002/gcc.22721

52. Sansregret L, Vanhaesebroeck B, Swanton C. Determinants and Clinical Implications of Chromosomal Instability in Cancer. *Nat Rev Clin Oncol* (2018) 15(3):139–50. doi: 10.1038/nrclinonc.2017.198

53. Ingham M, Schwartz GK. Cell-cycle Therapeutics Come of Age. *J Clin Oncol* (2017) 35(25):2949–59. doi: 10.1200/JCO.2016.69.0032

54. Merkel O, Taylor N, Prutsch N, Staber PB, Moriggl R, Turner SD, et al. When the Guardian Sleeps: Reactivation of the p53 Pathway in Cancer. *Mutat Res* (2017) 773:1–13. doi: 10.1016/j.mrrev.2017.02.003

55. Manning AL, Benes C, Dyson NJ. Whole Chromosome Instability Resulting From the Synergistic Effects of pRB and p53 Inactivation. *Oncogene* (2014) 33(19):2487–94. doi: 10.1038/onc.2013.201

56. Dariya B, Aliya S, Merchant N, Alam A, Nagaraju GP. Colorectal Cancer Biology, Diagnosis, and Therapeutic Approaches. *Crit Rev Oncog* (2020) 25 (2):71–94. doi: 10.1615/CritRevOncog.2020035067

57. Orr B, Compton DA. A Double-Edged Sword: How Oncogenes and Tumor Suppressor Genes can Contribute to Chromosomal Instability. *Front Oncol* (2013) 3:164. doi: 10.3389/fonc.2013.00164

58. Duijf PH, Benezra R. The Cancer Biology of Whole-Chromosome Instability. *Oncogene* (2013) 32(40):4727–36. doi: 10.1038/onc.2012.616

59. Cuomo M, Knebel A, Morrice N, Paterson H, Cohen P, Mittnacht S. P53-Driven Apoptosis Limits Centrosome Amplification and Genomic Instability Downstream of NPM1 Phosphorylation. *Nat Cell Biol* (2008) 10(6):723–30. doi: 10.1038/ncb1735

60. Van Loo P, Nordgard SH, Lingjærde OC, Russnes HG, Rye IH, Sun W, et al. Allele-Specific Copy Number Analysis of Tumors. *Proc Natl Acad Sci USA* (2010) 107(39):16910–5. doi: 10.1073/pnas.1009843107

61. Camacho N, Van Loo P, Edwards S, Kay JD, Matthews L, Haase K, et al. Appraising the Relevance of DNA Copy Number Loss and Gain in Prostate Cancer Using Whole Genome DNA Sequence Data. *PloS Genet* (2017) 13(9): e1007001. doi: 10.1371/journal.pgen.1007001

62. Taylor AM, Shih J, Ha G, Gao GF, Zhang X, Berger AC, et al. Genomic and Functional Approaches to Understanding Cancer Aneuploidy. *Cancer Cell* (2018) 33(4):676–89.e3. doi: 10.1016/j.ccell.2018.03.007

63. Anichini A, Tassi E, Grazia G, Mortarini R. The non-Small Cell Lung Cancer Immune Landscape: Emerging Complexity, Prognostic Relevance and Prospective Significance in the Context of Immunotherapy. *Cancer Immunol Immunother* (2018) 67(6):1011–22. doi: 10.1007/s00262-018-2147-7

64. Bassaganyas L, Pinyol R, Esteban-Fabró R, Torrens L, Torrecilla S, Willoughby CE, et al. Copy-number Alteration Burden Differentially Impacts Immune Profiles and Molecular Features of Hepatocellular Carcinoma. *Clin Cancer Res* (2020) 26(23):6350–61. doi: 10.1158/1078-0432.CCR-20-1497

65. Mermel CH, Schumacher SE, Hill B, Meyerson ML, Beroukhim R, Getz G. GISTIC2.0 Facilitates Sensitive and Confident Localization of the Targets of Focal Somatic Copy-Number Alteration in Human Cancers. *Genome Biol* (2011) 12(4). doi: 10.1186/gb-2011-12-4-r41

66. The Cancer Genome Atlas (TCGA). (2021). Available at: https://gdac.broadinstitute.org/ (Accessed 28 January 2021).

67. Luke JJ, Bao R, Sweis RF, Spranger S, Gajewski TF. Wnt/β-Catenin Pathway Activation Correlates With Immune Exclusion Across Human Cancers. *Clin Cancer Res* (2019) 25(10):3074–83. doi: 10.1158/1078-0432.CCR-18-1942

68. Kim HS, Cha H, Kim J, Park WY, Choi YL, Sun JM, et al. Genomic Scoring to Determine Clinical Benefit of Immunotherapy by Targeted Sequencing. *Eur J Cancer* (2019) 120:65–74. doi: 10.1016/j.ejca.2019.08.001

69. Hadi K, Yao X, Behr JM, Deshpande A, Xanthopoulakis C, Tian H, et al. Distinct Classes of Complex Structural Variation Uncovered Across Thousands of Cancer Genome Graphs. *Cell* (2020) 183(1):197–210.e32. doi: 10.1016/j.cell.2020.08.006

70. Cameron DL, Schroder J, Penington JS, Do H, Molania R, Dobrovic A, et al. GRIDSS: Sensitive and Specific Genomic Rearrangement Detection Using Positional De Bruijn Graph Assembly. *Genome Res* (2017) 27(12):2050–60. doi: 10.1101/gr.222109.117

71. Kim TM, Laird PW, Park PJ. The Landscape of Microsatellite Instability in Colorectal and Endometrial Cancer Genomes. *Cell* (2013) 155(4):858–68. doi: 10.1016/j.cell.2013.10.015

72. Palmieri G, Ascierto PA, Cossu A, Colombino M, Casula M, Botti G, et al. Assessment of Genetic Instability in Melanocytic Skin Lesions Through Microsatellite Analysis of Benign Nevi, Dysplastic Nevi, and Primary Melanomas Along With Their Metastases. *Melanoma Res* (2003) 13 (2):167–70. doi: 10.1097/00008390-200304000-00009

73. Hause RJ, Pritchard CC, Shendure J, Salipante SJ. Classification and Characterization of Microsatellite Instability Across 18 Cancer Types. *Nat Med* (2016) 22(11):1342–50. doi: 10.1038/nm.4191

74. Yan L, Zhang W. Precision Medicine Becomes Reality-Tumor Type-Agnostic Therapy. *Cancer Commun (Lond)* (2018) 38(1):6. doi: 10.1186/s40880-018-0274-3

75. Dudley JC, Lin MT, Le DT, Eshleman JR. Microsatellite Instability as a Biomarker for PD-1 Blockade. *Clin Cancer Res* (2016) 22(4):813–20. doi: 10.1158/1078-0432.CCR-15-1678

76. Le DT, Durham JN, Smith KN, Wang H, Bartlett BR, Aulakh LK, et al. Mismatch Repair Deficiency Predicts Response of Solid Tumors to PD-1 Blockade. *Science* (2017) 357(6349):409–13. doi: 10.1126/science.aan6733

77. Gelsomino F, Barbolini M, Spallanzani A, Pugliese G, Cascinu S. The Evolving Role of Microsatellite Instability in Colorectal Cancer: A Review. *Cancer Treat Rev* (2016) 51:19–26. doi: 10.1016/j.ctrv.2016.10.005

78. Yang Y, Wang D, Jin L, Wu G, Bai Z, Wang J, et al. Prognostic Value of the Combination of Microsatellite Instability and *BRAF* Mutation in Colorectal Cancer. *Cancer Manag Res* (2018) 10:3911–29. doi: 10.2147/CMAR.S169649

79. Murcia O, Juárez M, Rodríguez-Soler M, Hernández-Illán E, Giner-Calabuig M, Alustiza M, et al. Colorectal Cancer Molecular Classification Using BRAF, KRAS, Microsatellite Instability and CIMP Status: Prognostic Implications and Response to Chemotherapy. *PloS One* (2018) 13(9): e0203051. doi: 10.1371/journal.pone.0203051

80. Zhao H, Thienpont B, Yesilyurt BT, Moisse M, Reumers J, Coenegrachts L, et al. Mismatch Repair Deficiency Endows Tumors With a Unique Mutation Signature and Sensitivity to DNA Double-Strand Breaks. *Elife* (2014) 3: e02725. doi: 10.7554/eLife.02725

81. Richman S. Deficient Mismatch Repair: Read All About it. *Int J Oncol* (2015) 47(4):1189–202. doi: 10.3892/ijo.2015.3119

82. U.S. Food and Drug Administration. (2017). Available at: https://www.fda.gov/newsevents/newsroom/pressannouncements/ucm560167.htm.

83. Yoshino T, Pentheroudakis G, Mishima S, Overman MJ, Yeh KH, Baba E, et al. Jsco-ESMO-ASCO-JSMO-TOS: International Expert Consensus Recommendations for Tumor-Agnostic Treatments in Patients With Solid Tumors With Microsatellite Instability or NTRK Fusions. *Ann Oncol* (2020) 31:861–72. doi: 10.1016/j.annonc.2020.03.299

84. Mandal R, Samstein RM, Lee KW, Havel JJ, Wang H, Krishna C, et al. Genetic Diversity of Tumors With Mismatch Repair Deficiency Influences anti-PD-1 Immunotherapy Response. *Science* (2019) 364(6439):485–91. doi: 10.1126/science.aau0447

85. Petrelli F, Ghidini M, Ghidini A, Tomasello G. Outcomes Following Immune Checkpoint Inhibitor Treatment of Patients With Microsatellite Instability-High Cancers: A Systematic Review and Meta-Analysis. *JAMA Oncol* (2020) 6(7):1068–71. doi: 10.1001/jamaoncol.2020.1046

86. Hu X, Estecio MR, Chen R, Reuben A, Wang L, Fujimoto J, et al. Evolution of DNA Methylome From Precancerous Lesions to Invasive Lung Adenocarcinomas. *Nat Commun* (2021) 12(1):687. doi: 10.1038/s41467-021-20907-z

87. Thorstensen L, Lind GE, Løvig T, Diep CB, Meling GI, Rognum TO, et al. Genetic and Epigenetic Changes of Components Affecting the WNT Pathway in Colorectal Carcinomas Stratified by Microsatellite Instability. *Neoplasia* (2005) 7(2):99–108. doi: 10.1593/neo.04448

88. Molinari F, Signoroni S, Lampis A, Bertan C, Perrone F, Sala P, et al. BRAF Mutation Analysis is a Valid Tool to Implement in Lynch Syndrome Diagnosis in Patients Classified According to the Bethesda Guidelines. *Tumori* (2014) 100(3):315–20. doi: 10.1700/1578.17214

89. Guinney J, Dienstmann R, Wang X, de Reyniès A, Schlicker A, Soneson C, et al. The Consensus Molecular Subtypes of Colorectal Cancer. *Nat Med* (2015) 21(11):1350–6. doi: 10.1038/nm.3967

90. Yang D, Thangaraju M, Greeneltch K, Browning DD, Schoenlein PV, Tamura T, et al. Repression of IFN Regulatory Factor 8 by DNA Methylation is a Molecular Determinant of Apoptotic Resistance and Metastatic Phenotype in Metastatic Tumor Cells. *Cancer Res* (2007) 67:3301–9. doi: 10.1158/0008-5472.CAN-06-4068

91. Covre A, Coral S, Nicolay H, Parisi G, Fazio C, Colizzi F, et al. Antitumor Activity of Epigenetic Immunomodulation Combined With CTLA-4 Blockade in Syngeneic Mouse Models. *Oncoimmunology* (2015) 4(8): e1019978. doi: 10.1080/2162402X.2015.1019978

92. Jones PA, Ohtani H, Chakravarthy A, De Carvalho DD. Epigenetic Therapy in Immune-Oncology. *Nat Rev Cancer* (2019) 19(3):151–61. doi: 10.1038/s41568-019-0109-9

93. Alexandrov LB, Nik-Zainal S, Wedge DC, Aparicio SA, Behjati S, Biankin AV, et al. Signatures of Mutational Processes in Human Cancer. *Nature* (2013) 500:415–21. doi: 10.1038/nature12477

94. Roberts SA, Gordenin DA. Hypermutation in Human Cancer Genomes: Footprints and Mechanisms. *Nat Rev Cancer* (2014) 14:786–800. doi: 10.1038/nrc3816

95. Kandoth C, McLellan MD, Vandin F, Ye K, Niu B, Lu C, et al. Mutational Landscape and Significance Across 12 Major Cancer Types. *Nature* (2013) 502(7471):333–9. doi: 10.1038/nature12634

96. Kane DP, Shcherbakova PV. A Common Cancer-Associated DNA Polymerase ε Mutation Causes an Exceptionally Strong Mutator Phenotype, Indicating Fidelity Defects Distinct From Loss of Proofreading. *Cancer Res* (2014) 74(7):1895–901. doi: 10.1158/0008-5472.CAN-13-2892

97. Campbell BB, Light N, Fabrizio D, Zatzman M, Fuligni F, de Borja R, et al. Comprehensive Analysis of Hypermutation in Human Cancer. *Cell* (2017) 171:1042–1056.e10. doi: 10.1016/j.cell.2017.09.048

98. Tumini E, Barroso S, Calero CP, Aguilera A. Roles of Human POLD1 and POLD3 in Genome Stability. *Sci Rep* (2016) 6:38873. doi: 10.1038/srep38873

99. Esteban-Jurado C, Giménez-Zaragoza D, Muñoz J, Franch-Expósito S, Álvarez-Barona M, Ocaña T, et al. POLE and POLD1 Screening in 155 Patients With Multiple Polyps and Early-Onset Colorectal Cancer. *Oncotarget* (2017) 8(16):26732–43. doi: 10.18632/oncotarget.15810

100. Rosner G, Gluck N, Carmi S, Bercovich D, Fliss-Issakov N, Ben-Yehoyada M, et al. POLD1 and POLE Gene Mutations in Jewish Cohorts of Early-Onset Colorectal Cancer and of Multiple Colorectal Adenomas. *Dis Colon Rectum* (2018) 61(9):1073–9. doi: 10.1097/DCR.0000000000001150

101. Nicolas E, Golemis EA, Arora S. Pold1: Central Mediator of DNA Replication and Repair, and Implication in Cancer and Other Pathologies. *Gene* (2016) 590(1):128–41. doi: 10.1016/j.gene.2016.06.031

102. Wang C, Gong J, Tu TY, Lee PP, Fakih M. Immune Profiling of Microsatellite Instability-High and Polymerase ε (POLE)-Mutated Metastatic Colorectal Tumors Identifies Predictors of Response to anti-PD-1 Therapy. *J Gastrointest Oncol* (2018) 9:404–15. doi: 10.21037/jgo.2018.01.09

103. Snyder A, Makarov V, Merghoub T, Yuan J, Zaretsky JM, Desrichard A, et al. Genetic Basis for Clinical Response to CTLA-4 Blockade in Melanoma. *N Engl J Med* (2014) 371:2189–99. doi: 10.1056/NEJMoa1406498

104. Yadav M, Jhunjhunwala S, Phung QT, Lupardus P, Tanguay J, Bumbaca S, et al. Predicting Immunogenic Tumor Mutations by Combining Mass Spectrometry and Exome Sequencing. *Nature* (2014) 515:572–6. doi: 10.1038/nature14001

105. Waalkes A, Smith N, Penewit K, Hempelmann J, Konnick EQ, Hause RJ, et al. Accurate Pan-Cancer Molecular Diagnosis of Microsatellite Instability by Single-Molecule Molecular Inversion Probe Capture and High-Throughput Sequencing. *Clin Chem* (2018) 64(6):950–8. doi: 10.1373/clinchem.2017.285981

106. Palmieri G, Colombino M, Cossu A, Marchetti A, Botti G, Ascierto PA. Genetic Instability and Increased Mutational Load: Which Diagnostic Tool Best Direct Patients With Cancer to Immunotherapy? *J Transl Med* (2017) 15(1):17. doi: 10.1186/s12967-017-1119-6

107. Palmieri G, Casula M, Manca A, Palomba G, Sini MC, Doneddu V, et al. Genetic Instability Markers in Cancer. *Methods Mol Biol* (2020) 2055:133–54. doi: 10.1007/978-1-4939-9773-2_6

108. Hugo W, Zaretsky JM, Sun L, Song C, Moreno BH, Hu-Lieskovan S, et al. Genomic and Transcriptomic Features of Response to anti-PD-1 Therapy in Metastatic Melanoma. *Cell* (2016) 165:35–44. doi: 10.1016/j.cell.2016.02.065

109. Zaretsky JM, Garcia-Diaz A, Shin DS, Escuin-Ordinas H, Hugo W, Hu-Lieskovan S, et al. Mutations Associated With Acquired Resistance to PD-1 Blockade in Melanoma. *N Engl J Med* (2016) 375:819–29. doi: 10.1056/NEJMoa1604958

110. Shin DS, Zaretsky JM, Escuin-Ordinas H, Garcia-Diaz A, Hu-Lieskovan S, Kalbasi A, et al. Primary Resistance to PD-1 Blockade Mediated by JAK1/2 Mutations. *Cancer Discovery* (2017) 7(2):188–201. doi: 10.1158/2159-8290.CD-16-1223

111. Passiglia F, Galvano A, Castiglia M, Incorvaia L, Calò V, Listì A, et al. Monitoring Blood Biomarkers to Predict Nivolumab Effectiveness in NSCLC Patients. *Ther Adv Med Oncol* (2019) 11. doi: 10.1177/1758835919839928

112. Guibert N, Jones G, Beeler JF, Plagnol V, Morris C, Mourlanette J, et al. Targeted Sequencing of Plasma Cell-Free DNA to Predict Response to PD1 Inhibitors in Advanced non-Small Cell Lung Cancer. *Lung Cancer* (2019) 137:1–6. doi: 10.1016/j.lungcan.2019.09.005

113. Tan L, Sandhu S, Lee RJ, Li J, Callahan J, Ftouni S, et al. Prediction and Monitoring of Relapse in Stage III Melanoma Using Circulating Tumor DNA. *Ann Oncol* (2019) 30(5):804–14. doi: 10.1093/annonc/mdz048

114. Lee JH, Saw RPM, Thompson JF, Lo S, Spillane AJ, Shannon KF, et al. Pre-Operative ctDNA Predicts Survival in High Risk Stage III Cutaneous Melanoma Patients. *Ann Oncol* (2019) 30(5):815–22. doi: 10.1093/annonc/mdz075

115. Santiago-Walker A, Gagnon R, Mazumdar J, Casey M, Long GV, Schadendorf D, et al. Correlation of BRAF Mutation Status in Circulating-Free DNA and Tumor and Association With Clinical Outcome Across Four BRAFi and MEKi Clinical Trials. *Clin Cancer Res* (2016) 22(3):567–74. doi: 10.1158/1078-0432.CCR-15-0321

116. Palmieri G. Circulating Driver Gene Mutations: What is the Impact on Melanoma Patients' Management? *Ann Oncol* (2019) 30:669–71. doi: 10.1093/annonc/mdz090

117. Kasi PM. Mutational Burden on Circulating Cell-Free tumor-DNA Testing as a Surrogate Marker of Mismatch Repair Deficiency or Microsatellite Instability in Patients With Colorectal Cancers. *J Gastrointest Oncol* (2017) 8:747–8. doi: 10.21037/jgo.2017.06.05

118. Barata P, Agarwal N, Nussenzveig R, Gerendash B, Jaeger E, Hatton W, et al. Clinical Activity of Pembrolizumab in Metastatic Prostate Cancer With Microsatellite Instability High (MSI-H) Detected by Circulating Tumor DNA. *J Immunother Cancer* (2020) 8(2):e001065. doi: 10.1136/jitc-2020-001065

119. Chen EX, Jonker DJ, Loree JM, Kennecke HF, Berry SR, Couture F, et al. Effect of Combined Immune Checkpoint Inhibition vs Best Supportive Care Alone in Patients With Advanced Colorectal Cancer: The Canadian Cancer Trials Group Co.26 Study. *JAMA Oncol* (2020) 6(6):831–8. doi: 10.1001/jamaoncol.2020.0910

120. Cai Z, Wang Z, Liu C, Shi D, Li D, Zheng M, et al. Detection of Microsatellite Instability From Circulating Tumor DNA by Targeted Deep Sequencing. *J Mol Diagn* (2020) 22(7):860–70. doi: 10.1016/j.jmoldx.2020.04.210

18

Correlation between *In Vivo* Reflectance Confocal Microscopy and Horizontal Histopathology in Skin Cancer

Giuseppe Broggi[1], Anna Elisa Verzì[2], Rosario Caltabiano[1*], Giuseppe Micali[2] and Francesco Lacarrubba[2]

[1] Department of Medical, Surgical Sciences and Advanced Technologies "G.F. Ingrassia", Anatomic Pathology, University of Catania, Catania, Italy, [2] Dermatology Clinic, University of Catania, Catania, Italy

Correspondence:
Rosario Caltabiano
rosario.caltabiano@unict.it

In dermatopathological daily practice, vertical histopathology sections are classically used to analyze skin biopsies. Conversely, horizontal histopathological sections are currently used for the diagnosis of some types of alopecia. In the last years the morphological findings obtained by horizontal histopathology have been correlated to those obtained by *in vivo* reflectance confocal microscopy which provides the same "point of view" of the skin. This review paper emphasizes the strong matching and correlation between reflectance confocal microscopy images and horizontal histopathology in cutaneous neoplasms, further demonstrating the strong reliability of this innovative, non-invasive technique in the management of skin tumors.

Keywords: horizontal histopathology, reflectance confocal microscopy, skin cancer, correlation, horizontal histopathological sections

INTRODUCTION

One of the major application fields of dermatological research has always been the identification of new diagnostic tools capable of improving the diagnostic precocity and accuracy of skin neoplasms (1, 2). In the last decade, *in vivo* reflectance confocal microscopy (RCM) is gradually establishing itself as a non-invasive diagnostic technique for several skin diseases, being able to provide a horizontal high-resolution "point of view" of the skin, from the stratum corneum to the papillary dermis; horizontal skin images up to a 250 μm of maximum depth may be studied through this technique (3–6). The use of RCM in the diagnostic approach to many inflammatory and neoplastic skin diseases is still increasing, representing one of the major diagnostic aids in the dermatological clinical practice (7). However, the horizontal "point of view" provided by RCM does not allow an optimal correlation with classical histopathology that, as known, produces a full-thickness vertical overview of the skin (8, 9). Instead, horizontal histological sections (HHSs) allow a better correlation as they reflect the same skin plane observed by RCM (10).

The possibility of optimally comparing horizontal histopathology and RCM images represents a relatively new trend, and quite a few papers have been published in this field regarding both inflammatory and neoplastic disorders (11–17). The purpose of this review paper is to establish the "state of the art" on RCM and HHS findings in skin tumors, emphasizing how well horizontal histopathology reflects the images provided by RCM.

SQUAMOUS CELL CARCINOMA *IN SITU* (BOWEN'S DISEASE)

Squamous cell carcinoma *in situ* (SCCis) represents the earliest and non-invasive form of squamous cell carcinoma, in which, by definition, the neoplastic cells do not infiltrate the basement membrane and therefore lack distant metastatic potential (14). SCCis mainly affects photoexposed skin of elderly, and the head and neck are the most commonly affected sites (14). Clinically, SCCis arises in the form of flat/raised, reddish/brownish in color, often scaly, papules or plaques; due to the low specificity of the clinical presentation, further non-invasive diagnostic tools, such as dermoscopy and RCM, are often required to enhance the diagnostic accuracy of SCCis (14, 18). The detection of "red dots", representing glomerular vessels in the superficial dermis, is the most typical dermoscopic finding of SCCis (18). In addition, RCM has been also validated as useful diagnostic tool and its application in the dermatological practice has been supported by

the perfect matching with HHS found by our research group (14). SCCis shows the following RCM features (14) (**Figures 1A, C**): i) at the level of stratum corneum, highly refractive amorphous structures and sporadically polygonal, nucleated cells; ii) at the level of the stratum granulosum/spinosum, marked architectural disarray, consisting of keratinocytes highly variable in size, shape, and nuclear morphology; scattered bright dendritic cells may also be found; iii) at the level of the dermoepidermal junction, large rounded dark areas, corresponding to enlarged dermal papillae. Horizontal histopathology perfectly matches with the previous reported RCM findings (14) (**Figures 1B, D**): hyperkeratosis and parakeratosis are the histopathological causes of the refractive amorphous structures and the nucleated cells observed in the stratum corneum at RCM; the loss of architectural array visible in the stratum granulosum/spinosum at RCM reflects the presence of atypical keratinocytes with nuclei of variable size and shape along the entire thickness of epidermis; some S-100 positive, CD1a negative and Melan-A negative dendritic cells may be occasionally found scattered among the neoplastic cells; lastly, at the dermoepidermal junction, HHSs show enlarged dermal papillae containing glomeruloid capillary vessels, corresponding both to the rounded dark areas and to the "red

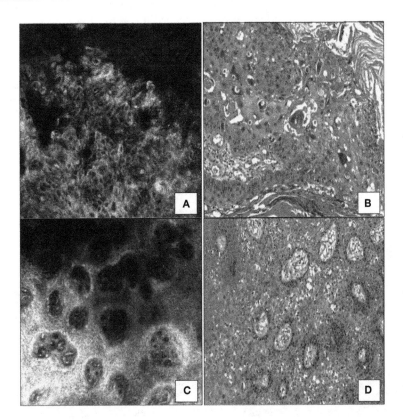

FIGURE 1 | Squamous cell carcinoma *in situ*. **(A)** RCM image at the stratum spinosum showing a marked loss of the normal honeycomb pattern (architectural disarray) due to the presence of markedly variable size, shape, and nuclear morphology keratinocytes. **(B)** Horizontal histopathology at the same level revealing neoplastic keratinocytes with high-grade nuclear atypia (hematoxylin and eosin; original magnification 400×). **(C)** RCM image at the dermoepidermal junction showing dilated blood vessels within enlarged edged dermal papillae. **(D)** Horizontal histopathology at the same level confirming the RCM finding (hematoxylin and eosin; original magnification 100×).

dots" observed at RCM and dermoscopy, respectively. Since the horizontal histopathology does not allow to evaluate the possible presence of dermal invasion, the concept that its use is only for the purpose of comparing it with the RCM findings, in order to further validate the diagnostic use of RCM, must be emphasized.

MYCOSIS FUNGOIDES WITH PATCH LESIONS

Mycosis fungoides (MF) is the most frequent T-cell lymphoma of the skin and seems pathogenetically related to a monoclonal T-cell receptor (TCR) gene rearrangement, leading to a monoclonal proliferation of cutaneous CD4-positive T lymphocytes (19, 20). Clinically, MF exhibits a higher predilection for dark skin (2:1) males (2:1) and, in its classical form, presents a slow-growing clinical course with a progressive shift from patches to plaques and, in final stages, tumors (19, 20). A variable combination of patches, plaques and tumors is frequently observed in MF with tumor lesions (20). Both clinical presentation and histopathology of MF are often non-specific, especially when it occurs in the form of patchy lesions, to such an extent that multiple biopsies are often necessary to obtain a definitive diagnosis (19, 21). RCM may improve the diagnostic accuracy of MF (13, 22, 23). In the upper portion of epidermis, epidermal disarray with disruption of the normal "honeycomb" appearance and sometimes hyporefractive areas, combined to the detection of small sized bright cells interspersed within epidermal layers are usually identifiable with RCM (13) (**Figure 2A**); the same bright cells are found at the dermoepidermal junction both inside and around dermal papillae, visible as round darker areas (13). RCM features of MF perfectly match with HHS (13): the presence of spongiosis, epidermotropic CD4-positive lymphocytes (**Figures 2B, C**) forming Pautrier's microabscesses and band-like distributed CD4-positive lymphocytes at dermoepidermal junction are the histopathological "mirror" of what is detectable with RCM. In

addition, the differential diagnosis with eczematous disorders can become more straightforward using RCM (13), that shows in the stratum spinosum widespread round, deeply dark areas, intercellular spaces and few mildly bright cells: these findings are confirmed by horizontal histopathology, displaying marked spongiotic features combined to a less conspicuous lymphocytic exocytosis than MF (13).

ECCRINE POROMA

Eccrine poroma (EP) is a sweat gland derived adnexal tumor, first described by Pinkus in 1956 (24), that clinically arises as a slow-growing, sometimes ulcerated, reddish, and firm in consistency nodule, mostly located to the acral regions (25, 26). Usually, EP has a benign clinical course, even if a malignant counterpart, called "porocarcinoma" and characterized by low distant metastatic potential, has been also described (27). EP usually occurs on photodamaged skin, mimicking cutaneous malignancies, such as basal cell carcinoma (BCC), squamous cell carcinoma (SCC) or malignant melanoma (MM) (25, 26). Although the definitive diagnosis of EP is still based on conventional histopathology, non-invasive techniques, including dermoscopy and RCM, allow ruling out malignant conditions, and to suspect a benign adnexal neoplasm (28, 29). Dermoscopically, EP usually presents milky red areas at the periphery of the lesion and a polymorphous vascular pattern in the center, including glomerular, flower-like and dotted vessels (30). RCM shows a uniformly well-circumscribed neoplasm, consisting of hyper-reflective clusters surrounded by a darker stromal component (28, 30). Neoplastic cells are bright and homogeneous in size and shape, with round and dark nuclei, and may be arranged around non-reflective rounded areas (28, 30). Deeper sections show a richly vascularized stroma intermingled with tumor nests (28, 30). RCM images of EP correspond well with HHS (28, 30): neoplastic cells are monomorphic, cuboid-shaped, arranged in

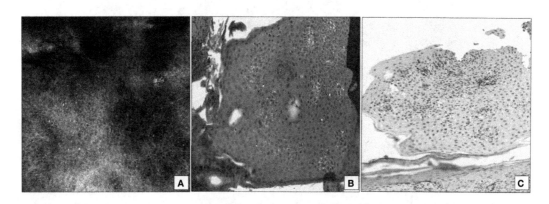

FIGURE 2 | Mycosis fungoides with patch lesions. **(A)** RCM at the stratum spinosum revealing a diffuse epidermal disarray with scattered small hyperreflective cells (epidermotropic lymphocytes). **(B)** Horizontal histopathology at the same level showing the presence of lymphocyte epidermotropism (hematoxylin and eosin; original magnification 400×). **(C)** Immunohistochemical staining for CD4 revealing the CD4-positive phenotype of epidermotropic T-lymphocytes (immunoperoxidase staining; original magnification 350×).

basaloid nests and occasionally forming round/slit-like ducts with eosinophilic material inside; these ducts strongly match with the non-reflective round dark areas visible with RCM and represent foci of ductal differentiation of EP. Bright uniformly shaped and sized cells interspersed within the tumor island or scattered in the upper dermis are often present at RCM in the pigmented variant of EP (28); these cells histologically correspond to melanocytes and melanophages, respectively. The presence of melanocytes in pigmented EP makes the differential diagnosis with MM mandatory: neoplastic melanocytes in MM are usually more irregularly shaped/ denditric or fusiform than those observed in pigmented EP (31, 32).

DISSEMINATED SUPERFICIAL ACTINIC POROKERATOSIS

Disseminated superficial actinic porokeratosis (DSAP) represents the most frequent variant of porokeratosis. It clinically presents as multiple scaly macules with a whitish central area surrounded by a slightly raised rim that mainly occurs on photoexposed regions (33). Dermoscopy frequently shows a double free edged scaly rim, whitish in color, representing the dermoscopic equivalent of the cornoid lamella, that is the histopathological hallmark of porokeratosis (34, 35). RCM may be useful in the diagnostic approach to DSAP, and its finding has been validated on the basis of the correlation with HHS (36). At RCM, architectural disarray with loss of the normal "honeycomb" pattern is observed in the center of the lesion (36); proceeding towards the periphery, a less refractile destructured area, containing more refractile amorphous substance (cornoid lamella) and surrounded by normal skin with regular "honeycomb" array, is found (36). HHS strongly matches with these RCM features and shows columns of parakeratosis

(cornoid lamella) combined with moderately atypical keratinocytes (36).

SOLITARY MASTOCYTOMA

The term "mastocytosis" includes a wide spectrum of diseases caused by a clonal proliferation of mast cell and affecting simultaneously or at different times several organs, including the skin, bone marrow, liver, spleen, and lymphatic system (37). Based on the involved organs, the World Health Organization identifies two different variants of mastocytosis: cutaneous mastocytosis, if the disease exclusively affects the skin, and systemic mastocytosis, if there are other organs affected, regardless of the skin. Furthermore, cutaneous mastocytosis may be clinically further subdivided into maculo-papular cutaneous mastocytosis, diffuse cutaneous mastocytosis, and cutaneous mastocytoma (38). The latter includes not only the cases when there is a single cutaneous lesion (solitary mastocytoma; SM), but also those in which up to three skin lesions are seen (38). Clinical presentation of SM is variable and ranges from brownish/reddish macules to papules, plaques and nodules, showing swelling spontaneously or after rubbing (Darier's sign). Zhang et al. (39) first described RCM findings of mastocytosis in a huge group of 200 patients, including all different clinical presentation; regardless of the specific variant examined; all cases showed similar RCM features: the absence of aggregates of bright element in the context of finely granular and edematous papillary dermis was a constant finding. Following these results, our group first described more specific RCM features of SM and correlated them with HSS for validation (15): in particular, the presence of enlarged dermal papillae, containing tortuous vessels and large, uniformly round-shaped, bright cells at the level of dermoepidermal junction (**Figure 3A**) perfectly matched with the finding of aggregates of round, CD117-positive mastocytes with granular cytoplasm located to dermal papillae on HHS (**Figure 3B**).

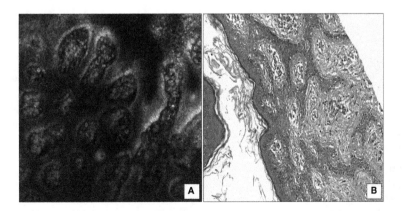

FIGURE 3 | Solitary mastocytoma. **(A)** RCM at the level of dermoepidermal junction showing multiple, large and rounded bright cells within dilated dermal papillae. **(B)** Horizontal histopathology at the same level revealing the presence of round mastocytes with pale and granular cytoplasm within dermal papillae (hematoxylin and eosin; original magnification 150×).

TABLE 1 | Correlation between reflectance confocal microscopy and horizontal histopathology in skin tumors: summary.

	Depth	RCM	HHS
SCCis (14)	Stratum Corneum Stratum granulosum/ spinosum	- Hyperrefractive amorphous structures - Polygonal, nucleated cells - Architectural disarray - Bright dendritic cells	- Hyperkeratosis - Parakeratosis - Large atypical keratinocytes - Langerhans cells (S-100 +, CD1a+, Melan-A -)
	Dermoepidermal junction	- Enlarged edged papillae with widened dermal papillae - Tortuouscapillary vessels	- Enlarged papillae with widened dermal papillae - Tortuouscapillary vessels
MF (13)	Upper epidermis	- Darker spots compared to the surrounding epidermis. - Epidermal disarray and presence of small bright cells	- Spongiosis - CD4-positive T-cellepidermotropism
	Dermoepidermal junction	- Small bright cells scattered within and among roundish hyporefractive areas (dermal papillae)	- CD4-positive lymphocytes infiltrating dermal papillae
EP (28, 30)	Epidermis	- Clusters of small, hyperrefractive and uniformly shaped cells with round dark nuclei surrounded by keratin - Parakeratosis	- Monomorphic basophilic neoplastic cells with large and round nuclei surrounded by amorphic keratin - Parakeratosis
	Dermis	- Larger and confluent cell clusters embedded in a denser and highly vascularized stroma- Neoplastic clusters arranged around darker hyporefractive rounded areas- Presence of bright, uniformly shaped and sized cells interspersed within tumor island or scattered in the upper dermis (pigmented variant)	- Increased tumor volume and denser and more vascularized stromal compartment - Intratumoral round or slit-like areas filled with eosinophilic substance (spots of ductal differentiation) - Intratumoral melanocytes or melanophages (pigmented variant)
DSAP (36)	Epidermis	- Architectural disarray with loss of the normal "honeycomb" pattern (central zone) - Hyperrefractive amorphous material (cornoid lamella) within hyporefractivedestructured areas, surrounded by skin with regular "honeycomb" pattern (peripheral zone)	- Columns of parakeratosis (cornoid lamella) combined with moderately atypical keratinocytes
SM (15)	Dermoepidermal junction	- Tortuous vessels and large, uniformly round-shaped, bright cells within enlarged dermal papillae	- Dermal papillae containing aggregates of round, CD117-positive mastocytes with granular cytoplasm
MTs (16, 17)	Dermoepidermal junction	- Atypical pigment network: proliferation of bright dendritic cells, forming "bridge" from epidermis to the superficial dermis (*in situ* melanoma) - Atypical pigment network: atypical nests of rounded and spindled hyperreflective melanocytes combined to an architectural disarray of dermal papillae and some bright cells or small dots within dermal papillae (*in situ* melanoma) - Hair follicles surrounded by multiple dendritic bright melanocytes and layers of keratinocytes filled at the periphery with rounded/ elongated hyperreflective melanocytes (lentigo maligna).	- Presence of atypical Melan-A-positive melanocytes surrounding dermal papillae and bulging into dermis (*in situ* melanoma) - Atypical melanocytes arranged in nests and presence of lymphocytes within dermal papillae (*in situ* melanoma) - Heavily pigmented keratinocytes of the basal layer of the epidermis combined with an increased number of junctional melanocytes (lentigo maligna).
	Upperdermis	- Dermoscopic globules: small nests of monomorphous non-atypical bright melanocytes non connected with epithelium in nevi and larger nests of pleomorphic neoplastic melanocytes in melanomas - Non-atypical peripheral pseudopods	- Small nests of non-atypical melanocytes in nevi and larger clusters of atypical neoplastic melanocytes in melanomas - peripheral confluent clusters of pigmented neoplastic melanocytes

RCM, reflectance confocal microscopy; HHS, horizontal histopathological section; SCCis, squamous cell carcinoma in situ; MF, mycosis fungoides; EP, eccrine poroma; DSAP, disseminated superficial actinic porokeratosis; SM, solitary mastocytoma; MTs, melanocytic tumours.

MELANOCYTIC TUMORS

While the introduction of dermoscopy has definitely represented a turning point in the diagnostic accuracy of melanocytic tumors, allowing the detection of some architectural patterns corresponding to specific histopathological features, in recent years RCM has emerged as a valid tool capable of providing architectural and morphological information at the cellular level (40–42); in particular, the combined use of dermoscopy and RCM proved to increase the accuracy for facial tumor detection, compared with RCM alone (43).

Braga et al. (17) compared RCM findings of melanocytic tumors and HHS. They selected four MMs and two benign nevi and compared specific dermoscopic patterns of cutaneous MM such as pigment network, irregular globules and pseudopods, and their benign counterparts, detectable in nevi, to RCM findings and both

vertical and horizontal histopathology. Regarding the pigment network, two melanomas showed two different types of atypical network: the first MM presented on RCM a proliferation of bright dendritic cells at the level of dermoepidermal junction, some of them protruding from the epidermis to the superficial dermis to form "bridges"; conventional vertical histopathology revealed an *in situ* melanoma, and HHS showed the same features observed on RCM, confirming the presence of many atypical Melan-A-positive melanocytes surrounding dermal papillae and bulging into dermis. RCM of the second MM with an atypical pigmented network showed at dermoepidermal junction atypical nests of both rounded and elongated hyperreflective melanocytes combined to an architectural disarray of dermal papillae and some bright cells or small dots within dermal papillae; vertical histopathology revealed an *in situ* melanoma, and RCM findings were confirmed by HHS showing pleomorphic melanocytes arranged in nests and presence of lymphocytes within dermal papillae. Based of RCM, Braga et al. (17) were also able to discriminate dermoscopic globules in nevi and melanomas on the basis of morphological atypia: both RCM and HHS showed small nests of monomorphous non-atypical bright melanocytes non-connected with epithelium in nevi and larger nests of pleomorphic neoplastic melanocytes in MMs. Lastly, pseudopods were not characterized by morphological atypia on RCM, corresponding to peripherally visible, confluent clusters of pigmented neoplastic melanocytes on horizontal histopathology. Navarrete-Dechent et al. (16) also matched the dermoscopic sign "circle within a circle" of lentigo maligna (presence of pigmentation within and around hair follicles) with its RCM and HHS: RCM revealed the presence of hair follicles surrounded by numerous dendritic bright melanocytes and layers of keratinocytes filled at the periphery with rounded/elongated hyperreflective melanocytes. HHS strongly overlapped with RCM, showing a high pigmentation of the keratinocytes of the basal layer of the epidermis combined with an increased number of junctional melanocytes.

As previously mentioned regarding SCCis, also for melanocytic tumors, the use of horizontal histopathology has only the purpose of validating the RCM application in clinical practice without replacing conventional histopathology as diagnostic gold standard.

DISCUSSION

In dermatology, the majority of skin specimens from biopsy or surgical procedures is analyzed using classical vertical histopathological sections, which represents the diagnostic gold standard. Horizontal histopathology is currently used for the diagnosis of some types of alopecia allowing a more correct visualization of follicular and perifollicular features (44).

More recently, HHS has been used to correlate with the morphological features obtained by RCM which provides the same transversal "point of view" of the skin. In particular, the strong matching and correlation between RCM images and HHS in skin tumors (**Table 1**), as shown in this review, further demonstrates the reliability of this innovative, non-invasive technique in the management of skin tumors. Based on such correlations, some considerations can be made: in SCCis and melanoma RCM may confirm the clinical suspect addressing the correct therapeutic approach; in clinically atypical SM, RCM evaluation may avoid biopsy or excision as it is generally self-resolving; in MF and DSAP, RCM is particularly useful for the selection of the best site for biopsy thus avoiding multiple biopsies often quite bothersome for the patient; a further application of RCM in skin tumors may consist in the early recognition of local recurrences after medical or surgical treatments of the disease (14).

AUTHOR CONTRIBUTIONS

All authors listed have made a substantial, direct and intellectual contribution to the work, and approved it for publication.

REFERENCES

1. Pehamberger H, Steiner A, Wolff K. In vivo epiluminescence microscopy of pigmented skin lesions. I. Pattern analysis of pigmented skin lesions. *J A m Acad Dermatol* (1987) 17:571–83. doi: 10.1016/s0190-9622(87)70239-4

2. Argenziano G, Soyer HP, Chimenti S, Talamini R, Corona R, Sera F, et al. Dermoscopy of pigmented skin lesions: results of a consensus meeting *via the Internet. J Am Acad Dermatol* (2003) 48:679–93. doi: 10.1067/mjd.2003.281

3. Ardigo M, Agozzino M, Franceschini C, Lacarrubba F. Reflectance Confocal Microscopy Algorithms for Inflammatory and Hair Diseases. *Dermatol Clin* (2016) 34:487–96. doi: 10.1016/j.det.2016.05.011

4. Lacarrubba F, Verzì AE, Pippione M, Micali G. Reflectance confocal microscopy in the diagnosis of vesicobullous disorders: case series with pathologic and cytologic correlation and literature review. *Skin Res Technol* (2016) 22:479–86. doi: 10.1111/srt.12289

5. Lacarrubba F, Boscaglia S, Nasca MR, Caltabiano R, Micali G. Grover's disease: dermoscopy, reflectance confocal microscopy and histopathological correlation. *Dermatol Pract Concept* (2017) 7:51–4. doi: 10.5826/dpc.0703a11

6. Lacarrubba F, Verzì AE, Ardigò M, Micali G. Handheld reflectance confocal microscopy for the diagnosis of molluscum contagiosum: histopathology and dermoscopy correlation. *Australas J Dermatol* (2017) 58:e123–5. doi: 10.1111/ajd.12511

7. Guitera P, Menzies SW, Longo C, Cesinaro AM, Scolyer RA, Pellacani G. In vivo confocal microscopy for diagnosis of melanoma and basal cell carcinoma using a two-step method: analysis of 710 consecutive clinically equivocal cases. *J Invest Dermatol* (2012) 132:2386–94. doi: 10.1038/jid.2012.172

8. Pellacani G, Longo C, Malvehy J, Puig S, Carrera C, Segura S, et al. In vivo confocal microscopic and histopathologic correlations of dermoscopic features in 202 melanocytic lesions. *Arch Dermatol* (2008) 144:1597–608. doi: 10.1001/archderm.144.12.1597

9. Soyer HP, Kenet RO, Wolf IH, Kenet BJ, Cerroni L. Clinicopathological correlation of pigmented skin lesions using dermoscopy. *Eur J Dermatol* (2000) 10:22–8.

10. Rezze GG, Scramim AP, Neves RI, Landman G. Structural correlations between dermoscopic features of cutaneous melanomas and histopathology using transverse sections. *Am J Dermatopathol* (2006) 28:13–20. doi: 10.1097/01.dad.0000181545.89077.8c

11. Verzì AE, Lacarrubba F, Caltabiano R, Broggi G, Musumeci ML, Micali G. Reflectance Confocal Microscopy Features of Plaque Psoriasis Overlap With Horizontal Histopathological Sections: A Case Series. *Am J Dermatopathol* (2019) 41:355–7. doi: 10.1097/DAD.0000000000001297

12. Lacarrubba F, Verzì AE, Caltabiano R, Broggi G, Di Natale A, Micali G. Discoid lupus erythematosus: Reflectance confocal microscopy features correlate with horizontal histopathological sections. *Skin Res Technol* (2019) 25:242–4. doi: 10.1111/srt.12636

13. Broggi G, Lacarrubba F, Verzì AE, Micali G, Caltabiano R. Confocal microscopy features of patch-stage mycosis fungoides and their correlation with horizontal histopathological sections. A Case Series. *J Cutan Pathol* (2019) 46:163–5. doi: 10.1111/cup.13384

14. Broggi G, Verzì AE, Lacarrubba F, Caltabiano R, Di Natale A, Micali G. Correlation between reflectance confocal microscopy features and horizontal histopathology in cutaneous squamous cell carcinoma in situ: A case series. *J Cutan Pathol* (2020) 47:777–80. doi: 10.1111/cup.13708

15. Verzì AE, Lacarrubba F, Caltabiano R, Dinotta F, Micali G. Reflectance confocal microscopy of solitary mastocytoma and correlation with horizontal histopathological sections. *Skin Res Technol* (2020). doi: 10.1111/srt.12902

16. Navarrete-Dechent C, Liopyris K, Cordova M, Busam KJ, Marghoob AA, Chen CJ. Reflectance Confocal Microscopic and En Face Histopathologic Correlation of the Dermoscopic "Circle Within a Circle" in Lentigo Maligna. *JAMA Dermatol* (2018) 154:1092–4. doi: 10.1001/jamadermatol.2018.2216

17. Braga JC, Macedo MP, Pinto C, Duprat J, Begnami MD, Pellacani G, et al. Learning reflectance confocal microscopy of melanocytic skin lesions through histopathologic transversal sections. *PLoS One* (2013) 8:e81205. doi: 10.1371/journal.pone.0081205

18. Ianoşi SL, Batani A, Ilie MA, Tampa M, Georgescu SR, Zurac S, et al. Non-invasive imaging techniques for the *in vivo* diagnosis of Bowen's disease: Three case reports. *Oncol Lett* (2019) 17:4094–101. doi: 10.3892/ol.2019.10079

19. Ahn CS, ALSayyah A, Sangüeza OP. Mycosis fungoides: an updated review of clinicopathologic variants. *Am J Dermatopathol* (2014) 36:933–48; quiz 949–51. doi: 10.1097/DAD.0000000000000207

20. Cerroni L. Mycosis fungoides-clinical and histopathologic features, differential diagnosis, and treatment. *Semin Cutan Med Surg* (2018) 37:2–10. doi: 10.12788/j.sder.2018.002

21. Mancebo SE, Cordova M, Myskowski PL, Flores ES, Busam K, Jawed SI, et al. Reflectance confocal microscopy features of mycosis fungoides and Sézary syndrome: correlation with histopathologic and T-cell receptor rearrangement studies. *J Cutan Pathol* (2016) 43:505–15. doi: 10.1111/cup.12708

22. Li W, Dai H, Li Z, Xu AE. Reflectance confocal microscopy for the characterization of mycosis fungoides and correlation with histology: a pilot study. *Skin Res Technol* (2013) 19:352–5. doi: 10.1111/srt.12049

23. Lacarrubba F, Ardigò M, Di Stefani A, Verzì AE, Micali G. Dermatoscopy and Reflectance Confocal Microscopy Correlations in Nonmelanocytic Disorders. *Dermatol Clin* (2018) 36:487–501. doi: 10.1016/j.det.2018.05.015

24. Goldman P, Pinkus H, Rogin JR. Eccrine poroma; tumours exhibiting features of the epidermal sweat duct unit. *AMA Arch Derm* (1956) 74:511–21. doi: 10.1001/archderm.1956.01550110055013

25. Chessa MA, Patrizi A, Baraldi C, Fanti PA, Barisani A, Vaccari S. Dermoscopic-Histopathological Correlation of Eccrine Poroma: An Observational Study. *Dermatol Pract Concept* (2019) 9:283–91. doi: 10.5826/dpc.0904a07

26. Ferrari A, Buccini P, Silipo V, De Simone P, Mariani G, Marenda S, et al. Eccrine poroma: a clinical-dermoscopic study of seven cases. *Acta Derm Venereol* (2009) 89:160–4. doi: 10.2340/00015555-0608

27. Parra O, Kerr DA, Bridge JA, Loehrer AP, Linos K. A case of YAP1 and NUTM1 rearranged porocarcinoma with corresponding immunohistochemical expression: Review of recent advances in poroma and porocarcinoma pathogenesis with potential diagnostic utility. *J Cutan Pathol* (2020) 48:95–101. doi: 10.1111/cup.13832

28. Tachihara R, Choi C, Langley RG, Anderson RR, González S. In vivo confocal imaging of pigmented eccrine poroma. *Dermatology* (2002) 204:185–9. doi: 10.1159/000057879

29. Moscarella E, Zalaudek I, Agozzino M, Vega H, Cota C, Catricalà C, et al. Reflectance confocal microscopy for the evaluation of solitary red nodules. *Dermatology* (2012) 224:295–300. doi: 10.1159/000339339

30. Schirra A, Kogut M, Hadaschik E, Enk AH, Haenssle HA. Eccrine poroma: correlation of reflectance confocal microscopy and histopathology of

horizontal sections. *J Eur Acad Dermatol Venereol* (2016) 30:e167–9. doi: 10.1111/jdv.13473

31. Langley RG, Rajadhyaksha M, Dwyer PJ, Sober AJ, Flotte TJ, Anderson RR. Confocal scanning laser microscopy of benign and malignant melanocytic skin lesions *in vivo*. *J Am Acad Dermatol* (2001) 45:365–76. doi: 10.1067/mjd.2001.117395

32. Busam KJ, Hester K, Charles C, Sachs DL, Antonescu CR, Gonzalez S, et al. Detection of clinically amelanotic malignant melanoma and assessment of its margins by *in vivo* confocal scanning laser microscopy. *Arch Dermatol* (2001) 137:923–9.

33. Gu CY, Zhang CF, Chen LJ, Xiang LH, Zheng ZZ. Clinical analysis and etiology of porokeratosis. *Exp Ther Med* (2014) 8:737–41. doi: 10.3892/etm.2014.1803

34. Errichetti E, Zalaudek I, Kittler H, Apalla Z, Argenziano G, Bakos R, et al. Standardization of dermoscopic terminology and basic dermoscopic parameters to evaluate in general dermatology (non-neoplastic dermatoses): an expert consensus on behalf of the International Dermoscopy Society. *Br J Dermatol* (2020) 182:454–67. doi: 10.1111/bjd.18125

35. Zaballos P, Puig S, Malvehy J. Dermoscopy of disseminated superficial actinic porokeratosis. *Arch Dermatol* (2004) 140:1410. doi: 10.1001/archderm.140.11.1410

36. Mazzeo M, Longo C, Manfreda V, Piana S, Bianchi L, Pellacani G, et al. Looking horizontally at disseminated superficial actinic porokeratosis: Correlations between in-vivo reflectance confocal microscopy and histopathology. *Skin Res Technol* (2020) 26:443–4. doi: 10.1111/srt.12802

37. Leung AKC, Lam JM, Leong KF. Childhood Solitary Cutaneous Mastocytoma: Clinical Manifestations, Diagnosis, Evaluation, and Management. *Curr Pediatr Rev* (2019) 15:42–6. doi: 10.2174/1573396315666181120163952

38. Matito A, Azaña JM, Torrelo A, Alvarez-Twose I. Cutaneous Mastocytosis in Adults and Children: New Classification and Prognostic Factors. *Immunol Allergy Clin North Am* (2018) 38:351–63. doi: 10.1016/j.iac.2018.04.001

39. Zhang G, Chen J, Liu X, Wang X. Concordance of reflectance confocal microscopy with histopathology in the diagnosis of mastocytosis: A prospective study. *Skin Res Technol* (2020) 26:319–21. doi: 10.1111/srt.12779

40. Longo C, Zalaudek I, Argenziano G, Pellacani G. New directions in dermatopathology: *in vivo* confocal microscopy in clinical practice. *Dermatol Clin* (2012) 30:799–814, viii. doi: 10.1016/j.det.2012.06.012

41. Scope A, Gill M, Benvenuto-Andrade C, Halpern AC, Gonzalez S, Marghoob AA. Correlation of dermoscopy with *in vivo* reflectance confocal microscopy of streaks in melanocytic lesions. *Arch Dermatol* (2007) 143:727–34. doi: 10.1001/archderm.143.6.727

42. Scope A, Benvenuto-Andrade C, Agero AL, Malvehy J, Puig S, Rajadhyaksha M, et al. In vivo reflectance confocal microscopy imaging of melanocytic skin lesions: consensus terminology glossary and illustrative images. *J Am Acad Dermatol* (2007) 57:644–58. doi: 10.1016/j.jaad.2007.05.044

43. Cinotti E, Fiorani D, Labeille B, Gonzalez S, Debarbieux S, Agozzino M, et al. The integration of dermoscopy and reflectance confocal microscopy improves the diagnosis of lentigo maligna. *J Eur Acad Dermatol Venereol* (2019) 33: e372–4. doi: 10.1111/jdv.15669

44. Palo S, Biligi DS. Utility of horizontal and vertical sections of scalp biopsies in various forms of primary alopecias. *J Lab Phys* (2018) 10:95–100. doi: 10.4103/JLP.JLP_4_17

19

Immune Checkpoint Inhibitor Induced Pericarditis and Encephalitis in a Patient Treated With Ipilimumab and Nivolumab for Metastatic Melanoma

Jorja Braden[1]* and Jenny H. Lee[1,2]

[1] Department of Medical Oncology, Chris O'Brien Lifehouse, Sydney, NSW, Australia, [2] Department of Biomedical Sciences, Macquarie University, Sydney, NSW, Australia

*Correspondence:
Jorja Braden
jorja.braden@melanoma.org.au

Immune checkpoint inhibitors (ICIs) have dramatically improved outcomes in melanoma. Common ICI toxicities have become familiar to clinicians; however, rare delayed toxicities remain challenging given the paucity of data with such presentations. We present the unique case of a 61-year-old with metastatic melanoma with two rare, delayed ICI-induced toxicities. After resection of a large symptomatic parietal metastases, this patient received two doses of combination ipilimumab and nivolumab. Five weeks following his second dose, he developed ICI-induced pericarditis with associated pericardial effusion and early signs of tamponade. Corticosteroids were not administered due to a concurrent cerebral abscess. Administration of colchicine, ibuprofen, judicious monitoring, and cessation of immunotherapy led to the complete resolution of the effusion over several weeks. Seven months following his last dose of immunotherapy, the patient developed ICI-associated grade four autoimmune encephalitis, presenting as status epilepticus. High-dose steroid initiation led to rapid clinical improvement. The patient remains in near-complete response on imaging with no recurrence of pericardial effusion and partial resolution of neurological symptoms. ICI-induced pericardial disease and encephalitis carry substantial mortality rates and prompt diagnosis and management is critical. Clinicians must therefore remain vigilant for these rare toxicities regardless of duration of drug exposure or time since cessation of therapy.

Keywords: immunotherapy, melanoma, immune-related adverse effects, pericarditis, encephalitis, delayed immune reaction

INTRODUCTION

The combination of immune checkpoint inhibitors (ICIs) ipilimumab and nivolumab have drastically improved outcomes for advanced melanoma patients with 5-year survival rates of 52% (1). This comes at the cost of increased rates of ICI-induced toxicities. The combination is associated with higher rates of a broad range of ICI-induced toxicities when compared to single-agent checkpoint inhibition, contributing to higher morbidity and mortality in these patients (1, 2). Severe ICI-induced pericarditis and encephalitis are exceedingly rare clinical entities accounting for far less than 1% of ICI toxicities and delayed events increase the rarity of such cases. With a paucity of data and a range of presentations, diagnosis and management remain a significant challenge. We report the case of a patient with two sequential rare ICI-associated toxicities of grade 3 pericarditis and grade 4 encephalitis presenting 1.5 months and 7.5 months after brief exposure to ipilimumab and nivolumab treatment for metastatic melanoma.

CASE PRESENTATION

A 61-year-old male was diagnosed with *de novo* metastatic melanoma in January 2020 after presenting with sudden onset left upper limb dyspraxia and confusion. Comorbidities included hemochromatosis and a distant history of meningococcal meningitis. Magnetic resonance imaging (MRI) brain demonstrated a large right parietal lesion. Computed tomography (CT) and positron emission tomography (PET) scan revealed left upper and lower lobe lung lesions, solitary liver lesion, and base of skull lesion. Histopathology confirmed BRAF/NRAS wild-type metastatic melanoma. He proceeded with resection of the right parietal lobe metastases in February followed by ipilimumab (3 mg/kg)/nivolumab (1 mg/kg) commencing in March (**Figure 1**).

MRI brain on the April 3 demonstrated intracranial recurrence with PET/CT confirming stable extracranial disease. A redo craniotomy was performed on April 8, complicated by the development of cerebral abscess and ventriculitis requiring burr hole and drainage. Cultures confirmed corynebacterium acnes and he commenced intravenous (IV) Cephalothin for a total of 12 weeks. Six weeks following his last dose of immunotherapy and while on IV antibiotics for his cerebral abscess, the patient developed severe peripheral edema, dyspnea, and tachycardia. Electrocardiograph (ECG) demonstrated sinus tachycardia, left axis deviation, and right bundle branch block. Transthoracic echocardiogram (TTE) revealed a new circumferential pericardial effusion with early signs of tamponade. Serial troponins remained normal, and cardiac MRI showed no

evidence of myocarditis. A diagnosis of ICI-induced pericarditis with associated pericardial effusion was made. The patient was commenced on aggressive diuresis, colchicine 500 mcg daily and ibuprofen 500 mg three times daily. The active decision to withhold high-dose corticosteroids was made given the patient's concomitant cerebral abscess. He was monitored with weekly echocardiograms by the treating cardiologist with gradual resolution of the pericardial effusion over 4 weeks. Immunotherapy was discontinued. In June 2020, the patient had a further recurrence of brain metastases. A third resection followed by stereotactic radiosurgery to the cavity were completed at that time.

Seven months following cessation of immunotherapy, the patient presented with sudden onset aphasia, left lower limb myoclonic jerks, and confusion. Further history revealed that the patient had developed subtle behavioral changes in the weeks prior. CT brain and angiogram showed no evidence of acute cerebrovascular event, infection, or intracranial disease progression. Laboratory results showed a normal CRP (0.7 m/L) and mild hyponatremia (129 mmol/L). An MRI brain revealed T2/FLAIR hyperintensity in the right mesotemporal lobe with differentials including encephalitis or postictal changes (**Figure 2**). Electroencephalogram (EEG) demonstrated lateralizing periodic discharges from the right temporal region. Empirical acyclovir was commenced following a lumbar puncture that demonstrated a mild elevation of protein 0.62 g/L, normal white cell count, negative bacterial/fungal cultures, and negative viral PCR panel. Despite up titration of antiepileptics, the patient continued to deteriorate with increasing confusion, fluctuating level of consciousness, persistent dysphasia, and development of visual hallucinations. Autoimmune encephalitis and antineuronal antibody panels were normal. ICI-induced encephalitis was considered the most likely diagnosis and methylprednisolone 500 mg IV/day was initiated, continued for 3 days, and followed by 2 days of 250 mg IV/day. There was a rapid and remarkable improvement in symptoms following steroid administration. A repeat EEG showed resolution of lateralizing periodic discharges from the right temporal region. He was discharged on 80 mg oral prednisone, which was slowly weaned over 2 months.

The patient has continued on surveillance since cessation of immunotherapy in April 2020. His most recent imaging in

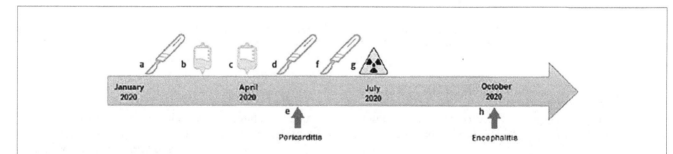

FIGURE 1 | Timeline of case report of patient with rare delayed immune-related toxicities. **(A)** February 14, 2020, first brain metastasis resection. **(B)** March 2020, first cycle ipilimumab/nivolumab. **(C)** April 4, second cycle ipilimumab/nivolumab. **(D)** April 8, second brain metastasis resection. **(E)** May 12, presentation with immune-related pericarditis. **(F)** June 24, third brain metastasis resection. **(G)** July 14, stereotactic radiosurgery of resection cavity. **(H)** Presentation with auto-immune encephalitis.

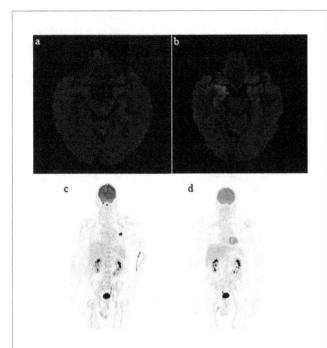

FIGURE 2 | Serial MRI brain showing development of encephalitis and serial PET/CT demonstrating the patient's durable response to immunotherapy. **(A)** MRI brain with gadolinium Sept 2, 2020—no abnormalities in medial temporal region. **(B)** MRI brain October 29, 2020 shows new T2/FLAIR hyperintensity in the right medial temporal lobes. **(C)** PET/CT March 2020. **(D)** PET CT March 2021.

March 2021 demonstrated an ongoing near-complete response of his metastatic melanoma. His pericarditis has not recurred with significant but partial neurological recovery from his grade 4 encephalitis.

DISCUSSION

Immune-related adverse events (irAEs) remain a major challenge, contributing to morbidity and mortality for melanoma patients. Immune-related cardiac toxicity and neurologic toxicities account for a high proportion of fatal immune-related toxicities (2). For the majority of patients, these irAEs occur early; however, a minority of patients will develop irAEs late in treatment or following treatment cessation (2, 3). The definition of a delayed autoimmune adverse event (DIRE) is varied in literature. The majority of clinical trials define delayed safety adverse events as greater than 90 days after discontinuation of immunotherapy and thus this timeframe has been used in several recent reviews to define DIREs (3). A review by Couey et al. (3) included a collation of 194 trials and 367 case reports and only identified 25 DIREs, 2 pericarditis, and no encephalitis cases, highlighting the exceptional rarity of these cases.

Immune-related pericardial disease is rare and variably reported in the literature. The incidence of pericardial disease reported in a recent pharmacovigilance study was reported at 0.36% with combination anti-PD1 and anti-CTLA4 (4). Immune-related pericardial disease has a wide variation in both onset and presentation and in some instances may well be under-reported due to the variability in severity. Such variation may lead to delayed diagnosis and treatment. This is a significant concern due to the relatively high mortality rates associated with immune-related cardiac toxicity. ICI-induced pericarditis has a fatality rate of 13% (5). Further to this, pericardial disease may be associated with myocarditis, which carries a significantly higher mortality rate reported as high as 65.6% in combination immunotherapy (4). Taking into account variability in the literature, pericardial disease is most often seen early during treatment with the majority of patients developing cardiac toxicities within the first month of commencement of immunotherapy (4, 6). Patients with symptomatic pericardial disease often present with chest pain, signs and symptoms of right heart failure, or tamponade (7). Essential investigations include ECG, cardiac biomarkers, and echocardiogram. Cardiac MRI is a critical investigation to assess for myocarditis and should be completed where possible given the mortality rates associated with myocarditis (4, 5). Performance of pericardiocentesis is highly varied among institutions' literature (5, 7) and should of course be balanced against the risks of this invasive procedure. Analysis of pericardial fluid can provide key diagnostic information. ICI-associated pericardial effusions commonly demonstrate a lymphocyte-rich infiltrate and the absence of malignant cells (5). As with most severe irAEs, high-dose corticosteroids are recommended; however, guidelines are based on limited case series. Cautiously selected patients may be suitable for management without high-dose corticosteroids *via* utilization of anti-inflammatories commonly employed for non-ICI-induced pericarditis, such as colchicine and ibuprofen. Such an approach is resource intensive as it requires close monitoring with serial TTEs and close cardiologist follow-up. On review of available literature, we identified two cases of ICI-induced pericarditis managed successfully without use of high-dose steroids. One case (5) was managed with therapeutic pericardiocentesis resulting in resolution of the effusion. The second case was successfully treated with colchicine and ibuprofen alone (8). This case highlights an approach that may be considered for patients with ICI-induced pericarditis where high dose steroids are contraindicated.

ICI-induced encephalitis is another extremely rare irAE with rates of 0.92% reported with combination immunotherapy (9, 10). ICI-induced encephalitis is reported to occur early during treatment with a median onset of 61 days reported in a large pharmacovigilance study by Johnson et al. (10). ICI-induced encephalitis typically presents with symptoms including altered mentation, speech disturbance, and altered level of consciousness (11). Diagnostic workup should be prioritized to exclude infectious etiologies. Diagnosis is often challenging given common overlapping toxicities. In this case, such overlapping toxicities included three cerebral metastasectomies, stereotactic radiotherapy, and a recent cerebral abscess. Key investigations for ICI-induced encephalitis include but are not limited to CT and MRI brain, EEG, LP with viral PCR and culture, autoimmune and paraneoplastic panels, serum inflammatory markers, and electrolytes (11). MRI changes typical of autoimmune encephalitis can include T2/FLAIR changes of the limbic system (11). CSF may show elevated white blood cell count and/or elevated protein levels. Prompt initiation of corticosteroids is crucial to decrease morbidity and mortality (12) in patients who develop ICI encephalitis with a mortality rate approaching 20% (2, 12).

Our case presented with ICI-induced encephalitis 7.5 months after cessation of immunotherapy. On review of the literature, we could identify only one other case of delayed ICI-induced encephalitis (13). Both cases were in patients who received treatment for prior brain metastases, responded rapidly to high-dose corticosteroids with partial neurological recovery in the short term. No medium- to long-term follow-up to assess ongoing neurological recovery was available for these cases.

CONCLUSION

Combination immunotherapy has a wide range of potentially fatal immune-related toxicities with both ICI-induced pericarditis and ICI-induced encephalitis contributing to a high proportion of these fatalities (2). This case highlights the challenges clinicians face with life-threatening toxicity emerging many months after treatment cessation. As ipilimumab and nivolumab become more frequently employed and with an increasing population of long-term survivors, this case emphasizes the importance of constant vigilance for such toxicities. Ongoing collaboration and research are needed to produce robust guidelines to support clinicians in managing these rare presentations.

ETHICS STATEMENT

Ethical review and approval was not required for the study on human participants in accordance with the local legislation and institutional requirements. The patients/participants provided their written informed consent to participate in this study. Written informed consent was obtained from the individual(s) for the publication of any potentially identifiable images or data included in this article.

AUTHOR CONTRIBUTIONS

All authors listed have made a substantial, direct, and intellectual contribution to the work and approved it for publication.

REFERENCES

1. Larkin J, Chiarion-Sileni V, Gonzalez R, Grob JJ, Rutkowski P, Lao CD, et al. Five-Year Survival With Combined Nivolumab and Ipilimumab in Advanced Melanoma. *N Engl J Med* (2019) 381(16):1535–46. doi: 10.1056/NEJMoa1910836

2. Wang DY, Salem JE, Cohen JV, Chandra S, Menzer C, Ye F, et al. Fatal Toxic Effects Associated With Immune Checkpoint Inhibitors: A Systematic Review and Meta-Analysis. *JAMA Oncol* (2018) 4(12):1721–8. doi: 10.1001/jamaoncol.2018.3923

3. Couey MA, Bell RB, Patel AA, Romba MC, Crittenden MR, Curti BD, et al. Delayed Immune-Related Events (DIRE) After Discontinuation of Immunotherapy: Diagnostic Hazard of Autoimmunity at a Distance. *J Immunother Cancer* (2019) 7(1):165. doi: 10.1186/s40425-019-0645-6

4. Salem JE, Manouchehri A, Moey M, Lebrun-Vignes B, Bastarache L, Pariente A, et al. Cardiovascular Toxicities Associated With Immune Checkpoint Inhibitors: An Observational, Retrospective, Pharmacovigilance Study. *Lancet Oncol* (2018) 19(12):1579–89. doi: 10.1016/S1470-2045(18)30608-9

5. Chen D-Y, Huang W-K, Wu C-C, Chang V, Chen J-S, Chuang C-K, et al. Cardiovascular Toxicity of Immune Checkpoint Inhibitors in Cancer Patients: A Review When Cardiology Meets Immuno-Oncology. *J Formosan Med Assoc* (2020) 119(10):1461–75. doi: 10.1016/j.jfma.2019.07.025

6. Canale ML, Camerini A, Casolo G, Lilli A, Bisceglia I, Parrini I, et al. Incidence of Pericardial Effusion in Patients With Advanced Non-Small Cell Lung Cancer Receiving Immunotherapy. *Adv Ther* (2020) 37(7):3178–84. doi: 10.1007/s12325-020-01386-y

7. Palaskas N, Morgan J, Daigle T, Banchs J, Durand JB, Hong D, et al. Targeted Cancer Therapies With Pericardial Effusions Requiring Pericardiocentesis Focusing on Immune Checkpoint Inhibitors. *Am J Cardiol* (2019) 123(8):1351–7. doi: 10.1016/j.amjcard.2019.01.013

8. Chahine J, Collier P, Maroo A, Tang WHW, Klein Allan L. Myocardial and Pericardial Toxicity Associated With Immune Checkpoint Inhibitors in Cancer Patients. *JACC: Case Rep* (2020) 2(2):191–9. doi: 10.1016/j.jaccas.2019.11.080

9. Larkin J, Chmielowski B, Lao CD, Hodi FS, Sharfman W, Weber J, et al. Neurologic Serious Adverse Events Associated With Nivolumab Plus Ipilimumab or Nivolumab Alone in Advanced Melanoma, Including a Case Series of Encephalitis. *Oncologist* (2017) 22(6):709–18. doi: 10.1634/theoncologist.2016-0487

10. Johnson DB, Manouchehri A, Haugh AM, Quach HT, Balko JM, Lebrun-Vignes B, et al. Neurologic Toxicity Associated With Immune Checkpoint Inhibitors: A Pharmacovigilance Study. *J Immunother Cancer* (2019) 7(1):134. doi: 10.1186/s40425-019-0617-x

11. Spain L, Walls G, Julve M, O'Meara K, Schmid T, Kalaitzaki E, et al. Neurotoxicity From Immune-Checkpoint Inhibition in the Treatment of Melanoma: A Single Centre Experience and Review of the Literature. *Ann Oncol* (2017) 28(2):377–85. doi: 10.1093/annonc/mdw558

12. Gkoufa A, Gogas H, Diamantopoulos PT, Ziogas DC, Psichogiou M. Encephalitis in a Patient With Melanoma Treated With Immune Checkpoint Inhibitors: Case Presentation and Review of the Literature. *J Immunother* (2020) 43(7):224–9. doi: 10.1097/CJI.0000000000000326

13. Shah N, Jacob J, Househ Z, Shiner E, Baird L, Soudy H, et al. Unchecked Immunity: A Unique Case of Sequential Immune-Related Adverse Events With Pembrolizumab. *J ImmunoTher Cancer* (2019) 7(1):247. doi: 10.1186/s40425-019-0727-5

20

Prognosis for Cutaneous Melanoma by Clinical and Pathological Profile

Alessandra Buja[1*], Andrea Bardin[1], Giovanni Damiani[2,3,4], Manuel Zorzi[5], Chiara De Toni[1], Riccardo Fusinato[1], Romina Spina[6], Antonella Vecchiato[6], Paolo Del Fiore[6], Simone Mocellin[6,7], Vincenzo Baldo[1], Massimo Rugge[5,8] and Carlo Riccardo Rossi[7]

[1] Department of Cardiologic, Vascular and Thoracic Sciences, and Public Health, University of Padua, Padua, Italy, [2] Clinical Dermatology, Istituto di Ricovero e Cura a Carattere Scientifico (IRCCS) Istituto Ortopedico Galeazzi, Milan, Italy, [3] Department of Biomedical, Surgical and Dental Sciences, University of Milan, Milan, Italy, [4] PhD Program in Pharmacological Sciences, Department of Pharmaceutical and Pharmacological Sciences, University of Padua, Padua, Italy, [5] Veneto Tumor Registry - Azienda Zero, Padova, Italy, [6] Surgical Oncology Unit, Veneto Institute of Oncology IOV-Istituto di Ricovero e Cura a Carattere Scientifico (IRCCS), Padova, Italy, [7] Department of Surgery, Oncology and Gastroenterology (DISCOG), University of Padua, Padova, Italy, [8] Department of Medicine DIMED, Surgical Pathology & Cytopathology Unit, University of Padova, Padova, Italy

*Correspondence:
Alessandra Buja
alessandra.buja@unipd.it

Introduction: Among white people, the incidence of cutaneous malignant melanoma (CMM) has been increasing steadily for several decades. Meanwhile, there has also been a significant improvement in 5-year survival among patients with melanoma. This population-based cohort study investigates the five-year melanoma-specific survival (MSS) for all melanoma cases recorded in 2015 in the Veneto Tumor Registry (North-Est Italian Region), taking both demographic and clinical-pathological variables into consideration.

Methods: The cumulative melanoma-specific survival probabilities were calculated with the Kaplan-Meier method, applying different sociodemographic and clinical-pathological variables. Cox's proportional hazards model was fitted to the data to assess the association between independent variables and MSS, and also overall survival (OS), calculating the hazard ratios (HR) relative to a reference condition, and adjusting for sex, age, site of tumor, histotype, melanoma ulceration, mitotic count, tumor-infiltrating lymphocytes (TIL), and stage at diagnosis.

Results: Compared with stage I melanoma, the risk of death was increased for stage II (HR 3.31, 95% CI: 0.94-11.76, p=0.064), almost ten times higher for stage III (HR 10.51, 95% CI: 3.16-35.02, p<0.001), and more than a hundred times higher for stage IV (HR 117.17, 95% CI: 25.30-542.62, p<0.001). Among the other variables included in the model, the presence of mitoses and histological subtype emerged as independent risk factors for death.

Conclusions: The multivariable analysis disclosed that older age, tumor site, histotype, mitotic count, and tumor stage were independently associated with a higher risk of death. Data on survival by clinical and morphological characteristics could be useful in modelling, planning, and managing the most appropriate treatment and follow-up for patients with CMM.

Keywords: melanoma, clinical characteristics, survival, epidemiology, cancer survival

INTRODUCTION

In recent decades, the incidence of cutaneous malignant melanoma (CMM) in white people has been increasing steadily (1, 2). Meanwhile, a significant improvement in CMM patients' 5-year overall survival has also been reported, and related mostly to the increasing prevalence of cancers detected in their earliest, "thinner" stage" (3, 4). Both the rising incidence of CMM (all stages), and changes in the treatment panorama (also including the advent of targeted therapies) prompt the collection of updated information which might re-orient both prevention efforts and diagnostic/therapeutic strategies.

Based on the natural history of CMM, a well-established set of clinicopathological variables has been significantly correlated with the clinical outcome of melanoma patients. Unfortunately, these data are often inconsistently recorded and/or scattered over different digital archives. This situation interferes with efforts to validate prognostic variables in the "real world" of large-scale population-based studies.

As for the stage-specific survival of CMM patients, most information comes from national cancer registries, and the USA American Surveillance, Epidemiology and End Results program (SEER) in particular (5). To the best of our knowledge, few registry-based studies on the stage-specific survival of CMM patients have been conducted in Italy or elsewhere in Europe in the last two decades (6-10).

The present study investigates the five-year melanoma-specific survival (MSS) for all cases of CMM recorded in 2015 in the resident population of a north-eastern Italian region (Veneto). Both demographic and clinical-pathological variables have been considered to measure their impact on patient survival in this cohort of CMM patients.

MATERIALS AND METHODS

Context

The Italian public national health service (NHS) is financed mainly by general taxation, and is largely managed on a regional basis. NHS policies are grounded on fundamental values of universality, free access, freedom of choice, pluralism in provision, and equity.

In the north-eastern Veneto region of Italy, the Regional Authority has endorsed a number of standardized Diagnostic Therapeutic Protocols (DTPs) for the clinical management of cancer patients. All DPTs have been edited by multidisciplinary task forces including dedicated experts belonging to the Regional Oncology Network (ROV).

This retrospective study on the outcome of CMM patients is based on clinico-pathological information recorded by the Veneto Cancer Registry in 2015 (11).

Study Participants and Data Collection

This retrospective population-based study involves a cohort of 1,279 incident cases of CMM diagnosed in the Veneto region in 2015 (resident population: 4,915,123). For each patient, the

following set of clinical-pathological features were considered: a) tumor site (lower limbs, upper limbs, head, hands/feet, trunk); b) CMM histological subtype (lentigo maligna, acral lentiginous, blue nevus, desmoplastic, nodular, superficial spreading, spitzoid); b) growth phase (radial *versus* vertical); c) histologically-proven ulceration (present *versus* absent); d) number of mitoses (categorized as 0-2 or >2) (12); e) tumor-infiltrating lymphocytes, ([TILs] absent *versus* present; f) TNM stage, as established by merging clinical and pathological information available at the time of patient enrolment (13).

Patients were grouped by age in the following brackets: < 40, 40-49, 50-59, 60-69,70-79, 80 years or more.

Statistical Analysis

The number of person-years in the cohort was calculated by taking the date of entry as the time when a tumor was diagnosed, and the date of exit as 31 December 2020 or the time of death or drop-out from follow-up, whichever came first. Patient deaths were considered in the overall survival (OS) analysis regardless of their cause, while only deaths caused by melanoma were considered in the analysis of MSS. The cumulative MSS rates were calculated with the Kaplan-Meier method using different sociodemographic and histopathologic features. Cox's proportional hazards model was fitted to the data to assess the association between both MSS and OS and the previously-detailed independent variables (except for growth type as this variable perfectly predicted the outcome). In the multivariate analysis, we grouped the less common histological categories (acral-lentiginous, blue nevus, desmoplastic, spitzoid) as "Other". A sensitivity analysis was performed, excluding stage IV patients from the multivariate analysis. The assumption of proportionality was accepted for all models. Statistical significance was ascertained using an alpha level of 0.05 and two-sided tests. All data analyses were run using the R statistical package (version 3.6.3; R Studio, Boston, MA).

Ethics

The data analysis was performed on anonymous aggregated data with no chance of individuals being identifiable. Ethical approval for the study was obtained from the Veneto Oncological Institute's Ethics Committee (n. 52/2016).

RESULTS

In 2015, the Veneto Cancer Registry 1,279 incident CMM-patient were registered at. **Table 1** shows patients' demographics (M/F: 1.13; median age: 58 years) and clinical-pathological profiles. Most of the invasive malignancies were diagnosed in the early stage (stage I: 71.8%). The mean follow-up was 1,670 ± 415 days.

Overall, the 5-year OS was 83.8% (95% CI: 81.8, 85.8) and it was higher for females (86.6%; 95% CI: 84.0, 89.4) than for males (81.2%; 95% CI: 78.4, 84.2). Five-year MSS was 92.5% (95% CI: 91.0, 94.0), with no significant survival advantage for females (93.6%; CI: 91.7, 95.6) over males (91.5%; CI: 89.4, 93.7).

TABLE 1 | Baseline characteristics of the study cohort (NOS, not otherwise specified; TILs, tumor infiltrating lymphocytes).

	Number (%)		Number (%)
All patients	1,279 (100)	**Mitotic count**	
Sex		0-2	798 (62.39)
Male	678 (53.0)	>2	252 (19.70)
Female	601 (47.0)	Not known	229 (17.91)
Age (years)		**TILs**	
<40	155 (12.1)	Present	927 (72.5)
40-49	252 (19.7)	Absent	189 (14.8)
50-59	252 (19.7)	Not known	163 (12.7)
60-69	257 (20.1)	**Tumor status (T)**	
70-79	217 (17)	T1	820 (64.1)
80+	146 (11.4)	T2	167 (13.1)
Tumor site		T3	126 (9.8)
Lower limbs	260 (20.33)	T4	98 (7.7)
Upper limbs	195 (15.25)	TX	14 (1.1)
Head	133 (10.40)	Not known	54 (4.2)
Hands/feet	56 (4.38)	**Nodal status (N)**	
Trunk	593 (46.36)	N0	1,119 (87.5)
Not known	42 (3.28)	N1	64 (5)
Histological subtype		N2	45 (3.5)
Superficial spreading melanoma	926 (72.40)	N3	31 (2.4)
Nodular melanoma	159 (12.43)	Not known	20 (1.6)
Lentigo maligna	28 (2.19)	**Metastasis status (M)**	
Acral-lentiginous melanoma	25 (1.95)	M0	1,225 (95.78)
Desmoplastic melanoma	4 (0.31)	M1	26 (2.03)
Blue nevus	1 (0.08)	Not known	28 (2.19)
Spitzoid melanoma	28 (2.19)	**TNM Stage (enrolment)**	
NOS Malignant melanoma	34 (2.66)	I	918 (71.8)
Growth phase		II	161 (12.6)
Horizontal	285 (22.3)	III	117 (9.1)
Vertical	701 (54.8)	IV	26 (2)
Not known	293 (22.9)	Not known	57 (4,5)
Ulceration		**Sentinel lymph node (*)**	
Yes	202 (15.8)	Performed	360 (0.45)
No	1,003 (78.4)	Not performed	86 (80.35)
Not known	74 (5.8)	Not known	2 (19.20)

(*) Only for patients with stage pT1b-pT4b and on stage I-II.

Figure 1 shows Kaplan-Meier MSS curves by TNM clinical-pathological staging at initial diagnosis, which had a strong impact on survival; T, N and M values are also reported. The 5-year MSS was 99.4% (95% CI: 98.9-100.0) for stage I, 82.6% (95% CI: 76.6-89.0) for stage II, 69.3% (95% CI: 61.0-78.7) for stage III, and only 23.0% (95% CI: 10.3-51.4) for stage IV.

Figures 2, **3** show the Kaplan-Meier MSS curves by each of the pathological variables considered at initial diagnosis (histological subtype, growth phase, mitotic index, ulceration, TILs). The 5-year MSS probability was 99.2% for the category 0-2 mitoses (95% CI: 98.6-99.8), and 76.2% (95% CI: 70.9-82.0) for more than 2 mitoses. Melanoma ulceration significantly affected the probability 5-year MSS (97.6%; 95%CI: 96.7-98.6 without ulceration *versus* 72.5%; 95% CI: 66.2-79.3). As for the tumor's growth phase, survival was better for cases described as RGP (radial growth phase) at diagnosis than for those described as VGP (vertical growth phase): the 5-year MSS probability was 100.0% (95%CI: 100.0-100.0) for the former, and 91.6% (95%CI: 89.6- 93.8) for the latter. TIL status (presence *versus* absence) was associated with a small, but significant impact on 5-year MSS probability(94.4%, 95%CI: 92.9-95.9 *versus* 90.5%, 95%CI: 86.4-

94.9, respectively). Finally, the survival analysis by histological subtype at diagnosis showed that nodular melanoma carried the worst 5-year MSS probability, at 70.3% (95%CI: 63.2-78.1). Superficial spreading melanoma had the highest 5-year MSS probability, at 96.9% (95% CI: 95.8-98.1). Intermediate survival probabilities were revealed for lentigo maligna melanoma (92.9%, 95% CI: 83.8-100.0).

Table 2 shows the results of Cox's regression model for MSS, adjusting for sex, age, histological subtype, ulceration, mitoses, site of tumor, stage at diagnosis and TILs. Compared with patients with a melanoma in stage I, the risk of death was increased for stage II (HR=3.31, 95% CI: 0.94-11.76, p=0.064), it was almost ten times higher for stage III (HR=10.51, 95% CI: 3.16-35.02, p<0.001), and it was more than a hundred times higher for stage IV (HR=117.17, 95% CI: 25.30-542.62, p<0.001). Superficial spreading melanoma carried a more than eleven times greater risk of death than lentigo maligna (HR=12.61, 95% CI: 1.42-112.02, p=0.023), and nodular melanoma a fourteen times higher risk (HR=15.04, 95% CI: 1.69-133.30, p=0.015). Sites of tumor involving the lower limbs, upper limbs and trunk had a better prognosis than those involving

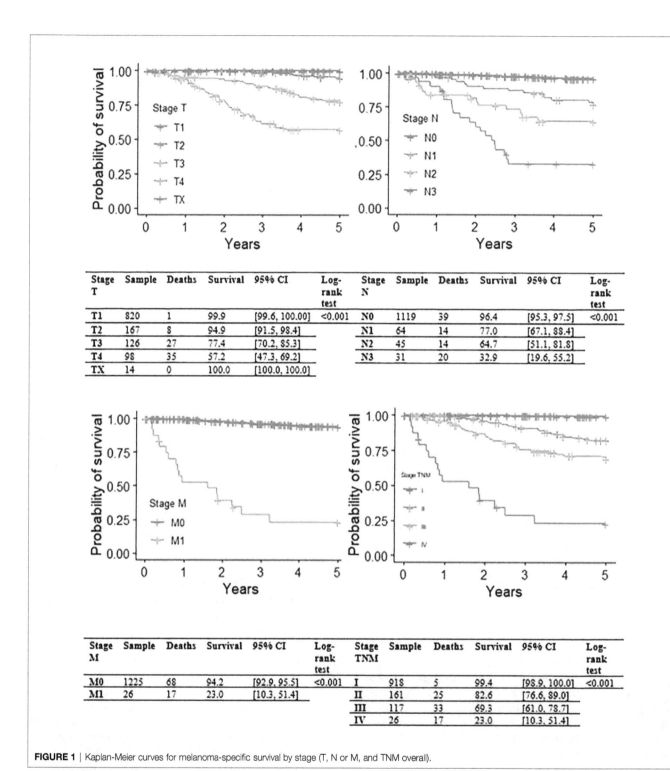

FIGURE 1 | Kaplan-Meier curves for melanoma-specific survival by stage (T, N or M, and TNM overall).

the hands and feet, with the difference reaching borderline statistical significance (p=0.058, p=0.083, p=0.066). Among the other variables included the model, the presence of mitoses emerged as an independent risk factor for death (HR=6.85, 95%CI: 2.21-21.28, p<0.001). The sensitivity analysis, excluding stage IV, generated much the same results as the previous model (data not shown). The analysis of overall survival produced similar results too, except that male sex coincided with a significantly worse prognosis (HR=1.75, % CI: 1.18-2.60, p=0.005).

DISCUSSION

In a population-based cohort of 1,279 incident CMM patients, this study focuses on the prognostic impact of both

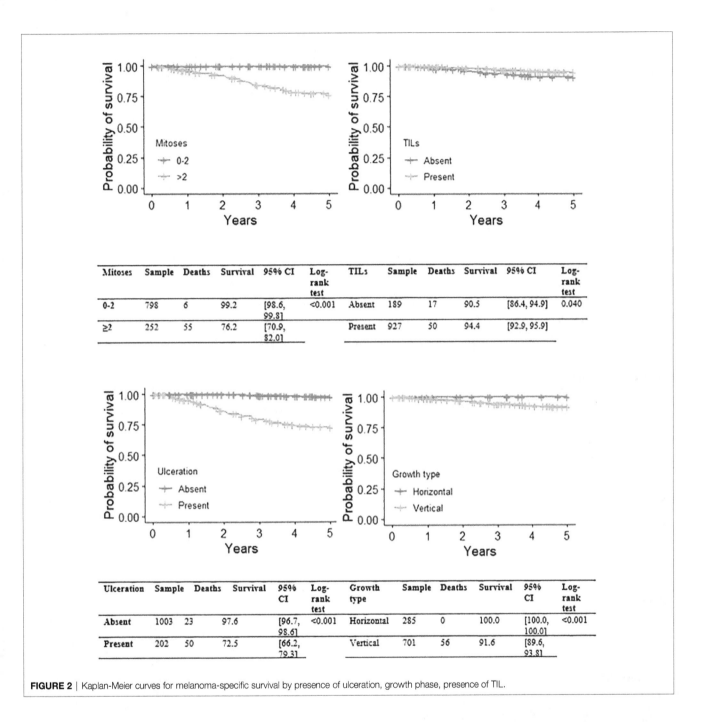

FIGURE 2 | Kaplan-Meier curves for melanoma-specific survival by presence of ulceration, growth phase, presence of TIL.

demographics and clinical-pathological variables, as recorded in a high-resolution Italian cancer registry.

The results obtained prompt two main types of consideration: one refers to the validation of the CMM-associated prognostic variables in a large cohort of consecutive patients; the other relates to the value of population-based trials for the purpose of updating/improving patient management based on a critical analysis of real-world clinical practice.

As regards the first point, the present results support the prognostic impact of (mostly) well-established clinical-pathological variables (6, 14, 15). In particular, the Kaplan-

Meier analysis showed that none of the RGP CMMs resulted in a melanoma-specific death within 5 years after the initial diagnosis (16). The present results also provide evidence to show that extra-nodal metastases from RGP CMMs are extremely rare (less than 3%), while almost all extra-nodal metastatic implants result from "vertically-growing" CMMs (17). Consistently with these findings, both the worst MSS rate and the highest risk of CMM-related death were associated with nodular CMMs. Based on the assumption that any greater risk associated with a nodular histology overlaps with the prognostic impact of a melanoma's thickness and ulceration, the American Joint Committee on

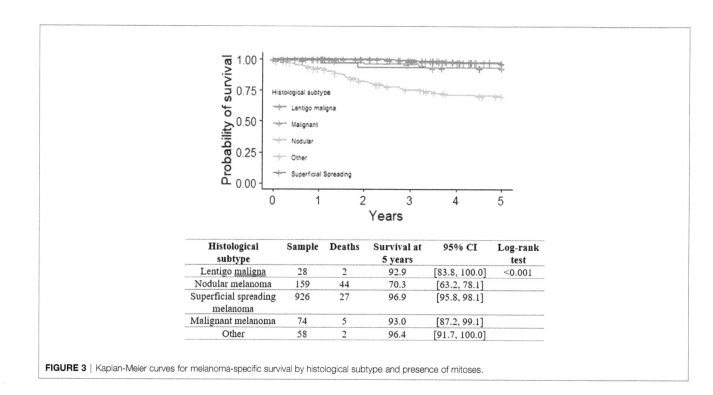

Histological subtype	Sample	Deaths	Survival at 5 years	95% CI	Log-rank test
Lentigo maligna	28	2	92.9	[83.8, 100.0]	<0.001
Nodular melanoma	159	44	70.3	[63.2, 78.1]	
Superficial spreading melanoma	926	27	96.9	[95.8, 98.1]	
Malignant melanoma	74	5	93.0	[87.2, 99.1]	
Other	58	2	96.4	[91.7, 100.0]	

FIGURE 3 | Kaplan-Meier curves for melanoma-specific survival by histological subtype and presence of mitoses.

TABLE 2 | Cox's regression analysis on cutaneous melanoma-specific survival patients, adjusting for sex, age, histological subtype, ulceration, mitotic count, CMM site, stage and TILs, as assessed at the patient's enrolment.

		HR	95% CI	P value
Sex	Female	1.00	–	–
	Male	1.67	0.87 - 3.21	0.120
Age	<40	1.00	–	–
	40-49	1.45	0.17 - 13.55	0.743
	50-59	2.19	0.24 - 20.32	0.489
	60-69	3.28	0.41 - 26.39	0.265
	70-79	7.95	1.02 - 61.91	0.048
	80 or more	3.58	0.43 - 29.79	0.238
CMM site	Hands/feet	1.00	–	–
	Lower limbs	0.34	0.11 - 1.04	0.058
	Upper limbs	0.34	0.10 - 1.15	0.083
	Head	1.83	0.62 - 5.40	0.272
	Hands/feet	1.00	–	–
	Trunk	0.39	0.15 - 1.06	0.066
CMM Histological subtype	Lentigo maligna	1.00	–	–
	Nodular m.	15.04	1.69 - 133.30	0.015
	Superficial spreading m.	12.61	1.42 - 112.02	0.023
	NOS cutaneous m.	6.07	0.46 - 79.67	0.170
	Others	3.26	0.16 - 67.66	0.444
CMM Ulceration	Present	1.00	–	–
	Absent	0.82	0.41 - 1.62	0.562
CMM Mitotic number	0-2	1.00	–	–
	>2	6.85	2.21 - 21.28	<0.001
CMM TILs	Absent	1.00	–	–
	Present	1.70	0.80 - 3.59	0.166
CMM TNM stage	I	1.00	–	–
	II	3.31	0.94 - 11.76	0.064
	III	10.51	3.16 - 35.02	<0.001
	IV	117.17	25.30 - 542.62	<0.001

CMM, cutaneous melanoma; NOS, not otherwise specified; TILs, tumor infiltrating lymphocytes; m, melanoma.
HR, hazard ratio; Assumption of proportionality: p-value 0.577.

Cancer (AJCC)'s staging system does not include the CMM subtype among the "discriminating" prognostic variables (14, 15). A recent analysis of the SEER cohort (18) nonetheless identifies the histological subtype as an independent predictor of survival, even after adjusting for CMM stage, thickness, ulceration, and mitotic index.

Previous studies found that the mitotic rate (more than neoplastic ulceration) is an independent prognostic factors in primary CMMs (irrespective of their thickness) (19–26). The present results associate a number of mitoses with a worse survival, further supporting the inclusion of the mitotic rate in the staging of thin, non-ulcerated CMMs.

A high-resolution cancer registry primarily needs to contain comprehensive, reliable, and accessible clinical information. All these conditions are hard to achieve, and the present study is no exception. In fact, our study suffered from the difficulty of assembling the necessary clinicopathological data, largely because of inconsistencies in the data format and/or their location in different digital repositories. The present study also suffers from a lack of important information on patients' socio-economic profiles and - even more important - data on the molecular biology profile of the malignancies considered (27). In this respect, the present study further supports the crucial importance of promoting standardized/synoptic formats in the recording of clinicopathological variables, as obtained by the main clinical actors involved in patient management (especially oncologists, radiologists, and clinical and surgical pathologists).

Inconsistencies in the recording of diagnostic procedures and the "scattering" of results in different datasets represent major limits to operative efforts to pursue the high-resolution cancer registration potentially capable of providing both clinicians and healthcare policy-makers with reliable information on the clinical management of CMM patients.

ETHICS STATEMENT

The studies involving human participants were reviewed and approved by Veneto Oncological Institute Ethics Committee (n 695/20.10.2016). Written informed consent for participation was not required for this study in accordance with the national legislation and the institutional requirements.

AUTHOR CONTRIBUTIONS

ABu and GD conceived the presented idea. MZ, RS, AV, PF, and SM collected the data, verified its accuracy, and developed the methods. CT verified the analyses. ABa, ABu, and RF wrote the draft. MR, VB, GD, and ABu. supervised the project and revised the draft. CR found the financial support for the project. All authors read and approved the final manuscript.

REFERENCES

1. Arnold M, Holterhues C, Hollestein LM, Coebergh JW, Nijsten T, Pukkala E, et al. Trends in Incidence and Predictions of Cutaneous Melanoma Across Europe Up to 2015. *J Eur Acad Dermatol Venereol* (2014) 28(9):1170–8. doi: 10.1111/jdv.12236
2. Jemal A, Saraiya M, Patel P, Cherala SS, Barnholtz-Sloan J, Kim J, et al. Recent Trends in Cutaneous Melanoma Incidence and Death Rates in the United States, 1992-2006. *J Am Acad Dermatol* (2011) 65(5 Suppl 1):S17–25.e1-3. doi: 10.1016/j.jaad.2011.04.032
3. Thomas L, Tranchand P, Berard F, Secchi T, Colin C, Moulin G. Semiological Value of ABCDE Criteria in the Diagnosis of Cutaneous Pigmented Tumors. *Dermatology* (1998) 197(1):11-7. doi: 10.1159/000017969
4. Leiter U, Keim U, Garbe C. Epidemiology of Skin Cancer: Update 2019. *Adv Exp Med Biol* (2020) 1268:123–39. doi: 10.1007/978-3-030-46227-7_6
5. Howlader N, Noone AM, Krapcho M, Miller D, Brest A, Yu M, et al. eds. *SEER Cancer Statistics Review, 1975-2018*. Bethesda, MD: National Cancer Institute (2021). Available at: https://seer.cancer.gov/csr/1975_2018/. based on November 2020 SEER data submission, posted to the SEER web site, April 2021.
6. Svedman FC, Pillas D, Taylor A, Kaur M, Linder R, Hansson J. Stage-Specific Survival and Recurrence in Patients With Cutaneous Malignant Melanoma in Europe - A Systematic Review of the Literature. *Clin Epidemiol* (2016) 8:109–22. doi: 10.2147/CLEP.S99021
7. Mandalà M, Imberti GL, Piazzalunga D, Belfiglio M, Labianca R, Barberis M, et al. Clinical and Histopathological Risk Factors to Predict Sentinel Lymph Node Positivity, Disease-Free and Overall Survival in Clinical Stages I-II AJCC Skin Melanoma: Outcome Analysis From a Single-Institution Prospectively Collected Database. *Eur J Cancer* (2009) 45(14):2537–45. doi: 10.1016/j.ejca.2009.05.034

8. Balzi D, Carli P, Giannotti B, Buiatti E. Skin Melanoma in Italy: A Population-Based Study on Survival and Prognostic Factors. *Eur J Cancer* (1998) 34 (5):699–704. doi: 10.1016/s0959-8049(97)10119-8
9. Cascinelli N, Bombardieri E, Bufalino R, Camerini T, Carbone A, Clemente C, et al. Sentinel and Nonsentinel Node Status in Stage IB and II Melanoma Patients: Two-Step Prognostic Indicators of Survival. *J Clin Oncol* (2006) 24 (27):4464–71. doi: 10.1200/JCO.2006.06.3198
10. Testori A, De Salvo GL, Montesco MC, Trifirò G, Mocellin S, Landi G, et al. Clinical Considerations on Sentinel Node Biopsy in Melanoma From an Italian Multicentric Study on 1,313 Patients (SOLISM-IMI). *Ann Surg Oncol* (2009) 16(7):2018–27. doi: 10.1245/s10434-008-0273-8
11. Guzzinati S, Zorzi M, Rossi CR, Buja A, Italiano I, Fiore AR, et al. High Resolution Registry of Melanoma and Care Pathways Monitoring in the Veneto Region, Italy. In: *ENCR Scientific Meeting*. Copenaghen. Available at: https://www.registrotumoriveneto.it/it/pubblicazioni/convegni/poster/101-2018/234-high-resolution-registry-of-melanoma-and-care-pathways-monitoring-in-the-veneto-region-italy (Accessed Last accessed July 2021).
12. Piñero-Madrona A, Ruiz-Merino G, Cerezuela Fuentes P, Martínez-Barba E, Rodríguez-López JN, Cabezas-Herrera J. Mitotic Rate as an Important Prognostic Factor in Cutaneous Malignant Melanoma. *Clin Transl Oncol* (2019) 21(10):1348–56. doi: 10.1007/s12094-019-02064-4
13. Edge SB, Compton CC. The American Joint Committee on Cancer: The 7th Edition of the AJCC Cancer Staging Manual and the Future of TNM. *Ann Surg Oncol* (2010) 17(6):1471–4. doi: 10.1245/s10434-010-0985-4
14. Amin MB, Greene FL, Edge SB, Compton CC, Gershenwald JE, Brookland RK, et al. The Eighth Edition AJCC Cancer Staging Manual: Continuing to Build a Bridge From a Population-Based to a More "Personalized" Approach to Cancer Staging. *CA Cancer J Clin* (2017) 67(2):93–9. doi: 10.3322/caac.21388
15. Balch CM, Buzaid AC, Soong SJ, Atkins MB, Cascinelli N, Coit DG, et al. New TNM Melanoma Staging System: Linking Biology and Natural History to

Clinical Outcomes. *Semin Surg Oncol* (2003) 21(1):43–52. doi: 10.1002/ssu.10020

16. Betti R, Agape E, Vergani R, Moneghini L, Cerri A. An Observational Study Regarding the Rate of Growth in Vertical and Radial Growth Phase Superficial Spreading Melanomas. *Oncol Lett* (2016) 12(3):2099–102. doi: 10.3892/ol.2016.4813

17. Elder D. Pathology of Melanoma. *Clin Cancer Res* (2006) 12(7):2308s–11s. doi: 10.1158/1078-0432.CCR-05-2504

18. Lattanzi M, Lee Y, Simpson D, Moran U, Darvishian F, Kim RH, et al. Primary Melanoma Histologic Subtype: Impact on Survival and Response to Therapy. *J Natl Cancer Inst* (2019) 111(2):180–8. doi: 10.1093/jnci/djy086

19. Barnhill RL, Katzen J, Spatz A, Fine J, Berwick M. The Importance of Mitotic Rate as a Prognostic Factor for Localized Cutaneous Melanoma. *J Cutan Pathol* (2005) 32(4):268–73. doi: 10.1111/j.0303-6987.2005.00310.x

20. Vollmer RT. Malignant Melanoma: A Multivariate Analysis of Prognostic Factors. *Pathol Annu* (1989) 24:383.

21. Donizy P, Kaczorowski M, Leskiewicz M, Zietek M, Pieniazek M, Kozyra C, et al. Mitotic Rate Is a More Reliable Unfavorable Prognosticator Than Ulceration for Early Cutaneous Melanoma: A 5-Year Survival Analysis. *Oncol Rep* (2014) 32(6):2735–43. doi: 10.3892/or.2014.3531

22. Evans JL, Vidri RJ, MacGillivray DC, Fitzgerald TL. Tumor Mitotic Rate Is an Independent Predictor of Survival for Nonmetastatic Melanoma. *Surgery* (2018) 164(3):589–93. doi: 10.1016/j.surg.2018.04.016

23. Thompson JF, Soong SJ, Balch CM, Gershenwald JE, Ding S, Coit DG, et al. Prognostic Significance of Mitotic Rate in Localized Primary Cutaneous Melanoma: An Analysis of Patients in the Multi-Institutional American Joint Committee on Cancer Melanoma Staging Database. *J Clin Oncol* (2011) 29(16):2199–205. doi: 10.1200/JCO.2010.31.5812

24. Kashani-Sabet M, Miller JR 3rd, Lo S, Nosrati M, Stretch JR, Shannon KF, et al. Reappraisal of the Prognostic Significance of Mitotic Rate Supports its Reincorporation Into the Melanoma Staging System. *Cancer* (2020) 126(21):4717–25. doi: 10.1002/cncr.33088

25. Tejera-Vaquerizo A, Pérez-Cabello G, Marínez-Leborans L, Gallego E, Oliver-Martínez V, Martín-Cuevas P, et al. Is Mitotic Rate Still Useful in the Management of Patients With Thin Melanoma? *J Eur Acad Dermatol Venereol* (2017) 31(12):2025–9. doi: 10.1111/jdv.14485

26. Damiani G, Buja A, Grossi E, Rivera M, De Polo A, De Luca G, et al. Use of an Artificial Neural Network to Identify Patient Clusters in a Large Cohort of Patients With Melanoma by Simultaneous Analysis of Costs and Clinical Characteristics. *Acta Derm Venereol* (2020) 100(18):adv00323. doi: 10.2340/00015555-3680

27. Rugge M. Gastric Cancer Risk: Between Genetics and Lifestyle. *Lancet Oncol* (2020) 21(10):1258–60. doi: 10.1016/S1470-2045(20)30432-0

21

Real Life Clinical Management and Survival in Advanced Cutaneous Melanoma: The Italian Clinical National Melanoma Registry Experience

Anna Crispo[1], Maria Teresa Corradin[2], Erika Giulioni[2], Antonella Vecchiato[3], Paolo Del Fiore[3], Paola Queirolo[4,5], Francesco Spagnolo[4], Vito Vanella[1], Corrado Caracò[1], Giulio Tosti[5], Elisabetta Pennacchioli[5], Giuseppe Giudice[6], Eleonora Nacchiero[6], Pietro Quaglino[7], Simone Ribero[7], Monica Giordano[8], Desire Marussi[8], Stefania Barruscotti[9], Michele Guida[10], Vincenzo De Giorgi[11], OccelliMarcella[12], Federica Grosso[13], Giuseppe Cairo[14], Alessandro Gatti[15], Daniela Massa[16], Laura Atzori[17], Nicola Calvani[18], Tommaso Fabrizio[19], Giuseppe Mastrangelo[20], Federica Toffolutti[21], Egidio Celentano[1], Mario Budroni[22], Sara Gandini[5], Carlo Riccardo Rossi[3,20], Alessandro Testori[9], Giuseppe Palmieri[23], Paolo A. Ascierto[1] and the Clinical National Melanoma Registry Study Group at the Italian Melanoma Intergroup*

[1] Istituto Nazionale Tumori IRCCS Fondazione G. Pascale, Napoli, Italy, [2] Dermatology Department, Azienda Sanitaria Friuli Occidentale, Pordenone, Italy, [3] Istituto Oncologico Veneto IOV - IRCCS, Padova, Italy, [4] IRCCS Ospedale Policlinico San Martino, Genova, Italy, [5] Istituto Europeo di Oncologia - IRCCS, Milano, Italy, [6] Plastic and Reconstructive Surgery Department, Università degli Studi di Bari Aldo Moro, Bari, Italy, [7] Clinica Dermatologica, Dipartimento di Scienze Mediche, Università di Torino, Torino, Italy, [8] Oncology Department, Ospedale Sant'Anna di Como, Como, Italy, [9] Fondazione I.R.C.C.S. Policlinico San Matteo, Pavia, Italy, [10] IRCCS Istituto Tumori "Giovanni Paolo II", Bari, Italy, [11] Dermatology Department, Università di Firenze, Firenze, Italy, [12] Oncology Department, Azienda ospedaliera Santa Croce e Carle, Cuneo, Italy, [13] Mesothelioma Unit, Azienda Ospedaliera SS Antonio e Biagio e Cesare Arrigo, Alessandria, Italy, [14] Oncology Department, ospedale "Vito Fazzi" di Lecce, Lecce, Italy, [15] ULSS 2 Marca Trevigiana Ospedale Ca' Foncello Treviso, Treviso, Italy, [16] Gruppo melanoma e tumori rari, Oncology Department, PO A Businco ARNAS G. Brotzu, Cagliari, Italy, [17] Dermatology Clinic, Department Medical Sciences and Public Health, University of Cagliari, Cagliari, Italy, [18] Oncology Department, Presidio Ospedaliero "Senatore Antonio Perrino", Brindisi, Italy, [19] IRCCS Centro di Riferimento Oncologico Basilicata, Rionero in Vulture, Italy, [20] Dermatology Clinic, Università degli studi di Padova, Padova, Italy, [21] Centro di Riferimento Oncologico di Aviano (CRO) IRCCS, Aviano (PN), Italy, [22] Registro Tumori Provincia di Sassari, Azienda Ospedaliera Universitaria Sassari, Sassari, Italy, [23] Istituto di Ricerca Genetica e Biomedica, CNR, Sassari, Italy

Correspondence:
Paolo A. Ascierto
paolo.ascierto@gmail.com;
p.ascierto@istitutotumori.na.it

Background: Cutaneous melanoma (CM) is one of the most aggressive types of skin cancer. Currently, innovative approaches such as target therapies and immunotherapies have been introduced in clinical practice. Data of clinical trials and real life studies that evaluate the outcomes of these therapeutic associations are necessary to establish their clinical utility. The aim of this study is to investigate the types of oncological treatments employed in the real-life clinical management of patients with advanced CM in several Italian centers, which are part of the Clinical National Melanoma Registry (CNMR).

Methods: Melanoma-specific survival and overall survival were calculated. Multivariate Cox regression models were used to estimate the hazard ratios adjusting for confounders and other prognostic factors.

Results: The median follow-up time was 36 months (range 1.2-185.1). 787 CM were included in the analysis with completed information about therapies. All types of immunotherapy showed a significant improved survival compared with all other therapies (p=0.001). 75% was the highest reduction of death reached by anti-PD-1 (HR=0.25), globally immunotherapy was significantly associated with improved survival, either for anti-CTLA4 monotherapy or combined with anti-PD-1 (HR=0.47 and 0.26, respectively) and BRAFI+MEKI (HR=0.62).

Conclusions: The nivolumab/pembrolizumab in combination of ipilimumab and the addition of ant-MEK to the BRAFi can be considered the best therapies to improve survival in a real-world-population. The CNMR can complement clinical registries with the intent of improving cancer management and standardizing cancer treatment.

Keywords: medical record systems, cutaneous melanoma, survival analysis, immunotherapy, ipilimumab

INTRODUCTION

Cutaneous melanoma (CM) is one of the most aggressive types of skin cancer. The incidence of CM has increased in Europe over the last years, and cohort studies suggest that the increasing trend of incidence will continue for at least the next 2 decades (1–3) Mortality rates have also increased in the last decades, especially in men, despite a clear decrease of Breslow tumor thickness in the USA and Europe (1, 4). In the USA, the raw mortality rates per 100,000 inhabitants per year increased from 2.8 to 3.1, with an estimate of 10,130 deaths from melanoma in 2016 (they were 8,650 in 2009) (1). In Italy, 12,300 new cases and over 2,000 deaths were estimated in 2019 (5, 6).

Surgery is currently the golden standard for patients with early stage CM, who represent only part of the global cases. The treatment of patients with advanced stage CM is more complex, as for decades no chemotherapy regimens have been found effective in prolonging survival. Currently, innovative approaches such as target therapies and immunotherapies have been introduced in clinical practice for the treatment of metastatic CM. Target therapies are based on the use of drugs targeting specific genetic alterations in candidate genes, blocking specific pathways implicated in the oncogenesis of melanoma (7). BRAF mutations represent currently the main molecular targets for melanoma treatment, as they involve approximately 50% of the cases, and identify patients who may benefit from treatment with BRAF inhibitors, like vemurafenib or dabrafenib (8–10). Recently, the combination of BRAFi drugs with MEK inhibitors showed improved oncological outcomes in comparison to monotherapies (70% one-year and 50% two-years survival), with a better safety profile (11–13).

Immuno-therapy enhances the immune system's T-cell response and indirectly affects cancer cells by stimulating the patient's immune system (14). Ipilimumab, a monoclonal antibody that blocks the activity of the CTLA-4, has shown a long-term survival in about 20% of the patients treated (15–17). Programmed death 1 (PD1) is a membrane receptor of tumor cells (its main ligand is PD-L1) that represents a powerful brake to the immune system's response and the target of specific inhibitors (nivolumab and pembrolizumab). Recently they have been introduced into clinical practice, as they were shown more effective than ipilimumab in terms of overall survival (OS) and toxicity (18, 19). Recent studies showed that the combination of anti-CTLA-4 and anti-PD-1 is more effective than monotherapy, but a higher incidence of high-grade adverse events was found (20). Combinations of targeted therapies and immunotherapies are currently investigated; the advantage of such combinations is that more than one anti-tumoral mechanism are employed against CM. Data of clinical trials and real life studies that evaluate the outcomes of these therapeutic associations are necessary to establish their clinical utility.

The aim of this study is to investigate the types of oncological treatments employed in the real-life clinical management of patients with advanced CM in several Italian centers which are part of the Clinical National Melanoma Registry (CNMR), and the oncological outcomes obtained.

MATERIALS AND METHODS

Patients and Data Collection

CNMR is the first clinical registry established in Italy in 2010. It collects data from a wide network of melanoma centers throughout the country with the aim to carry out clinical and therapeutic evaluations investigating geographical and policy differences and instruments for planning specific health interventions in different populations and areas, in order to optimize the clinical management and survival of CM patients. CNMR collects data of patients with a histologically confirmed diagnosis of primary CM treated in 38 Italian institutions (hospitals, research institutes, ecc.) participating in the network, as previously described (21). The AJCC7 staging was used. For the purposes of the present study, data of consecutive patients enrolled from January 2011 to December 2018 were considered (CNMR established in 2010 but the first year was spent for administrative approvement and ethical committee in each centers).

A diagram of the CNMR's organizational structure can be found in **Figure 1**.

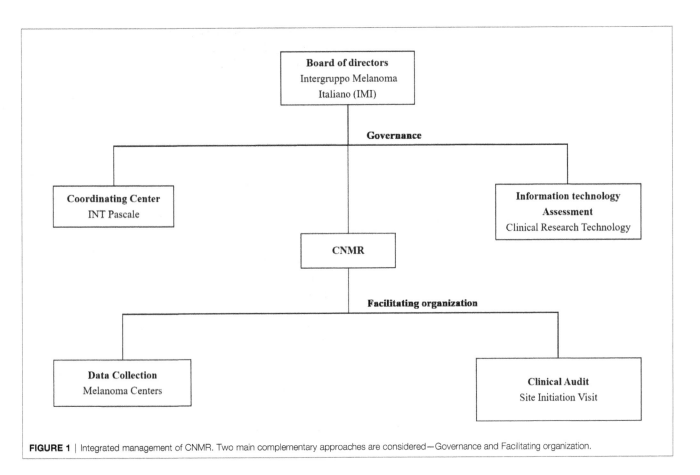

FIGURE 1 | Integrated management of CNMR. Two main complementary approaches are considered—Governance and Facilitating organization.

Data were collected *via* an electronic Case Report Form (eCRF), which was developed by the Clinical Research Technology S.r.l. group (Salerno, Italy) on its clinical platform 'eClinical'. 'eClinical' assigned an identification (ID) number to all the patients screened. The quality of the electronic data was verified through onsite clinical visits, undertaken periodically during the study. The eCRF was designed to collect information on sociodemographic, clinical, pathological and treatment variables. The first treatment was registered in all cases: local therapy (radiotherapy and electro-chemotherapy), systemic chemotherapy (platinum salts, dacarbazine, fotemustine), targeted therapy (BRAFi: vemurafenib/dabrafenib; BRAFI+MEKI: cobimetinib/trametinib), and immunotherapy (anti-CTLA4: ipilimumab, anti-PD-1: nivolumab/pembrolizumab; and anti-CTLA4 + anti-PD-1). Further information regarding the date of diagnosis, the duration of therapy, the date of the last follow-up, and the clinical status of the patients were also registered. Eligible patients for the survival analysis had histologically confirmed, unresectable stage III or stage IV metastatic melanoma (stage IIIB-IV) with an Eastern Cooperative Oncology Group (ECOG) performance status 0 or 3, and known BRAF mutation status.

Statistical Analysis

Descriptive statistics for the categorical data were reported. Pearson's Chi-squared was used to compare categorical variables. All patients were followed until 31 December 2018 or until the date of last visit, or death, whichever came first.

Melanoma-specific survival (MSS) was calculated from the date of initial adjuvant treatment to death for the disease and Overall survival (OS) until date of death from any cause. Patients who did not die were censored for OS on the last visit date available in the database. When the date of diagnosis was antecedent the beginning of the Melanoma Registry or the initial diagnosis was an early melanoma we considered the MSSurvival from the date of initial adjuvant treatment.

Kaplan-Meier curves and medians of OS and 95% CI are presented overall and by immunotherapy and target treatments. The Log-rank test compared curves by treatments (immunotherapy: anti-CTLA4, an-ti-PD-1 *vs.* no immunotherapy and no target therapy; BRAF: BRAFi, BRAFI+MEKI *vs.* no immunotherapy and no target therapy). Univariate and multivariable Cox regression models were used to estimate the hazard ratios adjusting for confounders and other prognostic factors.

All statistical tests were two-sided. P-values < 0.05 were considered significant. Statistical analyses were performed using statistical software SAS (version 9.02 for Windows), and Statistical Package for Social Science (SPSS) version 25 (SPSS inc., Chicago IL, USA).

RESULTS

Patients characteristics, sex, age, LDH, stage, BRAF execution and mutational status were reported in **Table 1**.

TABLE 1 | Tumor characteristics for Advanced Stage (IIIB-IIIC unresectable, IV).

	ADVANCED STAGE IIIB-IIIC (*unresectable*), IV N=787
Gender*	
Male	476 (60)
Female	307 (39)
missing	4 (1)
Age	
≤60 yrs	355 (45)
>60 yrs	432 (55)
BMI	
<25	315 (40)
≥25	386 (49)
missing	86 (11)
LDH	
Normal	479 (61)
Abnormal	43 (5)
Unknown	265 (34)
Initial Stage	
In situ	98 (12)
Stage I-II	297 (38)
Stage III	291 (37)
Stage IV	101 (13)
BRAF executed	
No	120 (15)
Yes	594 (76)
Not applicable	73 (9)
BRAF mutational status	
Mutant	322 (54)
Wild Type	269 (45.5)
unknown	3 (0.5)
Mutant	
BRAF V600	56 (17.4)
BRAF V600E	208 (64.6)
BRAF V600K	34 (10.6)
Other	24 (7.5)
Year BRAF executed	
<2013	498 (63)
≥2013	289 (37)

*4 patients did not report the gender.

Regarding to stage 12% had an initial diagnosis of "in situ", 38% had an early diagnosis (IA-IIC), 37% stage III and 13% had a confirmed advanced melanoma stage (IV). 76% was the percentage of BRAF executed in our sample and the incidence of BRAF mutations was slightly greater than 50% and 65% reported a BRAF V600E mutation most cases were analyzed after the year 2013 when target therapies were diffusely employed in clinical practice; in addition, more cases among those analyzed harbored stage IV tumors rather than stage IIIB-IIIC melanomas.

The median follow-up time was 36 months (range 1.2-185.1). Observed patients and percentage according to type of treatment were reported in **Table 2**; total death events (for all causes and deaths for the diseases) were reported and median Melanoma-specific survival (MSS) were calculated. As first line of treatment (choice), 41% of patients (n=319) received immunotherapy, 36% received BRAF-targeted therapies (n=285), 35% received chemotherapy (n=275) and 35% received local therapy (electrochemotherapy) (n=275). In details, among immunotherapy: 62% received ipilimumab (anti-CTLA4), 25% nivolumab/pebrolizumab (anti PD1), 13% the two combined. Among BRAF therapy: 69%

received BRAFi as monotherapy (vemurafenib/dabrafenib), about 31% received BRAFi+MEK combination treatment (vemurafenib/dabrafenib + cobimetinib/trametinib).

In the entire cohort the median overall melanoma-specific survival was 47 months (95% CI: 41-53), the lowest median survival was detected by patients treated by chemotherapy (33 months, 95% CI 27-38) as first option. Among immunotherapy the MSS globally was 50 months (95% CI 43-57), it varied from 47 months (95% CI 37-56) for ipilimumab (anti-CTLA4) to 70 months (95% CI 39-101) for nivolumab/pebrolizumab (anti-PD-1). Targeted therapy globally produced MSS of 44 months (95% CI 38-50), it varied from 40 months (95% CI 34-45) for BRAFi to 55 months (95% CI 49-61) for BRAFi+MEK (see **Table 3**).

Immunotherapy showed an improved survival compared with all other therapies (Chemotherapy, Local therapy and no targeted therapy) (p=0.001) (**Figure 2A**); for Ipilimumab and combined target therapy compared with all other therapies a slight significance were observed (p=0.05) (see **Figure 2B**). The highest survival (70 months; 95% CI 45-96) was reached by patients treated with Nivolumab/Pembrolizumab compared with combined target therapy and all other therapies (p=0.001) (see **Figure 2C**); Immunotherapy across strata showed an improved survival for anti-PD-1 and combined anti-PD-1 + anti-CTLA4 compared with Ipilimumab and all other therapies (p<0.0001) (see **Figure 2D**). The treatment-sequence did not show any significant difference (Immuno in 1st and Target in 2nd *vs*. Target in 1st and Immuno in 2nd line) (p=0.5) (see **Figure 2E**). A significant difference was observed between BRAF *vs*. BRAF with the addition of Cobimetinid/Trametinib (anti-MEK) (p=0.03) (see **Figure 2F**).

Multivariate Cox model hazard ratios were reported in **Table 4**: a significant increased risk of death was observed for abnormal LDH compared to normal (HR=1.94 95% CI 1.23-3.06); among the Target therapy a significant protective effect was observed for target therapy with the addition of Cobimetinid/Trametinib (BRAFI+MEKI) (HR=0.63 95% CI 0.42-0.94). All immunotherapy categories were significantly associated with a reduction of death: anti-PD-1 HR=0.25 (95% CI 0.15-0.43), anti-CTLA4 HR=0.47 (95% CI 0.33-0.67) and combined anti-PD-1+ anti-CTLA4 HR=0.26 (95% CI 0.15-0.47), respectively. The treatment-sequence was not associated to the risk of death (p=0.3).

DISCUSSION

In this study, we examined data of advanced melanoma in the Italian Clinical National Melanoma Registry (CNMR). CNMR does not have the typical aim of cancer registries to estimate incidence data, but as a clinical registry may collect data from the real world experience which is different from that coming from clinical studies which included selected patients (22, 23). Indeed, much of the existing research on advanced melanoma patients has been conducted in clinical trials settings among patients who meet stringent inclusion and exclusion criteria.

The analysis of the 787 patients from the advanced cohort showed some interesting results. As first, looking at the advanced patients' characteristics, a good percentage of them come from the initial stages more than from the high risk conditions.

TABLE 2 | Distribution of therapies and combined therapies in the cohort of advanced melanoma patients.

Indicator	Advanced Melanoma: IIIB-IIIC (unresectable), IV	
	Observed patients (n)	*(%)*
Patients eligible for analysis	787	(100)
Patients with at least one local treatment	275	(35)
No local treatment	512	
Patients with at least one chemotherapy	275	(35)
No chemotherapy	512	
Patients with at least one immunotherapy	319	(41)
Immunotherapy: ANTI-PD-1 (Nivolumab/Pebrolizumab)	*80 (25.1)*	
Immunotherapy: ANTI-CTLA4 (Ipilimumab)	*198 (62.1)*	
Immunotherapy: ANTI-PD-1 + ANTI-CTLA4	*41 (12.8)*	
No immunotherapy	468	
Patients with at least one target therapy (BRAFi, BRAFI+MEKI)	285	(36)
BRAFi: vemurafenib/dabrafenib	*198 (69.5)*	
BRAFI+MEKI: cobimetinib/trametinib	*87 (30.5)*	
No target therapy	502	
Numebr of Line-therapies		
Linel°	*233 (29.6)*	
Line I°+II°	*238 (30.2)*	
Linel°+II°+III°	*316 (40.2)*	

Indeed, 50% of advanced melanoma had an initial diagnosis of early stage that then developed into advanced one.

Unfortunately, the BRAF mutational status was not evaluated in all patients; indeed, the BRAF status has been documented in as much as 76% of these patients. An important consideration is that the CNMR collected data from December 2011 and the most important drug in the field of melanoma, like BRAF inhibitors, anti-CTLA4, anti-PD-1 were approved in the following years. Specifically ipilimumab was the first treatment to be approved, on February 2013, by AIFA (The Italian Medicines Agency). Vemurafenib and dabrafenib received approval on May 2013 and on October 2014 respectively as monotherapy, and on September 2016 and on January 2017 in combination with cobimetinib and trametinib respectively. Pembrolizumab was approved on May 2016 while nivolumab on 24 March 2016 (24). Moreover, the possibility to ask for the BRAF mutational status was probably related only to the centers which were participating to clinical studies or expanded access programs with such drugs.

Study strengths include a large sample size, many treatment options reported (immunotherapy such as anti-PD-1 or combination of anti-PD-1 and anti-CTLA-4, or targeted therapies) and this is the first study investigating oncological treatments in a real-life clinical settings in advanced melanoma in several Italian centers. Study limitations include a lack of information like the metastatic site and the collection of therapy data was not completely reported, therefore the evaluation of the combined treatment (chemotherapy and immunotherapy/chemotherapy and targeted therapy) was not possible.

Concerning the OS, with some limitations due to the time of data collection (before the approval and the use of anti-PD-1 and BRAF/MEK inhibitors, and the small number of patients considered), there are still some interesting findings. It is evident that the new therapies available had an important impact on the survival of these patients. Indeed, patients who practiced immunotherapy or target therapy performed better in terms of median survival than those who practiced local therapy and/or chemotherapy, considered for a long time the only standard of treatment for metastatic melanoma. The addition of the MEK inhibitor to the BRAF inhibitor significantly improved patient OS.

TABLE 3 | Results of the performance indicators on the quality of metastatic melanoma care – Univariate Analysis.

Long-term outcomes	Advanced Melanoma:IIIB-IIIC (unresectable), IV	
	Events[1] (n) DOD/DEAD	Median MSS (95% CI)
Melanoma-specific Survival (MSS) overall	314/353	*47 (41-53)*
Melanoma-specific Survival (MSS) of pts. with local treatment	132/147	*42 (35-48)*
Melanoma-specific Survival (MSS) of pts. with chemotherapy	151/163	*33 (27-38)*
Melanoma-specific Survival (MSS) of pts. with immunotherapy	126/137	*50 (43-57)*
MSS Immunotherapy: ANTI-PD-1 (Nivolumab/Pebrolizumab)	17/18	*70 (39-101)*
MSS Immunotherapy: ANTI-CTLA4 (Ipilimumab)	94/104	*47 (37-56)*
MSS Immunotherapy: ANTI-PD-1+ANTI-CTLA4	15/15	*58 (26-90)*
Melanoma-specific Survival (MSS) of pts. with target therapy	129/147	*44 (38-50)*
MSS BRAFi: vemurafenib/dabrafenib	91/107	*40 (34-45)*
MSS BRAFI+MEKI: cobimetinib/trametinib	38/40	*55 (49-61)*

[1]*Event: number of deaths of the disease (DOD)/number of deaths for all causes (DEAD).*

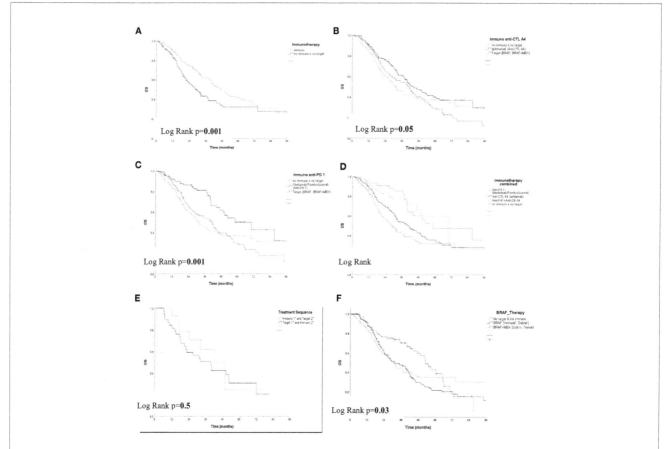

FIGURE 2 | Overall Survival (OS) in patients with IIIB-IIIC (UNRESECTABLE), IV by Therapy **(A–F)**. **(A)** Overall Survival (OS) Immunotherapy, **(B)** OS Immunotherapy: ANTI-CTL A4, **(C)** OS Immuno: ANTI-PD 1, **(D)** OS Immuno: ANTI-PD 1; ANTI-CTLA4; ANTI PD 1+ANTI-CTL A4, **(E)** OS Treatment Sequence:Immuno 1st, 2nd; Target 1st, 2nd; Target 1st & Immuno 2nd **(F)** OS BRAF *vs.* BRAFI+MEKI.

It seems that the greater advantage in terms of OS is in those patients who have performed immunotherapy lines, even compared to those who have performed target therapies. This finding could be explained by the fact that many patients received BRAF inhibitor therapy as single agent (69,5%), and only a minority had benefit from the addition of the MEK inhibitor. Indeed, we learned that disease progression during therapy with the BRAF inhibitor alone was often rapid and unresponsive to subsequent treatments (25); with the addition of MEK inhibitors, the fast progression from target therapy was reduced (26).

The data on the combination nivolumab + ipilimumab also appears intriguing, especially in terms of long survival; however, the low number of patients does not allow us to give definitive conclusions.

The correlation between survival and the LDH value is also consistent with the literature data. Analyzing the LDH values, there is an increased risk of death for patients with high LDH, compared to those with normal LDH, especially in the group of patients who received immunotherapy (HR = 2.45, p = 0.01)

We found that immunotherapy allows better results in terms of overall survival in patients with advanced melanoma, however in our analysis there is no statistically significant benefit of the

treatment-sequence variable (Immuno in 1st and Target in 2nd *vs.* Target in 1st and Immuno in 2nd line). In consideration of the retrospective analysis, the small number of patients who started with anti-PD-1, and the lack of patients who received the dual MAPK blockade, definitive conclusions cannot be made.

At the moment several combination studies of target and immunotherapies as well as protocols to establish the best sequential therapy are ongoing (27). Our study has several limitations. In fact, most patients received chemotherapy as a first systemic treatment for advanced disease, because more effective drugs such as BRAF/MEK inhibitors, anti-CTLA4 and anti-PD-1 inhibitors were approved subsequently in different years. In addition, many centers did not test all patients for BRAF, especially at the beginning.

CONCLUSIONS

Finally, this study shows that immunotherapy improves survival in advanced melanoma in a real-world population. The CNMR represents a set of data useful not only to plan the appropriate prevention measures but to better understand the effectiveness of

TABLE 4 | Multivariate Cox regression models for death.

Parameter/Category	Adjusted Multivariate Analysis[‡]		
	HR	95% CI	p
Gender			
Female	1[†]		
Male	1.121	0.898-1.398	0.314
Age			
≤60	1[†]		
>60	1.192	0.961-1.478	0.109
Area of enrollment in Italy[3]			
Center/South	1[†]		
North	0.981	0.778-1.238	0.873
Year BRAF executed[4]			
<2013	1[†]		
≥2013	1.06	0.837-1.355	0.609
LDH			
Normal	1.0[†]		
Abnormal	1.95	1.24-3.01	0.004
Unknown	0.97	0.95-1.53	0.09
Target therapy			
No Target and No Immuno therapy	1.0[†]		
BRAF	1.14	0.85-1.53	0.4
BRAFI+MEKI	0.623	0.42-0.94	0.02
Immunotherapy			
No Immuno and No Target therapy	1.0[†]		
ANTI-PD-1 (Nivolumab/Pebrolizumab)	0.25	0.147-0.43	<0.0001
ANTI-CTLA4 (Ipilimumab)	0.47	0.33-0.67	<0.0001
ANTI-PD-1+ ANTI-CTLA4	0.26	0.15-0.47	<0.0001
Treatment Sequence			
Immuno 1st and Target 2nd	1.0[†]		
Target 1st and Immuno 2nd	1.64	0.65-4.12	0.3

[†]Reference category; [‡]Multivariate Cox model adjusted for gender (male, female); age (≤60, >60); geographical area (North, Central-South);Year BRAF executed (≤2013, >2013); N. @ of therapies (1, 2, ≥3); Other therapies: Chemotherapy; Local and systemic therapy whenever.

anti-cancer treatments in a large unselected population from a real world experience. Furthermore, qualified data is essential and it is important that this information is constantly updated in order to maintain high levels of evidence.

The nivolumab/pembrolizumab and the combination of ipilimumab can be considered the best therapy to improve survival in a real-world-population. The CNMR can complement clinical registries with the intent of improving cancer management and standardizing cancer treatment.

DATA AVAILABILITY STATEMENT

The datasets presented in this study can be found in online repositories. The names of the repository/repositories and accession number(s) can be found below: http://imi.cr-technology.com/cnmr.

ETHICS STATEMENT

CNMR was approved by ethical committee of Istituto Nazionale dei Tumori Fondazione G. Pascale, protocol n.10/10, prot. CEI 537/10. The patients/participants provided their written informed consent to participate in this study.

CNMR GROUP

Maddalena Cespa, Fondazione I.R.C.C.S. Policlinico San Matteo Clinica Dermatologica, Pavia: **Rosachiara Forcignanò**, Azienda Ospedaliera Vito Fazzi, U.O. Di Oncologia, Lecce; **Gianmichele Moise**, Azienda Per I Servizi Sanitari N°2 Isontina Ospedale Di Gorizia Dipartimento Di Medicina , S.O.S. Di Dermatologia – Gorizia; **Maria Concetta Fargnoli**, Presidio Ospedaliero San Salvatore, U.O.S. Di Dermatologia Generale Ed Oncologica, L'Aquila; **Caterina Ferreli**, Università Degli Studi Di Cagliari - Azienda Ospedaliero Universitaria, Clinica Dermatologica, Cagliari; **Maria Grimaldi**, Istituto Nazionale dei Tumori Fondazione G. Pascale Napoli; **Guido Zannetti**, Azienda Ospedaliero-Universitaria Di Bologna Policlinico S. Orsola -Malpighi, Chirurgia Plastica, Bologna; **Saverio Cinieri**, Presidio Ospedaliero Antonio Perrino, U.O.C. Di Oncologia E Breast Unit, Brindisi; **Giusto Trevisan**, Ospedale Maggiore, Azienda Ospedaliera Universitaria Di Trieste, Clinica Dermatologica ,4° Piano (Palazzina Infettivi), Trieste; **Ignazio Stanganelli**, Ospedale S.Maria Delle Croci - Usl Di Ravenna, Centro Di Dermatologia Oncologica CPO/IRST, Ravenna; **Giovanna Moretti**, Azienda Ospedaliera Ospedali Riuniti Papardo-Piemonte S.C. Dermatologia Messina; **Francesca Bruder**, Ospedale Oncologico, Dipartimento Melanoma E Tumori Rari 5° Piano, Cagliari; **Luca Bianchi**, Azienda Ospedaliera Universitaria Policlinico Tor Vergata U.O.C. Dermatologia,

Roma; **Maria Teresa Fierro**, A.O.U. Città Della Salute E Della Scienza - P.O. San Lazzaro, S.C. Dermatolgia Torino; **Luigi Mascheroni**, Humanitas - Casa Di Cura San Pio X S.R.L., Chirurgia GeneraleMilano; **Salvatore Asero**, Azienda Ospedaliera Di Rilievo Nazionale E Di Alta Specializzazione Garibaldi-Nesima, U.O. Di Chirurgia Oncologica - Dip. Oncologia, Catania; **Caterina Catricalà**, Istituto Dermatologico San Gallicano IRCCS – IFO, UOC di Dermatologia Oncologica - Dipartimento Clinico-Sperimentale Di Dermatologia Oncologica Roma; **Stefania Staibano**, Azienda Ospedaliera Universitaria Federico II di Napoli, Scienze Biomorfologiche e Funzionali-Sezione Di Anatomia Patologica, Napoli; **Gaetana Rinaldi**, Azienda Ospedaliera Universitaria Policlinico `Paolo Giaccone`, Dipartimento Di Oncologia - U.O.C. Oncologia Medica, Palermo; **Riccardo Pellicano**, IRCCS Casa Sollievo Della Sofferenza, U.O.C. Dermatologia, San Giovanni Rotondo; **Laura Milesi**, Azienda Ospedaliera Papa Giovanni XXIII, USC Oncologia Medica, Bergamo; **Marilena Visini**, A.O. Di Lecco Presidio Ospedaliero Alessandro Manzoni, Oncologia Medica, Lecco; **Franco Di Filippo**, Istituto Nazionale Tumori Regina Elena IRCCS – IFO, Chirurgia Generale A, Roma; **Leonardo Zichichi**, Azienda Sanitaria Provinciale - Presidio Ospedaliero Di Trapani, U.O. C. Dermatologia, Casa Santa – Erice; **Maria Antonietta Pizzichetta**, Centro Di Riferimento Oncologico, Istituto Nazionale Tumori, Divisione Di Oncologia Medica C, Aviano; **Carmelo Iacono**, Azienda Ospedaliera Sanitaria 7 Ragusa - Ospedale Maria Paternò Arezzo, Dipartimento Di Oncologia, Ragusa; **Massimo Guidoboni**, I.R.S.T. Istituto Scientifico Romagnolo Per Lo Studio E La Cura Dei Tumori U.O. Immunoterapia E Terapia Cellulare Somatica, Meldola; **Giovanni Sanna**, Azienda Ospedaliero-Universitaria Di Sassari, Servizio Di Medicina Nucleare U.O. Di Oncologia Medica, Sassari; **Michele Maio**, Azienda Ospedaliera Universitaria Senese Ospedale Le Scotte U.O.C. Immunoterapia Oncologica, Siena; Michele Del Vecchio, Fondazione I.R.C.C.S. Istituto Nazionale Dei Tumori, S.C. Medicina Oncologica 1, Milano; **Lucia Lospalluti**, Azienda Sanitaria Locale BA - Ospedale Di Venere, U.O. Dermatologia, Carbonara Di Bari; **Rosanna Barbati**, Asl Roma C - Ospedale S.Eugenio , U.O. Dermatologia, Roma; **Leonardi Vita**, ARNAS Civico Palermo; **Annamaria Pollio**, Ospedale "A. Cardarelli" – Campobasso, U.O.C. di Anatomia Patologica; **Carlo Riberti**, Istituto di Chirurgia Plastica presso l'Arcispedale Sant'Anna, Ferrara.

AUTHOR CONTRIBUTIONS

Conceptualization, AC, GP, AT, and PA. Methodology, AC, VV, MB, SG, GP, and PA. Software, AC, and SG. Validation, AC, MC, AV, PF, PQ, FS, VV, CC, GT, GM, EC, MB, SG, AT, GP, and PA. Formal analysis, AC, VV, and SG. Investigation, MC, EG, AV, PF, PQ, FS, VV, CC, GT, EP, GG, EN, PQ, SR, MiG, DaM, SB, MoG, VG, MO, FG, GC, AG, DeM, LA, NC, TF, GM, FT, EC, MB, SG, CR, AT, and PA. Resources AC, VV, MB, SG, GP, and PA. Data curation, AC, VV, GP, and SG. Writing—original draft preparation, AC, MC, AV, PF, PQ, FS, VV, CC, GT, GM, EC, MB, SG, AT, GP, and PA. Writing—review and editing, AC, VV, GT, GM, EC, MB, SG, AT, GP, and PA. Visualization, AC, VV, SG, GP, and PA. Supervision, AC, VV, MB, SG, GP, and PA. Project administration, AC, VV, MB, SG, GP, and PA. Funding acquisition, CR, AT, and PA. All authors contributed to the article and approved the submitted version.

FUNDING

This research was funded by grants received from Bristol Myers Squibb (New York, NY, USA), GlaxoSmithKline (Brentford, UK) and Pierre Fabre Pharma. The funders were not involved in the study design, collection, analysis, interpretation of data, the writing of this article or the decision to submit it for publication.

ACKNOWLEDGMENTS

We would like to express our special thanks to Dr. Maurizio Montella († May 2, 2019) for his long-term contribution to the study and for his ideas and support of this current manuscript. The authors would like to thank the Intergruppo Melanoma Italiano (IMI), the Clinical Research Technology (CRT) and Dr. Giuseppe Porciello for graphical assistance.

REFERENCES

1. Bray F, Ferlay J, Soerjomataram I, Siegel RL, Torre LA, Jemal A. Global Cancer Statistics 2018: GLOBOCAN Estimates of Incidence and Mortality Worldwide for 36 Cancers in 185 Countries. *CA Cancer J Clin* (2018) 68 (6):394–424. doi: 10.3322/caac.21492

2. Hollestein LM, de Vries E, Nijsten T. Trends of Cutaneous Squamous Cell Carcinoma in the Netherlands: Increased Incidence Rates, But Stable Relative Survival and Mortality 1989-2008. *Eur J Cancer* (2012) 48:2046–53. doi: 10.1016/j.ejca.2012.01.003

3. de Vries E, Bray FI, Coebergh JW, Parkin DM. Changing Epidemiology of Malignant Cutaneous Melanoma in Europe 1953-1997: Rising Trends in Incidence and Mortality But Recent Stabilizations in Western Europe and Decreases in Scandinavia. *Int J Cancer* (2003) 107:119–26. doi: 10.1002/ijc.11360

4. Garbe C, Leiter U. Melanoma Epidemiology and Treands. *Clin Dermatol* (2009) 27:3–9. doi: 10.1016/j.clindermatol.2008.09.001

5. Crocetti E, Mallone S, Robsahm TE, Gavin A, Agius D, Ardanaz E, et al. Survival of Patients With Skin Melanoma in Europe Increases Further: Results of the EUROCARE-5 Study. *Eur J Cancer* (2015) 51(15):2179–90. doi: 10.1016/j.ejca.2015.07.039

6. Cossu A, Casula M, Cerasaccio R, Lissia A, Colombino M, Sini MC, et al. Epidemiology and Genetic Susceptibility of Malignant Melanoma in North Sardinia, Italy. *Eur J Cancer Prev* (2017) 26(3):263–7. doi: 10.1097/CEJ.0000000000000223

7. Ascierto PA and AIRTum Working Group and Working Group. In: *AssociazioneItaliana di Oncologia Medica, Associazione Italiana Registri Tumori, ed. I numeri del cancro in Italia.* (2018) p. 131–41.

8. Sini MC, Doneddu V, Paliogiannis P, Casula M, Colombino M, Manca A, et al. Genetic Alterations in Main Candidate Genes During Melanoma Progression. *Oncotarget* (2018) 9(9):8531–41. doi: 10.18632/oncotarget.23989

9. Palmieri G, Ombra M, Colombino M, Casula M, Sini M, Manca A, et al. Multiple Molecular Pathways in Melanomagenesis: Characterization of Therapeutic Targets. *Front Oncol* (2015) 5:183. doi: 10.3389/fonc.2015.00183

10. Chapman PB, Hauschild A, Robert C, Haanen JB, Ascierto PA, Larkin J, et al. Improved Survival With Vemurafenib in Melanoma With BRAF V600E Mutation. *N Engl J Med* (2011) J364(26):2507–16. doi: 10.1056/NEJMoa1103782

11. Hauschild A, Grob JJ, Demidov LV, Jouary T, Gutzmer R, Millward M, et al. Dabrafenib in BRAF-Mutated Metastatic Melanoma: A Multicentre, Open-Label, Phase 3 Randomised Controlled Trial. *Lancet* (2012) 380(9839):358–65. doi: 10.1016/S0140-6736(12)60868-X

12. Long GV, Flaherty KT, Stroyavskiy D, Gogas H, Levchenko, de Braud F, et al. Dabrafenib Plus Trametinib *Versus* Dabrafenib Monotherapy in Patients With Metastatic BRAFV600E/K-Mutant Melanoma: Long-Term Survival and Safety Analysis of a Phase 3 Study. *Ann Oncol* (2017) 28(7):1631–9. doi: 10.1093/annonc/mdx176

13. Robert C, Grob JJ, Stroyakovskiy D, Karaszewska B, Hauschild A, Levchenko E, et al. Five-Year Outcomes With Dabrafenib Plus Trametinib in Metastatic Melanoma. *N Engl J Med* (2019) 381(7):626–36. doi: 10.1056/NEJMoa1904059

14. Larkin J, Ascierto PA, Dréno B, Atkinson V, Liszkay G, Maio M, et al. Combined Vemurafenib and Cobimetinib in BRAF-Mutated Melanoma. *N Engl J Med* (2014) 371(20):1867–76. doi: 10.1056/NEJMoa1408868

15. Topalian SL, Stephen-Hodi F, Brahmer JR, Gettinger SN, Smith DC, McDermott DF, et al. Safety, Activity, and Immune Correlates of Anti-PD-1 Antibody in Cancer. *N Engl J Med* (2012) 366(26):2443–54. doi: 10.1056/NEJMoa1200690

16. Hodi FS, O'Day SJ, McDermott DF, Weber RW, Sosman JA, Haaner JB, et al. Improved Survival With Ipilimumab in Patients With Metastatic Melanoma. *N Engl J Med* (2010) 363(8):711–23. doi: 10.1056/NEJMoa1003466

17. Schadendorf D, Hodi FS, Robert C, Weber JS, Margolin K, Hamid O, et al. Pooled Analysis of Long-Term Survival Data From Phase II and Phase III Trials of Ipilimumab in Unresectable or Metastatic Melanoma. *J Clin Oncol* (2015) 33(17):1889–94. doi: 10.1200/JCO.2014.56.2736

18. Ascierto PA, Del Vecchio M, Robert C, Mackiewicz A, Chiarion-Sileni V, Arance A, et al. Ipilimumab 10 Mg/Kg *Versus* Ipilimumab 3 Mg/Kg in Patients With Unresectable or Metastatic Melanoma: A Randomised, Double-Blind, Multicentre, Phase 3 Trial. *Lancet Oncol* (2017) 18(5):611–22. doi: 10.1016/S1470-2045(17)30231-0

19. Schachter J, Ribas A, Long GV, Arance A, Grob JJ, Montier L, et al. Pembrolizumab *Versus* Ipilimumab for Advanced Melanoma: Final Overall Survival Results of a Multicentre, Randomised, Open-Label Phase 3 Study (KEYNOTE-006). *Lancet* (2017) 390(10105):1853–62. doi: 10.1016/S0140-6736(17)31601-X

20. Robert C, Long GV, Brady B, Dutriaux C, Maio M, Montier L, et al. Nivolumab in Previously Untreated Melanoma Without BRAF Mutation. *N Engl J Med* (2015) 372(4):320–30. doi: 10.1056/NEJMoa1412082

21. Larkin J, Chiarion-Sileni V, Gonzalez R, Grob JJ, Rutkowski P, Lao CD, et al. Five-Year Survival With Combined Nivolumab and Ipilimumab in Advanced Melanoma. *N Engl J Med* (2019) 381(16):1535–46. doi: 10.1056/NEJMoa1910836

22. Gandini S, Montella M, Ayala F, Benedetto L, Rossi CR, Vecchiato A, et al. Sun Exposure and Melanoma Prognostic Factors. *Oncol Lett* (2016) 4):2706–14. doi: 10.3892/ol.2016.4292

23. Jochems A, Schouwenburg MG, Leeneman B, Franken MG, van den Eertwegh AJ, Haanen JB, et al. Dutch Melanoma Treatment Registry: Quality Assurance in the Care of Patients With Metastatic Melanoma in the Netherlands. *Eur J Cancer* (2017) 72:156–65. doi: 10.1016/j.ejca.2016.11.021

24. Cowey CL, Liu FX, Boyd M, Aguilar KM, Krepler C. Real-World Treatment Patterns and Clinical Outcomes Among Patients With Advanced Melanoma: A Retrospective, Community Oncology-Based Cohort Study (A STROBE-Compliant Article). *Med (Baltimore)* (2019) 98(28):e16328. doi: 10.1097/MD.0000000000016328

25. *AIFA (Regime Di Rimborsabilita' E Prezzo Di Vendita Del Medicinale Nivolumab) - Autorizzata Con Procedura Centralizzata Europea Dalla Commissione Europea.* Gazzetta Ufficiale della Repubblica Italia n. 70 24-03-2016.

26. Pavlick AC, Fecher L, Ascierto PA, Sullivan RJ. Frontline Therapy for BRAF-Mutated Metastatic Melanoma: How Do You Choose, and Is There One Correct Answer? *Am Soc Clin Oncol Educ Book* (2019) 39:564–71. doi: 10.1200/EDBK_243071

27. Ascierto PA, Simeone E, Grimaldi AM, Curvietto M, Esposito E, Palmieri G, et al. Do BRAF Inhibitors Select for Populations With Different Disease Progression Kinetics? *J Transl Med* (2013) 11:61. doi: 10.1186/1479-5876-11-61

22

Melanoma in Adolescents and Young Adults: Evaluation of the Characteristics, Treatment Strategies and Prognostic Factors in a Monocentric Retrospective Study

Paolo Del Fiore [1*†], Irene Russo [1,2†], Beatrice Ferrazzi [3], Alessandro Dal Monico [4], Francesco Cavallin [5], Angela Filoni [1], Saveria Tropea [1], Francesco Russano [1], Claudia Di Prata [1], Alessandra Buja [6], Alessandra Collodetto [1], Romina Spina [1], Sabrina Carraro [1], Rocco Cappellesso [7], Lorenzo Nicolè [8,9], Vanna Chiarion-Sileni [10], Jacopo Pigozzo [10], Luigi Dall'Olmo [1,11], Marco Rastrelli [1,11], Antonella Vecchiato [1], Clara Benna [11], Chiara Menin [12], Daniela Di Carlo [13], Gianni Bisogno [13], Angelo Paolo Dei Tos [7], Mauro Alaibac [2‡] and Simone Mocellin [1,11‡]

[1] Soft-Tissue, Peritoneum and Melanoma Surgical Oncology Unit, Veneto Institute of Oncology - IOV IRCCS, Padua, Italy, [2] Division of Dermatology, Department of Medicine (DIMED), University of Padua, Padua, Italy, [3] Postgraduate School of Occupational Medicine, University of Verona, Verona, Italy, [4] Department of Medicine, University of Padua School of Medicine and Surgery, Padua, Italy, [5] Independent Statistician, Solagna, Italy, [6] Department of Cardiological, Thoracic, Vascular Sciences and Public Health, University of Padua, Padua, Italy, [7] Pathological Anatomy Unit, University Hospital of Padua, Padua, Italy, [8] Department of Medicine (DIMED), Unit of Pathology & Cytopathology, University of Padua, Padua, Italy, [9] Unit of Surgical Pathology & Cytopathology, Ospedale dell'Angelo, Mestre, Italy, [10] Melanoma Oncology Unit, Veneto Institute of Oncology IOV-IRCCS, Padua, Italy, [11] Department of Surgery, Oncology and Gastroenterology (DISCOG), University of Padua, Padua, Italy, [12] Immunology and Diagnostic Molecular Oncology Unit, Veneto Institute of Oncology IOV-IRCCS, Padua, Italy, [13] Hematology/Oncology Division, Department of Women's and Children's Health, University of Padua, Padua, Italy

*Correspondence:
Paolo Del Fiore
paolo.delfiore@iov.veneto.it
†These authors have contributed equally to this work
‡These authors share last authorship

The "Veneto Cancer Registry" records melanoma as the most common cancer diagnosed in males and the third common cancer in females under 50 years of age in the Veneto Region (Italy). While melanoma is rare in children, it has greater incidence in adolescents and young adults (AYA), but literature offers only few studies specifically focused on AYA melanoma. The aim of this study was to describe the characteristics, surgical treatment, and prognosis of a cohort of AYA melanoma in order to contribute to the investigation of this malignancy and provide better patient care. This retrospective cohort study included 2,752 Caucasian patients (702 AYA and 2,050 non-AYA patients) from the Veneto Region who were over 15 years of age at diagnosis, and who received diagnosis and/or treatment from our institutions between 1998 and 2014. Patients were divided in adolescents and youth (15-25 years), young adults (26-39 years) and adults (more than 39 years) for the analysis. We found statistically significant differences in gender, primary site, Breslow thickness, ulceration, pathologic TNM classification (pTNM) stage and tumor subtype among the age groups. Disease-specific survival and disease-free survival were also different among the age groups. Our findings suggest that the biological behavior of melanoma in young people is different to that in adults, but not such as to represent a distinct pathological entity. Additional and larger prospective studies should be performed to better evaluate potential biological and cancer-specific differences between AYAs and the adult melanoma population.

Keywords: melanoma, skin cancer, AYA, adolescent and young adult oncology, adolescent and young adult melanoma, survival, incidence, melanoma surgical treatment

1 INTRODUCTION

The incidence of melanoma is continuously increasing in both adult and pediatric population around the world (1, 2). Although melanoma is rare in pediatric patients, the risk of developing melanoma grows significantly in adolescents and young adults, and represents the second most common type of cancer in this age group (3–5). The literature on melanoma offers very few studies specifically addressing adolescents and young adults (AYA). Of note, previous studies presented clinical and prognostic differences between melanoma diagnosed in adolescents, young adults and adults (6, 7). Specific clinical practice guidelines for the treatment of melanoma in AYA do not exist, and current management is similar to melanoma in adults.

This study compared characteristics, surgical treatment, and prognosis in a cohort of melanoma patients according to the age at diagnosis, with the purpose of underling potential differences in terms of tumor characteristics and prognosis between melanoma in AYA and melanoma in adults (non-AYA).

2 MATERIALS AND METHODS

2.1 Study Design

This is a retrospective cohort study of patients who were diagnosed and/or treated for Melanoma of the skin between 1998-2014 at the Veneto Institute of Oncology (IOV) and at the University Hospital of Padua (UHP).

2.2 Material

The study included all 2,752 patients aged ≥15 years and living in the Veneto Region, who were diagnosed and/or treated for Primary Melanoma of the skin between 1998-2014 at the Veneto Institute of Oncology (IOV) and at the University Hospital of Padua (UHP). IOV and UHP are level III referral centers which are located in Northeastern Italy. Most patients are referred for diagnosis and/or first-line treatment, while some patients are referred for disease progression after being treated at local level II centers.

2.3 Diagnosis and Treatment

Melanoma was diagnosed according to the histopathology and immunohistochemistry of the lesion biopsy. Tumor stage was defined according to the eighth version of the American Joint Committee on Cancer (AJCC) staging system (8), effective from January 2018. All diagnoses before January 2018 were re-staged according to the last version of the staging system.

The surgical treatment included wide excision (WE) of the primary lesion, sentinel lymph node biopsy (SNB) and/or regional lymph node dissection. Patients with locoregional primary melanoma underwent WE, followed by complete lymph node dissection (LND) in clinical node-positive patients. Sentinel node biopsy was performed concurrently with WE in patients with primary lesions.

Follow-up visits were performed every three to four months for the first three years, every six months for up to five years, and every year thereafter.

Disease progression included regional recurrences, in-transit metastases, lymph node metastases, and distant metastases.

2.4 Data Collection

All data were extracted from a local database. Demographics included age at diagnosis, sex and family history, while tumor information included subtype of melanoma (such as acral lentiginous melanoma, lentigo maligna melanoma, nodular melanoma, superficial spreading melanoma, spitzoid melanoma, nevoid melanoma, pagetoid melanoma, polypoid melanoma, desmoplastic melanoma, minimal deviation melanoma and neurotropic melanoma) primary site, Breslow thickness, ulceration, mitotic rate, and pTNM stage.

Follow-up information was extracted from scheduled visits. Follow-up was calculated from the date of diagnosis to December 31, 2019. Disease-specific survival was calculated from date of diagnosis to date of disease-related death, or date of last visit/disease-unrelated death. Disease-free survival was calculated in patients with primary melanoma from date of diagnosis to date of recurrence, or date of last visit/death. Recurrence was defined as regional recurrences, in-transit metastases, lymph node metastases or distant metastases.

2.5 Statistical Analysis

Continuous data were summarized as median and interquartile range (IQR). The patient cohort was divided into three age groups: adolescents and youth (15-25 years), young adults (26-39 years) and adults (more than 39 years). Categorical data were compared between age groups using the Fisher's exact test, while the Kruskal-Wallis test was used for continuous data. Survival estimates were calculated using the Kaplan-Meier method and compared among age groups using log-rank test (unadjusted analysis) and Cox regression models with pTNM stage as additional independent variable (adjusted analysis). Effect sizes were reported as hazard ratio (HR) with 95% confidence interval (CI). The limited sample size and availability of immunohistochemistry data did not allow any meaningful multivariable analyses. All tests were two-sided and a p-value of less than 0.05 was considered statistically significant. Statistical analyses were performed using R software version 4.1 (R Foundation for Statistical Computing, Vienna, Austria) (9).

2.6 Ethics Considerations

The study was approved by the local Ethics Committee (number 2/2020). The study was conducted according to Helsinki Declaration principles, and all patients gave their consent to have their anonymized data used for scientific purpose.

3 RESULTS

3.1 Patients

This analysis included 2,752 Caucasian patients aged ≥15 years, involving 76 (2.8%) adolescents and youth (median 22 years, IQR 20-24), 626 (22.7%) young adults (median 34 years, IQR 31-37) and 2,050 (74.5%) adults (median 54 years, IQR 48-68). Patient characteristics according to age classes are outlined in

Table 1. Sex, primary tumor site, Breslow thickness, ulceration, number of mitoses, tumor stage and sub-type differed among the age classes.

3.2 Treatment of Primary Melanoma

All patients underwent WE, while SNB was performed in 1,412 patients and LND in 394. Treatment according to age classes is shown in Table 2. The number of excised sentinel lymph nodes (SLNs) differed among age classes, while the number of positive sentinel lymph nodes and the number of positive dissected lymph nodes were the same.

3.2.1 Disease-Specific Survival

Median follow-up was 96 months (IQR 60-132). Overall, 312 patients died from the disease, and 211 patients died due to other causes (18 patients were lost to follow-up). 5-year disease-

TABLE 1 | Patient and tumor characteristics in 2,752 patients aged ≥15 years and living in the Veneto Region who were diagnosed and/or treated for Melanoma of the skin between 1998-2014 at the Veneto Institute of Oncology and at the University Hospital of Padua (Italy): comparison between age classes (15-25 years, 26-39 years, 40 years or older).

	Adolescents and youth (15-25 years)	Young adults (26-39 years)	Adults (40 years or older)	p-value
N	76	626	2050	–
Sex:				<0.0001
Female	43 (56.6)	389 (62.1)	1010 (49.3)	
Male	33 (43.4)	237 (37.9)	1040 (50.7)	
Primary site:				0.0003
Acral	2 (2.6)	16 (2.6)	137 (6.7)	
Head/neck	2 (2.6)	32 (5.1)	150 (7.3)	
Upper limb	7 (9.2)	89 (14.2)	295 (14.4)	
Trunk	47 (61.8)	318 (50.8)	947 (46.2)	
Lower limb	18 (23.6)	171 (27.3)	521 (25.4)	
Breslow [ab]	0.63 (0.39-1.20)	0.57 (0.35-1.09)	0.75 (0.39-1.90)	<0.0001
Ulceration:				0.04
Absent	56 (73.7)	508 (81.1)	1561 (76.1)	
Present	16 (21.0)	100 (16.0)	435 (21.2)	
Unknown	4 (5.3)	18 (2.9)	54 (2.6)	
Mitotic rate(per mm^2) [ac]	1 (0-2)	1 (0-2)	2 (0-4)	0.02
pTNM stage:				0.0005
I	55 (72.4)	470 (75.1)	1387 (67.7)	
II	10 (13.1)	64 (10.2)	337 (16.4)	
III	11 (14.5)	90 (14.4)	326 (15.9)	
IV	0 (0.0)	2 (0.3)	0 (0.0)	
pT:				<0.0001
1a-b, 2a-b	64 (84.2)	534 (85.3)	1562 (76.2)	
3a-b, 4a-b	12 (15.8)	92 (14.7)	488 (23.8)	
pN:				0.63
0	65 (85.5)	536 (85.6)	1724 (84.1)	
1-3	11 (14.5)	90 (14.4)	326 (15.9)	
pM:		624 (99.7)		0.11
0	76 (100.0)	2 (0.3)	2050 (100.0)	
1a-d	0 (0.0)		0 (0.0)	
Subtype: [d]				<0.0001
ALM*	1 (1.5)	7 (.2)	72 (3.5)	
LMM*	0 (0.0)	2 (0.3)	37 (1.8)	
NM*	9 (12.7)	74 (12.9)	335 (16.3)	
SSM*	53 (74.6)	469 (81.6)	1541 (75.2)	
Other**	8 (11.2)	23 (4.0)	65 (3.2)	

Data expressed as n (%) or [a] median (IQR). Data not available in [b]70, [c]15, [d]56 patients. *ALM, Acral lentiginous melanoma; LMM, lentigo maligna melanoma; NM, nodular melanoma; SSM, superficial spreading melanoma. **Spitzoid Melanoma, Nevoid melanoma, pagetoid melanoma, polypoid melanoma, desmoplastic melanoma, minimal deviation melanoma and neurotropic melanoma.
The bold values are statistically significant.

TABLE 2 | Treatment of primary Melanoma of the skin in 2,752 patients aged ≥15 years and living in the Veneto Region who were diagnosed and/or treated for Melanoma between 1998-2014 at the Veneto Institute of Oncology and at the University Hospital of Padua (Italy): comparison between age classes (15-25 years, 26-39 years, 40 years or older).

	Adolescents and youth (15-25 years)	Young adults (26-39 years)	Adults (40 years or older)	p-value
N	76	626	2050	–
Patients who underwent WE	76 (100.0)	626 (100.0)	2050 (100.0)	-
Patient with positive SNB or clinical detection	10/75 (13.3)	83/612 (13.6)	272/2050 (13.3)	0.98
Excised sentinel nodes [a]	2 (2-4)	2 (1-3)	2 (1-3)	**0.002**
Positive sentinel nodes [a]	0 (0-0)	0 (0-0)	0 (0-0)	0.33
Positive dissected lymph node [a]	0 (0-6)	0 (0-1)	0 (1-3)	0.22

Data expressed as n (%) or [a] median (IQR). WE, Wide excision; SNB, sentinel lymph node biopsy. SNB was conducted in 41/76 adolescents, 324/626 young adults and 1047/2050 adults. Clinical detection: 0 adolescents, 9 young adults and 43 adults. Positive SNB: 10 adolescents, 74 young adults and 229 adults. Total lymphadenectomy: 10 adolescents, 83 young adults, 272 adults.
The bold values are statistically significant.

specific survival was 95% in patients aged 15-25 years, 95% in patients aged 26-39 years, and 90% in patients over 39 years (p<0.0001) (**Figure 1**). Adjusting for pTNM stage, patients aged 26-39 years had better disease-specific survival compared to patients over 39 years (HR 0.52, 95% CI 0.37 to 0.70; p<0.0001), while the difference between patients aged 15-25 years and patients over 39 years was not statistically significant (HR 0.46, 95% CI 0.19 to 1.12; p=0.09).

3.2.2 Disease-Free Survival

393 patients experienced a clinical event during follow-up: local recurrence in 56 patients, regional lymph node metastasis in 128, regional skin/in-transit in 130, and distant metastasis in 167.

5-year disease-free survival (i.e. survival until the occurrence of a clinical event or death/last visit) was 95% in patients aged 15-25

years, 91% in patients aged 26-39 years, and 87% in patients over 39 years (p=0.003) (**Figure 2**). Adjusting for pTNM stage, disease-free survival was better in patients aged 15-25 years (HR 0.42, 95% CI 0.19 to 0.95; p=0.04) and patients aged 26-39 years (HR 0.74, 95% CI 0.57 to 0.95; p=0.02) compared to patients over 39 years.

"Local recurrence"-free survival did not differ among age classes (p=0.20)

"Regional lymph node metastasis"- free survival differed among age classes (5-year survival: 98% in patients aged 15-25 years, 97% in patients aged 26-39 years, and 95% in patients aged over 39 years; p=0.02). Adjusting for pTNM stage, patients aged 26-39 years had better "regional lymph node metastasis"- free survival compared to patients over 39 years (HR 0.58, 95% CI 0.36 to 0.95; p=0.03), while the difference between patients aged 15-25 years and patients over 39 years was not statistically

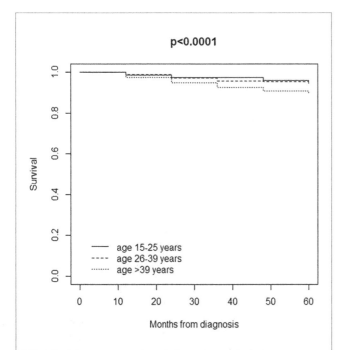

FIGURE 1 | Disease-specific survival in 2,734 patients (18 patients were lost to follow-up) aged ≥15 years and living in the Veneto Region who were diagnosed and/or treated for Melanoma between 1998-2014 at the Veneto Institute of Oncology and at the University Hospital of Padua (Italy): comparison between age classes (15-25 years, 26-39 years, 40 years or older).

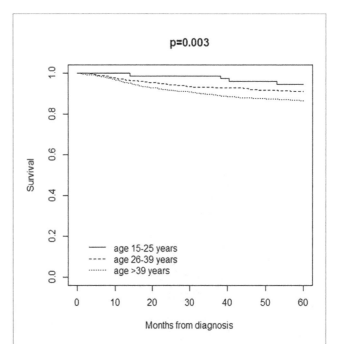

FIGURE 2 | Disease-free survival in 2,734 patients (18 patients were lost to follow-up) aged ≥15 years and living in the Veneto Region who were diagnosed and/or treated for Melanoma between 1998-2014 at the Veneto Institute of Oncology and at the University Hospital of Padua (Italy): comparison between age classes (15-25 years, 26-39 years, 40 years or older).

significant (HR 0.46, 95% CI 0.11 to 1.85; p=0.27)."Regional skin/in-transit" - free survival differed among age classes (5-year survival: 98% in patients aged 15-25 years, 98% in patients aged 26-39 years, 95% in patients aged over 39 years; p=0.003). Adjusting for pTNM stage, patients aged 26-39 years had better "regional skin/in-transit"- free survival compared to patients over 39 years (HR 0.44, 95% CI 0.26 to 0.75; p=0.002), while the difference between patients aged 15-25 years and patients over 39 years was not statistically significant (HR 0.42, 95% CI 0.10 to 1.72; p=0.23). "Distant metastasis" - free survival did not differ among age classes (p=0.06).

4 DISCUSSION

There is currently a lack of data with regard to melanoma features and outcomes in AYA. A distinction should be made between AYA and older adult cancer in disease biology, treatment efficacy, and psychosocial barriers to care for patients. Moreover, patients aged 15-25 are a sub-category of AYA which is trapped in a medical gray area and may receive cancer treatment from pediatric or adult oncologists. Although this may not be perceived as an important aspect, treatment regimens for pediatric and adult cancer can lead to significant survival differences (10).

Overall, we found some differences in epidemiological, clinical, histopathological and prognostic features between AYA and non-AYA melanoma patients. Furthermore, some differences between adolescents and young adults also emerged.

We found more female patients in the AYA group than in the non-AYA. Females represented 56.6% of adolescents and youth (15-25 years old) and 62.1% of young adults (26-39 years old), while the proportion of males and females was similar among older adults. This finding is consistent with available literature (3), and could be explained by both biological and behavioral gender differences between young male and female patients (11). A strong endogenous estrogen exposure, due to early menarche associated with UV exposure during childhood, seems to play a crucial role in cutaneous melanoma development, and may explain the higher occurrence of melanoma in young females than in males (11).

AYA melanoma presented higher involvement of the trunk, while non-AYA melanoma were more common in the acral region, head/neck and upper limbs. On the other hand, the occurrence in lower limbs was similar among the age groups. Adolescent subjects, compared to young adults, had less involvement of the head/neck and upper limbs, while the trunk was the main affected site. These data mirror what is already known in the literature, namely, that the most affected sites are the trunk and lower limbs in young people and the head/neck and upper limbs increases among adults (3). However, the involvement of the trunk, upper limbs and head/neck in young adults was more similar to older adults than adolescents.

We found a different distribution of histological subtypes of melanoma between AYAs and older adults. Superficial spreading melanoma (SSM) was more common in young adults than in adults, but less common in adolescents than in adults. Nodular

melanoma (NM), lentigo maligna melanoma (LMM) and acral lentiginous melanoma (ALM) were more common in adults. There was a considerable fraction of rare melanomas in adolescents these findings largely reflect what is known in the literature, namely, the greater presence of NM in older age, the presence of ALM almost exclusively in the elderly and rare melanomas in adolescent and young patients (12).

Moreover, we found that older adults were the subgroup with the worst pathological characteristics at the time of diagnosis. 21.2% of older adults presented ulceration, 32.3% had pTNM stage above the first, and the median Breslow thickness was 0.75 mm. At the time of diagnosis, melanoma in our cohort of patients was generally less advanced in AYAs than in adults. However, we found important differences between adolescents and young adults. Median Breslow thickness was 0.63 mm in adolescents and 0.57 mm in young adults; ulceration was found 21% in adolescents and 16% in young adults; a pTNM stage above the first was described in 27.6% of adolescents and in 24.9% of young adults. AYAs had lower Breslow thickness and lower pTNM stage at the time of diagnosis compared to adults, while there was no difference in regional lymph node involvement among age groups. Of note, adolescents had slightly worse stage characteristics than young adults.

It is important to emphasize that regional lymph node invasion (detected through positivity of the SNB or clinical positivity) was almost the same in the three age groups. Most pediatric melanoma studies suggested that the clinical history of melanoma in children and adolescents resembled that of adult disease (3, 4, 6, 7). As in adults, features such as ulceration, tumor thickness, and node involvement seemed to affect prognosis. Hence, in the absence of specific treatment guidelines, AYA melanoma is currently managed in the same way as non-AYA melanoma, though it is unclear whether it actually may have the same biological features as adult melanoma.

Data concerning the aggressiveness and prognosis of melanoma in AYAs are discordant in literature. Some studies reported that melanomas diagnosed in children and adolescents had higher Breslow thickness, greater tendency to regional lymph node invasion and, generally, a more advanced stage at the time of diagnosis compared to adults (13–17). On the other hand, it was also reported that young patients tended to have a better overall disease-specific survival than older adults (4, 15, 18).

In our study, disease-specific survival and disease-free survival were worse in older adults than in AYAs. Of note, most survival differences between younger and older age classes persisted after adjusting for tumor stage. This can be attributed to a diminished immune response with increased age, changes in host immune biology, and undertreatment due to medical comorbidities that may limit therapy with antineoplastic and biologic agents. The immune surveillance mechanism is one of the main factors which are hypothesized to account for better melanoma survival in the adolescents (19). Nonetheless, promoting skin cancer screening and public education (such as skin protection and self-examination awareness) is of utmost importance in patients of any age.

Regional lymph node metastasis-free survival and regional skin/in transit-free survival were different among age classes, with improved survival in young adults over adults, while the difference between adolescents and adults did not achieved statistical significance (likely due to the small number of adolescents in the study). Regional lymph node metastasis-free survival and regional skin/in transit-free survival have a substantial difference in survival regardless of patient's age and involve a different therapeutic strategy.

The findings of this study should be interpreted considering his strengths and limitations. The strengths involve the completeness of information regarding epidemiological, clinical, histopathological and prognostic features, and the follow-up duration (at least 5 years for all patients). The limitations include the retrospective nature of the study and the absence of data regarding the analysis of mutational profiles and medical treatments for advanced melanoma. Furthermore, the small number of adolescents (which reflects melanoma epidemiology) may limit the generalizability of the findings for this subgroup.

Nonetheless, our study highlighted a sub-category of AYA aged 15-25 which may receive cancer treatment from pediatric or adult oncologists, with potential difference in survival outcome (10). The proportion of stage II-III melanoma among such patients suggest the need for adequate communication about prevention and awareness. Future research may confirm our results and explore the most appropriate and effective ways of implementing educational interventions among AYA aged 15-25.

5 CONCLUSION

Our findings show that AYA melanoma does not represent a distinct pathological entity and however there are differences they do not require a different therapeutic strategy because AYA melanoma has a clinical outcome comparable or better than melanoma in adults.

ETHICS STATEMENT

The studies involving human participants were reviewed and approved by Il Comitato Etico per la Sperimentazione Clinica (CESC) IOV. Written informed consent to participate in this study was provided by the participants' legal guardian/next of kin.

AUTHOR CONTRIBUTIONS

Study concepts: PF, BF, AF, MA, and AV. Study design: PF, BF, CP, RS, and AC. Data acquisition: PF, VC, AB, AM, and JP. Quality control of data and algorithms: AM and FC. Data analysis and interpretation: PF, FC, AM, ST, FR, CB and MR. Statistical analysis: FC. Manuscript preparation: BF and PF. Manuscript editing: BF, PF, and IR. Manuscript review: FC, MA, SM, AB, VC-S, DC, GB, CM, and AD. All authors contributed to the article and approved the submitted version.

ACKNOWLEDGMENTS

The authors wish to thank "Piccoli Punti ONLUS" and "Fondazione Lucia Valentini Terrani" for their long-lasting support, as well as the Marco Possia family and Mr. Fabio Crivellaro for raising awareness on melanoma and skin cancer in young people.

REFERENCES

1. N Howlader, AM Noone, M Krapcho, D Miller, A Brest, M Yu, J Ruhl, Z Tatalovich, A Mariotto, DR Lewis, HS Chen, EJ Feuer, KA Cronin eds. *SEER Cancer Statistics Review, 1975-2017*. Bethesda, MD: National Cancer Institute (2020). Available at: https://seer.cancer.gov/csr/1975_2017/. based on November 2019 SEER data submission, posted to the SEER web site, April 2020.

2. Bray F, Ferlay J, Soerjomataram I, Siegel RL, Torre LA, Jemal A. Global Cancer Statistics 2018: GLOBOCAN Estimates of Incidence and Mortality Worldwide for 36 Cancers in 185 Countries [Published Correction Appears in CA Cancer J Clin. 2020 Jul;70(4):313]. *CA Cancer J Clin* (2018) 68(6):394–424. doi: 10.3322/caac.21492

3. Miller KD, Fidler-Benaoudia M, Keegan TH, Hipp HS, Jemal A, Siegel RL. Cancer Statistics for Adolescents and Young Adults, 2020. *CA Cancer J Clin* (2020) 70(6):443–59. doi: 10.3322/caac.216379.x

4. Bagnoni G, Fidanzi C, D'Erme AM, Viacava P, Leoni M, Strambi S, et al. Melanoma in Children, Adolescents and Young Adults: Anatomo-Clinical Features and Prognostic Study on 426 Cases. *Pediatr Surg Int* (2019) 35 (1):159–65. doi: 10.1007/s00383-018-4388-0

5. AIRTUM Working Group. CCM; AIEOP Working Group. Italian Cancer Figures, Report 2012: Cancer in Children and Adolescents. *Epidemiol Prev* (2013) 37(1 Suppl 1):1–225.

6. Indini A, Brecht I, Del Vecchio M, Sultan I, Signoroni S, Ferrari A, et al. Cutaneous Melanoma in Adolescents and Young Adults. *Pediatr Blood Cancer* (2018) 65(11):e27292. doi: 10.1002/pbc.27292

7. van der Kooij MK, Wetzels M, Aarts M, van den Berkmortel F, Blank CU, Boers-Sonderen MJ, et al. Age Does Matter in Adolescents and Young Adults Versus Older Adults With Advanced Melanoma; A National Cohort Study Comparing Tumor Characteristics, Treatment Pattern, Toxicity and Response. *Cancers (Basel)* (2020) 12(8):2072. doi: 10.3390/cancers12082072

8. Gershenwald JE, Scolyer RA. Melanoma Staging: American Joint Committee on Cancer (AJCC) 8th Edition and Beyond [Published Correction Appears in Ann Surg Oncol. 2018 Dec;25(Suppl 3):993-994]. *Ann Surg Oncol* (2018) 25 (8):2105–10. doi: 10.1245/s10434-018-6513-7

9. R Core Team. *R: A Language and Environment for Statistical Computing*. Vienna, Austria: R Foundation for Statistical Computing (2021).

10. Rizzari C, Putti MC, Colombini A, Casagranda S, Ferrari GM, Papayannidis C, et al. Rationale for a Pediatric-Inspired Approach in the Adolescent and Young Adult Population With Acute Lymphoblastic Leukemia, With a Focus

on Asparaginase Treatment. *Hematol Rep* (2014) 6(3):5554. doi: 10.4081/hr.2014.5554

11. Caroppo F, Tadiotto Cicogna G, Messina F, Alaibac M. Association Between Melanoma and Exposure to Sex Hormones in Puberty: A Possible Window of Susceptibility (Review). *Mol Clin Oncol* (2021) 14(4):66. doi: 10.3892/mco.2021.2228

12. Réguerre Y, Vittaz M, Orbach D, Robert C, Bodemer C, Mateus C, et al. Cutaneous Malignant Melanoma in Children and Adolescents Treated in Pediatric Oncology Units. *Pediatr Blood Cancer* (2016) 63(11):1922–7. doi: 10.1002/pbc.26113

13. Paradela S, Fonseca E, Pita-Fernández S, Kantrow SM, Diwan AH, Herzog C, et al. Prognostic Factors for Melanoma in Children and Adolescents: A Clinicopathologic, Single-Center Study of 137 Patients. *Cancer* (2010) 116 (18):4334–44. doi: 10.1002/cncr.25222

14. Mu E, Lange JR, Strouse JJ. Comparison of the Use and Results of Sentinel Lymph Node Biopsy in Children and Young Adults With Melanoma. *Cancer* (2012) 118(10):2700–7. doi: 10.1002/cncr.26578

15. Livestro DP, Kaine EM, Michaelson JS, Mihm MC, Haluska FG, Muzikansky A, et al. Melanoma in the Young: Differences and Similarities With Adult Melanoma: A Case-Matched Controlled Analysis. *Cancer* (2007) 110(3):614–24. doi: 10.1002/cncr.22818

16. Berg P, Lindelöf B. Differences in Malignant Melanoma Between Children and Adolescents. A 35-Year Epidemiological Study. *Arch Dermatol* (1997) 133 (3):295–7.

17. Howman-Giles R, Shaw HM, Scolyer RA, Murali R, Wilmott J, McCarthy SW, et al. Sentinel Lymph Node Biopsy in Pediatric and Adolescent Cutaneous Melanoma Patients. *Ann Surg Oncol* (2010) 17(1):138–43. doi: 10.1245/s10434-009-0657-4

18. Aldrink JH, Selim MA, Diesen DL, Johnson J, Pruitt SK, Tyler DS, et al. Pediatric Melanoma: A Single-Institution Experience of 150 Patients. *J Pediatr Surg* (2009) 44(8):1514–21. doi: 10.1016/j.jpedsurg.2008.12.003

19. Weiss SA, Han J, Darvishian F, Tchack J, Han SW, Malecek K, et al. Impact of Aging on Host Immune Response and Survival in Melanoma: An Analysis of 3 Patient Cohorts. *J Transl Med* (2016) 14(1):299. doi: 10.1186/s12967-016-1026-2

Early Exanthema upon Vemurafenib Plus Cobimetinib is Associated with a Favorable Treatment Outcome in Metastatic Melanoma: A Retrospective Multicenter DeCOG Study

Katharina C. Kähler[1*], Ralf Gutzmer[2], Friedegrund Meier[3,4], Lisa Zimmer[5], Markus Heppt[6], Anja Gesierich[7], Kai-Martin Thoms[8], Jochen Utikal[9,10], Jessica C. Hassel[11], Carmen Loquai[12], Claudia Pföhler[13], Lucie Heinzerling[6,14], Martin Kaatz[15], Daniela Göppner[16], Annette Pflugfelder[17], Ann-Sophie Bohne[1], Imke Satzger[2], Lydia Reinhardt[3,4], Jan-Malte Placke[5], Dirk Schadendorf[5] and Selma Ugurel[5]

[1] Department of Dermatology, University Hospital Schleswig-Holstein (UKSH), Kiel, Germany, [2] Department of Dermatology, University Hospital Hannover, Hannover, Germany, [3] Skin Cancer Center, National Center for Tumor Diseases, University Cancer Centre Dresden, Dresden, Germany, [4] Department of Dermatology, TU Dresden, University Hospital Carl Gustav Carus, Dresden, Germany, [5] Department of Dermatology, University Hospital Essen, German Cancer Consortium (DKTK), Essen, Germany, [6] Department of Dermatology, Universitätsklinikum Erlangen, Friedrich-Alexander University Erlangen-Nürnberg, Erlangen, Germany, [7] Department of Dermatology, University Hospital Würzburg, Würzburg, Germany, [8] Department of Dermatology, University Medical Center Göttingen, Göttingen, Germany, [9] Skin Cancer Unit, German Cancer Research Center (DKFZ), Heidelberg, Germany, [10] Department of Dermatology, Venereology and Allergology, University Medical Center Mannheim, Ruprecht-Karl University of Heidelberg, Mannheim, Germany, [11] Department of Dermatology, University Hospital Heidelberg, Heidelberg, Germany, [12] Department of Dermatology, University Hospital Mainz, Mainz, Germany, [13] Department of Dermatology, University Hospital Homburg, Homburg, Germany, [14] Department of Dermatology and Allergology, Ludwig-Maximilian University, München, Germany, [15] Department of Dermatology, SRH Waldklinikum, Gera, Germany, [16] Department of Dermatology, University Hospital Giessen, Gießen, Germany, [17] Department of Dermatology, University Hospital Tübingen, Tübingen, Germany

*Correspondence:
Katharina C. Kähler
kkaehler@dermatology.uni-kiel.de

Background: The combination of BRAF and MEK inhibitors has become standard of care in the treatment of metastatic BRAF V600-mutated melanoma. Clinical factors for an early prediction of tumor response are rare. The present study investigated the association between the development of an early exanthema induced by vemurafenib or vemurafenib plus cobimetinib and therapy outcome.

Methods: This multicenter retrospective study included patients with BRAF V600-mutated irresectable AJCC-v8 stage IIIC/D to IV metastatic melanoma who received treatment with vemurafenib (VEM) or vemurafenib plus cobimetinib (COBIVEM). The development of an early exanthema within six weeks after therapy start and its grading according to CTCAEv4.0 criteria was correlated to therapy outcome in terms of best overall response, progression-free (PFS), and overall survival (OS).

Results: A total of 422 patients from 16 centers were included (VEM, n=299; COBIVEM, n=123). 20.4% of VEM and 43.1% of COBIVEM patients developed an early exanthema.

In the VEM cohort, objective responders (CR/PR) more frequently presented with an early exanthema than non-responders (SD/PD); 59.0% versus 38.7%; p=0.0027. However, median PFS and OS did not differ between VEM patients with or without an early exanthema (PFS, 6.9 versus 6.0 months, p=0.65; OS, 11.0 versus 12.4 months, p=0.69). In the COBIVEM cohort, 66.0% of objective responders had an early exanthema compared to 54.3% of non-responders (p=0.031). Median survival times were significantly longer for patients who developed an early exanthema compared to patients who did not (PFS, 9.7 versus 5.6 months, p=0.013; OS, not reached versus 11.6 months, p=0.0061). COBIVEM patients with a mild early exanthema (CTCAEv4.0 grade 1-2) had a superior survival outcome as compared to COBIVEM patients with a severe (CTCAEv4.0 grade 3-4) or non early exanthema, respectively (p=0.047). This might be caused by the fact that 23.6% of patients with severe exanthema underwent a dose reduction or discontinuation of COBIVEM compared to only 8.9% of patients with mild exanthema.

Conclusions: The development of an early exanthema within 6 weeks after treatment start indicates a favorable therapy outcome upon vemurafenib plus cobimetinib. Patients presenting with an early exanthema should therefore be treated with adequate supportive measures to provide that patients can stay on treatment.

Keywords: melanoma, vemurafenib, cobimetinib, BRAF/MEK inhibition, skin toxicity, therapy outcome

INTRODUCTION

Melanoma patients treated with BRAF and MEK inhibitors frequently develop an exanthema, also referred to as "skin rash" by non-dermatologists. This exanthema is typically characterized by inflammatory macules and papules but may also present with pustules or urticae. Its first signs commonly show within the first four to six weeks after therapy start. In the pivotal COBRIM trial the incidence of a skin rash upon monotherapy with vemurafenib was reported to be around 67.5% and during combination therapy with vemurafenib/cobimetinib the incidence was slightly higher with 72.5% (1). However, the term "skin rash" covers a variety of cutaneous side effects and thus cannot be equated with exanthema. Studies of EGFR inhibitors demonstrated an association of skin rash development with an improved therapy outcome in various cancer entities including colorectal carcinoma, head-and-neck squamous cell carcinoma, non-small cell lung cancer, prostate cancer, gastro-esophageal cancer, pancreatic adenocarcinoma and cutaneous squamous cell carcinoma (2, 3). Thus, in these cancer entities patients presenting with a skin rash under EGFR inhibitor therapy are encouraged to continue this treatment with the prospect of an increased probability of a favorable treatment outcome. For BRAF and MEK inhibition in metastatic melanoma, so far, no correlation has been reported between treatment efficacy and outcome and the occurrence of cutaneous side effects.

The present study was aimed to investigate the frequency and severity of an early exanthema upon BRAF and MEK inhibition with vemurafenib alone or combined with cobimetinib and its association with therapy outcome in patients with metastatic melanoma.

PATIENTS AND METHODS

This multicenter retrospective study was initiated by the Dermatologic Cooperative Oncology Group (DeCOG), and undertaken with Ethics Committee approval (Hannover University Medical School, 1612-2012). Patients were identified for study inclusion at clinical centers of the DeCOG based on the following eligibility criteria: histologically proven diagnosis of melanoma, unresectable metastatic disease in stage III or IV following the American Joint Committee on Cancer version 8 (AJCCv8) criteria (4), detection of a BRAF V600 mutation in the tumor tissue, treatment with vemurafenib as a single agent (VEM) or as the combination of cobimetinib plus vemurafenib (COBIVEM) within a time frame of June 01, 2012 and April 30, 2018, either as per clinical trial or *via* prescription, and availability of follow-up data after treatment start including adverse events, response and survival. The patients were identified at the centers *via* their digital hospital information systems or by chart review, and the requested data were extracted from the respective patient files.

Data Collection

The requested data were collected on standardized electronic case report forms and merged in one central database for analysis. The data comprised patient demographics, BRAF V600 mutation subtype, sites of metastasis, overall performance status (OPS) graded by Eastern Cooperative Oncology Group (ECOG) criteria, and serum LDH activity, all at onset of VEM or COBIVEM therapy. For categorization of metastatic sites, we used the AJCCv8 M category by grouping by localization of metastases regardless of serum LDH activity. The used groups were (a) metastases to skin and/or lymph nodes (skin/LN), (b) metastases to the lung (lung),

(c) metastases to other organs (other organs), and (d) metastases to the brain (brain). Data on other systemic treatments received by the patients before VEM or COBIVEM were recorded as previous treatments. This pre-treatment was categorized into (a) regimens containing immune checkpoint inhibitors (checkpoint inhibition), and (b) regimens containing kinase inhibitors (BRAF/MEK inhibition). Collected data on the course and outcome of VEM or COBIVEM therapy included therapy duration, best response following RECIST criteria (5) categorizing into complete response (CR), partial response (PR), stable disease (SD), and progressive disease (PD), as well as progression-free (PFS) and overall survival (OS). Patients were grouped into either objective responders (CR +PR) or non-responders (SD+PD). An exanthema presenting within the first six weeks after start of VEM or COBIVEM therapy was considered as an early exanthema, regardless of its morphology (macular, papular, pustular, urticae). The severity of the exanthema was graded according to CTCAEv4.0 (grade 1, <10% body surface area (BSA); grade 2, 10-30% BSA; grade 3, 30-100% BSA; grade 4, 100% BSA and/or severe reduction of general condition; grade 5, death) (6).

Statistical Analysis

Data analysis was performed between January 01 and March 31, 2019. Survival (PFS, OS) was calculated from onset of VEM or COBIVEM until death or disease progression, respectively. If no such event occurred, the date of last patient contact was used as survival end point (censored observation). Survival curves, hazard ratios, and median survival times were calculated using the Kaplan–Meier method for censored failure time data. The log-rank test was used for comparison of survival probabilities between groups. Differences between groups were calculated using Fisher's exact test or Chi square test. P<0.05 was considered statistically significant.

RESULTS

Patient Characteristics and Early Exanthema

Data were collected of 422 patients at 16 clinical cancer centers in Germany. In total, 299 patients received VEM, 123 patients received COBIVEM. The patient flow is shown in **Figure 1**; detailed patient characteristics are presented in **Tables 1, 2**. An early exanthema occurring within the first 6 weeks after start of therapy occurred in 61 VEM patients (20.4%) (CTCAE grade 1, 62.3%; grade 2, 22.9%; grade 3, 11.4%; and grade 4, 3.2%) and in 53 COBIVEM patients (43.1%) (CTCAE grade 1, 28.3%; grade 2, 22.6%; grade 3, 45.2%; and grade 4, 3.7%). Representative patients from both cohorts are demonstrated in **Figure 2**. In the VEM cohort, most patient characteristics at therapy start were balanced between groups with and without occurrence of an early exanthema, besides patients' sex with females more often represented within the group of patients developing early exanthema than males (p=0.043; **Table 1**). In the COBIVEM cohort, the overall performance status at therapy start differed significantly between groups with and without occurrence of an

early exanthema with patients presenting at ECOG 0 being strongly over-represented in the group developing an early exanthema (p=0.0058; **Table 2**). Age or LDH were not identified to be an influencing factor for the incidence of early exanthema (p= 0.11, **Table 2**).

VEM and COBIVEM Therapy and Outcome

All patients started with the initial doses of 960 mg vemurafenib orally b.i.d. (VEM) or vemurafenib 960 mg orally b.i.d. plus cobimetinib 60 mg orally once daily (COBIVEM). Due to the occurrence of an early exanthema, 32.7% of VEM patients and 26.8% of COBIVEM patients had a dose reduction, and 11.4% of VEM and 5.7% of COBIVEM patients had a therapy discontinuation. At database closure on September 30, 2019, the median follow-up time was 21.6 months. 48.2% of the VEM patients and 30.1% of the COBIVEM patients had died. Of the patients alive, 27.4% were still on VEM treatment, and 30.8% on COBIVEM treatment.

As best overall response, 4.0% of VEM patients achieved a CR, 53.8% achieved a PR, 22.1% showed a SD, and 15.7% revealed a disease progression. 4.3% of the patients were not evaluable for treatment response due to other reasons. Patients presenting an early exanthema upon VEM revealed a superior therapy response with an objective response rate (CR+PR) of 59.0% in patients showing an early exanthema versus 38.7% in patients without this cutaneous reaction (p=0.0027; **Table 1**). In the patient cohort treated with COBIVEM, 10.6% of patients achieved a CR, 48.8% achieved a PR, 18.7% showed a SD, and 14.6% revealed disease progression. 7.3% of the patients were not evaluable for therapy response. Here again, patients showing an early exanthema upon treatment had a higher objective response rate than patients who did not (66.0% versus 54.3%; p=0.031; **Table 2**).

With regard to survival after therapy start, for patients treated with VEM median PFS and OS were not significantly different for patients with or without an early exanthema (6.9 versus 6.0 months, p=0.65; 11.0 versus 12.4 months, p=0.69 respectively, **Figures 3A, B**). Additionally, the respective Kaplan-Meier survival curves were almost identical in shape and were crossing each other repeatedly. In contrast, for patients treated with COBIVEM survival after therapy start was significantly better in patients presenting an early exanthema. Median PFS and OS were significantly prolonged in patients showing an early exanthema versus patients who did not (PFS, 9.7 versus 5.6 months, p=0.013; OS, not reached versus 11.6 months, p=0.0061; **Figures 4A, B**). With regard to the severity of the early exanthema, patients who developed a mild exanthema (CTCAE grade 1-2) had a superior outcome in terms of PFS and OS compared to patients who developed a severe (CTCAE grade 3-4) exanthema or patients who developed no exanthema (p=0.047, **Figures 4C, D**).

DISCUSSION

Vemurafenib is a selective inhibitor of V600-mutated BRAF, and was the first-in-class mitogen-activated protein (MAP) kinase

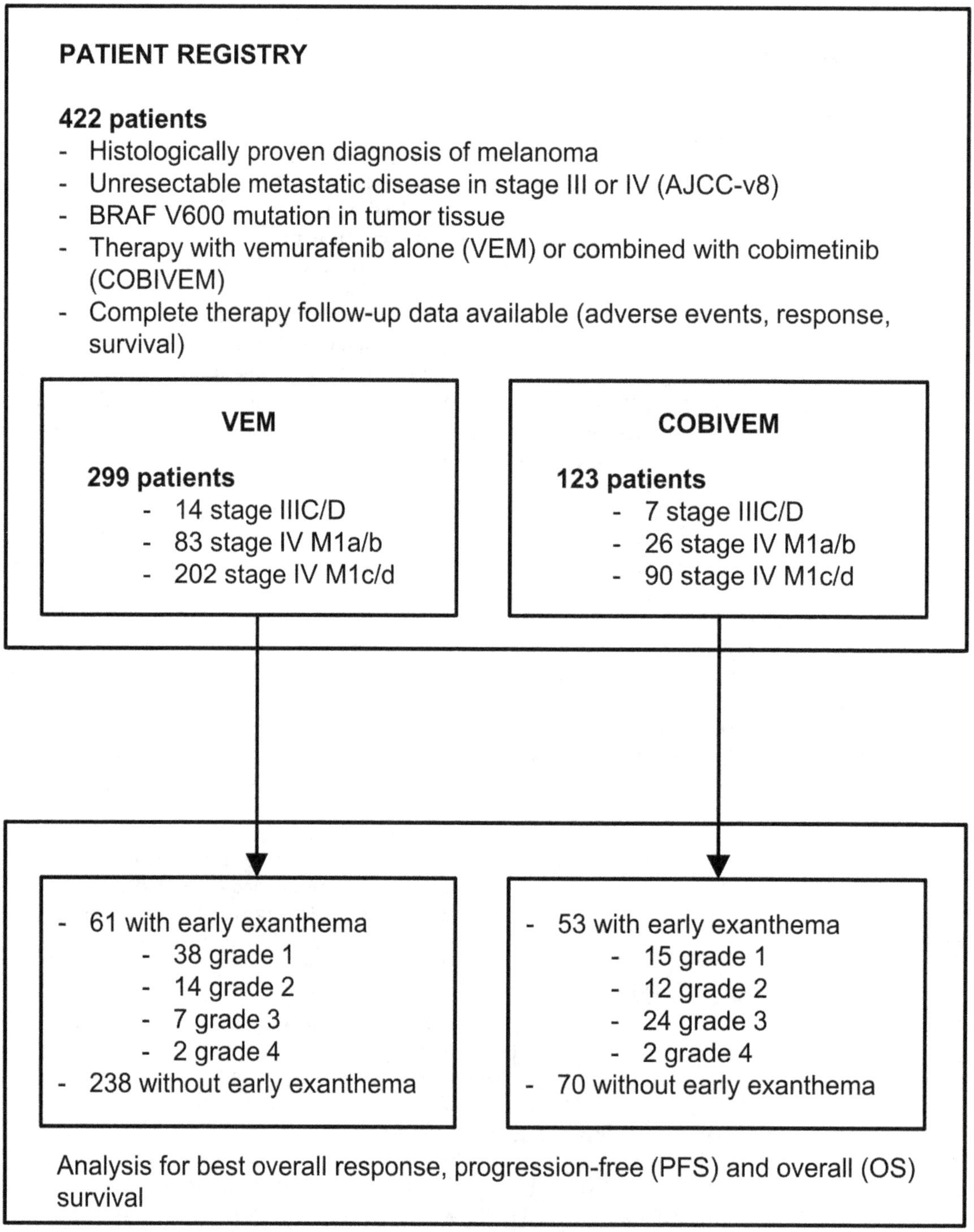

PATIENT REGISTRY

422 patients
- Histologically proven diagnosis of melanoma
- Unresectable metastatic disease in stage III or IV (AJCC-v8)
- BRAF V600 mutation in tumor tissue
- Therapy with vemurafenib alone (VEM) or combined with cobimetinib (COBIVEM)
- Complete therapy follow-up data available (adverse events, response, survival)

VEM

299 patients
- 14 stage IIIC/D
- 83 stage IV M1a/b
- 202 stage IV M1c/d

COBIVEM

123 patients
- 7 stage IIIC/D
- 26 stage IV M1a/b
- 90 stage IV M1c/d

- 61 with early exanthema
    - 38 grade 1
    - 14 grade 2
    - 7 grade 3
    - 2 grade 4
- 238 without early exanthema

- 53 with early exanthema
    - 15 grade 1
    - 12 grade 2
    - 24 grade 3
    - 2 grade 4
- 70 without early exanthema

Analysis for best overall response, progression-free (PFS) and overall (OS) survival

FIGURE 1 | Schematic presentation of the study patient flow into patient registry. Patient inclusion criteria and grading of the early exanthemas was performed according to CTCAEv4.0 (grade 1, <10% body surface area (BSA); grade 2, 10-30% BSA; grade 3, 30-100% BSA; grade 4, 100% BSA and/or severe reduction of general condition).

pathway inhibitor approved for the treatment of melanoma (7). Subsequently, the combination therapy of vemurafenib together with the MEK inhibitor cobimetinib was approved for metastatic melanoma due to the significant prolongation of survival times shown by clinical trial data (1, 8). Nevertheless, predictive markers of the treatment outcome of either vemurafenib monotherapy or vemurafenib plus cobimetinib combination therapy are rare and most often characterized by low

Early Exanthema Upon Vemurafenib Plus Cobimetinib Is Associated With a Favorable Treatment Outcome...

197

TABLE 1 | Patients treated with vemurafenib (VEM).

	Total n=299 (100%)	Early exanthema n=61 (100%)	No early exanthema n=238 (100%)	P-value	Relative risk
Patient characteristics at therapy start					
Sex					
male	164 (54.8%)	26 (42.6%)	138 (58.0%)		
female	135 (45.2%)	35 (57.4%)	100 (42.0%)	**0.043**	1.64
Age at treatment onset					
≤65 years	199 (66.6%)	39 (63.9%)	160 (67.2%)		
>65 years	100 (33.4%)	22 (36.1%)	78 (32.8%)	0.65	1.12
Localisation of primary					
skin	248 (82.9%)	50 (82.0%)	198 (83.2%)		
occult (MUP)	51 (17.1%)	11 (18.0%)	40 (16.8%)	0.85	1.07
Pre-treatment in stage III/IV					
no	169 (56.5%)	30 (49.2%)	139 (58.4%)		
yes	130 (43.5%)	31 (50.8%)	99 (41.6%)	0.25	1.34
BRAF/MEK inhibition	0 (0.0%)	0 (0.0%)	0 (0.0%)		
checkpoint inhibition	25 (8.4%)	6 (9.8%)	19 (8.0%)		
chemotherapy	127 (42.5%)	30 (49.2%)	87 (36.6%)		
Serum LDH					
normal (≤ULN)	150 (50.2%)	30 (49.2%)	120 (50.4%)		
elevated (>ULN)	149 (49.8%)	31 (50.8%)	118 (49.6%)	0.89	1.04
OPS (ECOG)					
0	177 (59.2%)	39 (63.9%)	138 (58.0%)		
≥1	110 (36.8%)	15 (24.6%)	95 (39.9%)	0.088	0.62
not specified	12 (4.0%)	7 (11.5%)	5 (2.1%)		
Stage (sites of metastasis)					
IIIC/D (skin/LN)	14 (4.7%)	8 (13.1%)	6 (2.5%)		
IV M1a (skin/LN)	46 (15.4%)	6 (9.8%)	40 (16.8%)		
IV M1b (lung)	37 (12.4%)	4 (6.6%)	33 (13.9%)		
IV M1c/d (other organ/brain)	202 (67.6%)	43 (70.5%)	159 (66.8%)	0.15	
BRAF V600 mutation status					
V600E	169 (56.5%)	34 (55.7%)	135 (56.7%)		
V600K	24 (8.0%)	5 (8.2%)	19 (8.0%)		
V600D	1 (0.3%)	0 (0.0%)	1 (0.4%)		
not further specified	105 (35.1%)	22 (36.1%)	83 (34.9%)	0.96	
Therapy outcome					
Best overall response					
CR	12 (4.0%)	3 (4.9%)	9 (3.8%)		
PR	161 (53.8%)	33 (54.1%)	128 (53.8%)		
SD	66 (22.1%)	15 (24.6%)	51 (21.4%)		
PD	47 (15.7%)	6 (9.8%)	41 (17.2%)		
NE	13 (4.3%)	4 (6.6%)	9 (3.8%)		
objective response (CR + PR)	128 (42.8%)	36 (59.0%)	92 (38.7%)	**0.0027**	**2.12**
Disease progression	207 (69.2%)	47 (77.0%)	160 (67.2%)		
Median PFS	6.3 months	6.9 months	6.0 months	0.65	HR=1.08
Death	144 (48.2%)	33 (54.1%)	111 (46.6%)		
Median OS	12.0 months	11.0 months	12.4 months	0.69	HR=1.09

The given patient characteristics refer to the start of vemurafenib (VEM) therapy. Percentages are given per column. Stage categories refer to the AJCCv8 classification system. Pre-treatment describes systemic therapies received by the patient for inoperable stage III or IV disease (non-adjuvant) prior to VEM therapy. Patient groups with and without early exanthema were compared by Fisher's exact test or Chi square test; results are given by p-values, relative risks or hazard ratios. MUP, melanoma of unknown primary; LDH, lactate dehydrogenase; ULN, upper limit of normal; OPS, overall performance status; CR, complete response; PR, partial response; SD, stable disease; PD, progressive disease; NE, not evaluable. Bold means statistically significant.

specificity. Elevated serum LDH, as well as multiple organ involvement by metastases were shown to be associated with a less favorable treatment outcome of BRAF/MEK inhibition (9). However, these parameters are likewise associated with a poor treatment outcome upon immune checkpoint inhibition (10). Thus, other biomarkers associated with treatment outcome are urgently required to indicate a patient's individual probability to benefit from vemurafenib/cobimetinib therapy. Optimally, these markers are detectable immediately before treatment start. However, biomarkers which become evident shortly after treatment start like cutaneous adverse events may also be of great help.

So far, only one retrospective analysis showed a possible correlation between the cutaneous side effects panniculitis and vitiligo-like lesions and the treatment outcome upon the BRAF plus MEK inhibitor combination dabrafenib and trametinib (11). Another retrospective case series showed a correlation between different cutaneous and extra-cutaneous adverse events including vitiligo, erythema nodosum, uveitis and keratitis sicca and the treatment outcome upon BRAF inhibitors either administered alone or in combination with MEK inhibitors (12). However, all these adverse events were reported in patients under BRAF/MEK inhibition, but at low frequencies and thus are of

TABLE 2 | Patients treated with cobimetinib plus vemurafenib (COBIVEM).

	Total n=123 (100%)	Early exanthema n=53 (100%)	No early exanthema n=70 (100%)	P-value	Relative risk
Patient characteristics at therapy start					
Sex					
male	69 (56.1%)	27 (50.9%)	42 (60.0%)		
female	54 (43.9%)	26 (49.1%)	28 (40.0%)	0.36	1.23
Age at treatment onset					
≤65 years	88 (71.5%)	42 (79.2%)	46 (65.7%)		
>65 years	35 (28.5%)	11 (20.8%)	24 (34.3%)	0.11	0.66
Localisation of primary					
skin	108 (87.8%)	47 (88.7%)	61 (87.1%)		
occult (MUP)	15 (12.2%)	6 (11.3%)	9 (12.9%)	1.0	0.92
Pre-treatment in stage III/IV					
no	55 (44.7%)	24 (45.3%)	31 (44.3%)		
yes	68 (55.3%)	29 (54.7%)	39 (55.7%)	1.0	0.98
BRAF/MEK inhibition	43 (34.9%)	12 (22.6%)	31 (44.3%)		
checkpoint inhibition	44 (35.8%)	17 (32.1%)	27 (38.6%)	0.36	1.38
Serum LDH					
normal (≤ULN)	72 (58.5%)	31 (58.5%)	41 (58.6%)		
elevated (>ULN)	51 (41.5%)	22 (41.5%)	29 (41.4%)	1.0	1.0
OPS (ECOG)					
0	83 (67.5%)	42 (79.2%)	41 (58.6%)		
≥1	38 (30.9%)	9 (17.0%)	29 (41.4%)	**0.0058**	0.47
not specified	2 (1.6%)	2 (3.8%)	0 (0.0%)		
Stage (sites of metastasis)					
IIIC/D (skin/LN)	7 (5.7%)	1 (1.9%)	6 (8.6%)		
IV M1a (skin/LN)	13 (10.6%)	7 (13.2%)	6 (8.6%)		
IV M1b (lung)	13 (10.6%)	8 (15.1%)	5 (7.1%)		
IV M1c/d (other organ/brain)	90 (73.1%)	37 (69.8%)	53 (75.7%)	0.18	
BRAF V600 mutation status					
V600E	92 (74.8%)	39 (73.6%)	53 (75.7%)		
V600K	15 (12.2%)	6 (11.3%)	9 (12.9%)		
V600R	2 (1.6%)	1 (1.9%)	1 (1.4%)		
V600D	1 (0.8%)	1 (1.9%)	0 (0.0%)		
K601E	1 (0.8%)	0 (0.0%)	1 (1.4%)		
not further specified	12 (9.8%)	6 (11.3%)	6 (8.6%)	0.79	
Therapy outcome					
Best overall response					
CR	13 (10.6%)	8 (15.1%)	5 (7.1%)		
PR	60 (48.8%)	27 (50.9%)	33 (47.1%)		
SD	23 (18.7%)	8 (15.1%)	15 (21.4%)		
PD	18 (14.6%)	3 (5.7%)	15 (21.4%)		
NE	9 (7.3%)	7 (13.2%)	2 (2.9%)		
objective response (CR + PR)	73 (59.3%)	35 (66.0%)	38 (54.3%)	**0.031**	1.79
Disease progression	77 (62.6%)	30 (56.6%)	47 (67.1%)		
Median PFS	7.3 months	9.7 months	5.6 months	**0.013**	HR=0.55
Death	37 (30.1%)	7 (13.2%)	30 (42.9%)		
Median OS	not reached	not reached	11.6 months	**0.0061**	HR=0.39

The given patient characteristics refer to the start of cobimetinib plus vemurafenib (COBIVEM) therapy. Percentages are given per column. Stage categories refer to the AJCCv8 classification system. Pre-treatment describes systemic therapies received by the patient for inoperable stage III or IV disease (non-adjuvant) prior to COBIVEM therapy. Patient groups with and without early exanthema were compared by Fisher's exact test or Chi square test; results are given by p-values, relative risks or hazard ratios. MUP, melanoma of unknown primary; LDH, lactate dehydrogenase; ULN, upper limit of normal; OPS, overall performance status; CR, complete response; PR, partial response; SD, stable disease; PD, progressive disease; NE, not evaluable.
Bold means statistically significant.

little use as predictive markers of treatment response in the majority of patients treated with BRAF/MEK inhibitors.

In contrast, exanthema is a common adverse event in patients treated with BRAF/MEK inhibitors (13). In clinical trials, 15.7% of patients treated with encorafenib/binimetinib developed a low grade rash/maculopapular rash (high grade 1%). Additional 3.1% showed an acneiform exanthem (high grade 0%). 27.7% of patients treated with dabarafenib/trametinib developed a low

grade rash/maculopapular rash (high grade 1.5%). Additional 6.6% showed an acneiform exanthema (high grade 0%). The combination of vemurafenib/cobimetinib induced in 56.3% of patients a low grade rash/maculopapular rash (high grade 12.6%). Additional 13.8% showed an acneiform exanthema (high grade 2.4%). Important to acknowledge is the fact, that non-dermatologists do not differentiate between the common term rash and the specific characteristics of e.g. a maculopapular

Early Exanthema Upon Vemurafenib Plus Cobimetinib Is Associated With a Favorable Treatment Outcome...

199

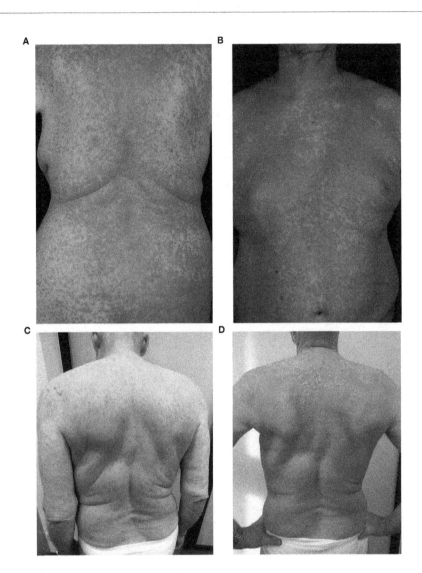

FIGURE 2 | Representative patients from the study cohorts showing an early exanthema defined as onset within 6 weeks upon start of vemurafenib **(A)** or vemurafenib plus cobimetinib **(B)**, both grade 4 according to CTCAEv4.0. **(C)** Exanthem during vemurafenib and cobimetinib **(D)** follow-up after 4 weeks of topical and systemic steroids.

exanthema or acneiform exanthema (13). Additionally, in clinical trials the onset of exanthema is not specified, so the reported incidence of exanthema does not give further information about the rate of early exanthemas within the first weeks of treatment initiation. Moreover, an exanthema develops early during treatment, most often within the first four to six weeks of treatment, and is easily detectable by an inspection of the patient's skin (13). These advantages render the detection of an early exanthema as a useful indicator of a favorable treatment outcome.

Interestingly, in the VEM cohort, females were more often represented within the group of patients developing early exanthema than males (p=0.043; **Table 1**). This has also been demonstrated to be a known risk factor for rash induced by BRAF/MEK inhibitors in the metaanalysis of Hopkins et al. (14).

This early exanthema is usually treated by a dose reduction of the BRAF/MEK inhibitors in combination with topical steroids and only in rare, severe cases with systemic steroids. Due to their early exanthema, 32.7% of VEM patients and 26.8% of COBIVEM patients needed a dose reduction.

Indeed, in our study we found that the occurrence of an exanthema within the first six weeks of treatment was significantly associated with an improved response rate and a prolonged survival in terms of PFS and OS in patients treated with COBIVEM. In patients treated with VEM, the development of an early exanthema was correlated with an improved objective response, but did not show an association to an improved survival.

Possible reasons for this differential impact on survival remain to be elucidated. First it should be mentioned that the early exanthema during COBIVEM and other BRAF/MEK

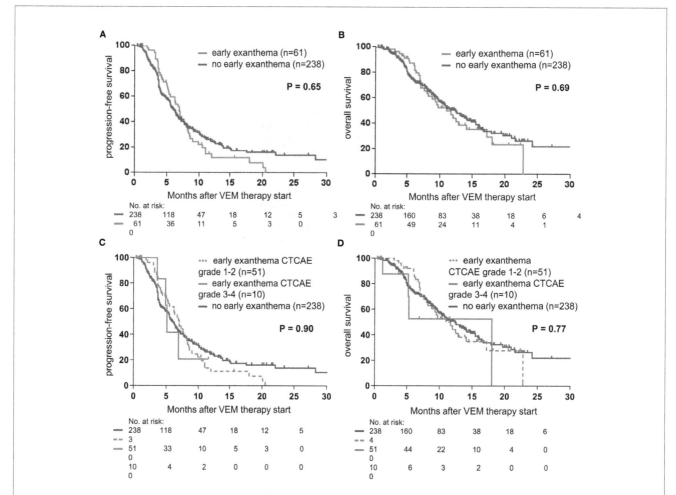

FIGURE 3 | Kaplan-Meier curves showing the probability of progression-free **(A, C)**, and overall survival **(B, D)**, of metastatic melanoma patients treated with vemurafenib (VEM; n=299). Survival curves are displayed for patients with or without presentation of early exanthema upon treatment. Censored observations are indicated by vertical bars. P-values were calculated using the log rank test.

combination therapies has to be differentiated from the acneiform rash induced specifically by MEK inhibitor monotherapies. This acneiform rash commonly occurs later during treatment, most often between week 6 and 12 after treatment start, and has a well-defined causal mechanism (13). The early exanthema developing within the first six weeks of COBIVEM treatment might be induced by the immune activation described for MEK inhibition therapies. It has been demonstrated that COBIVEM as well as dabrafenib plus trametinib therapy induces a type I interferon response in keratinocytes which acts proinflammatory and antineoplastically (15). In histopathology analysis, a slight basal layer vacuolization, dermal edema and a superficial dermal perivascular lymphocyte and eosinophil infiltrate was described (16). Also, it has been demonstrated that a pre-treatment with MEK inhibitors enhances immune responses, tumor-infiltrating T cells, and an immune-stimulating tumor microenvironment (17).

Interestingly, patients developing a mild exanthema revealed a stronger benefit from COBIVEM therapy than patients with a severe exanthema or patients without any exanthema. This

finding might be explained by the fact that of the patients who developed a severe exanthema, 18.7% underwent a dose reduction of COBIVEM and 4.9% completely discontinued the treatment, compared to only 8.1% of patients who developed a mild exanthema that needed a dose reduction and 0.8% that discontinued the treatment. In contrast, it has been shown that dose reductions of BRAF/MEK inhibitors due to early toxicity in the first 28 days are significantly associated with improved survival, progression free survival and response (18, 19). However, following our present results, patients developing an early exanthema upon COBIVEM are patients with a high probability of a favorable therapy outcome and should thus be supported to continue treatment with COBIVEM. This support can be provided by an adequate therapeutic management of the exanthema, e.g. by the use of topical corticosteroids and/or anti-pruritics.

In conclusion, our results indicate that the development of an early exanthema upon BRAF/MEK inhibition with COBIVEM is a surrogate marker of a favorable therapy outcome in metastatic

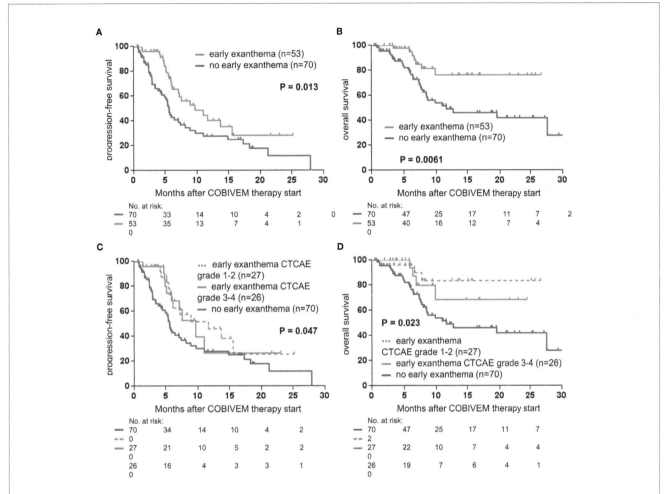

FIGURE 4 | Kaplan-Meier curves showing the probability of progression-free **(A, C)** and overall survival **(B, D)** of metastatic melanoma patients treated with vemurafenib plus cobimetinib (COBIVEM; n=123). Survival curves are displayed for patients with or without presentation of early exanthema upon treatment. Censored observations are indicated by vertical bars. P-values were calculated using the log rank test.

melanoma patients. Thus, patients presenting with an early exanthema under COBIVEM therapy should be treated with adequate supportive measures to provide that patients can stay on treatment. As a limitation, our findings result from a retrospective analysis and should therefore be confirmed in prospective clinical trials or registries.

ETHICS STATEMENT

The studies involving human participants were reviewed and approved by Ethics Committee approval (Hannover University Medical School, 1612-2012). Written informed consent for participation was not required for this study in accordance with the national legislation and the institutional requirements.

AUTHOR CONTRIBUTIONS

SU and KK contributed to conception and design of the study. All authors contributed to the acquisition pf data. SU organized the database. SU and KK performed the statistical analysis. KK wrote the first draft of the manuscript. SU and KK wrote sections of the manuscript. All authors contributed to the article and approved the submitted version.

ACKNOWLEDGMENTS

We wish to thank all patients participating in this study, as well as their families and caregivers.

REFERENCES

1. Dréno B, Ribas A, Larkin J, Ascierto PA, Hauschild A, Thomas L, et al. Incidence, Course, and Management of Toxicities Associated With Cobimetinib in Combination With Vemurafenib in the coBRIM Study. *Ann Oncol* (2017) 28(5):1137–44. doi: 10.1093/annonc/mdx040

2. Abdel-Rahman O, Fouad M. Correlation of Cetuximab-Induced Skin Rash and Outcomes of Solid Tumor Patients Treated With Cetuximab: A Systematic Review and Meta-Analysis. *Crit Rev Oncol Hematol* (2015) 93 (2):127–35. doi: 10.1016/j.critrevonc.2014.07.005

3. Sonnenblick A, de Azambuja E, Agbor-Tarh D, Bradbury I, Campbell C, Huang Y, et al. Lapatinib-Related Rash and Breast Cancer Outcome in the ALTTO Phase III Randomized Trial. *J Natl Cancer Inst* (2016) 108(8):djw037. doi: 10.1093/jnci/djw037

4. Gershenwald JE, Scolyer RA, Hess KR, Sondak VK, Long GV, Ross MI, et al. For Members of the American Joint Committee on Cancer Melanoma Expert Panel and the International Melanoma Database and Discovery Platform. Melanoma Staging: Evidence-based Changes in the American Joint Committee on Cancer Eighth Edition Cancer Staging Manual. *CA Cancer J Clin* (2017) 67(6):472–92. doi: 10.3322/caac.21409

5. Therasse P, Arbuck SG, Eisenhauer EA, Wanders J, Kaplan RS, Rubinstein L, et al. New Guidelines to Evaluate the Response to Treatment in Solid Tumors. European Organization for Research and Treatment of Cancer, National Cancer Institute of the United States, National Cancer Institute of Canada. *J Natl Cancer Inst* (2000) 92(3):205–16. doi: 10.1093/jnci/92.3.205

6. National Cancer Institute Enterprise Vocabulary Services. *Criteria for Adverse Events (Ctcae)* . Available at: https://evs.nci.nih.gov/ftp1/CTCAE/CTCAE_4.03/ CTCAE_4.03_2010-06-14_QuickReference_5x7.pdf (Accessed May 14, 2020).

7. Chapman PB, Hauschild A, Robert C, Haanen JB, Ascierto P, Larkin J, et al. Brim-3 Study Group. Improved Survival With Vemurafenib in Melanoma With BRAF V600E Mutation. *N Engl J Med* (2011) 364(26):2507–16. doi: 10.1056/NEJMoa1103782

8. Ascierto PA, McArthur GA, Dréno B, Atkinson V, Liszkay G, Di Giacomo AM, et al. Cobimetinib Combined With Vemurafenib in Advanced BRAF (V600)-mutant Melanoma (coBRIM): Updated Efficacy Results From a Randomised, Double-Blind, Phase 3 Trial. *Lancet Oncol* (2016) 17(9):1248–60. doi: 10.1016/S1470-2045(16)30122-X

9. Petrelli F, Ardito R, Merelli B, Lonati V, Cabiddu M, Seghezzi S, et al. Prognostic and Predictive Role of Elevated Lactate Dehydrogenase in Patients With Melanoma Treated With Immunotherapy and BRAF Inhibitors: A Systematic Review and Meta-Analysis. *Melanoma Res* (2019) 29(1):1–12. doi: 10.1097/CMR.0000000000000520

10. Hodi FS, Chiarion-Sileni V, Gonzalez R, Grob JJ, Rutkowski P, Cowey CL, et al. Nivolumab Plus Ipilimumab or Nivolumab Alone Versus Ipilimumab Alone in Advanced Melanoma (CheckMate 067): 4-Year Outcomes of a Multicentre, Randomised, Phase 3 Trial. *Lancet Oncol* (2018) 19(11):1480–92. doi: 10.1016/S1470-2045(18)30700-9

11. Consoli F, Manganoni AM, Grisanti S, Petrelli F, Venturini M, Rangoni G, et al. Panniculitis and Vitiligo Occurring During BRAF and MEK Inhibitors Combination in Advanced Melanoma Patients: Potential Predictive Role of Treatment Efficacy. *PloS One* (2019) 14(4):e0214884. doi: 10.1371/journal.pone.0214884

12. Ben-Betzalel G, Baruch EN, Boursi B, Steinberg-Silman Y, Asher N, Shapira-Frommer R, et al. Possible Immune Adverse Events as Predictors of Durable Response to BRAF Inhibitors in Patients With BRAF V600-Mutant Metastatic Melanoma. *Eur J Cancer* (2018) 101:229–35. doi: 10.1016/j.ejca.2018.06.030

13. Heinzerling L, Eigentler TK, Fluck M, Hassel JC, Heller-Schenck D, Leipe J, et al. Tolerability of BRAF/MEK Inhibitor Combinations: Adverse Event Evaluation and Management. *ESMO Open* (2019) 4(3):e000491. doi: 10.1136/ esmoopen-2019-000491

14. Hopkins AM, Rathod AD, Rowland A, Kichenadasse G, Sorich MJ. Risk Factors for Severe Rash With Use of Vemurafenib Alone or in Combination With Cobimetinib for Advanced Melanoma: Pooled Analysis of Clinical Trials. *BMC Cancer* (2020) 20:157. doi: 10.1186/s12885-020-6659-0

15. Lulli D, Carbone ML, Pastore S. The MEK Inhibitors Trametinib and Cobimetinib Induce a Type I Interferon Response in Human Keratinocytes. *Int J Mol Sci* (2017) 18(10):2227. doi: 10.3390/ijms18102227

16. Naqash AR, File DM, Ziemer CM, Whang YE, Landman P, Googe PB, et al. Cutaneous Adverse Reactions in B-RAF Positive Metastatic Melanoma Following Sequential Treatment With B-RAF/MEK Inhibitors and Immune Checkpoint Blockade or Vice Versa. A Single-Institutional Case-Series. *J Immunother Cancer* (2019) 7(1):4. doi: 10.1186/s40425-018-0475-y

17. Kuske M, Westphal D, Wehner R, Schmitz M, Beissert S, Praetorius C, et al. Immunomodulatory Effects of BRAF and MEK Inhibitors: Implications for Melanoma Therapy. *Pharmacol Res* (2018) 136:151–9. doi: 10.1016/j.phrs. 2018.08.019

18. Hopkins AM, Van Dyk M, Rowland A, Sorich MJ. Effect of Early Adverse Events on Response and Survival Outcomes of Advanced Melanoma Patients Treated With Vemurafenib or Vemurafenib Plus Cobimetinib: A Pooled Analysis of Clinical Trial Data. *Pigment Cell Melanoma Res* (2019) 32(4):576–83. doi: 10.1111/pcmr.12773

19. Lewis K, Hauschild A, Larkin J, Ribas A, Flaherty KT, McArthur GA, et al. Effect of Concomitant Dosing With Acid-Reducing Agents and Vemurafenib Dose on Survival in Patients With BRAF^{V600} Mutation-Positive Metastatic Melanoma Treated With Vemurafenib ± Cobimetinib. *Eur J Cancer* (2019) 116:45–55. doi: 10.1016/j.ejca.2019.05.002

24

Identification of Therapeutic Targets and Prognostic Biomarkers among Integrin Subunits in the Skin Cutaneous Melanoma Microenvironment

Yeltai Nurzat[†], Weijie Su[†], Peiru Min, Ke Li, Heng Xu[*] and Yixin Zhang[*]

Department of Plastic and Reconstructive Surgery, Shanghai Ninth People's Hospital, Shanghai JiaoTong University School of Medicine, Shanghai, China

*Correspondence:
Heng Xu
xuh1990@gmail.com
Yixin Zhang
zhangyixin6688@hotmail.com

[†]These authors have contributed equally to this work and share first authorship

The roles of different integrin alpha/beta (ITGA/ITGB) subunits in skin cutaneous melanoma (SKCM) and their underlying mechanisms of action remain unclear. Oncomine, UALCAN, GEPIA, STRING, GeneMANIA, cBioPortal, TIMER, TRRUST, and Webgestalt analysis tools were used. The expression levels of ITGA3, ITGA4, ITGA6, ITGA10, ITGB1, ITGB2, ITGB3, ITGB4, and ITGB7 were significantly increased in SKCM tissues. The expression levels of ITGA1, ITGA4, ITGA5, ITGA8, ITGA9, ITGA10, ITGB1, ITGB2, ITGB3, ITGB5, ITGB6 and ITGB7 were closely associated with SKCM metastasis. The expression levels of ITGA1, ITGA4, ITGB1, ITGB2, ITGB6, and ITGB7 were closely associated with the pathological stage of SKCM. The expression levels of ITGA6 and ITGB7 were closely associated with disease-free survival time in SKCM, and the expression levels of ITGA6, ITGA10, ITGB2, ITGB3, ITGB6, ITGB7, and ITGB8 were markedly associated with overall survival in SKCM. We also found significant correlations between the expression of integrin subunits and the infiltration of six types of immune cells (B cells, CD8+ T cells, CD4+T cells, macrophages, neutrophils, and dendritic cells). Finally, Gene Ontology (GO) enrichment analysis and Kyoto Encyclopedia of Genes and Genomes (KEGG) pathway analysis were performed, and protein-protein interaction (PPI) networks were constructed. We have identified abnormally-expressed genes and gene regulatory networks associated with SKCM, improving understanding of the underlying pathogenesis of SKCM.

Keywords: biomarkers, integrin subunit family, melanoma, skin cutaneous melanoma, cancer genome atlas

INTRODUCTION

Skin cutaneous melanoma (SKCM) is one of the most aggressive and lethal skin cancers (1). In the past decade, incidence of SKCM has increased rapidly worldwide (1). Hence, SKCM poses a major global threat to human health. Recently, associations between molecular biological biomarkers and tumor prognosis during the development of SKCM have elicited great interest. However, our understanding of the etiology and pathogenesis of SKCM could be improved, and more effective prognostic biomarkers are required.

Integrins are glycosylated heterodimers composed of non-covalently bound α and β subunits (2). Specific integrin subunits are known to be closely associated with various tumors, including gallbladder cancer and breast cancer, etc. (3–5). The diversity of integrin function in tumors may be related to differences in the integrin domains. Therefore, we speculate that different integrin subunits may play a role in several biological processes underlying SKCM.

Several comprehensive scientific reviews of the molecular factors underlying SKCM biology, SKCM drug target mechanisms (6), and SKCM prognosis have been published. However, studies clarifying the role of integrins in SKCM are relatively scarce. In the present study, we evaluate the utility of abnormally-expressed integrin subunits as biomarkers in SKCM. In addition, we employ bioinformatics tools for analyzing the underlying mechanisms by which different integrin subunits affect SKCM. Our overall aim is to identify potential biological targets in the integrin subunit family which can be used as biomarkers in SKCM.

MATERIALS AND METHODS

ONCOMINE

The ONCOMINE Database is a multi-functional website based on the Cancer Genome Atlas (TCGA) tumor database (7). Here, we used ONCOMINE to analyze the differentially expressed integrins subunits using a threshold limited by P value<0.05, Fold change ≥2. The specific referencing steps are as follows: the filter of Analysis Type: Cancer vs. Normal Analysis; the filter of Cancer Type: Cutaneous Melanoma; the filter of Data Type: mRNA. The data was order by: over-expression: Gene Rank.

UALCAN

UALCAN (http://ualcan.path.uab.edu/index.html) is an integrated data-mining platform facilitating comprehensive analyses of the cancer transcriptome (8). The functionalities of UALCAN including identifying biomarkers, analyzing expression profile, analyzing gene correlation, and survival analysis (9). In this study, UALCAN database was used to analyze the expression of target genes in primary SKCM, metastasis SKCM and normal samples. The sample information of UALCAN was derived from the TCGA

Abbreviations: SKCM, skin cutaneous melanoma; AJCC, American Joint Committee on Cancer.

database, and it used the TCGA-Assembler (10) to download the RNA-Seq data of 31 tumors in the TCGA database. RNA-Seq data were obtained for 'Primary Solid Tumor' and 'Solid Tissue Normal' for each cancer, and the tumor staging in UALCAN was based on the pathological tumor staging data of the American Joint Committee on Cancer (AJCC), which divided the samples into different stages (8). Data visualization was conducted by Highcharts (Highsoft AS Highcharts, http://www.highcharts.com/), a JavaScript library from Highsoft AS (8).

GEPIA

Developed by Gepia Zefang Tang, is a website that analyzes RNA sequence expression databases based on the TCGA and GTEX projects. Using a deconvolution strategy, it can present cell type information combined with clinical data to help us explore the relationship between cell proportion and prognosis (11). The cancer data of GEPIA was collected from TCGA or GTEx, and the tumor staging definition in GEPIA was based on the pathological tumor staging data of the American Joint Committee on Cancer (AJCC) (12, 13). For the calculation methods of survival analysis, the python package lifeline (https://github.com/CamDavidsonPilon/lifelines) was used for the survival analysis (11). Here, we mainly used the Multiple Gene Analysis module for analyzing the expression of integrins in SKCM at different pathological stages, and correlations between integrin subunit expression and overall survival and disease-free survival.

STRING

String is a website that can analyze the interaction relationship between genes. In order to understand the interaction relationship between integrin genes in this study, we used STRING website to build a PPI network. Each gene is represented by nodes in the network, and the strength and connections in the network are represented by the color and thickness of the lines.

GeneMANIA

GeneMANIA is a website for reprocessing PPI network maps (14). GeneMANIA can perform cluster analysis on nodes in the PPI network graph by collecting hundreds of data sets from GEO, Biogrid, Pathway Commons and I2D, so as to provide biological function analysis of each gene in the PPI network graph (14).

CBioPortal

CBioPortal (http://www.cbioportal.org) is a website used to analyze and visualize cancer genomics data (15). Cbioportal collected the data of 126 tumor genomic studies from TCGA data, based on which cBioPortal can detect the genetic variation, gene network and co-expression of target genes in SKCM (9). Here, we analyzed the gene variation of integrins in SKCM using cBioPortal.

TIMER

TIMER is a website that analyzes the relationship between tumor purity and immune cell infiltration. Specifically, TIMER can explore the correlation between the degree of infiltration of immune cells in tumor microenvironment and clinical results, somatic mutations, gene expression and somatic copy number changes (16). By collecting the gene expression information of different tumors in the TCGA database, TIMER inferred the abundance of tumor-infiltrated immune cells in the gene expression profile using deconvolution method (17). In this study, the relationship between immune cell infiltration and integrin subunit in SKCM was investigated by using the "gene" module in TIMER.

Trrust

TRRUST (https://www.grnpedia.org/trrust/) is a curated database of human and mouse transcriptional regulatory networks. TRRUST is useful as a tool in predicting these transcriptional regulatory networks (18). Here, TRRUST was used to identify the relationships between selected integrin subunit genes and other target genes.

Webgestalt

WebGestalt is a website for gene enrichment analysis based on David database. Through the use of WebGestalt, we can quickly visualize the results of the enrichment analysis of DAVID, and at the same time, we can also visualize the results of KEGG pathway (19, 20).

RESULTS

1. Aberrant Expression of Integrin Subunits in SKCM Patients

Firstly, we used the ONCOMINE database to compare the expression profiles of integrin subunits in cutaneous melanoma patients and control groups (**Figure 1** and **Table 1**). The results reveal that the transcription levels of ITGA3, ITGA4, ITGA6, ITGA10, ITGB1, ITGB2, ITGB3, ITGB4, and ITGB7 in Cutaneous Melanoma samples were significantly increased (compared with normal control samples). These results were compiled from several sources. According to Riker et al., the transcription levels of ITGA4, ITGA10, ITGB1, ITGB2, and ITGB7 in SKCM patients were significantly increased (compared with normal skin tissue), with fold changes of 3.224, 2.074, 3.525, 3.968, and 2.84 respectively (21). Haqq et al. reported that the transcription level of ITGB3 in melanoma patients was significantly increased (compared with normal skin tissue), with a fold change of 3.147 (22). Talatov et al. reported that the transcription levels of ITGA3, ITGA6, and ITGB4 in cutaneous melanoma were significantly increased (compared with normal tissue), with fold changes of 14.807, 16.226, and 10.644 (23). The significant differences in the expression levels of other integrin subunits were not observed between SKCM patients and normal patients. For specific sample information, please refer to the references mentioned in **Table 1**.

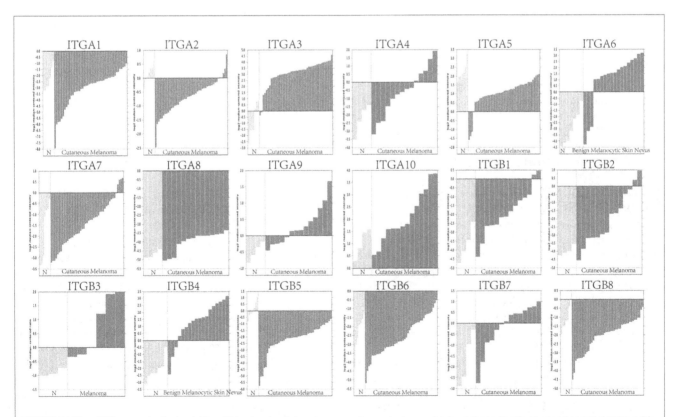

FIGURE 1 | The mRNA expression levels of different integrin subunits in cutaneous melanoma/melanoma/benign melanocytic skin nevus and normal skin tissue (N). The t-test statistic provided in ONCOMINE reflects the magnitude of the difference between the groups. Each bar represents the gene expression of one sample. The p value was set at 0.05.

TABLE 1 | Aberrant expression of integrin subunits in SKCM patients.

GENE	CANCER TYPE	FOLD CHANGE	p-value	t-test	Reference	PMID
ITGA3	Cutaneous Melanoma vs. Normal	14.807	9.58E-05	7.105	Talantov Melanoma	PMID: 16243793
ITGA4	Cutaneous Melanoma vs. Normal	3.224	0.013	2.75	Riker Melanoma	PMID: 18442402
ITGA6	Benign Melanocytic Skin Nevus vs. Normal	16.226	1.71E-05	5.491	Talantov Melanoma	PMID: 16243793
ITGA10	Cutaneous Melanoma vs. Normal	2.074	0.015	2.55	Riker Melanoma	PMID: 18442402
ITGB1	Cutaneous Melanoma vs. Normal	3.525	0.011	2.983	Riker Melanoma	PMID: 18442402
ITGB2	Cutaneous Melanoma vs. Normal	3.968	3.61E-04	4.213	Riker Melanoma	PMID: 18442402
ITGB3	Melanoma vs. Normal	3.147	0.006	3.681	Haqq Melanoma	PMID: 15833814
ITGB4	Benign Melanocytic Skin Nevus vs. Normal	10.644	2.76E-03	7.278	Talantov Melanoma	PMID: 16243793
ITGB7	Cutaneous Melanoma vs. Normal	2.84	0.043	2.21	Riker Melanoma	PMID: 18442402

To further validate the above results, we assessed the expression levels of different integrin subunits in primary SKCM samples and metastatic SKCM samples with UALCAN. Our analysis revealed that the transcriptional levels of ITGA1 ($p = 6.89 \times 10^{-7}$), ITGA4 ($p = 6.27 \times 10^{-8}$), ITGA5 ($p = 6.30 \times 10^{-5}$), ITGA8 ($p = 6.40 \times 10^{-4}$), ITGA9 ($p = 3.24 \times 10^{-3}$), ITGA10 ($p = 1.06 \times 10^{-3}$), ITGB1 ($p = 1.22 \times 10^{-6}$), ITGB2 ($p < 1 \times 10^{-12}$), ITGB3 ($p = 5.61 \times 10^{-4}$), ITGB5 ($p = 1.74 \times 10^{-3}$), and ITGB7 ($p = 3.15 \times 10^{-11}$) in metastatic SKCM tissues were significantly increased compared with primary SKCM tissues (**Figure 2**). Whereas, the expression level of ITGB6 ($p = 1.18 \times 10^{-2}$) in metastatic SKCM tissue was decreased compared with primary SKCM tissue (**Figure 2**). All other comparisons do not meet our threshold by p value<0.05 and fold change ≥ 2.

Lastly, to clarify the clinical significance of the observed changes in integrin subunit expression, we analyzed the correlations between integrin subunit expression and the pathological stage of SKCM using GEPIA. The analysis revealed that ITGA1 ($p = 0.000326$), ITGA4 ($p = 1.1 \times 10^{-5}$), ITGB1 ($p = 0.0213$), ITGB2 ($p = 5.78 \times 10^{-5}$), ITGB6 ($p = 0.00257$), and ITGB7 ($p = 0.00017$) were notably associated with the pathological stage of SKCM (**Figure 3**). To clarify the gene expression rank of integrin subunit gene expression, we analyzed the expression levels of these genes in SKCM tissue using the GEPIA website (**Figure 4**). The results reveal that the expression level of ITGB1 in SKCM patients was highest among the integrin genes of interest.

2. The Prognostic Value of Integrin Subunits in SKCM Patients

We next investigated correlations between integrin subunit expression levels and patient prognosis using GEPIA. The results of this analysis reveal that integrin subunit expression and disease-free survival time in SKCM patients are related. Two of these correlations — those involving ITGA6 and ITGB7 — were statistically significant (**Figure 5**). We next analyzed the associations between integrin subunit expression levels and overall survival in SKCM patients. The results reveal that the expression levels of ITGA6, ITGA10, ITGB2, ITGB3, ITGB6, ITGB7, and ITGB8 were remarkably correlated with overall survival in SKCM patients (**Figure 6**).

3. Relationship Between Integrin Subunit Expression and Immune Cell Infiltration

Tumor immune microenvironment (TIME) refers to the mutual environment composed of tumor cells and their surrounding immune cells. Evidence is accumulating to suggest that immune cell infiltration is closely related with cancer occurrence and resistance, and the degree of immune cell infiltration can evaluate the effectiveness of clinical tumor immunotherapy (16, 24). If the expression of the gene in SKCM TIME is related to the infiltration of immune cells and tumor purity, it is suggested that the gene may become a target of tumor immunotherapy. To further explore the function of integrin subunits in SKCM, the immune effects of integrin subunits were analyzed using the TIMER website (**Figures 7** and **8**).

The expression of *ITGA4, ITGA8, ITGB2, ITGB7* and *ITGB8* was correlated with the infiltration of all types immune cell and tumor purity in the SKCM TIME. *ITGA5* was related with tumor purity, B cell, Macrophage cell, Neutrophil cell, and Dendritic cell invasion in SKCM TIME. The expression of *ITGA1* and *ITGA9* was correlated with the infiltration of all types immune cell in the SKCM TIME, but not tumor purity. The expression of *ITGA2* was correlated with the infiltration of CD8+/CD4+ T cell, Macrophage cell, Neutrophil cell and Dendritic cell in SKCM patients. *ITGA6, ITGB1* and *ITGB3* was correlated with B cell, CD8+ T cell, Macrophage cell, Neutrophil cell and Dendritic cell infiltration. *ITGA10* was associated with CD4+/CD8+ T cell, Macrophage cell and Neutrophil cell infiltration. *ITGB5* was related with the invasion of CD4+ T cell, Macrophage cell, Neutrophil cell and Dendritic cell. *ITGB8* was correlated with CD8+ T cell, B cell and Neutrophil cell invasion.

4. Integrin Subunit Genetic Alteration and Protein Interaction Network in 1SKCM Patients

Firstly, we explored genetic alterations in the integrin subunit family in SKCM using the cBioportal website. The results of this analysis reveal that *ITGA1, ITGA2, ITGA3, ITGA4, ITGA5, ITGA6, ITGA7, ITGA8, ITGA9, ITGA10, ITGB1, ITGB2, ITGB3, ITGB4, ITGB5, ITGB6, ITGB7,* and *ITGB8* were changed in 6%, 3%, 3%, 8%, 5%, 3%, 5%, 7%, 4%, 7%, 1.6%, 3%, 4%, 8%, 2.1%, 4%, 1.9%, and 6% of the queried SKCM samples, respectively (**Figure 9A**). Next a PPI network of the integrin subunit family was constructed to explore possible interactions. A PPI network with 18 nodes and 152 edges was constructed using STRING (**Figure 9B**). According to the statistical results reported by the String website, the P-value of PPI enrichment was <1.0e-16. Further analysis using GeneMANIA revealed that the above-mentioned integrin subunits were mainly involved in extracellular matrix

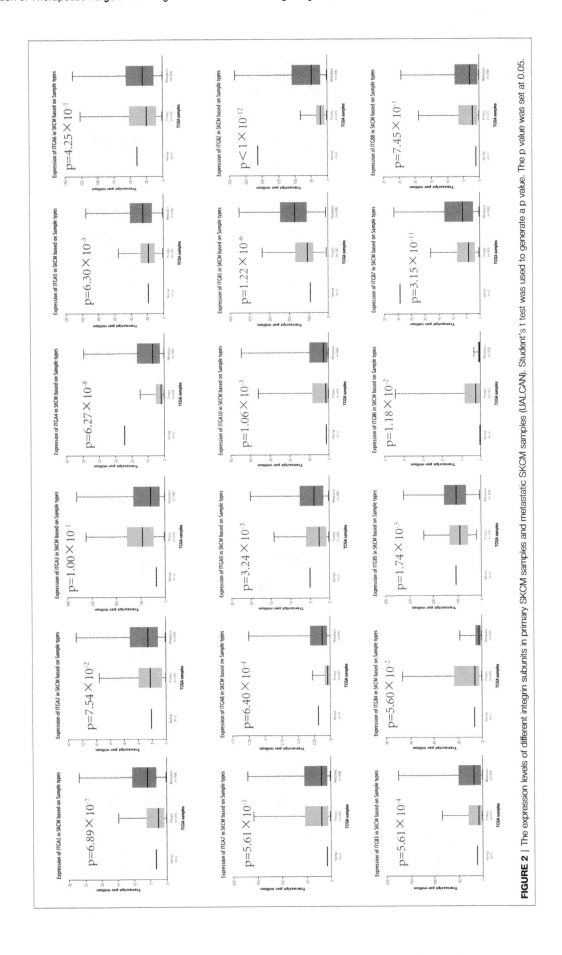

FIGURE 2 | The expression levels of different integrin subunits in primary SKCM samples and metastatic SKCM samples (UALCAN). Student's t test was used to generate a p value. The p value was set at 0.05.

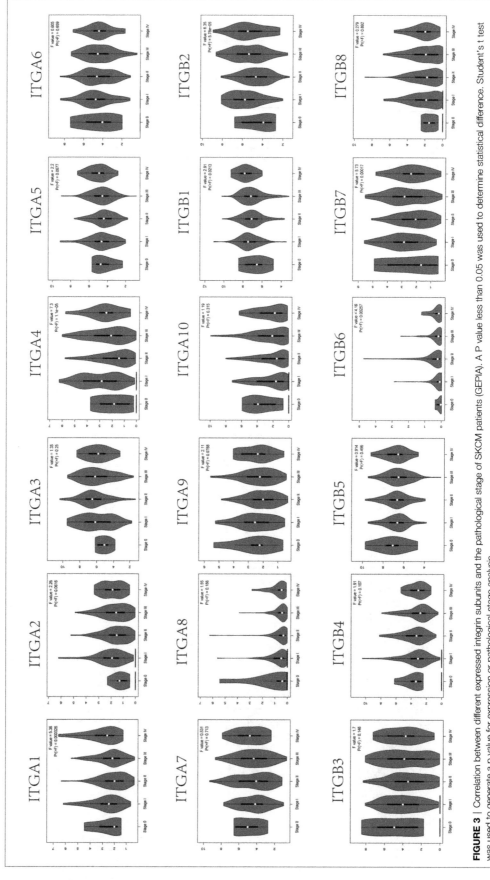

FIGURE 3 | Correlation between different expressed integrin subunits and the pathological stage of SKCM patients (GEPIA). A P value less than 0.05 was used to determine statistical difference. Student's t test was used to generate a p value for expression or pathological stage analysis.

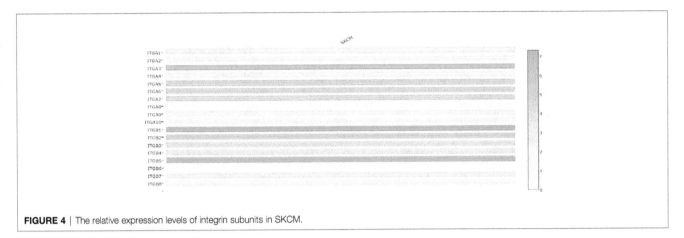

FIGURE 4 | The relative expression levels of integrin subunits in SKCM.

organization, extracellular structure organization, integrin complex, receptor complex, and leukocyte migration (**Figure 9C**). To further corroborate these observations, we used STRING to analyze the top 48 most interacting neighboring genes associated with 18 integrin subunits. The results demonstrate that ALB, CBL, CBY1, CD247, CDC25C, CTGF, EGF, EGFR, ERBB2, ERBB3, ERBB4, FBN1, FLNA, FN1, GRB2, ICAM1, ICAM3, ICAM5, ILK,IRS1, ITGA1, ITGA10, ITGA2, ITGA2B, ITGA3, ITGA4, ITGA5, ITGA6, ITGA7, ITGA8, ITGA9, ITGAL, ITGAM, ITGAV, ITGAX, ITGB1, ITGB1BP1, ITGB2, ITGB3, ITGB4, ITGB5, ITGB6, ITGB7, ITGB8, NPNT, NTRK1, NTRK2, PCSK9, PIK3R1, PIK3R2, PLEC, PXN, RAF1, SHC1, SMAD2, SOS1, SRC, TGFB1, TGFBR1, TGFBR2, TLN1, VEGFA, VTN, VWF, YWHAB, YWHAG, YWHAH, and YWHAZ are all involved in either the regulation or function of integrin subunit family members in SKCM patients (**Figure 9D**).

5. Gene Ontology and KEGG Pathway Analysis of Integrin Subunits in SKCM Patients

Go and KEGG pathway analysis for 18 integrin subunits and top 48 most interacting neighboring genes was performed using the Webgestalt website (**Figures 9E, F**). In the KEGG pathway analysis, the top 5 pathways identified were ECM-receptor interaction, arrhythmogenic right ventricular cardiomyopathy, hypertrophic cardiomyopathy, dilated cardiomyopathy, and focal adhesion. In the GO enrichment analysis, the results pertaining to biological processes were response to stimulus, biological regulation, and cell communication. For the results pertaining to the analysis of cellular components, the top five cellular components were membrane, protein-containing complex, vesicle, extracellular space, and endomembrane system. For the results pertaining to the analysis of molecular function, the top 5 molecular functions were protein binding, ion binding, molecular transducer activity, transferase activity, and nucleic acid binding.

DISCUSSION

Recent studies indicate that ITGA1 is associated with melanoma proliferation *via* the regulation of miR-3065-5p (25). In addition,

as a mediator of cell-cell and cell-matrix adhesion, ITGA1 was differentially expressed in melanoma samples (26). In the present study, we found that ITGA1 expression levels in SKCM tissues are correlated with different stages of SKCM and with migration in SKCM. ITGA1 protein mediate the adhesion of extracellular matrix proteins (27). We hypothesized that ITGA1 protein in SKCM promote the adhesion of melanocytes to the epidermal basement membrane (28), thus affecting the metastasis of SKCM. Besides, we found a positive correlation between the expression of *ITGA1* and infiltration of all types of immune cell, but not tumor purity (**Figure 7**). Therefore, the effect of ITGA1 in tumor immune therapy may need further verification.

ITGA2 plays a role in melanoma by regulating the expression GTSE1, thereby restoring the epithelial-to-mesenchymal transition in SKCM (29). However, according to our results, the increased expression of ITGA2 may only be related to the infiltration of some immune cells, and this infiltration of immune cells does not lead to the reduction of tumor purity in SKCM TIME, suggesting that the infiltration of immune cells may not play a decisive role in SKCM.

Schumacher et al. reported that flocculating material observed around melanoma cells or nests contains basal membrane protein components, particularly ITGA3 (30). In line with previous research, we found that ITGA3 expression in SKCM tissues was significantly increased (in comparison with non-tumor tissue). Moreover, it is worth mentioning that ITGA3 has most biological functions compared with other integrin subunits, suggesting that it may play a central role in integrin subunits gene clusters (**Figure 9C**).

ITGA4 is closely related to the occurrence and development of melanoma, and ITGA4 can promote the metastasis of melanoma by promoting the aggregation of melanoma cells in the lymphatic system (31). J. Zhao et al. reported that ITGA4 down-regulation inhibits the adhesion and migration of melanoma cells *in vitro* and *in vivo* (32). The immunomodulatory mechanism of ITGA4 in melanoma has also been reported in previous studies. Geherin et al. reported that IL-10+ B1 cells are part of the skin immune system and require α4β1 integrin for homing into the skin (33). In addition, Kobayashi et al. reported that IL-10+ B1a B cells suppress melanoma tumor immunity by inhibiting Th1 cytokine production in tumor-infiltrating CD8+ T cells (34). According to

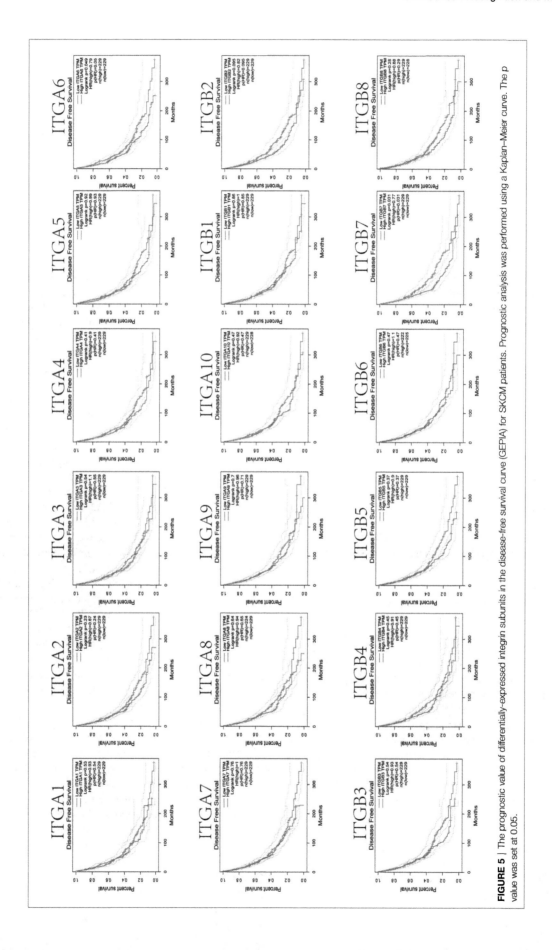

FIGURE 5 | The prognostic value of differentially-expressed integrin subunits in the disease-free survival curve (GEPIA) for SKCM patients. Prognostic analysis was performed using a Kaplan–Meier curve. The p value was set at 0.05.

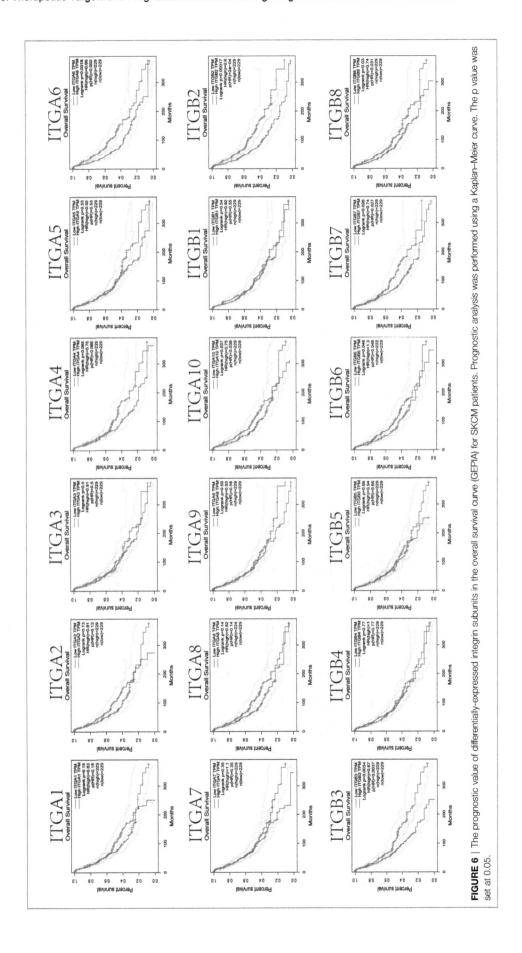

FIGURE 6 | The prognostic value of differentially-expressed integrin subunits in the overall survival curve (GEPIA) for SKCM patients. Prognostic analysis was performed using a Kaplan–Meier curve. The p value was set at 0.05.

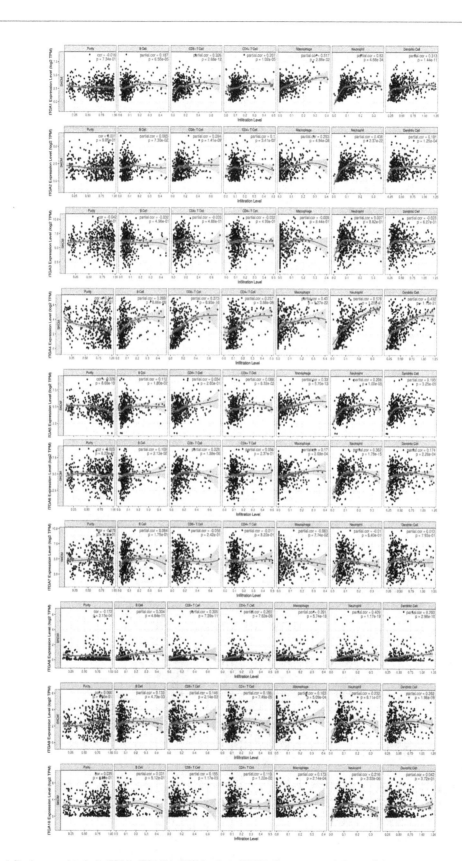

FIGURE 7 | Immune infiltration associated with ITGA1 – ITGA10 in SKCM patients (TIMER). Spearman correlation coefficient was used for statistical analysis. A P value less than 0.05 was used to determine statistical difference.

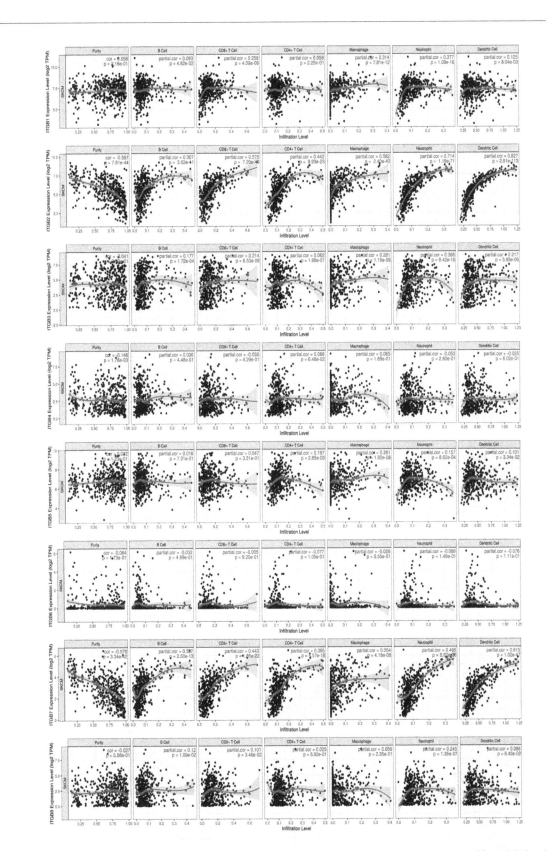

FIGURE 8 | Immune infiltration associated with ITGB1 – ITGB8 in SKCM patients (TIMER). Spearman correlation coefficient was used for statistical analysis. A P value less than 0.05 was used to determine statistical difference.

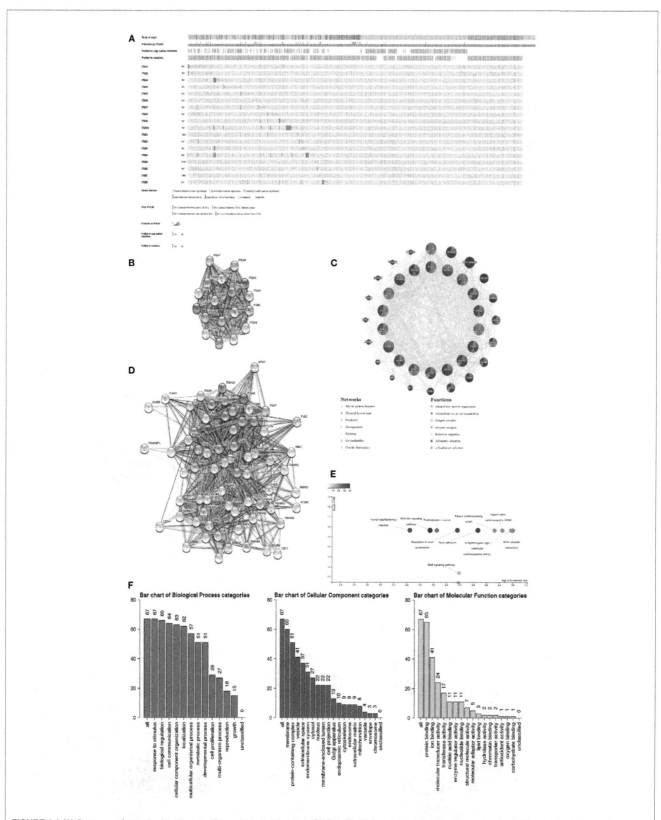

FIGURE 9 | **(A)** Summary of genetic alterations in different integrin subunits in SKCM. **(B, C)** Protein-protein interaction network of different integrin subunits. **(D)** Gene-gene interaction network of different integrin subunits and 48 most frequently altered neighboring genes. **(E, F)** Enrichment analysis of different integrin subunits and 48 most frequently altered neighboring genes in SKCM (Webgestalt). **(E)** Bar plot of KEGG enriched terms. **(F)** Bar plot of GO enrichment in biological process terms, cellular component terms, and molecular function terms.

our results, we speculated that the differentially expressed ITGA4 may recruit immune cells by effecting leukocyte migration, reduce the percentage of melanoma cells in SKCM TIME by affecting cell matrix adhesion in SKCM TIME, and ultimately affect the metastasis and tumor stage of SKCM (**Figures 7** and **9C**).

ITGA5 forms a receptor for extracellular fibronectin, which known to be involved in the formation of malignant tumor cells and tumor vascular systems (35). ITGA5 is known to play a role in melanoma by regulating miR-148b (36). Combined with our results, we hypothesized that ITGA5 may affect the infiltration of immune cells and tumor purity in SKCM TIME by regulating leukocyte migration (**Figures 7** and **9C**).

Specific ITGA6 variants were reported to be associated with a decreased risk of melanoma, and Luo et al. reported that ITGA6 can be considered a prognostic gene for uveal melanoma (37, 38). We also found that abnormally expressed ITGA6 is a potential prognostic biomarker in SKCM, and we speculate that missense mutation is one of the main reasons for the abnormal expression of ITGA6 (**Figure 9A**).

ITGA8 is a transmembrane cell surface receptor belonging to the alpha integrin family (39). To date, several studies have linked ITGA8 and tumorigenesis (40, 41). In addition, anti-ITGA8 therapies have been reported to play a role in the treatment of lupus and other glomerular diseases (42). Tumor cells express antigens that mediate recognition by CD8+ T cells and the infiltration of CD8+ T cells in SKCM TIME is a very important part of immunotherapy (43). Combined with our results, we speculated that interference against ITGA8 expression could effectively increase the infiltration of CD8+ T cells in SKCM TIME and reduce the percentage of tumor cells in SKCM, which is a potential target of SKCM targeted therapy (**Figure 7**).

Several studies have reported a close association between ITGA9 and cell adhesion, proliferation, and migration (44). Changes in ITGA9 expression levels affect the interaction between tumor cells and the extracellular matrix (45). *ITGA9* is a host gene for various long non-coding RNAs, including LncCCAT1 and HOXA11-AS. Therefore, proliferation, apoptosis, metastasis of melanoma cells may be modulated *via* regulation of *ITGA9*-related non-coding RNAs (46, 47). In the present study *ITGA9* was positively correlated with the invasion of several immune cells in SKCM TIME, but not tumor purity (**Figure 7**). Combined with our results and previous reports, we suggest that ITGA9 in SKCM may mediate cell-cell communication between cancer cells and their microenvironment by influencing the formation of integrin and receptor complexes, and ultimately effect SKCM metastasis and progression (**Figure 9C**) (48).

ITGA10 is a transmembrane glycoprotein involved in cell adhesion and integrin-mediated signaling pathways (49). ITGA10 is associated with various cancers development and metastasis, and variants in *ITGA10* are associated with changes of melanoma risks (50). In the present study, we found that ITGA10 expression was up-regulated in SKCM tissues (in comparison with control tissues), and this abnormal expression of ITGA10 may be the results of amplification mutations or the missense mutations (**Figure 9A**).

Previous studies have confirmed the correlation between ITGB1 expression and SKCM metastasis (51). In line with previous studies, we report aberrant ITGB1 expression in SKCM, and we reveal that ITGB1 expression is closely associated with SKCM metastasis by effecting cell migration (**Figure 2**) (52).

According to a bioanalysis conducted by Jun Zhu et al., ITGB2 was one of the top hub genes in malignant melanoma, and its expression was related to overall survival and disease-free survival (53). Combined with our results, we believe that ITGB2 is one of the integrin subunits most closely related to SKCM. ITGB2 plays a variety of roles in integrin complex, including extracellular matrix formation, Integrin complex formation, leukocyte migration, etc. Through the above functions, the highly expressed ITGB2 can effectively recruit T cells in SKCM TIME and reduce the purity of tumor cells in SKCM, so the overexpression of ITGB2 may effectively improve the effectiveness of immunotherapy against SKCM and improve the overall survival rate.

ITGB3 may play a vital role in the treatment of melanoma. Inhibition of ITGB3-SRC-STAT3 pathway activation can sensitize tumor-repopulating cells to the effects of IFN-α, and enhance the overall efficacy of melanoma treatment (54). In addition, the ADAR1-ITGB3 network may also play a central role in acquisition of an invasive phenotype in metastatic melanoma (55, 56). Transcription of ITGB3 gene induces the expression of NME1, a metastatic suppressor, in melanoma (57). According to our results, we hypothesized that the abnormal expression of ITGB3 in SKCM suggesting its value as a prognostic marker.

ITGB4 and ITGA6 are heterodimeric cambium adhesin receptors. ITGB4 has a long cytoplasmic domain and has unique cytoskeleton and signaling functions (58, 59). In addition, a mutation in ITGB4 has been identified in a metastasis sample taken from acral melanoma patients (60). The findings presented here are consistent with this previous research. In particular, ITGB4 expression was significantly increased in SKCM tissues compared with non-tumor tissues (**Figure 1**).

ITGB5, which is located between 13:133161078 and 13:139609422 in the SSC13Q41 region, encodes the integrin β5 subunit, and this coordinates with the αV subunit to produce the integrin αVβ5 (61). Reports concerning the role of ITGB5 in melanoma are scarce.

ITGB6 is extensively involved in wound healing and the pathogenesis of a variety of diseases, including fibrosis and cancer (62). Previous studies have identified abnormal expression of ITGB6 in SK-Mel-28 human melanoma cells (63). In line with previous findings, we demonstrate here that ITGB6 expression was positively associated with SKCM tumor stage (**Figure 3**).

There are only a few reports concerning ITGB7 expression in melanoma and its potential role. However, we found that ITGB7 was not only abnormally expressed in SKCM, but also correlated with the prognosis of SKCM. The expression of ITGB7 in SKCM TIME was positively correlated with immune cell infiltration and negatively correlated with tumor purity. integrin subunits target therapy such as etrolizumab may play a role in the treatment of SKCM by mediated the infiltration of immune cells, of course, this needs further trial verification.

As for ITGA7 and ITGB8, there have been few reports confirming their connection to SKCM, and we did not find meaningful results in our study, we prefer to leave this question open.

Integrins form a heterodimer with α subunit and β subunit, and there is an intimate connection between integrin α subunits and β subunits (**Figure 9B**). Considering the biological functions of integrin subunits family and the results of our gene enrichment analysis (**Figures 9E, F**), we believe that integrin subunits family, which are mainly distributed in cell membrane and protein-containing complex, may affect protein-binding in SKCM by participating in biological processes such as cell communication, cellular component organization and response to stimulus and other biological processes. Further, these biological functions of the integrin family may also be inseparable from 48 genes (**Figure 9D**) that interact with them.

CONCLUSION

In conclusion, ITGA4, ITGB2 and ITGB7 was identified as novel biomarkers which may assist in the design of new immunotherapeutic drugs and server as diagnostic biomarkers.

However, there are several limitations with our research. Firstly, *in vivo* and *in vitro* research should be conducted to verify our results. Secondly, this research was conducted mainly based on public databases. As we have not explained all the statistics and code information used in these databases in detail, this may cause some confusion in non-specialist readers.

AUTHOR CONTRIBUTIONS

YN and WS carried out the experiment and wrote the manuscript with support from PM and KL, HX, and YZ helped supervise the project and conceived the original idea. All authors contributed to the article and approved the submitted version.

REFERENCES

1. Bertolotto C. Melanoma: From Melanocyte to Genetic Alterations and Clinical Options. *Scientifica* (2013) 2013:635203. doi: 10.1155/2013/635203
2. Valero MC, Huntsman HD, Liu J, Zou K, Boppart MD. Eccentric Exercise Facilitates Mesenchymal Stem Cell Appearance in Skeletal Muscle. *Plos one* (2012) 7:e29760. doi: 10.1371/journal.pone.0029760
3. Zhang H, Cui X, Cao A, Li X, Li L. ITGA3 Interacts With VASP to Regulate Stemness and Epithelial-Mesenchymal Transition of Breast Cancer Cells. *Gene* (2020) 734:144396. doi: 10.1016/j.gene.2020.144396
4. Brooks DL, Schwab LP, Krutilina R, Parke DN, Sethuraman A, Hoogewijs D, et al. ITGA6 Is Directly Regulated by Hypoxia-Inducible Factors and Enriches for Cancer Stem Cell Activity and Invasion in Metastatic Breast Cancer Models. *Mol Cancer* (2016) 15:26. doi: 10.1186/s12943-016-0510-x
5. Bhandari A, Xia E, Zhou Y, Guan Y, Xiang J, Kong L, et al. ITGA7 Functions as a Tumor Suppressor and Regulates Migration and Invasion in Breast Cancer. *Cancer Manag Res* (2018) 10:969–76. doi: 10.2147/cmar.S160379
6. Kobayashi T, Matsumoto S, Shimizu K, Miyake M, Maeda S, Hamaguchi Y, et al. Discrepancy in Responses to Dabrafenib Plus Trametinib Combination Therapy in Intracranial and Extracranial Metastases in Melanoma Patients. *J Dermatol* (2021) 48:e82–82e83. doi: 10.1111/1346-8138.15677
7. Rhodes DR, Yu J, Shanker K, Deshpande N, Varambally R, Ghosh D, et al. ONCOMINE: A Cancer Microarray Database and Integrated Data-Mining Platform. *Neoplasia* (2004) 6:1–6. doi: 10.1016/s1476-5586(04)80047-2
8. Chandrashekar DS, Bashel B, Balasubramanya SAH, Creighton CJ, Ponce-Rodriguez I, Chakravarthi B, et al. UALCAN: A Portal for Facilitating Tumor Subgroup Gene Expression and Survival Analyses. *Neoplasia* (2017) 19:649–58. doi: 10.1016/j.neo.2017.05.002
9. Zhou X, Peng M, He Y, Peng J, Zhang X, Wang C, et al. CXC Chemokines as Therapeutic Targets and Prognostic Biomarkers in Skin Cutaneous Melanoma Microenvironment. *Front Oncol* (2021) 11:619003. doi: 10.3389/fonc.2021.619003
10. Zhu Y, Qiu P, Ji Y. TCGA-Assembler: Open-Source Software for Retrieving and Processing TCGA Data. *Nat Methods* (2014) 11:599–600. doi: 10.1038/nmeth.2956
11. Tang Z, Kang B, Li C, Chen T, Zhang Z. GEPIA2: An Enhanced Web Server for Large-Scale Expression Profiling and Interactive Analysis. *Nucleic Acids Res* (2019) 47:W556–60. doi: 10.1093/nar/gkz430

12. Human genomics. The Genotype-Tissue Expression (GTEx) Pilot Analysis: Multitissue Gene Regulation in Humans. *Science* (2015) 348:648–60. doi: 10.1126/science.1262110
13. Weinstein JN, Collisson EA, Mills GB, Shaw KR, Ozenberger BA, Ellrott K, et al. The Cancer Genome Atlas Pan-Cancer Analysis Project. *Nat Genet* (2013) 45:1113–20. doi: 10.1038/ng.2764
14. Warde-Farley D, Donaldson SL, Comes O, Zuberi K, Badrawi R, Chao P, et al. The GeneMANIA Prediction Server: Biological Network Integration for Gene Prioritization and Predicting Gene Function. *Nucleic Acids Res* (2010) 38: W214–20. doi: 10.1093/nar/gkq537
15. Cerami E, Gao J, Dogrusoz U, Gross BE, Sumer SO, Aksoy BA, et al. The Cbio Cancer Genomics Portal: An Open Platform for Exploring Multidimensional Cancer Genomics Data. *Cancer Discov* (2012) 2:401–4. doi: 10.1158/2159-8290.Cd-12-0095
16. Li T, Fan J, Wang B, Traugh N, Chen Q, Liu JS, et al. TIMER: A Web Server for Comprehensive Analysis of Tumor-Infiltrating Immune Cells. *Cancer Res* (2017) 77(21):e108–10. doi: 10.1158/0008-5472.Can-17-0307
17. Li T, Fu J, Zeng Z, Cohen D, Li J, Chen Q, et al. TIMER2.0 for Analysis of Tumor-Infiltrating Immune Cells. *Nucleic Acids Res* (2020) 48:W509–509W514. doi: 10.1093/nar/gkaa407
18. Han H, Cho JW, Lee S, Yun A, Kim H, Bae D, et al. TRRUST V2: An Expanded Reference Database of Human and Mouse Transcriptional Regulatory Interactions. *Nucleic Acids Res* (2018) 46:D380–6. doi: 10.1093/nar/gkx1013
19. Zhang B, Kirov S, Snoddy J. WebGestalt: An Integrated System for Exploring Gene Sets in Various Biological Contexts. *Nucleic Acids Res* (2005) 33:W741–8. doi: 10.1093/nar/gki475
20. Wang J, Vasaikar S, Shi Z, Greer M, Zhang B. WebGestalt 2017: A More Comprehensive, Powerful, Flexible and Interactive Gene Set Enrichment Analysis Toolkit. *Nucleic Acids Res* (2017) 45:W130–7. doi: 10.1093/nar/gkx356
21. Riker AI, Enkemann SA, Fodstad O, Liu S, Ren S, Morris C, et al. The Gene Expression Profiles of Primary and Metastatic Melanoma Yields a Transition Point of Tumor Progression and Metastasis. *BMC Med Genomics* (2008) 1:13. doi: 10.1186/1755-8794-1-13
22. Haqq C, Nosrati M, Sudilovsky D, Crothers J, Khodabakhsh D, Pulliam BL, et al. The Gene Expression Signatures of Melanoma Progression. *Proc Natl Acad Sci USA* (2005) 102:6092–7. doi: 10.1073/pnas.0501564102

23. Talantov D, Mazumder A, Yu JX, Briggs T, Jiang Y, Backus J, et al. Novel Genes Associated With Malignant Melanoma But Not Benign Melanocytic Lesions. *Clin Cancer Res* (2005) 11:7234–42. doi: 10.1158/1078-0432.CCR-05-0683

24. Kobayashi T, Hamaguchi Y, Hasegawa M, Fujimoto M, Takehara K, Matsushita T. B Cells Promote Tumor Immunity Against B16F10 Melanoma. *Am J Pathol* (2014) 184:3120–9. doi: 10.1016/j.ajpath.2014.07.003

25. Palkina N, Komina A, Aksenenko M, Moshev A, Savchenko A, Ruksha T. miR-204-5p and miR-3065-5p Exert Antitumor Effects on Melanoma Cells. *Oncol Lett* (2018) 15:8269–80. doi: 10.3892/ol.2018.8443

26. Cioanca AV, Wu CS, Natoli R, Conway RM, McCluskey PJ, Jager MJ, et al. The Role of Melanocytes in the Human Choroidal Microenvironment and Inflammation: Insights From the Transcriptome. *Pigment Cell Melanoma Res* (2021). doi: 10.1111/pcmr.12972

27. Hynes RO. Integrins: Bidirectional, Allosteric Signaling Machines. *Cell* (2002) 110:673–87. doi: 10.1016/s0092-8674(02)00971-6

28. Pinon P, Wehrle-Haller B. Integrins: Versatile Receptors Controlling Melanocyte Adhesion, Migration and Proliferation. *Pigment Cell Melanoma Res* (2011) 24:282–94. doi: 10.1111/j.1755-148X.2010.00806.x

29. Xu T, Ma M, Chi Z, Si L, Sheng X, Cui C, et al. High G2 and S-Phase Expressed 1 Expression Promotes Acral Melanoma Progression and Correlates With Poor Clinical Prognosis. *Cancer Sci* (2018) 109:1787–98. doi: 10.1111/cas.13607

30. Schumacher D, Schaumburg-Lever G. Ultrastructural Localization of Alpha-3 Integrin Subunit in Malignant Melanoma and Adjacent Epidermis. *J Cutan Pathol* (1999) 26:321–6. doi: 10.1111/j.1600-0560.1999.tb01853.x

31. Rebhun RB, Cheng H, Gershenwald JE, Fan D, Fidler IJ, Langley RR. Constitutive Expression of the Alpha4 Integrin Correlates With Tumorigenicity and Lymph Node Metastasis of the B16 Murine Melanoma. *Neoplasia* (2010) 12:173–82. doi: 10.1593/neo.91604

32. Zhao J, Qi Q, Yang Y, Gu HY, Lu N, Liu W, et al. Inhibition of Alpha(4) Integrin Mediated Adhesion was Involved in the Reduction of B16-F10 Melanoma Cells Lung Colonization in C57BL/6 Mice Treated With Gambogic Acid. *Eur J Pharmacol* (2008) 589:127–31. doi: 10.1016/j.ejphar.2008.04.063

33. Geherin SA, Gómez D, Glabman RA, Ruthel G, Hamann A, Debes GF. IL-10+ Innate-Like B Cells Are Part of the Skin Immune System and Require α4β1 Integrin To Migrate Between the Peritoneum and Inflamed Skin. *J Immunol* (2016) 196:2514–25. doi: 10.4049/jimmunol.1403246

34. Kobayashi T, Oishi K, Okamura A, Maeda S, Komuro A, Hamaguchi Y, et al. Regulatory B1a Cells Suppress Melanoma Tumor Immunity *via* IL-10 Production and Inhibiting T Helper Type 1 Cytokine Production in Tumor-Infiltrating CD8(+) T Cells. *J Invest Dermatol* (2019) 139:1535–44.e1. doi: 10.1016/j.jid.2019.02.016

35. Feng C, Jin X, Han Y, Guo R, Zou J, Li Y, et al. Expression and Prognostic Analyses of ITGA3, ITGA5, and ITGA6 in Head and Neck Squamous Cell Carcinoma. *Med Sci Monit* (2020) 26:e926800. doi: 10.12659/msm.926800

36. Quirico L, Orso F, Esposito CL, Bertone S, Coppo R, Conti L, et al. Axl-148b Chimeric Aptamers Inhibit Breast Cancer and Melanoma Progression. *Int J Biol Sci* (2020) 16:1238–51. doi: 10.7150/ijbs.39768

37. Lenci RE, Rachakonda PS, Kubarenko AV, Weber AN, Brandt A, Gast A, et al. Integrin Genes and Susceptibility to Human Melanoma. *Mutagenesis* (2012) 27:367–73. doi: 10.1093/mutage/ger090

38. Karhemo PR, Ravela S, Laakso M, Ritamo I, Tatti O, Mäkinen S, et al. An Optimized Isolation of Biotinylated Cell Surface Proteins Reveals Novel Players in Cancer Metastasis. *J Proteomics* (2012) 77:87–100. doi: 10.1016/j.jprot.2012.07.009

39. Wu J, Cheng J, Zhang F, Luo X, Zhang Z, Chen S. Estrogen Receptor α Is Involved in the Regulation of ITGA8 Methylation in Estrogen Receptor-Positive Breast Cancer. *Ann Transl Med* (2020) 8:993. doi: 10.21037/atm-20-5220

40. Matsushima S, Aoshima Y, Akamatsu T, Enomoto Y, Meguro S, Kosugi I, et al. CD248 and Integrin Alpha-8 Are Candidate Markers for Differentiating Lung Fibroblast Subtypes. *BMC Pulm Med* (2020) 20:21. doi: 10.1186/s12890-020-1054-9

41. Talbot JC, Nichols JT, Yan YL, Leonard IF, BreMiller RA, Amacher SL, et al. Pharyngeal Morphogenesis Requires Fras1-Itga8-Dependent Epithelial-Mesenchymal Interaction. *Dev Biol* (2016) 416:136–48. doi: 10.1016/j.ydbio.2016.05.035

42. Scindia Y, Deshmukh U, Thimmalapura PR, Bagavant H. Anti-Alpha8 Integrin Immunoliposomes in Glomeruli of Lupus-Susceptible Mice: A Novel System for Delivery of Therapeutic Agents to the Renal Glomerulus in Systemic Lupus Erythematosus. *Arthritis Rheum* (2008) 58:3884–91. doi: 10.1002/art.24026

43. Yan K, Lu Y, Yan Z, Wang Y. 9-Gene Signature Correlated With CD8(+) T Cell Infiltration Activated by IFN-Gamma: A Biomarker of Immune Checkpoint Therapy Response in Melanoma. *Front Immunol* (2021) 12:622563. doi: 10.3389/fimmu.2021.622563

44. Zhang J, Na S, Liu C, Pan S, Cai J, Qiu J. MicroRNA-125b Suppresses the Epithelial-Mesenchymal Transition and Cell Invasion by Targeting ITGA9 in Melanoma. *Tumour Biol* (2016) 37:5941–9. doi: 10.1007/s13277-015-4409-8

45. Xu TJ, Qiu P, Zhang YB, Yu SY, Xu GM, Yang W. MiR-148a Inhibits the Proliferation and Migration of Glioblastoma by Targeting ITGA9. *Hum Cell* (2019) 32:548–56. doi: 10.1007/s13577-019-00279-9

46. Fan J, Kang X, Zhao L, Zheng Y, Yang J, Li D. Long Noncoding RNA CCAT1 Functions as a Competing Endogenous RNA to Upregulate ITGA9 by Sponging MiR-296-3p in Melanoma. *Cancer Manag Res* (2020) 12:4699–714. doi: 10.2147/cmar.S252635

47. Xu Y, Zhang J, Zhang Q, Xu H, Liu L. Long Non-Coding RNA HOXA11-AS Modulates Proliferation. Apoptosis Metastasis EMT Cutaneous Melanoma Cells Partly *via* miR-152-3p/ITGA9 Axis. *Cancer Manag Res* (2021) 13:925–39. doi: 10.2147/cmar.S281920

48. Peng Y, Wu D, Li F, Zhang P, Feng Y, He A. Identification of Key Biomarkers Associated With Cell Adhesion in Multiple Myeloma by Integrated Bioinformatics Analysis, Apoptosis, Metastasis and EMT in Cutaneous Melanoma Cells Partly *via* miR-152-3p/ITGA9 Axis. *Cancer Cell Int* (2020) 20:262. doi: 10.1186/s12935-020-01355-z

49. Hamaia SW, Luff D, Hunter EJ, Malcor JD, Bihan D, Gullberg D, et al. Unique Charge-Dependent Constraint on Collagen Recognition by Integrin Alpha10beta1. *Matrix Biol* (2017) 59:80–94. doi: 10.1016/j.matbio.2016.08.010

50. Lasić V, Kosović I, Jurić M, Racetin A, Čurčić J, Šolić I, et al. GREB1L, CRELD2 and ITGA10 Expression in the Human Developmental and Postnatal Kidneys: An Immunohistochemical Study. *Acta Histochem* (2021) 123:151679. doi: 10.1016/j.acthis.2021.151679

51. Menefee DS, McMasters A, Pan J, Li X, Xiao D, Waigel S, et al. Age-Related Transcriptome Changes in Melanoma Patients With Tumor-Positive Sentinel Lymph Nodes. *Aging (Albany NY)* (2020) 12:24914–39. doi: 10.18632/aging.202435

52. El-Hachem N, Habel N, Naiken T, Bziouche H, Cheli Y, Beranger GE, et al. Uncovering and Deciphering the Pro-Invasive Role of HACE1 in Melanoma Cells. *Cell Death Differ* (2018) 25:2010–22. doi: 10.1038/s41418-018-0090-y

53. Zhu J, Hao S, Zhang X, Qiu J, Xuan Q, Ye L. Integrated Bioinformatics Analysis Exhibits Pivotal Exercise-Induced Genes and Corresponding Pathways in Malignant Melanoma. *Front Genet* (2020) 11:637320. doi: 10.3389/fgene.2020.637320

54. Li Y, Song Y, Li P, Li M, Wang H, Xu T, et al. Downregulation of RIG-I Mediated by ITGB3/c-SRC/STAT3 Signaling Confers Resistance to Interferon-α-Induced Apoptosis in Tumor-Repopulating Cells of Melanoma. (2020) 8:e000111. doi: 10.1136/jitc-2019-000111

55. Nemlich Y, Baruch EN, Besser MJ, Shoshan E, Bar-Eli M, Anafi L, et al. ADAR1-Mediated Regulation of Melanoma Invasion. *Nat Commun* (2018) 9:2154. doi: 10.1038/s41467-018-04600-2

56. Nemlich Y, Besser MJ, Schachter J, Markel G. ADAR1 Regulates Melanoma Cell Invasiveness by Controlling Beta3-Integrin *via* microRNA-30 Family Members. *Am J Cancer Res* (2018) 8:2677–86.

57. Leonard MK, Novak M, Snyder D, Snow G, Pamidimukkala N, McCorkle JR, et al. The Metastasis Suppressor NME1 Inhibits Melanoma Cell Motility *via* Direct Transcriptional Induction of the Integrin Beta-3 Gene. *Exp Cell Res* (2019) 374:85–93. doi: 10.1016/j.yexcr.2018.11.010

58. Sung JS, Kang CW, Kang S, Jang Y, Chae YC, Kim BG, et al. ITGB4-Mediated Metabolic Reprogramming of Cancer-Associated Fibroblasts. *Oncogene* (2020) 39:664–76. doi: 10.1038/s41388-019-1014-0

59. Li M, Jiang X, Wang G, Zhai C, Liu Y, Li H, et al. ITGB4 Is a Novel Prognostic Factor in Colon Cancer. *J Cancer* (2019) 10:5223–33. doi: 10.7150/jca.29269

60. Abramov IS, Emelyanova MA, Ryabaya OO, Krasnov GS, Zasedatelev AS, Nasedkina TV. Somatic Mutations Associated With Metastasis in Acral Melanoma. *Mol Biol (Mosk)* (2019) 53:648–53. doi: 10.1134/S0026898419040025

62. Meecham A, Marshall JF. The ITGB6 Gene: Its Role in Experimental and Clinical Biology. *Gene* (2020) 5:100023. doi: 10.1016/j.gene.2019.100023

63. Klein A, Capitanio JS, Maria DA, Ruiz IR. Gene Expression in SK-Mel-28 Human Melanoma Cells Treated With the Snake Venom Jararhagin. *Toxicon* (2011) 57:1–8. doi: 10.1016/j.toxicon.2010.09.001

61. Zhang LY, Guo Q, Guan GF, Cheng W, Cheng P, Wu AH. Integrin Beta 5 Is a Prognostic Biomarker and Potential Therapeutic Target in Glioblastoma. *Front Oncol* (2019) 9:904. doi: 10.3389/fonc.2019.00904

25

Merkel Cell Carcinoma: Evaluation of the Clinico-Pathological Characteristics, Treatment Strategies and Prognostic Factors in a Monocentric Retrospective Series (n=143)

Marco Rastrelli[1,2†], Paolo Del Fiore[1*†], Irene Russo[1,3†], Jacopo Tartaglia[3], Alessandro Dal Monico[3], Rocco Cappellesso[4], Lorenzo Nicolè[5,6], Luisa Piccin[7], Alessio Fabozzi[8], Bernardo Biffoli[9], Claudia Di Prata[1], Beatrice Ferrazzi[10], Luigi Dall'Olmo[1,2], Antonella Vecchiato[1], Romina Spina[1], Francesco Russano[1], Elisabetta Bezzon[11], Sara Cingarlini[12], Renzo Mazzarotto[13], Alessandro Parisi[14], Giovanni Scarzello[14], Jacopo Pigozzo[7], Tito Brambullo[9], Saveria Tropea[1], Vincenzo Vindigni[9], Franco Bassetto[9], Daniele Bertin[15], Michele Gregianin[15], Angelo Paolo Dei Tos[4,16], Francesco Cavallin[17], Mauro Alaibac[3‡], Vanna Chiarion-Sileni[7‡] and Simone Mocellin[1,2‡]

[1] Soft-Tissue, Peritoneum and Melanoma Surgical Oncology Unit, Veneto Institute of Oncology (IOV)-IRCCS, Padua, Italy, [2] Department of Surgery, Oncology and Gastroenterology (DISCOG), University of Padua, Padua, Italy, [3] Division of Dermatology, Department of Medicine (DIMED), University of Padua, Padua, Italy, [4] Pathological Anatomy Unit, University Hospital of Padua, Padua, Italy, [5] Department of Medicine, University of Padua School of Medicine and Surgery, Padua, Italy, [6] Unit of Surgical Pathology & Cytopathology, Ospedale dell'Angelo, Mestre, Italy, [7] Melanoma Oncology Unit, Veneto Institute of Oncology (IOV)-IRCCS, Padua, Italy, [8] Oncology Unit 3, Veneto Institute of Oncology (IOV)-IRCCS, Padua, Italy, [9] Clinic of Plastic Surgery, Department of Neuroscience, Padua University Hospital, University of Padua, Padua, Italy, [10] Postgraduate School of Occupational Medicine, University of Verona, Verona, Italy, [11] Radiology Unit, Department of Imaging and Medical Physics, Istituto Oncologico Veneto (IOV) IRCSS, Padua, Italy, [12] Oncology Section, Department of Oncology, Verona University and Hospital Trust, Verona, Italy, [13] Department of Radiotherapy, Ospedale Civile Maggiore, Azienda Ospedaliera Universitaria Integrata Verona, Verona, Italy, [14] Radiotherapy Unit, Veneto Institute of Oncology, Istituto Oncologico Veneto (IOV)-IRCCS, Padua, Italy, [15] Radiotherapy and Nuclear Medicine Unit, Oncological Institute of Veneto IOV-IRCCS, Padua, Italy, [16] Department of Medicine (DIMED), Surgical Pathology Unit, University of Padua, Padua, Italy, [17] Independent Statistician, Solagna, Italy

*Correspondence:
Paolo Del Fiore
paolo.delfiore@iov.veneto.it

† These authors have contributed equally to the work

‡ These authors share last authorship

Background: Merkel cell carcinoma (MCC) is a rare neuroendocrine tumor of the skin. The incidence of the disease has undergone a significant increase in recent years, which is caused by an increase in the average age of the population and in the use of immunosuppressive therapies. MCC is an aggressive pathology, which metastasizes early to the lymph nodes. These characteristics impose an accurate diagnostic analysis of the regional lymph node district with radiography, clinical examination and sentinel node biopsy. In recent years, there has been a breakthrough in the treatment of the advanced pathology thanks to the introduction of monoclonal antibodies acting on the PD-1/PD-L1 axis. This study aimed to describe the clinico-pathological characteristics, treatment strategies and prognostic factors of MCC.

Methods: A retrospective cohort study was conducted involving 143 consecutive patients who were diagnosed and/or treated for MCC. These patients were referred to the Veneto Institute of Oncology IOV-IRCCS and to the University Hospital of Padua (a third-level center) in the period between December 1991 and January 2020. In the majority of cases, diagnosis took place at the IOV. However, some patients were diagnosed elsewhere and subsequently referred to the IOV for a review of the diagnosis or to begin specific therapeutic regimens.

Results: 143 patients, with an average age of 71 years, were affected mainly with autoimmune and neoplastic comorbidities. Our analysis has shown that age, autoimmune comorbidities and the use of therapy with immunomodulating drugs (which include corticosteroids, statins and beta-blockers) are associated with a negative prognosis. In this sense, male sex is also a negative prognostic factor.

Conclusions: Autoimmune and neoplastic comorbidities were frequent in the studied population. The use of drugs with immunomodulatory effects was also found to be a common feature of the population under examination. The use of this type of medication is considered a negative prognostic factor. The relevance of a multidisciplinary approach to the patient with MCC is confirmed, with the aim of assessing the risks and benefits related to the use of immunomodulating therapy in the individual patient.

Keywords: Merkel cell cancer, Merkel carcinoma, Merkel treatment strategies, non-melanoma skin cancer (NMSC), skin cancer

INTRODUCTION

Merkel cell carcinoma (MCC) is a rare and highly aggressive malignancy of the skin (1–4). MCC usually presents itself as a rapidly growing pink to red-violet indurated plaque or nodule on sun-damaged skin, most commonly on the head and neck and less frequently on the trunk and extremities (5, 6). Lesions are often asymptomatic and ulceration is uncommon (5, 6). Male predominance is reported and the median age at diagnosis is 75-80 years (7, 8). Risk factors include older age, fair skin, ultraviolet (UV) exposure, immunosuppression, previous malignancies and Merkel Cell Polyomavirus (MCPyV) infection (9). The acronym AEIOU has been coined to encapsulate the main clinical features associated with MCC: asymptomatic, expanding rapidly, immunosuppressed, older than age 50 and UV-exposed (10).

The diagnosis of MCC is based on histopathological and immunohistochemical findings. Histologically, MCC is characterized by dermal and/or subcutaneous nodules or sheets of small, undifferentiated, round-to-oval cells with a vesicular nucleus and scanty cytoplasm (11). The characteristic immunohistological profile demonstrates positive staining with cytokeratins, notably AE1/AE3, CAM5.2, and CK20, and neuroendocrine markers such as chromogranin, synaptophysin, CD56, and NSE (9).

MCC is characterized by a high rate of local recurrence and nodal metastasis, a high mortality rate, and a deep psychological impact (12). The treatment regimen depends on the stage of the disease and includes surgery, radiation, chemotherapy, and/or immunotherapy (4, 7, 13). Surgical treatment consists of a wide excision of the primary lesion, sentinel lymph node biopsy, and/or regional lymph node dissection. Adjuvant radiotherapy may be offered after surgery. Metastatic or inoperable disease could be managed with chemotherapy and/or immunotherapy (4, 13).

There is considerable evidence suggesting that the dysfunction of the immune system contributes significantly to disease progression. This implies that therapies acting on the immune system can prove to be effective in slowing down disease progression (14). Overexpression of PD-L1 is observed in many tumors, including MCC, and allows the tumor to escape immune surveillance which normally enables the immune system to recognize and eliminate any abnormal cell (15). Therefore, the blockage of the interaction between PD-1 and its ligand allows the reactivation of T cells and an effective recruitment of the adaptive immune response. Some monoclonal antibodies capable of acting on this axis are avelumab (anti-PD-L1) and pembrolizumab (anti-PD-1). Both drugs have shown significant clinical efficacy in patients with stage IV MCC and, therefore, they are used as first-line treatment in this subpopulation of patients (16, 17).

Although significant progress has been made in understanding the molecular mechanisms underlying the development of this neoplasm, the characterization of the prognostic factors still remains limited. The importance of this aspect is enhanced by the high mortality rate of MCC and its deep psychological impact on the patient (18).

This study aims to contribute to current literature on MCC by providing an update on consecutive cases of MCC at our institution. This paper describes the demographic, clinical, and diagnostic characteristics of MCC and the therapeutic approach that had a significant prognostic impact.

MATERIAL AND METHODS

Study Design

A retrospective cohort study was conducted involving 143 consecutive patients who were diagnosed and/or treated for MCC. These patients were referred to the Veneto Institute of Oncology IOV-IRCCS and to the University Hospital of Padua (a tertiary care facility) in the period between December 1991 and January 2020. In the majority of cases, diagnosis took place at the IOV. However, some patients were diagnosed elsewhere and subsequently referred to the IOV for a review of the diagnosis or to begin specific therapeutic regimens.

Diagnosis and Treatment

All diagnoses were based on the histopathologic and immunohistochemical examination of the primary tumor. The stage of the disease was determined using the indicators provided by the Eighth edition of the AJCC staging system (19). Performed surgical treatments include wide excision (WE), a treatment performed on the primary lesion; sentinel lymph node biopsy (SNB), typically performed at the same time as the excision of the primary lesion; dissection of the lymph node basin, draining the region of the primary lesion (CLND).

CLND was performed on patients who reported a positive outcome to SNB and on subjects with clinically or radiologically evident lymph node involvement. SNB was performed routinely on all patients with a negative clinical examination of the regional lymph nodes. SNB was omitted in patients whose performance status was so compromised that adequate surgical treatment could not be performed.

The decision on whether to perform radiotherapy and/or chemotherapy was based on specific information concerning individual patient characteristics. The predominant factor influencing this decision was the stage of the disease based on the AJCC system. Possible radiotherapy settings were as follows: adjuvant, in patients who had already undergone surgical treatment for the lesion and/or CLND; neoadjuvant, before carrying out the surgical treatment; palliative, in the case of distant dissemination.

Conventional chemotherapy was reserved for stage IV patients classified in accordance with the AJCC system. Immunotherapy with monoclonal antibodies was also reserved for patients with metastatic disease: to date, this treatment is used as first-line treatment for stage IV patients. Some patients were treated with conventional chemotherapy for first-line treatment and only subsequently referred for immunotherapy.

Patients were subjected to a stringent follow-up regimen for the detection of early disease progression or relapse. Patients were typically seen once every six months for the first five years, then once every twelve months.

Any disease progression was recorded in the database. Disease progression was defined as the onset of distant, lymph node and in-transit metastases or local disease recurrence.

Data Collection

All data were retrieved from a local prospectively maintained database and entered in a dedicated data sheet for final checks and data analysis.

Study data included demographics, tumor characteristics, comorbidity information including autoimmune and neoplastic comorbidities, and the Charlson Comorbidity Index (20), details on treatment (WE, SNB, CLND, radiotherapy, chemotherapy, and immunotherapy) and prognosis.

Particular attention was paid to the tumor's immuno-histochemical characteristics, as immunohistochemical analysis was performed for most patients. Neuroendocrine and epithelial markers (such as CK20, NSE, Synaptophysin, Chromogranin, AE1/AE3, MNF 116, and Cam 5.2) were included in the database.

Overall survival was calculated from the date of diagnosis to the date of death, or the patient's last available visit. Disease-specific survival was calculated from the date of diagnosis to the date of death caused by MCC, or to the date of the last available visit/death not caused by the disease. Finally, disease-free survival was calculated in patients with primitive MCC from the date of diagnosis to the date on which the first relapse arose, or to the date of the last available visit/death.

Statistical Analysis

Categorical data were summarized as n (%), and compared using the Chi Square test and Fisher's exact test. Continuous data were reported as medians and interquartile ranges (IQR), and compared using the Mann-Whitney test. Survival curves were estimated using the Kaplan-Meier method and compared by means of the log-rank test. The association between clinically relevant variables and survival was evaluated using Cox regression models and reported as a Hazard Ratio (HR) with a 95% confidence interval (95% CI). The association between survival and chemotherapy was not considered, because chemotherapy was reserved for patients with metastatic disease and was thus a proxy of severe disease rather than a risk factor associated with reduced survival. The limited sample size did not allow any meaningful multivariable analyses. All tests were two-sided and a p-value below 0.05 was considered statistically significant. Statistical analysis was performed using R 4.0 (R Foundation for Statistical Computing, Vienna, Austria) (21).

RESULTS

Patients

The analysis included 143 patients (median age at diagnosis 71 years; 74 males and 69 females). Patient characteristics are outlined in **Table 1**. Most of the patients examined presented a primary lesion (110 patients, 77%), while 13 patients presented non-primary lesions (9 metastatic patients, and 4 disease recurrences). With regard to the initial clinical staging, 48% of patients were stage III (the most commonly attributed stage), 27% stage I, 15% stage II, and 10% stage IV. Limbs were the most common location of the lesion (57%), followed by the head/neck

TABLE 1 | Characteristics of 143 patients who had a diagnosis of MCC between December 1991 and January 2020.

		All patients	Non-primary tumors	Primary tumors
	N patients	143	33	110
Demographics	Age at diagnosis, years[a]	71 (63-79)	71 (63-76)	71 (62-79)
	Sex:			
	Female	69 (55)	13 (19)	56 (81)
	Male	64 (45)	20 (27)	54 (73)
	Family history of cancer:			
	No	37 (26)	7 (21)	30 (27)
	Yes	15 (10)	4 (12)	11 (10)
	Information not available	91 (64)	22 (67)	69 (63)
Merkel cell Carcinoma	Presentation:			
	Primary	110 (77)	0 (0)	110 (100)
	Occult primary	24 (17)	24 (73)	0 (0)
	Metastatic	5 (3)	5 (15)	0 (0)
	Recurrence	4 (3)	4 (12)	0 (0)
	Tumor size:			
	≤2 cm	38 (27)	0	38 (35)
	>2 cm	105 (73)	33 (100)	72 (65)
	Anatomic location:			
	Head/neck	32 (23)	1 (3)	31 (28)
	Extremities	82 (57)	11 (33)	71 (65)
	Trunk/buttocks	29 (20)	21 (64)	8 (7)
	Tumor stage:			
	I	38 (27)	0 (0)	38 (35)
	II	22 (15)	1 (3)	21 (19)
	III	68 (48)	25 (76)	43 (39)
	IV	15 (10)	7 (21)	8 (7)
Comorbidity	Age-adjusted Charlson comorbidity index[a]	4 (2-5)	3 (2-4)	4 (2-5)
	Neoplastic comorbidity:			
	No	109 (76)	28 (85)	81 (74)
	Yes	34 (24)	5 (15)	29 (16)
	Autoimmune comorbidity:			
	No	104 (73)	22 (67)	82 (75)
	Organ-specific	14 (10)	3 (9)	11 (10)
	Systemic	12 (8)	4 (12)	8 (7)
	Both	13 (9)	4 (12)	9 (8)
Drugs	Immunomodulatory:			
	No	84 (59)	20 (61)	64 (58)
	Yes	59 (41)	13 (39)	46 (42)
	Statins:			
	No	120 (84)	27 (82)	93 (85)
	Yes	23 (16)	6 (18)	17 (15)
Immunohistochemistry	Immunohistochemistry availability, N patients	99	21	78
	CK20: expression	74/99 (75)	17/21 (81)	57/78 (73)
	NSE: expression	26/99 (26)	3/21 (14)	23/78 (29)
	Synaptophysin: expression	82/99 (83)	18/21 (86)	64/78 (82)
	Chromogranin: expression	68/99 (69)	14/21 (67)	54/78 (69)
	AE1 AE3: expression	17/99 (17)	4/21 (19)	13/78 (17)
	MNF 116: expression	32/99 (32)	6/21 (29)	26/78 (33)
	CAM 5.2: expression	33/99 (33)	8/21 (38)	25/78 (32)

Data expressed as n (%) or [a]median (IQR).

area (23%), and the trunk/buttocks (20%). Immunohistochemical analysis of the bioptic material was performed in 99 patients (69.23% of the total). The most commonly detected immunohistochemical markers were cytokeratin 20 (in 75% of lesions), synaptophysin (83%), NSE (26%), chromogranin (69%), AE1/AE3 (17%), MNF 116 (32%), and CAM 5.2 (33%). The male sex was associated with worse disease-free survival. Neoplastic comorbidities were found in 24% of patients and autoimmune comorbidities in 27% (the most frequently encountered were Type 1 diabetes mellitus, rheumatoid, or psoriatic arthritis). Specifically, 6% of patients were affected by hematological neoplasms (mainly Non-Hodgkin's Lymphoma, chronic lymphocytic Leukemia, and Myeloproliferative or Myelodysplastic syndromes). Many of the patients examined were on immunomodulatory medications (59 patients, 41%), while 23 patients (16%) were using statins. The most commonly used immunomodulatory drugs were corticosteroids (16 patients, 11%) and beta-blockers (23 patients, 16%).

Treatment

Figure 1 summarizes the treatment strategy for MCC patients in this study.

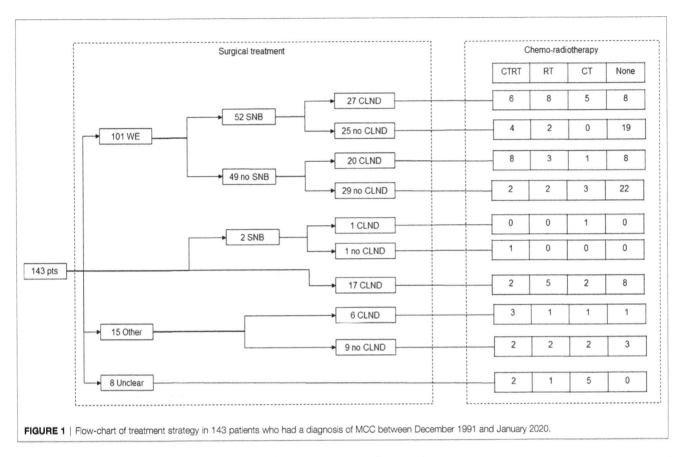

FIGURE 1 | Flow-chart of treatment strategy in 143 patients who had a diagnosis of MCC between December 1991 and January 2020.

Wide excision (WE) was the most common treatment for the primary lesion (101 patients, 71%). Of these, 52 patients also underwent SNB. Two patients underwent direct sentinel lymph node biopsy and 17 CLND. Fifteen patients underwent other treatments (such as wide resection and locoregional perfusion of the limb), while 8 patients were treated at other centers and it was not possible to retrieve their surgical details.

Following SNB, CLND identified a median of 1 positive lymph node (IQR 0-6). CLND was also performed in 5 patients with negative SNLB (median 3 positive lymph nodes, IQR 0-5).

Radiotherapy was administered to 54 patients (in 35 of the patients who received radiotherapy, the intent was adjuvant) and chemotherapy to 50 patients. Of these, 17 patients were treated using monoclonal antibodies acting on the PD-1/PD-L1 axis (avelumab or pembrolizumab).

Survival

The median follow-up in 128 stage I-III patients was 31 months (IQR 15-62). Thirty-seven patients died from the disease and 19 patients died from other causes. The five-year overall survival rate was 62-59-50% in patients with stage I-II-III ($p = 0.21$). The five-year disease-specific survival rate was 69-74-58% in patients with stage I-II-III ($p = 0.31$). (**Figure 2**). Univariate analyses of overall survival and disease-specific survival are shown in **Table 2**. Impaired overall survival was associated with older age (HR 1.03, 95% CI 1.00-1.06) and a higher Charlson Comorbidity Index (HR 1.16, 95% CI 1.01-1.33). Impaired disease-specific survival was associated with the presence of autoimmune

comorbidities (HR 2.00, 95% CI 1.03-3.91) and the use of immunomodulatory drugs (HR 2.94, 95% CI 1.52-5.67).

SNB was found to be positive in 19 patients and negative in 24 patients who received SNB concurrently with WE. Patients with positive SNB had worse overall survival rate (HR 4.44, 95% CI 1.15-17.16; $p = 0.03$) and disease-specific survival (HR 3.96, 95% CI 1.00-15.72; $p = 0.04$) with respect to patients with negative SNB. In the same subgroup, having 3 or more positive lymph nodes at CLND was not associated with a worse overall survival rate (HR 1.77, 95% CI 0.68-4.61; $p = 0.24$) or disease-specific survival (HR 3.09, 95% CI 0.97-9.88; $p = 0.06$) when compared to patients with 2 or less positive lymph nodes.

At the time of the analysis, 43 of the 102 stage I-III patients with primary disease relapsed (43%). Local recurrence was observed in 11 patients, in-transit metastases in 4 patients, lymph node metastases in 15 patients, and distant metastases in 13 patients. The five-year recurrence-free survival rate was 43% (**Figure 3**). A univariate analysis of recurrence-free survival is shown in **Table 3**. Impaired disease-free survival was associated with receiving immunomodulatory drugs (HR 2.51, 95% CI 1.36-4.57; $p = 0.003$) and radiotherapy (HR 2.74, 95% CI 1.50-5.03; $p = 0.001$). Among stage I-III patients with primary disease who received SNB concurrently with WE, recurrence-free survival was not associated with the positivity of SNB (HR 1.00, 95% CI 0.38-2.65; $p = 0.99$). In the same subgroup, having three or more positive LNs at CLND was not associated with recurrence-free survival (HR 2.05, 95% CI 0.85 to 4.94; $p = 0.11$) with respect to having two or less positive LNs at CLND.

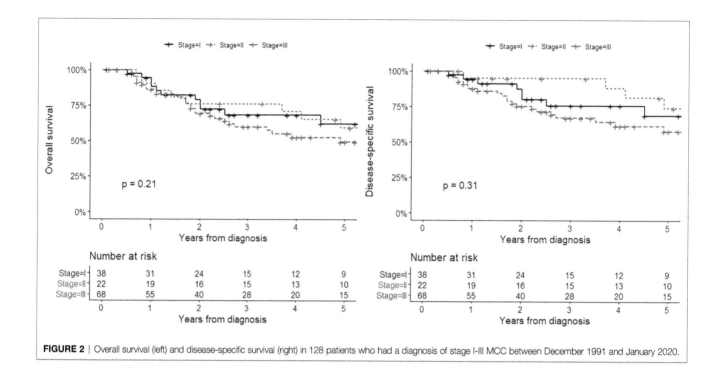

FIGURE 2 | Overall survival (left) and disease-specific survival (right) in 128 patients who had a diagnosis of stage I-III MCC between December 1991 and January 2020.

TABLE 2 | Univariate analysis of overall survival and disease-specific survival in 128 patients who had a diagnosis of stage I-III MCC between December 1991 and January 2020.

	Overall survival		Disease-specific survival	
	HR (95% CI)	p-value	HR (95% CI)	p-value
Primary vs. non primary tumor	1.02 (0.54 to 1.90)	0.96	1.05 (0.50 to 2.30)	0.90
Age at diagnosis	1.03 (1.00 to 1.06)	0.04	1.00 (0.97 to 1.03)	0.90
Male vs. female	1.69 (0.98 to 2.91)	0.06	2.24 (1.14 to 4.41)	**0.02**
Anatomic location:				
Head/neck vs. extremities	1.15 (0.59 to 2.22)	0.67	1.62 (0.74 to 3.56)	0.23
Trunk/buttocks vs. extremities	1.35 (0.70 to 2.59)	0.37	1.81 (0.83 to 3.97)	0.14
Tumor size: >2 cm vs. ≤2 cm	1.57 (0.81 to 3.05)	0.18	1.42 (0.64 to 3.10)	0.39
Tumor stage: III vs. I-II	1.61 (0.93 to 2.77)	0.09	1.67 (0.86 to 3.25)	0.13
Age-adjusted Charlson comorbidity index	1.16 (1.01 to 1.33)	0.03	1.12 (0.94 to 1.33)	0.21
Neoplastic comorbidity: yes vs. no	0.93 (0.49 to 1.76)	0.82	1.13 (0.53 to 2.39)	0.76
Autoimmune comorbidity: yes vs. no	1.43 (0.79 to 2.59)	0.23	2.00 (1.03 to 3.91)	**0.04**
Immunomodulatory drugs:				
Corticosteroids vs. no drugs	1.46 (0.68 to 3.15)	0.33	2.19 (0.93 to 5.17)	0.07
Beta blockers and statins v. no drugs	1.10 (9.53 to 2.23)	0.79	1.94 (0.89 to 4.26)	0.09
CK20: expression vs. absence	1.46 (0.68 to 3.12)	0.34	1.85 (0.77 to 4.47)	0.17
NSE: expression vs. absence	0.69 (0.31 to 1.52)	0.35	0.75 (0.32 to 1.75)	0.50
Synaptophysin: expression vs. absence	2.02 (0.77 to 5.30)	0.15	1.63 (0.61 to 4.34)	0.33
Chromogranin: expression vs. absence	1.13 (0.54 to 2.35)	0.75	1.72 (0.70 to 4.22)	0.24
AE1 AE3: expression vs. absence	0.43 (0.10 to 1.84)	0.26	0.26 (0.04 to 1.94)	0.19
MNF 116: expression vs. absence	0.96 (0.46 to 2.01)	0.92	0.93 (0.41 to 2.10)	0.86
CAM 5.2: expression vs. absence	1.15 (0.58 to 2.27)	0.69	0.90 (0.42 to 1.93)	0.78
Radiotherapy: yes vs. no	1.46 (0.85 to 2.51)	0.17	2.01 (1.07 to 3.99)	**0.03**

The bold values are statistically significant.

DISCUSSION

This study provides an update on MCC consecutive cases treated at our institution, confirming previous findings (18) in a larger sample of patients (143 v. 90). The prognostic features found in this study are explained below.

Therapy performed using immunomodulatory drugs was one of the main factors associated with worsened prognosis. 59 patients (41% of the total) were on immunomodulatory drug therapy, a category that does not only include drugs used in the treatment of autoimmune or inflammatory diseases (such as corticosteroids, azathioprine, or tacrolimus), but also other drugs

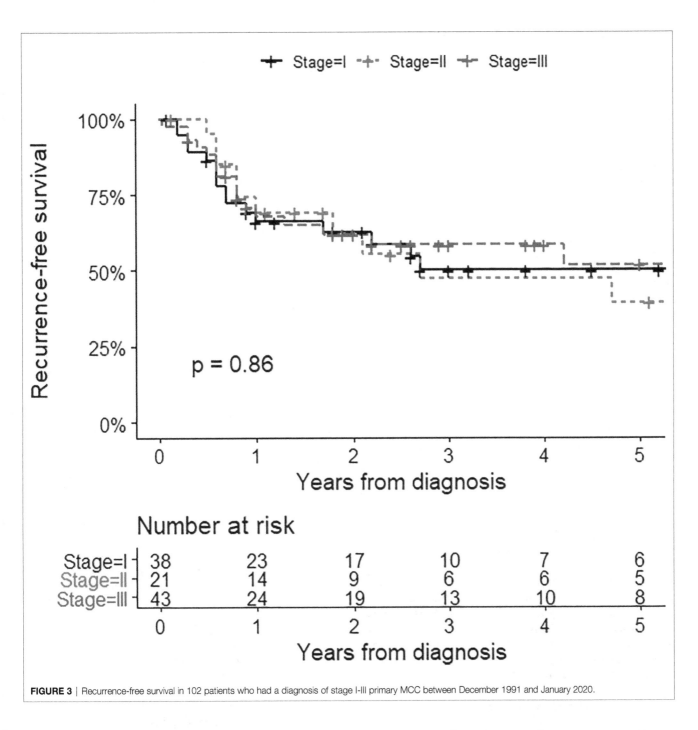

FIGURE 3 | Recurrence-free survival in 102 patients who had a diagnosis of stage I-III primary MCC between December 1991 and January 2020.

exerting an effect on the immune system. Among these, we included statins and beta blockers. From the analysis of the literature, emerges the immuno-modulating role of pharmacological agents such as beta-blockers and statins. As for HMG-CoA reductase inhibitors, their non-LDL-c lowering properties could be involved in immunomodulation. This effect could occur both through mevalonate pathway-dependent and independent mechanisms. Then, statins are able to interfering with the expression of MHC molecules and to inducing lymphocyte class switch. These effects could determine an increased incidence of Merkel cell carcinoma in patients who

chronically use these drugs. Furthermore, many evidences supporting an immune-modulating role of beta-blocking agents. In fact, adrenaline promotes the activation of the immune system against cancer cells by activating NK cells through signaling of the beta-2 adrenergic receptor. Finally, the beta-blockers could promote the expression of CD107a and HLA-DR on cytotoxic T cells (22–24). We propose these pharmacological effects could determine a state of sub-clinical immunomodulation (a phenomenon distinct from the immunosuppression which is seen, for example, in transplant patients) which, could cause an increased incidence of Merkel

TABLE 3 | Factors associated with recurrence-free survival among patients with primary stage I-III MCC.

	Recurrence-free survival	
	HR (95% CI)	p-value
Age at diagnosis	1.01 (0.98 to 1.03)	0.58
Male vs. female	1.33 (0.74 to 2.42)	0.34
Anatomic location:		
Head/neck vs. extremities	0.85 (0.42 to 1.70)	0.64
Trunk/buttocks vs. extremities	1.07 (0.93 to 3.07)	0.90
Tumor size: >2 cm vs. ≤2 cm	0.98 (0.53 to 1.82)	0.95
Tumor stage III vs. I-II	0.86 (0.47 to 1.59)	0.65
Age-adjusted Charlson comorbidity index	1.09 (0.92 to 1.27)	0.35
Neoplastic comorbidity: yes vs. no	1.07 (0.53 to 2.10)	0.87
Autoimmune comorbidity: yes vs. no	1.06 (0.98 to 1.14)	0.17
Immunomodulatory drugs:		
Corticosteroids vs. no drugs	1.02 (0.39 to 2.65)	0.97
Beta blockers and statins v. no drugs	2.53 (1.27 to 5.05)	**0.008**
CK20: expression vs. absence	1.16 (0.53 to 2.57)	0.71
NSE: expression vs. absence	0.75 (0.34 to 1.63)	0.47
Synaptophysin: expression vs. absence	1.71 (0.65 to 4.51)	0.28
Chromogranin: expression vs. absence	1.19 (0.55 to 2.58)	0.66
AE1 AE3: expression vs. absence	0.60 (0.18 to 1.99)	0.41
MNF 116: expression vs. absence	0.94 (0.45 to 2.00)	0.88
CAM 5.2: expression vs. absence	0.62 (0.28 to 1.38)	0.24
Radiotherapy: yes vs. no	2.74 (1.50 to 5.03)	**0.001**

The bold values are statistically significant.

cell carcinoma. The use of drugs with immunomodulatory effects was found to be associated with worse disease-specific survival. This association is in line with the data reported in the literature (25). In fact, in this subpopulation of patients, one could hypothesize the presence of an iatrogenic immunosuppression which could justify worsened survival. It is known that immunocompromised patients are characterized by a worse prognosis than immunocompetent patients (26, 27). Based on this observation, it might be advantageous to review the patient's therapeutic regimen and weigh the potential benefits in order to reduce the extent of iatrogenic immunosuppression and consequently improve the prognosis.

The expression of epithelial and neuroendocrine immunohistochemical markers (CK20, NSE, Synaptophysin, Chromogranin, AE1/AE3, MNF 116, and Cam 5.2) did not appear to be significantly correlated with survival outcome, unlike the previous study where the lack of CK20 expression in immunohistochemical markers was associated with better survival (18).

The presence of a high number of comorbidities (expressed by the Charlson Comorbidity Index) correlates with reduced survival. These data are in line with the already existing international literature (28). The relatively high proportion of MCC patients with hematologic malignancies is consistent with the evidence described by other investigators, who report a percentage of about 5% of patients affected by these comorbidities (29). This association might find a potential explanation in the putative cell of origin of MCC from B-cell precursors (30) and/or the presence of immunological changes (often subclinical) in patients affected by chronic lymphocytic leukemia and other lymphoproliferative disorders (30). Although the origin of MCC cells from pre/pro B-cells appears unlikely,

given the lack of experimental evidence regarding the fact that these cells are able to assume a phenotype similar to MCC (31), it is not possible to define with certainty the main factor underlying the described association.

Although the literature analysis reveals the presence of an association between the number of positive lymph nodes following CLND and survival (32, 33), such an association did not emerge in the present study. Data in the literature concerning the association between SNB positivity and survival are discordant (33). The present study showed a clear association between SNB positivity and a worse prognosis. This data testifies to the importance of adequate treatment of the regional lymph nodes (with CLND and/or radiotherapy, often combined) in this subpopulation of patients.

As for comorbidities, patients with autoimmune conditions are characterized by a worse prognosis, probably due to the intake of immunomodulatory drugs (18).

Radiation therapy was linked to reduced survival; however, this association could be influenced by the fact that patients undergoing radiotherapy are characterized by a more advanced stage (18% of patients presented with a clinical stage <II and 72% with a stage> II) of disease (lymph node or distant metastases) (8).

In our study we confirm the data present in the literature relating to Merkel cell tumor, which define the typical age of the patient, the localization of the tumor and the expression of epithelial and neuroendocrine markers.

CONCLUSION

Autoimmune and neoplastic comorbidities were frequent in the studied population. The use of drugs with immunomodulatory effects was also found to be a common feature of the population under examination. The use of this type of medication is considered a negative prognostic factor. The relevance of a multidisciplinary approach to the patient with MCC is confirmed, with the aim of assessing the risks and benefits related to the use of immunomodulating therapy in the individual patient.

Strengths and Weaknesses of the Study

The strengths of this study include the large monocentric sample and the importance attributed to the analysis of comorbidities. This experience has allowed us to validate almost all previous prognostic features and to design a future national collaborative study.

Limitations are related to the lack of data regarding the diagnosis of certain patients and their therapy (missing data about expression of immunohistochemical markers, type and intent of clinical treatment). This study, in fact, took place over a very long period (from 1991 to 2020), which is why several data routinely recorded today (such as the expression of immunohistochemical markers) were not available for patients who were enrolled in the early stages. It is also necessary to consider the diagnostic and therapeutic heterogeneity characterizing such a prolonged period.

ETHICS STATEMENT

The studies involving human participants were reviewed and approved by Ethics Committee of the Veneto Institute of Oncology (Approval No. 0015918 CESC-IOV) on 21 September 2020. The patients/participants provided their written informed consent to participate in this study.

AUTHOR CONTRIBUTIONS

Study concepts: PF, IR, MR, JT, RC, and LN. Study design: PF, FC, MR, MA, and SM. Data acquisition: PF, FC, BF, BB, FR, RS, DB, ADM, AF, LP, ST, EB, SC, and RM. Quality control of data and algorithms: PF and FC Data analysis and interpretation: PF, FC, and SM. Statistical analysis: FC. Manuscript preparation: PF, IR, JT, and FC. Manuscript editing: PF, FC, SM, LD, and MR. Manuscript review: SM, MR, VC-S, JP, TB, AF, FB, MG, AD, RC, MA and RM. All authors contributed to the manuscript's revision, and read and approved the submitted version.

ACKNOWLEDGMENTS

The authors thank "Piccoli Punti ONLUS", Mr. Giuseppe Valentini, and "Fondazione Lucia Valentini Terrani" for their long-lasting support.

REFERENCES

1. Patel P, Hussain K. Merkel Cell Carcinoma. *Clin Exp Dermatol* (2020) 46 (5):814–9. doi: 10.1111/ced.14530

2. Becker JC, Stang A, Hausen AZ, Fischer N, DeCaprio JA, Tothill RW, et al. Epidemiology, Biology and Therapy of Merkel Cell Carcinoma: Conclusions From the EU Project IMMOMEC. *Cancer Immunol Immunother* (2018) 67 (3):341–51. doi: 10.1007/s00262-017-2099-3

3. Fitzgerald TL, Dennis S, Kachare SD, Vohra NA, Wong JH, Zervos EE. Dramatic Increase in the Incidence and Mortality From Merkel Cell Carcinoma in the United States. *Am Surg* (2015) 81(8):802–6. doi: 10.1177/000313481508100819

4. Rastrelli M, Del Fiore P, Buja A, Vecchiato A, Rossi CR, Chiarion Sileni V, et al. A Therapeutic and Diagnostic Multidisciplinary Pathway for Merkel Cell Carcinoma Patients. *Front Oncol* (2020) 10:529. doi: 10.3389/fonc.2020.00529

5. Becker JC, Kauczok CS, Ugurel S, Eib S, Bröcker EB, Houben R. Merkel Cell Carcinoma: Molecular Pathogenesis, Clinical Features and Therapy. *J Dtsch Dermatol Ges* (2008) 6(9):709–19. doi: 10.1111/j.1610-0387.2008.06830.x. English, German.

6. Llombart B, Monteagudo C, López-Guerrero JA, Carda C, Jorda E, Sanmartín O, et al. Clinicopathological and Immunohistochemical Analysis of 20 Cases of Merkel Cell Carcinoma in Search of Prognostic Markers. *Histopathology* (2005) 46(6):622–34. doi: 10.1111/j.1365-2559.2005.02158.x

7. Ezaldein HH, Ventura A, DeRuyter NP, Yin ES, Giunta A. Understanding the Influence of Patient Demographics on Disease Severity, Treatment Strategy, and Survival Outcomes in Merkel Cell Carcinoma: A Surveillance, Epidemiology, and End-Results Study. *Oncoscience* (2017) 4:106–14. doi: 10.18632/oncoscience.358

8. Harms KL, Healy MA, Nghiem P, Sober AJ, Johnson TM, Bichakjian CK, et al. Analysis of Prognostic Factors From 9387 Merkel Cell Carcinoma Cases Forms the Basis for the New 8th Edition AJCC Staging System. *Ann Surg Oncol* (2016) 23(11):3564–71. doi: 10.1245/s10434-016-5266-4

9. Becker JC, Stang A, DeCaprio JA, Cerroni L, Lebbé C, Veness M, et al. Merkel Cell Carcinoma. *Nat Rev Dis Primers* (2017) 3:17077. doi: 10.1038/nrdp.2017.77

10. Heath M, Jaimes N, Lemos B, Mostaghimi A, Wang LC, Peñas PF, et al. Clinical Characteristics of Merkel Cell Carcinoma at Diagnosis in 195 Patients: The AEIOU Features. *J Am Acad Dermatol* (2008) 58(3):375–81. doi: 10.1016/j.jaad.2007.11.020

11. Walsh NM, Cerroni L. Merkel Cell Carcinoma: A Review. *J Cutan Pathol* (2021) 48(3):411–21. doi: 10.1111/cup.13910

12. Becker JC. Merkel Cell Carcinoma. *Ann Oncol* (2010) 21 Suppl 7:vii81–5. doi: 10.1093/annonc/mdq366

13. Lebbe C, Becker JC, Grob JJ, Malvehy J, Del Marmol V, Pehamberger H, et al. Diagnosis and Treatment of Merkel Cell Carcinoma. European Consensus-Based Interdisciplinary Guideline. *Eur J Cancer* (2015) 51(16):2396–403. doi: 10.1016/j.ejca.2015.06.131

14. Behr DS, Peitsch WK, Hametner C, Lasitschka F, Houben R, Schönhaar K, et al. Prognostic Value of Immune Cell Infiltration, Tertiary Lymphoid Structures and PD-L1 Expression in Merkel Cell Carcinomas. *Int J Clin Exp Pathol* (2014) 7(11):7610–21.

15. Santarpia M, Karachaliou N. Tumor Immune Microenvironment Characterization and Response to Anti-PD-1 Therapy. *Cancer Biol Med* (2015) 12(2):74–8. doi: 10.7497/j.issn.2095-3941.2015.0022

16. Nghiem PT, Bhatia S, Lipson EJ, Kudchadkar RR, Miller NJ, Annamalai L, et al. PD-1 Blockade With Pembrolizumab in Advanced Merkel-Cell Carcinoma. *N Engl J Med* (2016) 374(26):2542–52. doi: 10.1056/NEJMoa1603702

17. D'Angelo SP, Hunger M, Brohl AS, Nghiem P, Bhatia S, Hamid O, et al. Early Objective Response to Avelumab Treatment is Associated With Improved Overall Survival in Patients With Metastatic Merkel Cell Carcinoma. *Cancer Immunol Immunother* (2019) 68(4):609–18. doi: 10.1007/s00262-018-02295-4

18. Rastrelli M, Ferrazzi B, Cavallin F, Chiarion Sileni V, Pigozzo J, Fabozzi A, et al. Prognostic Factors in Merkel Cell Carcinoma: A Retrospective Single-

Center Study in 90 Patients. *Cancers (Basel)* (2018) 10(10):350. doi: 10.3390/cancers10100350

19. Gershenwald JE, Scolyer RA. Melanoma Staging: American Joint Committee on Cancer (AJCC) 8th Edition and Beyond [Published Correction Appears in Ann Surg Oncol. 2018 Dec;25(Suppl 3):993-994]. *Ann Surg Oncol* (2018) 25 (8):2105–10. doi: 10.1245/s10434-018-6513-7

20. Charlson ME, Pompei P, Ales KL, MacKenzie CR. A New Method of Classifying Prognostic Comorbidity in Longitudinal Studies: Development and Validation. *J Chronic Dis* (1987) 40(5):373–83. doi: 10.1016/0021-9681 (87)90171-8

21. R Core Team. *R: A Language and Environment for Statistical Computing.* Vienna, Austria: R Foundation for Statistical Computing (2020).

22. Sahi H, Koljonen V, Böhling T, Neuvonen PJ, Vainio H, Lamminpää A, et al. Increased Incidence of Merkel Cell Carcinoma Among Younger Statin Users. *Cancer Epidemiol* (2012) 36(5):421–4. doi: 10.1016/j.canep.2012.05.006

23. Dehnavi S, Sohrabi N, Sadeghi M, Lansberg P, Banach M, Al-Rasadi K, et al. Statins and Autoimmunity: State-Of-the-Art. *Pharmacol Ther* (2020) 214:107614. doi: 10.1016/j.pharmthera.2020.107614

24. Chung JF, Lee SJ, Sood AK. Immunological and Pleiotropic Effects of Individual β-Blockers and Their Relevance in Cancer Therapies. *Expert Opin Investig Drugs* (2016) 25(5):501–5. doi: 10.1517/13543784.2016.1164141

25. Paulson KG, Iyer JG, Blom A, Warton EM, Sokil M, Yelistratova L, et al. Systemic Immune Suppression Predicts Diminished Merkel Cell Carcinoma-Specific Survival Independent of Stage. *J Invest Dermatol* (2013) 133(3):642–6. doi: 10.1038/jid.2012.388

26. Kempf W, Mertz KD, Hofbauer GF, Tinguely M. Skin Cancer in Organ Transplant Recipients. *Pathobiology* (2013) 80(6):302–9. doi: 10.1159/000350757

27. Engels EA, Frisch M, Goedert JJ, Biggar RJ, Miller RW. Merkel Cell Carcinoma and HIV Infection. *Lancet* (2002) 359(9305):497–8. doi: 10.1016/S0140-6736(02)07668-7

28. Austin SR, Wong YN, Uzzo RG, Beck JR, Egleston BL. Why Summary Comorbidity Measures Such As the Charlson Comorbidity Index and Elixhauser Score Work. *Med Care* (2015) 53(9):e65–72. doi: 10.1097/MLR.0b013e318297429c

29. Miller RW, Rabkin CS. Merkel Cell Carcinoma and Melanoma: Etiological Similarities and Differences [Published Correction Appears in Cancer Epidemiol Biomarkers Prev 1999 May;8(5):485]. *Cancer Epidemiol Biomarkers Prev* (1999) 8(2):153–8.

30. Tadmor T, Aviv A, Polliack A. Merkel Cell Carcinoma, Chronic Lymphocytic Leukemia and Other Lymphoproliferative Disorders: An Old Bond With Possible New Viral Ties. *Ann Oncol* (2011) 22(2):250–6. doi: 10.1093/annonc/

31. Kervarrec T, Samimi M, Guyétant S, Sarma B, Chéret J, Blanchard E, et al. Histogenesis of Merkel Cell Carcinoma: A Comprehensive Review. *Front Oncol* (2019) 9:451. doi: 10.3389/fonc.2019.00451

32. Cheraghlou S, Agogo GO, Girardi M. Evaluation of Lymph Node Ratio Association With Long-Term Patient Survival After Surgery for Node-Positive Merkel Cell Carcinoma. *JAMA Dermatol* (2019) 155(7):803–11. doi: 10.1001/jamadermatol.2019.0267

33. Thompson JF, Hruby G. The Role of Sentinel Lymph Node Biopsy in Patients With Merkel Cell Carcinoma: Uncertainty Prevails. *Ann Surg Oncol* (2014) 21 (5):1517–9. doi: 10.1245/s10434-014-3587-8

Permissions

The contributors of this book come from diverse backgrounds, making this book a truly international effort. This book will bring forth new frontiers with its revolutionizing research information and detailed analysis of the nascent developments around the world.

We would like to thank all the contributing authors for lending their expertise to make the book truly unique. They have played a crucial role in the development of this book. Without their invaluable contributions this book wouldn't have been possible. They have made vital efforts to compile up to date information on the varied aspects of this subject to make this book a valuable addition to the collection of many professionals and students.

This book was conceptualized with the vision of imparting up-to-date information and advanced data in this field. To ensure the same, a matchless editorial board was set up. Every individual on the board went through rigorous rounds of assessment to prove their worth. After which they invested a large part of their time researching and compiling the most relevant data for our readers.

The editorial board has been involved in producing this book since its inception. They have spent rigorous hours researching and exploring the diverse topics which have resulted in the successful publishing of this book. They have passed on their knowledge of decades through this book. To expedite this challenging task, the publisher supported the team at every step. A small team of assistant editors was also appointed to further simplify the editing procedure and attain best results for the readers.

Apart from the editorial board, the designing team has also invested a significant amount of their time in understanding the subject and creating the most relevant covers. They scrutinized every image to scout for the most suitable representation of the subject and create an appropriate cover for the book.

The publishing team has been an ardent support to the editorial, designing and production team. Their endless efforts to recruit the best for this project, has resulted in the accomplishment of this book. They are a veteran in the field of academics and their pool of knowledge is as vast as their experience in printing. Their expertise and guidance has proved useful at every step. Their uncompromising quality standards have made this book an exceptional effort. Their encouragement from time to time has been an inspiration for everyone.

The publisher and the editorial board hope that this book will prove to be a valuable piece of knowledge for researchers, students, practitioners and scholars across the globe.

List of Contributors

Siwei Bi, Ying Cen and Junjie Chen
Department of Burn and Plastic Surgery, West China Hospital, Sichuan University, Chengdu, China

Shanshan Chen and Beiyi Wu
West China School of Medicine, Sichuan University, Chengdu, China

Daniela Russo, Silvia Varricchio, Gennaro Ilardi, Francesco Martino, Rosa Maria Di Crescenzo, Sara Pignatiello, Massimo Mascolo and Stefania Staibano
Pathology Unit, Department of Advanced Biomedical Sciences, University of Naples "Federico II", Naples, Italy

Massimiliano Scalvenzi and Claudia Costa
Dermatology Unit, Department of Clinical Medicine and Surgery, University of Naples "Federico II", Naples, Italy

Francesco Merolla
Department of Medicine and Health Sciences "V.Tiberio", University of Molise, Campobasso, Italy

Salvatore Crisafulli, Ylenia Ingrasciotta and Claudio Guarneri
Department of Biomedical and Dental Sciences and Morphofunctional Imaging, University of Messina, Messina, Italy

Lucrezia Bertino
Department of Clinical and Experimental Medicine, University of Messina, Messina, Italy

Andrea Fontana
Unit of Biostatistics, Fondazione IRCCS Casa Sollievo della Sofferenza, San Giovanni Rotondo, Italy

Fabrizio Calapai
Department of Chemical, Biological, Pharmaceutical and Environmental Sciences, University of Messina, Messina, Italy

Massimiliano Berretta
Department of Clinical and Experimental Medicine, Section of Infectious Diseases, University of Messina, Messina, Italy

Gianluca Trifirò
Department of Diagnostics and Public Health, University of Verona, Verona, Italy

Rafał Czepczyński and Jolanta Szczurek
Department of Endocrinology, Metabolism and Internal Diseases, Poznan University of Medical Sciences, Poznań, Poland
Department of Nuclear Medicine, Affidea, Poznań, Poland

Jacek Mackiewicz
Department of Medical and Experimental Oncology, Poznan University of Medical Sciences, Poznań, Poland

Marek Ruchała
Department of Endocrinology, Metabolism and Internal Diseases, Poznan University of Medical Sciences, Poznań, Poland

Gabriella Brancaccio, Elvira Moscarella and Giuseppe Argenziano
Dermatology Unit, University of Campania "Luigi Vanvitelli", Naples, Italy

Federico Pea
Department of Medicine, University of Udine, Udine, Italy
Institute of Clinical Pharmacology, Azienda Ospedaliero-Universitaria Santa Maria Della Misericordia, Azienda Sanitaria Universitaria Friuli Centrale, Udine, Italy

Hiroki Hashimoto, Yumiko Kaku-Ito, Masutaka Furue and Takamichi Ito
Department of Dermatology, Graduate School of Medical Sciences, Kyushu University, Fukuoka, Japan

Maria Paola Belfiore, Alfonso Reginelli, Anna Russo, Gaetano Maria Russo, Maria Paola Rocco, Marilina Ferrante, Antonello Sica and Salvatore Cappabianca
Department of Precision Medicine, University of Campania Luigi Vanvitelli, Naples, Italy

Elvira Moscarella
Dermatology Unit, University of Campania Luigi Vanvitelli, Naples, Italy

Roberto Grassi
Italian Society of Medical Radiology (SIRM) Foundation, Milan, Italy

Emmanuele Venanzi Rullo, Maria Grazia Maimone, Massimiliano Berretta and Giuseppe Nunnari
Unit of Infectious Disease, Department of Clinical and Experimental Medicine, University of Messina, Messina, Italy

Francesco Fiorica
Department of Radiation Oncology and Nuclear Medicine, State Hospital "Mater Salutis" Azienda Unità Locale Socio Sanitaria (AULSS) 9, Legnago, Italy

Manuela Ceccarelli
Unit of Infectious Disease, Department of Clinical and Experimental Medicine, University of Messina, Messina, Italy
Unit of Infectious Disease, Department of Clinical and Experimental Medicine, University of Catania, Catania, Italy

Claudio Guarneri
Unit of Dermatology, Department of Biomedical and Dental Sciences and Morphofunctional Imaging, University of Messina, Messina, Italy

Hanlin Zhang, Qingyue Zheng, Keyun Tang, Rouyu Fang, Yuchen Wang and Qiuning Sun
Department of Dermatology, Peking Union Medical College Hospital, Chinese Academy of Medical Sciences, Peking Union Medical College, Beijing, China

Giuseppina Rosaria Umano, Giulia Delehaye, Letizia Trotta and Alfonso Papparella
Department of Woman, Child and General and Specialized Surgery, University of Campania "Luigi Vanvitelli", Naples, Italy

Maria Elena Errico and Vittoria D'Onofrio
Department of Pathology, Azienda Ospedaliera di Rilievo Nazionale (AORN) Santobono Pausilipon, Pediatric Hospital, Naples, Italy,

Claudio Spinelli and Silvia Strambi
Pediatric, Adolescent and Young Adults Surgery Division, Department of Surgical, Medical, Pathological, Molecular and Critical Area, University of Pisa, Pisa, Italy

Renato Franco, Giuseppe D'Abbronzo and Andrea Ronchi
Pathology Unit, Department of Mental and Physical Health and Preventive Medicine, University of Campania "Luigi Vanvitelli", Naples, Italy

Antonella Vecchiato and Angela Filoni
Surgical Oncology Unit, Veneto Institute of Oncology IOV - IRCCS, Padua, Italy

Carlo Riccardo Rossi
Surgical Oncology Unit, Veneto Institute of Oncology IOV - IRCCS, Padua, Italy
Department of Surgery, Oncology and Gastroenterology (DISCOG), University of Padua, Padua, Italy

Rocco Cappellesso
Surgical Pathology and Cytopathology Unit, Department of Medicine (DIMED), University of Padua, Padua, Italy

Andrea Grego and Clara Benna
Department of Surgery, Oncology and Gastroenterology (DISCOG), University of Padua, Padua, Italy

Alessio Rotondi
Department of Medicine (DIMED), University of Padua, Padua, Italy

Franco Bassetto
Clinic of Plastic Surgery, Department of Neuroscience, Padua University Hospital, University of Padua, Padua, Italy

Jacopo Pigozzo and Vanna Chiarion Sileni
Melanoma Oncology Unit, Veneto Institute of Oncology IOV-IRCCS, Padua, Italy

Qingyue Zheng, Hanlin Zhang and Yuanzhuo Wang
Department of Dermatology, Peking Union Medical College Hospital, Chinese Academy of Medical Sciences and Peking Union Medical College, Beijing, China
Eight-year MD Program, Peking Union Medical College, Beijing, China

Jiarui Li
Department of Medical Oncology, Peking Union Medical College Hospital, Chinese Academy of Medical Sciences and Peking Union Medical College, Beijing, China

Shu Zhang
Department of Dermatology, Peking Union Medical College Hospital, Chinese Academy of Medical Sciences and Peking Union Medical College, Beijing, China

Gerardo Ferrara
Anatomic Pathology Unit, Macerata General Hospital, Macerata, Italy

Anne L. Ryan
Department of Haematology, Oncology and Bone Marrow Transplant, Perth Children's Hospital, Perth, WA, Australia

Charlotte Burns
Children's Cancer Centre, The Royal Children's Hospital, Melbourne, VIC, Australia

Aditya K. Gupta and Geoff B. McCowage
Cancer Centre for Children, The Children's Hospital at Westmead, Westmead, NSW, Australia

Ruvishani Samarasekera and David S. Ziegler
Kids Cancer Centre, Sydney Children's Hospital, Randwick, NSW, Australia

Maria L. Kirby
Department of Haematology/Oncology, Women's and Children's Hospital, Adelaide, SA, Australia

Frank Alvaro
Department of Haematology/Oncology, John Hunter Children's Hospital, Newcastle, NSW, Australia

Peter Downie
Children's Cancer Centre, The Royal Children's Hospital, Melbourne, VIC, Australia
Department of Haematology/Oncology, Monash Children's Hospital, Melbourne, VIC, Australia

Stephen J. Laughton
Starship Blood and Cancer Centre, Starship Children's Hospital, Auckland, New Zealand

Siobhan Cross
Children's Haematology/Oncology Centre, Christchurch Hospital, Christchurch, New Zealand

Timothy Hassall
Department of Haematology/Oncology, Queensland Children's Hospital, Brisbane, QLD, Australia

Jordan R. Hansford
Children's Cancer Centre, The Royal Children's Hospital, Melbourne, VIC, Australia
Murdoch Children's Research Institute; Department of Pediatrics, University of Melbourne, Melbourne, VIC, Australia

Rishi S. Kotecha
Department of Haematology, Oncology and Bone Marrow Transplant, Perth Children's Hospital, Perth, WA, Australia
Telethon Kids Cancer Centre, Telethon Kids Institute, Perth, WA, Australia
Curtin Medical School, Curtin University, Perth, WA, Australia

Nicholas G. Gottardo
Department of Haematology, Oncology and Bone Marrow Transplant, Perth Children's Hospital, Perth, WA, Australia
Telethon Kids Cancer Centre, Telethon Kids Institute, Perth, WA, Australia

Yiyi Feng, Xin Song and Renbing Jia
Department of Ophthalmology, Ninth People's Hospital, Shanghai Jiao Tong University School of Medicine, Shanghai Key
Laboratory of Orbital Diseases and Ocular Oncology, Shanghai, China

Riccardo Pampena and Stefania Borsari
Centro Oncologico ad Alta Tecnologia Diagnostica, Azienda Unità Sanitaria Locale - IRCCS di Reggio Emilia, Reggio Emilia, Italy

Michela Lai and Caterina Longo
Centro Oncologico ad Alta Tecnologia Diagnostica, Azienda Unità Sanitaria Locale - IRCCS di Reggio Emilia, Reggio Emilia, Italy
Department of Dermatology, University of Modena and Reggio Emilia, Modena, Italy

Giovanni Paolino
Unit of Dermatology, IRCCS Ospedale San Raffaele, Milano, Italy
Clinica Dermatologica, La Sapienza University of Rome, Rome, Italy

Anna Maria Cesinaro
Department of Pathological Anatomy, Modena University Hospital, Modena, Italy

Gabriele Parisi, Mattia Benati, Silvana Ciardo, Francesca Farnetani, Sara Bassoli and Giovanni Pellacani
Department of Dermatology, University of Modena and Reggio Emilia, Modena, Italy

Giuseppe Palmieri, Carla Maria Rozzo, Antonella Manca and Marina Pisano
Institute of Genetic and Biomedical Research (IRGB), National Research Council (CNR), Sassari, Italy

Maria Colombino, Milena Casula and Maria Cristina Sini
Institute of Biomolecular Chemistry (ICB), National Research Council (CNR), Sassari, Italy

Valentina Doneddu, Panagiotis Paliogiannis and Antonio Cossu
Department of Medical, Surgical, and Experimental Sciences, University of Sassari, Sassari, Italy

Giuseppe Broggi and Rosario Caltabiano
Department of Medical, Surgical Sciences and Advanced Technologies "G.F. Ingrassia", Anatomic Pathology, University of Catania, Catania, Italy

Anna Elisa Verzì, Giuseppe Micali and Francesco Lacarrubba
Dermatology Clinic, University of Catania, Catania, Italy

Jorja Braden
Department of Medical Oncology, Chris O'Brien Lifehouse, Sydney, NSW, Australia

Jenny H. Lee
Department of Medical Oncology, Chris O'Brien Lifehouse, Sydney, NSW, Australia
Department of Biomedical Sciences, Macquarie University, Sydney, NSW, Australia

Alessandra Buja, Andrea Bardin, Vincenzo Baldo, Chiara De Toni and Riccardo Fusinato
Department of Cardiologic, Vascular and Thoracic Sciences, and Public Health, University of Padua, Padua, Italy

Giovanni Damiani
Clinical Dermatology, Istituto di Ricovero e Cura a Carattere Scientifico (IRCCS) Istituto Ortopedico Galeazzi, Milan, Italy
Department of Biomedical, Surgical and Dental Sciences, University of Milan, Milan, Italy
PhD Program in Pharmacological Sciences, Department of Pharmaceutical and Pharmacological Sciences, University of Padua, Padua, Italy

Manuel Zorzi
Veneto Tumor Registry - Azienda Zero, Padova, Italy

Romina Spina
Surgical Oncology Unit, Veneto Institute of Oncology IOV-Istituto di Ricovero e Cura a Carattere Scientifico (IRCCS), Padova, Italy

Simone Mocellin
Surgical Oncology Unit, Veneto Institute of Oncology IOV-Istituto di Ricovero e Cura a Carattere Scientifico (IRCCS), Padova, Italy
Department of Surgery, Oncology and Gastroenterology (DISCOG), University of Padua, Padua, Italy

Massimo Rugge
Veneto Tumor Registry - Azienda Zero, Padova, Italy
Department of Medicine DIMED, Surgical Pathology & Cytopathology Unit, University of Padova, Padova, Italy

Anna Crispo, Vito Vanella, Corrado Caracò, Egidio Celentano and Paolo A. Ascierto
Istituto Nazionale Tumori IRCCS Fondazione G. Pascale, Napoli, Italy

Maria Teresa Corradin and Erika Giulioni
Dermatology Department, Azienda Sanitaria Friuli Occidentale, Pordenone, Italy

Antonella Vecchiato
Istituto Oncologico Veneto IOV - IRCCS, Padova, Italy

Paola Queirolo
IRCCS Ospedale Policlinico San Martino, Genova, Italy
Istituto Europeo di Oncologia - IRCCS, Milano, Italy

Francesco Spagnolo
IRCCS Ospedale Policlinico San Martino, Genova, Italy

Giulio Tosti, Elisabetta Pennacchioli and Sara Gandini
Istituto Europeo di Oncologia - IRCCS, Milano, Italy

Giuseppe Giudice and Eleonora Nacchiero
Plastic and Reconstructive Surgery Department, Università degli Studi di Bari Aldo Moro, Bari, Italy

Pietro Quaglino and Simone Ribero
Clinica Dermatologica, Dipartimento di Scienze Mediche, Università di Torino, Torino, Italy

Monica Giordano and Desire Marussi
Oncology Department, Ospedale Sant'Anna di Como, Como, Italy

Stefania Barruscotti and Alessandro Testori
Fondazione I.R.C.C.S. Policlinico San Matteo, Pavia, Italy

Michele Guida
IRCCS Istituto Tumori "Giovanni Paolo II", Bari, Italy

Vincenzo De Giorgi
Dermatology Department, Università di Firenze, Firenze, Italy

OccelliMarcella
Oncology Department, Azienda ospedaliera Santa Croce e Carle, Cuneo, Italy

Federica Grosso
Mesothelioma Unit, Azienda Ospedaliera SS Antonio e Biagio e Cesare Arrigo, Alessandria, Italy

Giuseppe Cairo
Oncology Department, ospedale "Vito Fazzi" di Lecce, Lecce, Italy

Alessandro Gatti
ULSS 2 Marca Trevigiana Ospedale Ca' Foncello Treviso, Treviso, Italy

Daniela Massa
Gruppo melanoma e tumori rari, Oncology Department, PO A Businco ARNAS G. Brotzu, Cagliari, Italy

Laura Atzori
Dermatology Clinic, Department Medical Sciences and Public Health, University of Cagliari, Cagliari, Italy

Nicola Calvani
Oncology Department, Presidio Ospedaliero "Senatore Antonio Perrino", Brindisi, Italy

Tommaso Fabrizio
IRCCS Centro di Riferimento Oncologico Basilicata, Rionero in Vulture, Italy

Giuseppe Mastrangelo
Dermatology Clinic, Università degli studi di Padova, Padova, Italy

Federica Toffolutti
Centro di Riferimento Oncologico di Aviano (CRO) IRCCS, Aviano (PN), Italy

Mario Budroni
Registro Tumori Provincia di Sassari, Azienda Ospedaliera Universitaria Sassari, Sassari, Italy

Angela Filoni, Alessandra Collodetto and Sabrina Carraro
Soft-Tissue, Peritoneum and Melanoma Surgical Oncology Unit, Veneto Institute of Oncology - IOV IRCCS, Padua, Italy

Alessandro Dal Monico
Department of Medicine, University of Padua School of Medicine and Surgery, Padua, Italy

Vanna Chiarion-Sileni
Melanoma Oncology Unit, Veneto Institute of Oncology IOV-IRCCS, Padua, Italy

Luigi Dall'Olmo, Marco Rastrelli and Simone Mocellin
Soft-Tissue, Peritoneum and Melanoma Surgical Oncology Unit, Veneto Institute of Oncology - IOV IRCCS, Padua, Italy
Department of Surgery, Oncology and Gastroenterology (DISCOG), University of Padua, Padua, Italy

Clara Benna
Department of Surgery, Oncology and Gastroenterology (DISCOG), University of Padua, Padua, Italy,

Chiara Menin
Immunology and Diagnostic Molecular Oncology Unit, Veneto Institute of Oncology IOV-IRCCS, Padua, Italy

Daniela Di Carlo and Gianni Bisogno
Hematology/Oncology Division, Department of Women's and Children's Health, University of Padua, Padua, Italy

Katharina C. Kähler, Ann-Sophie Bohne
Department of Dermatology, University Hospital Schleswig-Holstein (UKSH), Kiel, Germany

Ralf Gutzmer and Imke Satzger
Department of Dermatology, University Hospital Hannover, Hannover, Germany

Friedegrund Meier and Lydia Reinhardt
Skin Cancer Center, National Center for Tumor Diseases, University Cancer Centre Dresden, Dresden, Germany
Department of Dermatology, TU Dresden, University Hospital Carl Gustav Carus, Dresden, Germany

Lisa Zimmer, Jan-Malte Placke, Dirk Schadendorf and Selma Ugurel
Department of Dermatology, University Hospital Essen, German Cancer Consortium (DKTK), Essen, Germany

Markus Heppt
Department of Dermatology, Universitätsklinikum Erlangen, Friedrich-Alexander University Erlangen-Nürnberg, Erlangen, Germany

Anja Gesierich
Department of Dermatology, University Hospital Würzburg, Würzburg, Germany

Kai-Martin Thoms
Department of Dermatology, University Medical Center Göttingen, Göttingen, Germany

Jochen Utikal
Skin Cancer Unit, German Cancer Research Center (DKFZ), Heidelberg, Germany
Department of Dermatology, Venereology and Allergology, University Medical Center Mannheim, Ruprecht-Karl University of Heidelberg, Mannheim, Germany

Jessica C. Hassel
Department of Dermatology, University Hospital Heidelberg, Heidelberg, Germany

Carmen Loquai
Department of Dermatology, University Hospital Mainz, Mainz, Germany

Claudia Pföhler
Department of Dermatology, University Hospital Homburg, Homburg, Germany

Lucie Heinzerling
Department of Dermatology, Universitätsklinikum Erlangen, Friedrich-Alexander University Erlangen-Nürnberg, Erlangen, Germany
Department of Dermatology and Allergology, Ludwig-Maximilian University, München, Germany

Martin Kaatz
Department of Dermatology, SRH Waldklinikum, Gera, Germany

Daniela Göppner
Department of Dermatology, University Hospital Giessen, Gießen, Germany

Annette Pflugfelder
Department of Dermatology, University Hospital Tübingen, Tübingen, Germany

Yeltai Nurzat, Weijie Su, Peiru Min, Ke Li, Heng Xu and Yixin Zhang
Department of Plastic and Reconstructive Surgery, Shanghai Ninth People's Hospital, Shanghai JiaoTong University School of Medicine, Shanghai, China

Paolo Del Fiore, Claudia Di Prata, Antonella Vecchiato, Romina Spina, Francesco Russano and Saveria Tropea
Soft-Tissue, Peritoneum and Melanoma Surgical Oncology Unit, Veneto Institute of Oncology (IOV)-IRCCS, Padua, Italy
Department of Surgery, Oncology and Gastroenterology (DISCOG), University of Padua, Padua, Italy

Irene Russo
Soft-Tissue, Peritoneum and Melanoma Surgical Oncology Unit, Veneto Institute of Oncology (IOV)-IRCCS, Padua, Italy
Division of Dermatology, Department of Medicine (DIMED), University of Padua, Padua, Italy

Jacopo Tartaglia, Alessandro Dal Monico and Mauro Alaibac
Division of Dermatology, Department of Medicine (DIMED), University of Padua, Padua, Italy

Lorenzo Nicolè
Department of Medicine, University of Padua School of Medicine and Surgery, Padua, Italy
Unit of Surgical Pathology & Cytopathology, Ospedale dell'Angelo, Mestre, Italy

Luisa Piccin, Jacopo Pigozzo and Vanna Chiarion-Sileni
Melanoma Oncology Unit, Veneto Institute of Oncology (IOV)-IRCCS, Padua, Italy

Alessio Fabozzi
Oncology Unit 3, Veneto Institute of Oncology (IOV)-IRCCS, Padua, Italy

Bernardo Biffoli, Tito Brambullo, Vincenzo Vindigni and Franco Bassetto
Clinic of Plastic Surgery, Department of Neuroscience, Padua University Hospital, University of Padua, Padua, Italy

Beatrice Ferrazzi
Postgraduate School of Occupational Medicine, University of Verona, Verona, Italy

Elisabetta Bezzon
Radiology Unit, Department of Imaging and Medical Physics, Istituto Oncologico Veneto (IOV) IRCSS, Padua, Italy

Sara Cingarlini
Oncology Section, Department of Oncology, Verona University and Hospital Trust, Verona, Italy

Renzo Mazzarotto
Department of Radiotherapy, Ospedale Civile Maggiore, Azienda Ospedaliera Universitaria Integrata Verona, Verona, Italy

Alessandro Parisi and Giovanni Scarzello
Radiotherapy Unit, Veneto Institute of Oncology, Istituto Oncologico Veneto (IOV)-IRCCS, Padua, Italy

Daniele Bertin and Michele Gregianin
Radiotherapy and Nuclear Medicine Unit, Oncological Institute of Veneto IOV-IRCCS, Padua, Italy

Angelo Paolo Dei Tos
Pathological Anatomy Unit, University Hospital of Padua, Padua, Italy
Department of Medicine (DIMED), Surgical Pathology Unit, University of Padua, Padua, Italy

Francesco Cavallin
Independent Statistician, Solagna, Italy

Index

Printed in the USA
CPSIA information can be obtained
at www.ICGtesting.com
JSHW050003260324
59877JS00005B/44